Readings in
Health Care
Ethics

READINGS IN HEALTH CARE ETHICS

edited by
Elisabeth Boetzkes and Wilfrid J. Waluchow

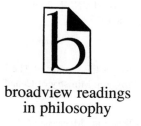

broadview readings
in philosophy

Canadian Cataloguing in Publication Data

Main entry under title:
Readings in health care ethics

ISBN 1-55111-258-2

1. Medical ethics   I. Boetzkes, Elisabeth Airini.   II. Waluchow, Wilfrid J., 1953-   .

R724.R435   2000   174'.2   C00-930520-3

The publisher has made every attempt to locate the authors of the copyrighted material or their heirs and assigns, and would be grateful for information that would allow correction of any errors or omissions in subsequent editions of the work.

Broadview Press, Ltd.
is an independent, international publishing house, incorporated in 1985

North America
Post Office Box 1243, Peterborough, Ontario, Canada K9J 7H5
3576 California Road, Orchard Park, New York, USA 14127
TEL: (705) 743-8990; FAX (705) 743-8353;
E-MAIL: customerservice@broadviewpress.com

United Kingdom and Europe
Thomas Lyster, Ltd.,
Units 3 & 4a, Ormskirk Industrial Park, Burscough Rd, Ormskirk,
Lancashire L39 2YW Tel: (1695) 575112; Fax: (1695) 570120;
E-Mail: books@tlyster.co.uk

Australia
St. Clair Press, Post Office Box 287, Rozelle, NSW 2039
TEL: (612) 818-1942; FAX: (612) 418-1923

www.broadviewpress.com

Broadview Press gratefully acknowledges the support of The Book Publishing Industry Development Program, Ministry of Canadian Heritage, Government of Canada.

Typesetting and assembly: True to Type Inc., Mississauga, Canada

Printed in Canada

TABLE OF CONTENTS

CHAPTER ONE

INTRODUCTION

ETHICAL RESOURCES FOR DECISION-MAKING

(1) MORAL PHILOSOPHY

The current prominence enjoyed by health care ethics is due, in no small measure, to the impact of biochemistry and improved technology. There is much more that can be done for (or to) patients than could ever be done before. New technological possibilities raise all sorts of questions which never had to be faced in the past. At one time the question "What *should* be done?" may have been more or less equivalent to the question "What *can* be done?" Whether or not this was true in the past, it is clearly not true now. To take one example: medicine is now able to keep people alive on respirators and other life-support mechanisms in situations where many question the propriety of doing so. If someone is irreversibly comatose, it may be that we *can* keep her alive. But whether we *should* utilize scarce resources to do so is another question altogether. This is only one example of the many decisions that arise in health care ethics. How can philosophy help?

Decision-making has always had a moral dimension, and many ethical decisions are extremely difficult. Moral philosophers are not moral experts capable of providing ready-made answers when difficult or intransigent moral conflicts arise. Rather, they perform more modest tasks: clarifying the terms of moral debate, scrutinizing distinctions to see if they stand up to rational examination, assessing the validity and cogency of arguments, and examining the fit between moral practice and moral principles and values.

Moral philosophers are of course also concerned sometimes with defending their own moral theories and convictions, particularly when they detect unwarranted, dogmatic beliefs. But a student unaccustomed to the ways of the moral philosopher will often find the philosopher's arguments a trifle strange. The moral philosopher will often seek to defend or justify the obvious—e.g., that it is morally wrong intentionally to deceive a patient about the dangerous side-effects of an experimental drug the patient is being asked to take, or that it is wrong deliberately to enrol mentally competent patients in clinical trials without their consent. At other times the moral philosopher will offer arguments which *question* the obvious. She might even try to defend a position which strikes others as patently false—e.g., that elderly people have less right to scarce medical resources than younger people or that other animals have less claim to moral consideration than do humans. The main reason for these strange activities of the moral philosopher lies in his chief motivation, expressed in a maxim propounded by the ancient Greek philosopher Socrates. According to Socrates, the unexamined life is not worth living. Socrates and other moral philosophers always want to know *why* we should believe the things we do, even those things which we firmly and passionately believe to be true. Many of our moral beliefs just seem right to us. We've never had occasion to question them or to ask ourselves why we hold them. Yet if pushed to articulate the grounds or bases of our moral beliefs, we are often unable to provide them. And even if we do manage to come up with something, we often find that our grounds do not stand up well to critical scrutiny. It may seem obvious that no patient should be enroled in a clinical drug trial without the prior consent of the patient or a person entitled to give consent on the patient's behalf. This principle, P, helps to explain why we would condemn a physician/experimenter who, without first gaining informed consent, tried out a new drug on a group of patients in their thirties who had lung cancer but were otherwise normal adults.

But now ask whether principle P stands up to rational scrutiny. Imagine that you are on an Ethics Review Board at a University Hospital and that a project in which principle P seems to be compromised comes before the Board for approval. The situation is as follows.

Babies are sometimes born with a hypotensive condition for which potentially life-saving medication is immediately required. Your hospital has routinely used two types of medication to combat this condition, some physicians preferring the one drug, X, others the second, Y. Both X and Y seem effective, but they operate in different ways. It is also unclear whether X or Y is preferable in terms of degree of efficacy or severity of potential side-effects. The doctors want to clear up these uncertainties and ascertain whether X or Y is better. A trial is proposed in which all new-born babies with hypotension will be randomly allocated to receive either X or Y. The study protocol calls for "double blinding." That is, no one, including the doctors and nurses in the neonatal ward who will be administering the medication, will know to which group any particular baby has been assigned. There is only one hitch. Hypotension is not a condition which can be predicted before birth. Therefore it is not feasible to gain consent from parents before their baby is born. It is also not feasible, in most cases, to gain consent after birth when it becomes apparent that medication for hypotension is immediately required. As a consequence, the researcher suggests the following. If the parents are available, they will be asked to consent to enrolment of their baby in the study. If they object, their baby will then receive whichever of X or Y the attending physician happens to prefer. If they consent to their baby's participation, then the baby will be enroled in the study and assigned, randomly and blindly, either to the group receiving X or to the group receiving Y. As for those babies whose parents are unavailable when the necessity for immediate medication becomes apparent, they will be enroled in the study *without consent*. The parents of these babies will be contacted, however, as soon as possible and asked for consent to the continued enrolment of their baby. Should there be any objections at this stage, the choice of the baby's medication will then fall into the hands of the attending physician who will exercise his discretion in choosing X or Y.

Given that both X and Y are standard drugs in common use at the hospital, that parents are given the choice of opting out as soon as they can be

reached, and that the proposed procedure for gaining consent is the only feasible one under the circumstances, it seems reasonable, and ethical, to permit temporary enrolment in the study without the parents' consent. But then doesn't this show that principle P must be rejected, or at least modified in some way? If so, what might the alternative be? We need to develop a moral theory for distinguishing cases where *prior* consent is vital from special cases in which it may not be necessary. It is here that the moral philosopher might be of some help. He might be able to supply an ethical theory upon the basis of which it is possible to support a reasonable alternative to P.

The family of activities pursued by the moral philosopher is prompted largely by a desire for clarity of thought and integrity of action—by Socrates's maxim that the unexamined life is not worth living. The student of moral philosophy must be prepared to approach the subject with the correct frame of mind, with a willingness to challenge the obvious and to consider seriously both the questionable and the unfamiliar. Should she do so, there is much of value that can be gleaned from the study of health care ethics.

One final point about the role of the moral philosopher. Moral philosophy is not the moral conscience of society. On the contrary, moral philosophers should be viewed as partners with the rest of the citizenry in worrying through troublesome moral questions. Moral philosophers are not out simply to criticize for moral failure—except perhaps when blind dogma rules moral practice, where the lives we lead do remain largely unexamined. Most important of all, perhaps, is the following point. To raise or consider a moral question is not necessarily to imply that there is something inherently immoral or unethical going on. The questions which arise in health care ethics are difficult ones, and those who disagree with us or are generally perplexed do not necessarily have any less moral integrity than we do.

(2) MORALITY VERSUS ETHICS

Moral persons are equally distributed in all walks of life. As noted earlier, morality is always of relevance, but no one can claim to be a moral expert. Ethics or ethical theory is another matter. Ethical theory, as opposed to morality, is the systematic, critical study of the basic underlying principles, values, and concepts utilized in thinking about moral life. Ethics, so understood, is something the average person concerns himself with only infrequently, if ever. But this is not true of moral philosophers or ethicists. They are primarily concerned with ethical theory. They have developed concepts, theories, and techniques of argument which can often be of use to non-philosophers in finding their way through the tangled moral issues to which the practice of medicine often gives rise. We would do well, then, to consider the general ethical theories of some of the most influential moral philosophers of Western civilization. This we will do in later sections. First, a few thoughts on the nature and role of ethical theories.

(3) LEVELS OF MORAL RESPONSE

Consider the question "Why do you oppose abortion?" As put to an opponent of abortion, this question can trigger different types of responses.

(a) *The Expressive Level*

At the most primitive level the answer is likely to be: "Because abortion is repugnant" or "I hate the very thought of killing a fetus." These responses are unanalyzed expressions or feelings which, in themselves, do not constitute any kind of justification or reason for opposing abortion. This is not to deny that feelings are relevant to morality or that moral convictions are often accompanied by strong emotions. It is simply to say that the mere fact that one feels a certain way about an action or practice in no way constitutes an adequate justification for making moral pronouncements on it.

(b) *The Pre-reflective Level*

At the next level of response, justification is offered by reference to values, rules, and principles—i.e., norms—accepted uncritically. Most often it is offered by reference to what we will call, somewhat loosely, a "conventional" norm. Such a standard may be expressed in a legal rule, in one of society's conventionally accepted values, in a religious pronouncement, or in a professional code of ethics. At this level of response one's opposition to abortion might take the following form: "I disapprove of

abortion because my priest informs me that it is morally wrong" or "I disapprove of treating patients without their consent because this is prohibited by the professional code governing my national Medical Association."

It is a defining feature of the pre-reflective level of response that its conventional norms are uncritically accepted and acted upon. We don't stop to think why we should act or base our judgments upon the conventional norms or if they are good standards to adopt. Assuming that the conventional norms are good ones, any ensuing behaviour may be classified as conventionally moral or ethical, but it is important to realize that it is a species of externally directed behaviour. It is the blind following of standards or norms set by someone else. As noted, this is not necessarily bad. Sometimes conventional norms are capable of reasoned defence and can be fully justified morally. Sometimes there is even good moral reason to follow conventional rules just because they are conventionally accepted. Conventional norms can help to foster common understandings and serve to ground justified expectations in others concerning how we will conduct ourselves. Sometimes it is crucial to know that other people will be playing by the same rules that we are. Imagine what it would be like if there were no conventionally agreed rules governing the making of promises. We would never be certain whether a promise had been made or whether its author considered it binding.

It is a serious mistake, however, to think that morality is exhausted by conventional norms alone or that moral justification *ends* with the invocation of a conventional rule. The norms must always be subject to critical moral scrutiny. Perhaps there are much better rules which we should try to persuade others to adopt. Or perhaps existing conventions are morally objectionable. That X is generally accepted as morally right never, in itself, entails that X is morally right. Slavery was at one time widely accepted as morally correct. Slavery was, and always will be, morally wrong nonetheless. It is quite possible that practices currently sanctioned by conventional morality should likewise be modified or rejected. Morality requires eternal vigilance: we must always be prepared to think about the justification of what we are about to do.

(c) The Reflective Level

At this level of response our moral judgments are not based entirely on conventional norms blindly accepted, but on principles, rules and values to which we ourselves consciously subscribe and with regard to which we, as rational moral agents, are prepared to offer reasoned moral defence. It is possible of course that the norms to which we subscribe at the reflective level are in fact norms conventionally accepted as well. They might, for instance, be those which have found their way into a professional code (e.g. the CNA or CMA Codes of Ethics) by which one is expected to abide. The point is that at the reflective level of moral response we must be prepared to consider questions of justification. We must not blindly accept the conventional norms but be prepared to consider for ourselves whether they are justified, or whether other, perhaps wholly novel, norms are those by which people should lead their lives.

At the reflective level, opposition to abortion may now take the form: "I oppose abortion because the fetus's right to life takes precedence over the woman's right to control her own reproductive processes." Here a reason is given—a basis or ground for the moral judgment is provided. The complexity and sophistication of the reflective level of response is evident from the presence of competing judgments and the plausible bases for them. One can imagine, as a reply to the above, the following retort: "Abortion is morally permissible because the rights of *actual* persons (pregnant women) take precedence over the rights of *potential* persons (fetuses)." As this example illustrates, ethics at the reflective level admits of few easy answers!

Of the three levels considered, the reflective level is the one at which most of the discussion in the present book takes place. This is so despite grounds for misgivings about the possibilities for full resolution of moral controversies at the reflective level. Reflection does not guarantee agreement. As will be evident throughout this book, moral reflection often yields *a* defensible position, but rarely yields the *only* defensible position. Not only do people feel differently at the expressive level, and uncritically favour different conventional rules at the pre-reflective level, they also often reach different conclusions at the reflective level. It is important to stress, once again, that there are no moral experts and that at each level, including the reflective one, we are often met with genuine dilemmas and competing bases for moral belief. Arriving at unassailable moral judgments is difficult, and some think impossible, not only because there are different levels of moral response, but also because people approach moral questions with very different perspectives.

(4) A Variety of Perspectives

The different approaches that moral agents take to moral questions may be illustrated by distinguishing between three ways in which the term "know" can be used.

(i) Sometimes the claim to know amounts to nothing more than a claim to feel sure or certain. This yields no more than a subjective, psychological criterion. While emotionally reassuring, a feeling of certainty is not a reliable mark of bona fide moral judgments. Others with different, even opposing, moral views may feel just as strongly that they are right. One who claims to know, and tries to add as a warrant that he just feels certain about what he believes, offers no warrant at all. His certainty is no more a warrant than the certainty with which many people at one time believed slavery to be morally justified.

(ii) Next the claim to know may be reduced to: "The position I hold is the one for which the best reasoned justification seems possible." Such a claim acknowledges the requirement of reasoned defence and that the position held may not be the only defensible one. It recognizes that rational people of good will and integrity may reasonably disagree about moral matters and that no one can claim, with absolute certainty, to have *the right* answer.

(iii) The third use of "know" is much stronger than the second and, according to many moral philosophers, quite unwarranted. It is equivalent to: "I know my view is the right one, and anyone who disagrees with me suffers from moral blindness, error or misunderstanding." Leaving aside the question of whether, in moral life, there are ever uniquely correct solutions to moral issues, the degree of self-assurance echoed in the above claim amounts to sheer audacity and arrogance. Even a commitment to the notion that there is "a final truth" in ethics should be accompanied by the acknowledgment that in practice we must often operate in humility with only partial knowledge and approximations to the truth. Moral progress is possible at both the social and the personal levels. Just as we believe that a society's practices can improve morally, as when slavery was abandoned, we should always believe that our own personal practices and beliefs can be improved, usually by listening to what others, whose opinions we respect, have to say.

Misgivings about the ethical enterprise may go even deeper than the foregoing comments suggest. There are profound philosophical disputes about the status of ethics itself—about whether moral judgments are in the end capable of full justification. Three of the more extreme difficulties are as follows.

(a) The Issue of Verification

The problem of verification in the context of moral judgments may be illustrated by reference to the following scenario. Apple Mary is sitting in the downtown Hamilton market selling her produce. Suddenly a furtive-looking character sneaks up behind her and clubs her. As she falls to the ground, her assailant scoops up her purse and vanishes.

Imagine two witnesses commenting as follows:

A. Did you see that?
B. I did.
A. What a dreadful thing to happen in our town.
B. I agree.
A. What that man did was terribly wrong.
B. I didn't see anything wrong.
A. How can you possibly say that?
B. Easily. Let's go over carefully what happened.
A. Let's do that.
B. I saw Apple Mary sitting at her stall. I saw a man creep up behind her. I saw him lift a club and bring it down on her head. I saw Mary slump to the ground and her assailant take off with her purse. I didn't see anything wrong.

The clue to the dispute between A and B is to be found in the ambiguity of the word "see." Of course B is correct if by "see" we mean physical seeing. We do not see the wrong in the way we see arms raised, clubs

wielded, and purses snatched. Moral seeing is more like "seeing that" (making a judgment) than seeing with our eyes. We see *that* assault is wrong. We see *that* stealing is wrong. Moral insights are expressed in the form of judgments which are not verifiable empirically in the way that observational statements are. Rather they are substantiated by reference to principles, rules, or values which serve as their ground or warrant. According to the first ethical theory we will examine, as well as one version of the second, we justify our actions in terms of the following schemata:

principles

↓

rules

↓

actions or judgements

The contemplated action, or a moral judgment concerning it, falls under a rule, and the rule, in turn, conforms to a higher-order principle. By contrast, the third routine we will consider involves identifying principles specifying "prima facie duties," and in situations of conflicting prima facie duties, determining which takes precedence. But more on this later. The point to be stressed at this stage is that we do not see moral properties in the way we see the club which hit Apple Mary. Moral judgments are not open to empirical verification—indeed, they cannot be substantiated by way of a universally agreed routine or procedure. There are a plurality of competing theories on how our moral judgments are to be substantiated. Most, but not all, may be mapped onto the above schemata.

(b) A Plurality of Ethical Systems

The existence of a plurality of different approaches to the justification of moral judgments may be a cause for dismay. It is one thing to be made aware that the morality of our actions is not open to empirical verification; it is quite another to learn that different ethical theories prescribe quite different routines to be utilized in moral reasoning. It would certainly be simpler if there were only one theory and one routine. The only problems then remaining would be problems of casuistry (i.e., application of rules or principles to particular cases). But philosophers have yet to discover an ethical theory upon which all reasonable people agree, and as we have already seen, there are those who believe that no such theory will ever be found. As the understanding we have of ourselves and the world around us increases, we should expect our ethical theories to change, and we hope, progress. In this particular respect, ethics is no different from science where change and progress are routinely accepted as inevitable. The best we can do at present is to engage in the pursuit of a defensible ethical theory and try to learn as much as we can from those who have done so in the past. There is much to be learned from the theorists whose views will be outlined below.

(c) *The Limits of Justification*

If one were to adopt, for example, a rule-based moral stance, the prescribed routine for justifying moral judgments would be more or less clear. It might be difficult to tell precisely what action the theory required of us in a particular case, but it would be reasonably clear how to go about trying to answer that question. Two rule-based approaches are discussed below—that of Immanuel Kant, and that of an important strain of utilitarianism. For Kant, as we shall see, an action is morally obligatory if it conforms to a rule and the rule, in turn, conforms to a principle which Kant calls the Categorical Imperative. For a rule-utilitarian there is an analogous procedure. Our actions must conform to a rule, and the rule must conform to the principle of utility: actions must facilitate the greatest possible degree of good for the greatest possible number. For fully committed utilitarians or Kantians, justification is limited to judgments made within the prescribed framework. We inquire, "Does the action in question conform to the rule and the rule to the (appropriate) principle?" If the answer is affirmative, the morality of the action is settled and we know what the theory prescribes as the right thing to do.

It is possible, of course, for a rule-utilitarian to raise questions about Kant's Categorical Imperative or for a Kantian to challenge the principle of utility. This involves raising questions concerning the validity of the frameworks themselves. In such cases what we have is a deeply philosophical dispute, the kind

of dispute which is a primary concern of ethical theorists. Utilitarians and Kantians will marshal philosophical arguments which challenge the validity of the other's ethical theory. They will do so even when it is clear what actions the opposing frameworks require of us in particular cases, or even when the different frameworks prescribe exactly the same actions. The two theorists may agree on *what* we should do but disagree about *why* we should do it. Again, the reason is clear: the philosopher is concerned to understand why we should do certain things and refrain from doing others.

External philosophical questions concerning the validity of ethical frameworks are best dealt with in books devoted exclusively to ethical theory. This is not such a book. In what follows we shall outline five competing frameworks and only briefly mention some of the many external, philosophical questions which have been raised about them. Some students will likely feel a strong affinity for one of the five theories discussed below, but most will find something of value in each one. This is not surprising. Four of the theories to be examined reflect currents of thought which have dominated western culture in recent centuries, and the fifth is expressive of a powerful contemporary movement of thought. For those strongly inclined to think that one of the theories represents the truth of the matter, the old adage should be borne in mind: "Those who live in glass houses should not throw stones." External challenges to other systems should be seasoned with a measure of caution and humility and the recognition that questions of morality and ethics are ones upon which reasonable people of good will and integrity do often disagree.

They should also be informed by the wisdom of John Stuart Mill's observation that "conflicting doctrines, instead of one being true and the other false, [often] share the truth between them, and the nonconforming opinion is needed to supply the remainder of the truth of which the received doctrine embodies only a part."[1]

Given these profound difficulties with the ethical enterprise, the student may wonder why we should bother at all with an introduction to ethical theory. Why not just get on with an analysis of the various specific, moral issues that arise in the practice of health care, issues like prescribing birth control pills to minors or screening fetuses for genetic defects? One response is that we are not warranted in dropping ethical theory altogether simply because it has difficulties. Quantum physics is fraught with theoretical difficulties too, but it would be silly to give it up entirely because of this. Another response is that there are valuable lessons to be learned from the ways in which some of the greatest thinkers within our cultural history have seriously and systematically approached ethical issues. These are thinkers whose formulations have been extremely influential and whose theories provide the frameworks within which current ethical disputes are argued. One cannot get too far in modern moral debate without encountering some appeal to the concept of utility or to the value of individual autonomy. These concepts are the cornerstones of the theories of Mill and Kant respectively.

(5) SOME BASIC CONCEPTS

Before turning to examine the theories of Kant, Mill, Ross, Aristotle, and the feminists, let us consider some basic terminology that is employed by ethical theorists. This terminology will be introduced by way of noting several distinctions.

First we should distinguish between *judgments of obligation* and *judgments of value*. Judgments of obligation concern what we ought to do. In expressing such judgments, we use sentences like: "You *ought* to take all steps to save human life"; "Your overriding *duty* was to protect the interests of your patient, not her fetus"; "You were under an obligation to honour your patient's wishes"; "It wasn't right to proceed without consent"; "He had a right to your best clinical judgment." All these judgments have to do directly with our conduct, with how we should behave.

Judgments of value, by contrast, are not directly related to action. These are judgments not about the right thing to do but about what is *good* or has *value*. For instance the judgments that freedom is a good thing for human beings to enjoy, and that pleasure is the only thing of ultimate or intrinsic worth are judgments of value. They don't tell us what it is right to do. For this we need a judgment of obligation. Under some ethical theories a judgment of obligation is

dependent on, and follows directly from, a judgment of value. If an ethical theory does hold that judgments of obligation are dependent in this way, then it is what philosophers call a *teleological* or *consequentialist* theory of obligation. A teleological theory of obligation posits one and only one fundamental obligation and that is to maximize the good consequences and minimize the bad consequences of our actions. In so far as we need to know, under such theories, which consequences are good so that we can maximize them and which are bad so that we can minimize them, it is easy to see why a teleological theory of obligation presupposes a *theory of value*. Such a theory will provide us with the basis for justifying our judgments of value and thus ultimately our judgments of obligation.

The duty to maximize the good and minimize the bad consequences of our actions is the only fundamental duty under a teleological theory of obligation. On such a theory, then, any other obligations by which we feel bound, such as the obligation to honour our agreements or to tell the truth, are secondary and derivable from this one primary obligation. Mill's utilitarianism, as we shall see, is a teleological theory of obligation. In his view, all questions concerning what we ought to do are ultimately based on the principle of utility which requires that we maximize what is intrinsically good, namely, happiness or pleasure, and minimize what is intrinsically bad, unhappiness or pain. We have a duty to tell the truth, Mill would argue, but only because truth-telling is (normally) prescribed by the principle of utility.

In contrast to teleological theories of obligation there are those which are non-teleological. These we call *deontological theories* of obligation. Deontological theories of obligation essentially deny what teleological theories assert. They deny that we have one and only one fundamental duty, which is to maximize the good and minimize the bad consequences of our actions. There are basically two forms which this denial can take. First, a theory may suggest that the good and bad consequences of our actions have absolutely no bearing whatsoever on whether they are morally right or wrong. Such a strong deontological theory of obligation can operate wholly independently of any theory of value. We needn't know, as we do with teleological theories of obligation, what the good is if we are to know what we ought to do. The reason is simple: our obligation does not in any way involve the maximization of good consequences. Our duty is not to maximize what is ultimately of value and so we needn't have a theory of value which tells us what that is. Kant, as we shall see, appears to have held a strong deontological theory. Kant is notorious for suggesting that the rightness or wrongness of our actions is totally independent of whether or not they maximize good consequences. According to Kant, a judgment of obligation, like the judgment that health-care professionals must never withhold the truth from their patients, is in no way justified in terms of consequences. It is justified if and only if it meets the Categorical Imperative test which ignores consequences altogether.

A deontological theory of obligation need not, however, follow Kant's lead and claim that the consequences of our actions are completely irrelevant to their rightness or wrongness. There is a second kind of deontological theory which makes the weaker claim that good and bad consequences are not always the only things of moral importance. We have other ultimate obligations in addition to our duty to maximize the good and minimize the bad consequences of our actions. According to Ross, for example, the principle of beneficence, which requires promoting the good of others in our actions, is only one of many ultimate principles defining our moral obligations. Others include the obligation to be grateful for benefits given and the duty to be fair to other people. In Ross's view, we sometimes have a duty to be grateful even when neglecting this duty would on that occasion lead to the best consequences overall. Some actions, such as displays of gratitude are right, regardless of their consequences. Other actions, such as instances of unfairness, are sometimes wrong, even when they lead to good consequences.

Unlike Kant and Mill, then, Ross suggests that we have many fundamental obligations. The duty to be grateful and the duty to be fair are ultimate obligations which are not based on any moral basic principle of obligation. This clearly separates Ross from Kant and Mill. We frequently have a duty to be fair, Mill would urge, but this is because being fair nor-

mally maximizes the balance of good over bad consequences. Ross will have none of this. For him the duty to be fair is just as ultimate as the duty to maximize good consequences. We have many basic obligations and these cannot be reduced to any of the others. Ross's theory of obligation, insofar as it is not based on a single, fundamental principle defining a single, fundamental obligation is a *pluralist theory of obligation*. A pluralist theory of obligation, put simply, is one which does not posit a single, fundamental obligation upon which all other secondary obligations are based. A *monistic theory of obligation*, by contrast, does posit one such obligation. A utilitarian will be happy to talk of obligations to tell the truth or to be fair to others in our dealings with them. He will simply add that we have these obligations because fairness and truth-telling usually lead, in the end and all things considered, to the best consequences. Hence his theory is monistic. So too is Kant's.

To sum up, teleological theories of obligations are all logically dependent on theories of value. Some deontological theories of obligation are also dependent on a theory of value. Strong deontological theories such as Kant's exclude, as irrelevant, questions about the good or bad consequences of our actions (i.e. the value or disvalue to be realized in them). They therefore have no need of a theory of value. But most deontological theories do have such a need, since most deontological theories are pluralistic. Most are like Ross's in espousing principles which direct us, but not exclusively, to the good and bad consequences of our actions.

When we turn to theories of value, we find that these too may be categorized as either monistic or pluralistic. A *monistic theory of value*, as one might expect, posits one and only one thing, or characteristic of things, as being of value for its own sake. It posits, in other words, only one thing or characteristic as *intrinsically valuable*. Hedonism is one influential type of monistic theory of value. On this view, pleasure is the only thing which is valuable for its own sake. Anything else we value, say money or health, is valuable only *instrumentally*, as a means to the pleasure it brings. Classical utilitarianism, of the form espoused by Mill and his teacher Jeremy Bentham, is hedonistic. But it needn't be. Utilitarians who agree on a theory of obligation may divide on their theories of value. G.E. Moore, for instance, was a utilitarian like Mill. But unlike Mill, Moore espoused a *pluralistic theory of value* which saw pleasure as only one of many things of intrinsic value. Knowledge and aesthetic experience are among many other things worthy of pursuit for their own sakes.[2] If one holds a pluralistic theory of value, then one is faced with a difficulty: what to do in situations where two or more values conflict or cannot be pursued together. If freedom from manipulation and freedom from disease are both intrinsically valuable, then doctors may have to decide somehow between allowing their patients complete freedom of choice concerning their own medical treatment (thus risking bad decisions) and leading their patients to make what they, the doctors, think is the right choice. The question arises, however, whether it is possible to compare such very different values. Is comparing freedom from manipulation with freedom from disease, so as to see which is of greater value or importance in the circumstances, something that can be done rationally? Is an attempt to compare these two values a bit like trying to compare apples with oranges?

If, on the other hand, we adopt a monistic theory of value, we may seem to rid ourselves of such problems. We only have to compare, say, one pleasure with the next. But there are serious difficulties even here. How does one compare one person's pleasure with that of another, especially if those persons are as different as Bill Clinton and Pope John Paul II?

Monistic theories of value face another objection of some importance. According to many people there are numerous things in the world of ultimate, irreducible value. Friendship, for example, seems to be compromised if an attempt is made to reduce its value to the pleasure it brings. As will be seen, the attempt to place "value" on human lives and welfare is fraught with such difficulties. Some of these will be explored later in discussions concerning the propriety of utilizing "quality of life" as a criterion for decisions involving health care.

(6) FIVE TYPES OF ETHICAL THEORY

Here follows a brief survey of five major types of ethical theory. The main reason for including the theories of Kant and Mill is that their contributions have dominated western moral thought since the scientific revolution. Kant strove to establish ethics as a purely rational enterprise while Mill believed that an objective standard of right and wrong could be discovered in the methods of the empirical sciences. If the rightness of our actions depends on the pleasure and pain they produce, then we ought to be able to estimate their rightness by empirical observation, measurements, and induction. Mill's utilitarianism is an ancestor of modern theories of cost-benefit analysis, which are assuming an ever-increasing role in controversies surrounding the allocation of money to various forms of health care.

Between them Kant and Mill zero in on the roles played respectively by intention and consequences in shaping our moral responses. One cannot get very far in discussions of ethics without paying deference to the Kantian notions of autonomy and universalizability, or the injunction to treat human beings as ends in themselves and not merely as means. Similarly one cannot ignore Mill's emphasis on protecting and promoting human happiness or well-being.

W.D. Ross's contribution to ethics is invaluable not only for its reaction to Kant and Mill, but because, in certain crucial respects, it seems more accurately to reflect the ordinary thinking and practice of moral agents than the more systematic reflections of professional moral philosophers. This is particularly evident in Ross's opposition to Kant's and Mill's reductionism in moral theory. Ross was unwilling to subscribe to a monistic theory of obligation. While acknowledging the powerful contributions of Kant and Mill to ethical theory, Ross resists elevating either the Categorical Imperative or the principle of utility to the status of a foundational first principle from which all other moral principles, rules, and judgments follow. In coming to grips with the moral issues considered in this text, it will be difficult to escape making reference to Ross's notion of *prima facie* duty.

Contemporary ethical theorists have expressed renewed interest in the ethical writings of the ancient Greek philosopher, Aristotle. Among Aristotle's many contributions to the history of ethical thought is his doctrine of the mean. As we will see below, Aristotle attempts to isolate a number of virtues which we can more or less express or display in our lives when we aim for the *golden mean* between undesirable extremes. For example, we display the virtue courage when, in conducting our lives, we successfully steer clear of the extremes of cowardliness and foolhardiness. Courage is the mean between these two vices, and a courageous person is one whose character and (developed) dispositions lead him to act in neither a foolhardy nor a cowardly manner.

Those who are impressed with the immense complexity of moral life, and with the difficulties encountered when we try to articulate rules and principles to cover all cases, may find enormous potential in the Aristotelian approach. It is a consequence of Aristotle's conception of the moral life that there are no hard and fast rules or principles to tell us whether and to what extent our conduct approximates the relevant mean and is therefore virtuous. There are also no hard and fast rules to tell us what to do when our situation involves more than one virtue, as when our beneficence inclines us towards treating someone who would object were she informed about the matter, but our wish to be an honest person leads us in the other direction. In addressing moral questions we are not asking for rules which tell us what to do on some particular occasion. Rather, we are asking ourselves what kind of person we would be, what kinds of virtues we would display, were we to conduct our lives in a particular manner. And to these types of questions there are almost never uniquely correct answers. Perhaps in this respect Aristotle's theory more accurately reflects our moral experience, and the humility of which we have spoken above.

Finally, we have included a section on feminist perspectives. Feminist writings in health care ethics have been characterized as much by the *approach* taken to ethical theory as by any distinctive set of principles, rules, or values. Most varieties of feminist ethics are marked by a heightened concern for the personal and social *contexts* in which ethical decisions are made, and by the ways in which traditional ethical theory, with its attempt to discover universal, and therefore necessarily abstract, moral norms, ignores the context in which decisions are made. Of particular concern to most feminists is the perceived failure of mainstream ethical theory to appreciate the context of oppressed individuals, like women and the socially vulnerable, and the various ways in which their legitimate concerns and interests are ignored, undervalued, or suppressed.

(a) Utilitarianism

As noted above, utilitarianism is an ethical theory founded on the belief that the right action is that which facilitates the greatest possible degree of good for all those affected by the action. It is a monistic theory in that it posits a single fundamental obligation upon which all other secondary obligations are based. And it is a teleological theory in that it rests on a theory of value. In the context of this introduction we will largely ignore the different theories of value espoused by utilitarians, and concentrate instead on what they have to say about obligation.

Essentially there are two different kinds of utilitarianism, act and rule utilitarianism. Act utilitarianism (AU) defines the rightness or wrongness of individual actions in terms of the good or bad consequences realized by those actions themselves. In other words, AU defines the rightness or wrongness of an action in terms of its "utility" and "disutility." The term "utility" stands for whatever it is that is intrinsically valuable under the utilitarian's theory of value, "disutility" for whatever is thought to be intrinsically bad. According to John Stuart Mill, "actions are right in proportion as they tend to promote happiness; wrong as they tend to produce the reverse of happiness."[3] For him "utility" means happiness, and "disutility" unhappiness. Mill went on to identify happiness with pleasure and unhappiness with pain. Hence, Mill may be characterized as a *hedonistic* utilitarian, one on whose theory of value pleasure is the only thing of intrinsic worth. But a utilitarian need not make this identification, nor need he define utility in terms of happiness. Some utilitarians think it best to define utility in terms of the satisfaction of our actual preferences, while others would have us look to satisfy preferences we would have were we fully informed and rational. Regardless of the theory of value with which it is associated, however, AU always makes the following claim:

AU: An act is right if and only if there is no other action I could have done instead which either (a) would have produced a greater balance of utility over disutility; or (b) would have produced a smaller balance of disutility over utility.

We must add (b) to account for those unfortunate situations where whatever we do we seem to cause more disutility than utility—where we're damned if we do and damned if we don't. In short, AU tells us to act always so as to bring about the best consequences we can, and sometimes that means trying to make the best of a bad situation.

AU was made famous in modern times by Mill and Bentham, at a time when it was quite natural for many people to think that some individuals simply count more than others. There were some who thought that members of the aristocracy, the Church, or a particular race were in some sense more worthy or superior than others and were therefore deserving of special consideration or privilege. The utilitarians were part of a social revolution which would have none of this. In the famous words of Bentham, "each is to count for one, none to count for more than one." In other words, according to utilitarians, *all* those affected by my actions should count *equally* in my deliberations concerning my moral obligations. The happiness of the King is to count equally with the equal happiness of the shop clerk. Mill put this important point in the following way:

> I must again repeat what the assailants of utilitarianism seldom have the justice to acknowledge, that the happiness which forms the utilitarian standard of what is right in conduct is *not* the agent's own happiness but that of all concerned. As between others, utilitarianism requires him to be as *strictly impartial as a disinterested benevolent spectator.*[4]

So built into AU is a commitment to equality and impartiality. We are to be concerned equally and impartially with the happiness or welfare, i.e. utility, of all those, including ourselves, who might be affected by our actions. On these grounds alone, AU is a very appealing theory. What could be better than to be sure that I always maximize, not my own happiness or that of my friends, but the happiness of all those people affected by my actions whoever they might be? What more could morality require?

Despite its inherently desirable features, many philosophers have come to find serious difficulties with AU. These have led some utilitarians to opt for an alternative form of the theory. One of the more serious difficulties for AU revolves around *special duties* and *special relationships*. These include duties of loyalty, of fidelity, and familial obligations. The latter rest in part on the special relationships which arise out of family ties and require some degree of partiality and special concern towards family members. It would be wrong, some think, to be impartial between friends and family, on the one hand, and perfect strangers on the other. It would be equally wrong to be impartial between one's patient and others who might benefit from the knowledge to be gained from using one's patient in an experiment. The importance of personal relationships in the moral evaluation of conduct is often stressed by feminists who reject the "impartiality" required by utilitarianism. In their view, treating everyone the same would be equivalent to treating them all as strangers.

Let us centre on promises to illustrate some of the most serious difficulties facing AU. Suppose I am a doctor and that a dear friend, Monica, comes to my clinic concerned that she might have AIDS. Monica has been unfaithful to her husband, Jack, whom I have also known for years. Our friendships go a long way back and are a continual source of happiness for all of us. Recent media discussions of the AIDS "epidemic" have got Monica worried. In order to ease her concern, I run the appropriate tests and determine that Monica has not been exposed to the HIV virus (the cause of AIDS). She is extremely relieved. Now she can continue her affair without worry. Her partner had a similar test done recently and so they are both clean. As Monica leaves my office she announces with a smile that of course she fully expects me to keep quiet about the test and the ongoing affair. Under no circumstances must Jack ever find out. She points out that as her physician I owe her a duty of confidentiality, a duty which is even stronger in this case, given our long friendship.

Upon reflection, however, I begin to wonder whether my duty does ultimately lie in confidentiality. I add up the utilities and disutilities involved for all affected by my decision, including not only Jack and Monica but their two young children and Monica's sexual partner. I correctly conclude that overall utility would be maximized, on balance, if I told Jack about the affair. He's a very reasonable and forgiving person and would likely be able to keep the marriage on the rails, something which would be of benefit to the entire family. As for Monica's partner, he will likely experience no difficulty in finding another sexual partner. As a consequence of my valid, act-utilitarian reasoning, I betray the confidence, despite my apparent duty as a physician and a friend. I consider it my moral obligation to maximize utility, even at the expense of harming a dear friend and violating a trust which has been placed in me.

Some philosophers believe that examples such as this show that AU takes promises, commitments, special relationships of trust, and so on, far too lightly. Indeed, some think it makes such factors totally irrelevant. This is because AU is a monistic theory of obligation which posits one and only one obligation—to maximize utility. Future consequences are all that count. Past commitments and special relationships are irrelevant.

A defender of AU, on the other hand, will likely reply that I have simply failed to consider all the relevant consequences. Of crucial importance here is not simply the fact that a marriage may be saved and a potentially destructive affair stopped, but also that my action will almost certainly destroy at least one valuable relationship (my friendship with Monica) which, in the long run, would add significantly to the utility I am able to bring about in my future actions. There is also the possibility that my betrayal will become common knowledge, thus threatening my role as a physician who can be trusted. Without my patients' trust, how can I practice medicine effectively? And if I cannot practice medicine effectively, how am I going to promote utility in my role as a doctor? Of course there's also the possibility that my action will weaken the public's trust of physicians in general—an even more disastrous possibility, viewed from the perspective of AU. All of these indirect consequences of breaking the agreement, when put into the balance, tip the scales in favour of keeping quiet. Those who think that AU takes special relationships and commitments far too lightly have simply ignored all the long-range, indirect effects of doing so.

So the defender of AU has a fairly forceful reply to such counter-examples to his theory of obligation. We should always be sure to ask, when a critic provides such an example: Have all the relevant consequences, long-range and indirect as well as immediate and direct, been accounted for? In all likelihood, they have not been. This is true whether we are talking about breaking confidences or violating autonomy.

Philosophers are fairly industrious when it comes to thinking up counter-examples to ethical theories. Having met replies such as the above, they have altered their counter examples to get rid of those convenient indirect, long-range effects upon which the defence is based. Some have dreamt up the *Desert Island Promise Case*, a version of which now follows.

> You and a friend are alone on a deserted island. Your friend is dying and asks you to see to it when you are rescued that the elder of her two children receives the huge sum of money your friend has secretly stashed away. You now are the only other person who knows of its existence. You solemnly promise to fulfil your friend's final request and she passes away secure in the knowledge that her last wish is in good hands. Upon rescue you are faced with a dilemma. The elder child turns out to be a lazy lout who squanders to no good end—even his own pleasure—whatever money he has. Even when he has lots of money to spend he still ends up being miserable and causing misery to other people. Your friend's younger child, however, is an aspiring researcher in dermatology. She is on the brink of uncovering a solution to the heartache of psoriasis, but will fail unless she receives financial backing. All her applications for grants have unjustly been denied and she has been left in desperation. As a good act utilitarian, you reason that utility would obviously be maximized if your solemn word to your dying friend were broken and you gave the money to the younger daughter. Think of all the utility that would be realized, all the suffering that would be alleviated! Compare this with the very little utility and considerable disutility that would result were you to give the money to the elder son.

Notice that in this case all the indirect, long-range consequences to which appeal was made in Monica's case are absent. No one will know that the promise is being broken and there are no valuable, utility-enhancing relationships in jeopardy. Your friend is dead. There seems little doubt in this situation that the promise should be broken according to AU—this is your moral obligation. But surely, the opponent will argue, this cannot be so. Solemn promises to dying friends, regardless of the good consequences which might be realized by breaking them, must be kept, except perhaps where disaster would result from keeping them. That it seems in such cases to give no weight at all to such promises shows that AU is a faulty theory of obligation. Solemn promises should weigh heavily—and independently of good consequences. Hence AU cannot be an adequate theory.

So promises and other such special commitments pose difficulties for AU. Free riders do too. Suppose there is a temporary but serious energy shortage in your community. All private homes and businesses have been requested to conserve electricity and gas. Private homes are to keep their thermostats no higher than 15 degrees centigrade and all businesses are temporarily to cut production by one-half. If everyone helps out in this way an overload which would prove disastrous will be avoided. Being a good act utilitarian, and knowing the tendencies of your neighbours, you reason as follows. "I know that everyone else will pay scrupulous attention to the government's request. So the potential disaster will be averted regardless of what I do. It will make no difference whatsoever if I run my production lines at two-thirds capacity. The little bit of extra electricity we use will have no negative effect at all. Of course if everyone ran at two-thirds, then disaster would result. But I know this is not going to happen and so the point is irrelevant. As for my employees, they will see a reduction and assume that the cut was to one-half, so no one will know but me. Using two-thirds, then, will in no way prove harmful, but it will make a considerable amount of difference to my balance sheet. The extra production will enable the company to show a much higher profit this year. All things considered, then, it is morally permissible, indeed, my moral obligation, to run at two-thirds. This is what AU tells me that I should do."

Imagine the moral outrage which would result were your acting on this line of reasoning to become

common knowledge. If the case seems far-fetched, consider how an analogous line of reasoning could be employed to justify extra diagnostic tests for a patient. Were you to pursue the recommended conduct, you would be labeled a "free rider," one who rides freely while others shoulder the burdens necessary for all to prosper. Your actions would be thought most unfair to all those who had willingly sacrificed their best interests, or the interests of their patients, for the good of everyone concerned. All this despite your efforts to maximize the utility of your actions.

In response to these (and similar) sorts of objections, some utilitarians have developed an alternative to AU. Consider further what would be said if your free riding came to light. The likely response would be to say: "Sure, no one is harmed if you use the extra electricity or prescribe the extra diagnostic tests. But imagine what would happen if everyone did what you are doing. Imagine if that became the norm. Disaster would result!" This request: "Imagine what would happen if everybody did that" has great **probative** force for many people. If *not everyone* could do what I propose to do without serious harm resulting, then many are prepared to say that it would be wrong for *anyone* to do it, and hence wrong for me to do it. In response to the force of this intuition, some utilitarians have developed a very different variety of their theory called *rule utilitarianism* (RU). On this version the rightness or wrongness of an action is not to be judged by its consequences. Rather, it is to be judged by the consequences of everyone's adopting a *general rule* under which the action falls.

As an introduction to RU, consider a case outlined by John Rawls in his famous paper "Two Concepts of Rules."[5] Rawls has us imagine that we are a sheriff in the deep American south. The rape of a white woman has taken place and although the identity of the rapist is unknown, it is clear that the offender was black. The predominantly white and racially **bigoted** community is extremely agitated over the incident and great social unrest is threatening. Riots are about to break out and many innocent, and possibly some not so innocent, people will be killed. If you were able to identify and arrest the rapist, the unrest would undoubtedly subside; but unfortunately you have no leads, other than the fact that the rapist was black. It occurs to you that you do not really need the actual culprit to calm things down. Why not simply concoct a case against a randomly chosen black man who has no alibi and have him arrested? The crowd will be placated, and although one innocent man will suffer, many innocent lives will be saved.

Rawls uses this example to illustrate an apparent weakness in AU and how RU allows one to overcome it. The consequences of framing the (possibly) innocent black are far better (or less bad), in terms of utility, than allowing the riot to occur. Hence, AU seems to require the frame, a course of action which is clearly unjust. Of course the defender of AU has several tricks up his sleeve at this point. He can once again appeal to the possible indirect effects of the frame. Suppose the lie came to light. Terrible social paranoia and unrest would result; people would no longer trust the judicial system and would wonder constantly whether they might be next. Indirect consequences such as these, the defender of AU will argue, clearly outweigh any short-term, direct benefits. But Rawls suggests that we consider a different question than the one AU would have us ask. We are to consider whether a general rule which permits the framing of innocent persons could possibly figure in a moral code general acceptance of which would result in the maximization of utility. If it could not (which is surely the case), then the proposed frame is morally impermissible. Since no such general rule could find its way into an acceptable moral code, largely for the reasons mentioned above in the parenthetical aside, an action in accordance with that rule would be morally wrong. Hence it would be morally wrong on RU to frame the possibly innocent black, even if the consequences of that particular action would be better than those of the alternatives. We are not morally required, on RU, to perform actions which individually would maximize utility. Rather we are to perform actions which accord with a set of rules whose general observance would maximize utility. Actions are judged according to whether they conform with acceptable rules; only the rules themselves are judged in terms of utility. The essence of RU is expressed in the following claim:

RU: An act is morally right if and only if it conforms with a set of rules whose general observance would maximize utility.

One extremely important difference between RU and AU is worth stressing. It is quite possible, on RU, to be required to perform an action which does not, on that particular occasion, maximize utility. Observance of the best set of general rules does not, on each individual occasion, always lead to the best consequences. Of course it *generally* does, but there are exceptions. This is something the defender of RU seems willing to live with for the sake of overall, long-term utility gains and the ability to deal with desert-island promises, free riders, and so on.

RU is not without its difficulties, however. Some utilitarians claim, for example, that RU really does violate the spirit of utilitarianism and amounts to "rule worship."[6] If the ideal behind utilitarianism is the maximization of utility, then should we not be able to deviate from the generally acceptable rules when doing so will serve to maximize utility? If the defender of RU allows exceptions to be made in such cases, then he runs the risk of collapsing his RU into AU. The rules would no longer hold any special weight or authority in our moral decisions. We would end up following the rules when it is best to do so and depart from them when that seems best.[7] In each case we seem led to do what AU requires, namely, maximize the utility of our individual actions. If, on the other hand, the defender of RU holds fast and says we must *never* deviate from rules which generally advance utility but sometimes do not, then the charge of rule worship comes back to plague the utilitarian.

A second problem facing RU can be summed up in an example. Suppose it were true that the best set of rules for the circumstances of our society would place an obligation on first-born children to provide for their elderly parents. I, the younger of two sons, reason that I therefore have no obligation whatsoever to provide for my elderly parents, even though I know that my elder brother is unwilling to provide more than the 50 per cent he thinks we each ought to provide. My parents end up living a life of abject poverty on only 50 per cent of what they need to sustain themselves. Something seems clearly wrong here. Our obligations, it would seem, cannot be entirely a function of an *ideal code* which may never in fact be followed by anyone except me. We seem to require, in an acceptable moral theory, some recognition of how other people are behaving, what rules they are in fact following. The rules they are following may be perfectly acceptable but not ideal, in which case I should perhaps follow them too. This is as true in medicine as it is elsewhere. Serious harm might result were an idealistic physician to act according to an ideal code, general observance of which would maximize utility, when no one else was prepared to do so. Perhaps here the excuse, "But no one else is willing to do it" carries some weight.

To sum up, there are significant differences between AU and RU and neither theory is free from difficulty. AU requires that we always seek, on each particular occasion, to maximize utility. It has difficulties with, among other things, free riders, desert-island promises, and sheriffs tempted by good consequences to commit injustice. RU tells us to perform actions that conform to a set of rules general observance of which would lead to the best consequences overall. This theory seems to provide solutions to many of the problems plaguing AU but it does so only at the expense of introducing new puzzles of its own. It must somehow provide a bridge between the best ideal code and the actual beliefs, practices, and accepted rules of one's society, all the while steering a course between rule worship and a straightforward reduction to AU.

(b) Deontological Ethics: Immanuel Kant

Kant, like Mill, proposes a monistic theory of obligation. Unlike that of Mill, however, the theory is thoroughly non-consequentialist. It denies that the possible consequences of our actions are what determine their rightness or wrongness. According to Kant,

> An action done from duty has its moral worth, not in *the purpose* [i.e. the consequences] to be attained by it, but in the maxim in accordance with which it is decided upon; it depends, therefore, not on the realization of the object of the action, but solely on the *principle of volition* [the maxim] in accordance with which, irrespective

of all objects of the faculty of desire [i.e. pleasure, happiness, preferences] the action has been performed.[8]

In this remark we see clearly that Kant espouses a deontological theory of obligation. The morality of an action is determined not by its consequences but by the maxim, the general principle, to which it conforms. Its moral worth lies not in the happiness or pleasure it produces, but in the kind of action it is. Let's try to clarify this point.

A key notion in Kant's theory is the notion of a maxim. By this technical term Kant means a general rule or principle which specifies what it is I conceive myself as doing and my reason for doing it. For example, suppose I decide to tell a lie in order to avoid distress to my patient. The maxim of my action could be expressed in the following way: "Whenever I am able to avoid distress to my patient by lying, I shall do so." This maxim makes plain that I conceive myself as lying and that my reason is the avoidance of a patient's distress. It makes plain that I consider the avoidance of such distress as a *sufficient reason* to lie. Were I to act on my maxim I would in effect be expressing my commitment to a general rule which extends in its scope beyond the particular situation in which I find myself. In supposing that the avoidance of patient distress is a sufficient reason in that situation to lie, I commit myself to holding that in any other situation just like it, i.e. any other case in which a lie would serve to avoid a patient's distress, I should tell a lie. This *generalizability of reasons* and maxims can perhaps be illustrated through an example involving a non-moral judgment.

Suppose you and I are baseball fans.

I say to you, "The Toronto Blue Jays are a good baseball team because their team batting average is about .260 and the average ERA among their starting pitchers is under 3.50."

You reply, "What is your opinion of the Montreal Expos?"

I say, "They are a lousy team."

You reply, "But their team batting average is also about .260 and the average ERA among their starters is 3.40."

I am stuck here in a logical inconsistency. I must either modify my earlier assessment of the Blue

Jays—say that they too are a lousy team—or admit that the Expos are also a good team. By citing my reasons for judging the Blue Jays a good ball team, I commit myself to a general maxim that *any* baseball team with a team batting average of over .260 and whose starting rotation has an ERA of below 3.50 is a good baseball team. If I don't agree with the implications of that general maxim, e.g. I still think the Expos are a bad ball team, then logical consistency demands that I reject or modify the maxim. Perhaps I will add that in addition to a team batting average of over .260 and a ERA among starting pitchers of under 3.5, a good baseball team must have several "clutch" players. I would add this if I thought that the absence of clutch players explains why the Expos, unlike the Blue Jays, are not a good team. Of course I could make this alteration only if I thought the Blue Jays did have at least a few clutch players.

So my maxim that whenever I can avoid distress to my patient by lying I shall do so, insofar as it expresses a general reason, applies to other situations similar to the one in which I initially act upon it. But this is not the full extent of my commitment. If avoiding patient distress really is a sufficient reason for *my* telling a lie, then it must also be a sufficient reason for *anyone else* who finds herself in a situation just like mine. According to Kant, and virtually all moral philosophers, acting upon a maxim commits me, as a rational moral agent, to a *universal* moral rule governing all persons in situations just like mine (in the relevant respects). I must be prepared to accept that a sufficient reason for me is a sufficient reason for anyone else in precisely my situation. This is the force of the first formulation of Kant's Categorical Imperative we are about to consider. If I think some other person in a position to avoid patient distress by lying should not tell the lie, then I must either retract my earlier maxim or specify some relevant difference between our situations, as I did when I tried to show that the Expos are a bad baseball team despite their strong team batting average and pitching staff.

(i) The Categorical Imperative, first formation: logical consistency

Acting for reasons, that is, acting rationally (which is required, according to Kant if we are to be moral),

commits me to universal rules or maxims which I must be prepared to accept. Kant expresses this point in terms of my capacity to will that my personal maxim should become a *universal law*. According to the first formulation of the Categorical Imperative, the fundamental principle of obligation in Kant's monistic system, "I ought never to act except in such a way that *I can also will that my maxim should become a universal law*."[9] Later he writes, "*Act as if the maxim of your action were to become through your will a universal law of nature*."[10] According to Kant, immoral maxims and the immoral actions based upon them can never, under any conceivable circumstances, pass the Categorical Imperative test. This is not, as we shall now see, because the consequences of general observance of an immoral maxim would be undesirable in terms of utility. Rather it is because the state of affairs in which the maxim is observed as a universal law is *logically impossible* or *inconceivable*—it involves us in contradiction.

Some states of affairs simply cannot exist, in the strongest sense of "cannot." The state of affairs in which I am, at one and the same time, Rob's father *and* Rob's son is logically impossible. It cannot exist: Were I for some strange reason to will that this state of affairs exist, my will, Kant would say, would contradict itself. It would be willing inconsistent, contradictory things: that I am Rob's father and son at one and the same time. Now consider a case actually discussed by Kant. Suppose that a man

finds himself driven to borrowing money because of need. He well knows that he will not be able to pay it back; but he sees too that he will get no loan unless he gives a firm promise to pay it back within a fixed time. He is inclined to make such a promise; but he has still enough conscience to ask "Is it not unlawful and contrary to duty to get out of difficulties in this way?" Supposing, however, he did resolve to do so, the maxim of his action would run thus, "Whenever I believe myself short of money, I will borrow money and promise to pay it back, though I know that this will never be done." Now this principle of self-love or personal advantage is perhaps quite compatible with my own entire future welfare; only there remains the question "Is it right?" I therefore transform the demand of self love into a universal law and frame my question thus, "How would things stand if my maxim became a universal law?" I then see straight away that this maxim can never rank as a universal law of nature and be self-consistent, but must necessarily contradict itself. For the universality of a law that every one believing himself to be in need can make any promise he pleases with the intention not to keep it would make promising, and the very purpose of promising, itself impossible, since no one would believe he was being promised anything, but would laugh at utterances of this kind as empty shams.[11]

It is important to be clear exactly what Kant is saying in this passage. He is not objecting to insincere promises on the ground that they will cause others to lose confidence in us and mean that we will jeopardize the valuable consequences of future promises. Nor is he arguing that false promises contribute to a general mistrust of promises and the eventual collapse of a valuable social practice. These are all *consequentialist* considerations which, according to the deontologist Kant, are totally irrelevant to questions of moral obligation. His point is a very different one. He is suggesting that a state of affairs in which everyone in need makes false promises is incoherent. There is a *contradiction* because, on the one hand, everyone in need *would* borrow on false promises. They would be following the maxim "as a law of nature," with the same regularity as the planets observe Kepler's laws of planetary motion. Yet on the other hand, in this very same state of affairs no one *could* borrow on a false promise, because if such promises were always insincere, no one would be stupid enough to lend any money. Promising requires trust on the part of the promisee, but in the state of affairs contemplated there just couldn't be any, and so promises of the sort in question would simply be impossible. Hence, any attempt to will, as a universal law of nature, the maxim "Whenever I believe myself short of money, I will borrow money and promise to pay it back, though I know that this will never be done," lands us in contradiction. "I ... see straight away that this maxim can never rank as a universal law of nature and be self-consistent, but must necessarily contradict itself."[12]

With Kant, then, we have a moral test of our actions which does not lie in an assessment of their consequences. Nor does the test lie in weighing the consequences of adopting a general rule which licences those actions. Rather, the test considers the logical coherence of the universalized maxim upon which I personally propose to act. Whether this test successfully accounts for all of our moral obligations is highly questionable. Is there anything incoherent in the state of affairs in which everyone kills his neighbour if she persists in playing her stereo at ear-piercing levels? Such a state of affairs might be highly *undesirable* (though some days I really do wonder) but it seems perfectly possible or conceivable. Yet killing off annoying neighbours seems hardly the right thing to do.

(ii) The Categorical Imperative, second formulation: Don't Just Use People

Kant provided two further formulations of his Categorical Imperative. He thought these versions equivalent to the first, though it is difficult to see why Kant thought this to be so. The equivalence question needn't concern us here however. The additional formulations bring to light two important principles which many people find highly appealing and which may prove helpful in dealing with some of the problems discussed later in this text.

According to Kant, if I act only on maxims which could, without contradiction, serve as universal laws I will never treat people as *mere means* to my ends. The Categorical Imperative requires that I "Act in such a way that [I] always treat humanity, whether in [my] own person or in the person of any other, never simply as a means, but always at the same time as an end."[13] In more common terms, we should never just *use* people. The emphasis here is on the *intrinsic worth* and *dignity* of rational creatures. I treat rational beings as ends in themselves if I respect in them the same value I discover in myself, namely, my freedom to determine myself to action and to act for reasons which I judge for myself. As Kant observes, there can be nothing more dreadful to a rational creature than that his actions should be subject to the will of another. I treat others as mere things rather than as persons, subject them to my will in the way I do a tool, if I fail to respect their dignity. This principle has an important role to play in assessing, for example, the therapeutic relationship, the requirement of informed, valid consent to medical experimentation, and requests for physician-assisted suicide.

(iii) The Categorical Imperative, third formulation: Autonomous Agents

Kant's third formulation of the Categorical Imperative seems closely tied to the second. In effect, it spells out what it is in rational agents which gives them their dignity and worth. It requires that we treat others as *autonomous* agents, capable of self-directed, rational action. The capacity to rise above the compelling forces of desire, self-interest, and physical necessity, to act freely on the basis of *reasons*, is what gives rational beings their dignity and worth. To treat a person as an end in herself, then, is to respect her autonomy and freedom. It rules out various kinds of manipulative practices and paternalistically motivated behaviours. In a case involving asbestos poisoning at Johns Manville,[14] company doctors neglected to tell workers the alarming results of their medical tests. This was rationalized on the ground that there was nothing that could be done to curb the disease anyway, and so the workers were better off not knowing. Such paternalistic conduct clearly violated Kant's Categorical Imperative. It failed to respect the autonomy and dignity of the asbestos workers. Of course the conduct might have been fully justified by AU, though this point is open to argument. Whether in the long run such deceptions serve to maximize utility is perhaps questionable.

With Kant we have a clear alternative to the monistic, teleological theory of obligation provided by the act and rule utilitarians. Kant's theory is clearly deontological and is at the very least monistic in its intent. Kant attempts to ground all our obligations on one fundamental principle: the Categorical Imperative. As we have seen, Kant provides three formulations of this principle, though it is difficult to see how they are exactly equivalent. In any event, we may view Kant as requiring that we ask the following three questions:

1. Could I consistently will, as a universal law, the personal maxim upon which I propose to act?
2. Would my action degrade other rational agents or myself by treating them or myself as a mere means?
3. Would my action violate the autonomy of some rational agent, possibly myself?

Should any of these three questions yield the wrong answer, my moral obligation is to refrain from acting on my personal maxim.

(c) Ethical Pluralism: W.D. Ross

As we noted above, W.D. Ross's contribution to ethics is valuable both for its reaction to what some see as the reductionism of Kant and Mill, and because it seems more accurately to reflect the ordinary thinking and practice of moral agents than the more systematic reflections of professional moral philosophers.

Ross's theory of obligation arose mainly out of his dissatisfaction with utilitarian theories. While Ross's main target was G.E. Moore, his criticisms are relevant to utilitarianism in general, particularly AU. According to Ross, utilitarianism in all of its guises grossly oversimplifies the moral relationships between people. As we have seen, utilitarianism is, in the end, concerned solely with the maximization of utility. Our concern should rest exclusively with the overall consequences of our actions, or the rules under which we perform them. In Ross's view, morality should acknowledge the importance of consequences, but not exclusively. Utilitarianism errs in thinking that consequences are all that matter, in thinking that "the only morally significant relationship in which my neighbours stand to me is that of being possible beneficiaries [or victims] of my action."[15] It errs, in other words, in being a monistic, teleological theory of obligation. Ross proposes instead a pluralistic theory of obligation which recognizes several, irreducible moral relationships and principles. In addition to their role as possible beneficiaries of my actions, my fellow human beings "may also stand to me in the relation of promisee to promiser, of creditor to debtor, of wife to husband, of child to parent, of friend to friend, of fellow countryman to fellow countryman, and the like."[16] "The like" no doubt includes the relation of doctor to patient, doctor to nurse, experimenter to subject and so on, relationships which are integral to the healthcare professions and which are ignored only at the cost of moral confusion.

In Ross's view, utilitarianism not only oversimplifies the moral relationships in which we stand to others, it also distorts the whole basis of morality by being thoroughly teleological in orientation. On utilitarian theories we must always be *forward-looking* to the future consequences of our actions or rules. But sometimes, Ross urges, morality requires that we look *backwards* to what has occurred in the past. There is significance, for example, in the sheer fact that a promise has been made, a promise which has moral force independent of any future good consequences that might arise from keeping it. This moral force explains why we should normally keep promises made to dying friends even if utility would be maximized were we to break them. A promise itself, because of the *kind* of action it is, has a moral force which is totally independent of its consequences. Teleological theories, because they ignore such features and are entirely forward-looking, distort morality. *Promises, contracts, commitments* to serve a certain role, *agreements, loyalty, friendship* and so on, all have moral force, and all can give rise to obligations and responsibilities independently of good or bad consequences.

Ross provides us, then, with a pluralistic, deontological theory of obligation. In this theory we find a plurality of ultimate principles, only some of which are consequentialist in orientation. According to Ross, each of these principles specifies a *prima facie* duty or obligation. These are duties which we must fulfil *unless* we are also, in the circumstances, subject to another, competing prima facie duty of greater weight. We have a prima facie duty to tell the truth, which means that we must always tell the truth unless a more stringent duty applies to us and requires a falsehood. An example from Kant helps to illustrate this feature nicely.

Kant is notorious for arguing that the Categorical Imperative establishes an unconditional duty always to tell the truth. He has us consider a case where a murderer comes to our door asking for the whereabouts of his intended victim. Should we tell him the truth, that the victim is seeking refuge in our house, and thereby become accomplices in his murder? Both AU and RU would undoubtedly licence a lie under such extraordinary circumstances, but according to Kant the Categorical Imperative does not. The duty to tell the truth is unconditional, despite the consequences of its observance. "To be truthful (honest) in all declarations ... is a sacred and absolutely commanding decree of reason, limited by no expediency."[17] According to Ross's theory this is not so. Kant's case is clearly one where our prima facie duty to be truthful is overridden or outweighed by more stringent duties to our friend.

Ross's list of prima facie duties provides a helpful classification of some of the various duties and morally significant relationships recognized in our everyday moral thinking. There are:

1. Duties resting on previous actions of our own. These include:
   (a) duties of *fidelity* arising from explicit or implicit promises;
   (b) duties of *reparation*, resting on previous wrongful acts of ours and requiring that we compensate, as best we can, the victims of our wrongful conduct.
2. Duties resting on the services of others; duties of *gratitude* which require that we return favour for favour.
3. Duties involving the *fair* distribution of goods; duties of *justice*, which require fair sharing of goods to be distributed.
4. Duties to improve the condition of others; duties of *beneficence* (which in part form the basis of utilitarian theories of obligation).
5. Duties to improve our own condition; duties of *self-improvement*.
6. Duties not to injure others; duties of *non-maleficence*.[18]

Ross's list of duties is by no means exhaustive, and no doubt many would quarrel with some of the duties Ross has included. For instance, it might be questioned whether duties of self-improvement belong on a list of *moral* duties. It is plausible to suppose that moral duties arise only in our relationships with other people; that the demands of morality govern inter-personal relationships only. Allowing one's talents to lie unused or allowing one's health to deteriorate may be imprudent or foolish, but is it immoral? Perhaps it is if others, say our children, are depending on us. But in this case it is not a moral duty of self-improvement which is violated but rather the duty of beneficence and possibly that of non-maleficence.

Another questionable entry on Ross's list is the duty to be grateful. If someone does me a favour, is it true that I am required, as a matter of duty, to be grateful? Is gratitude something that can be subject to duty, or is it rather something that must be freely given, given not out of a sense of duty but out of genuine, heartfelt goodwill? If a favour is done with the sense that something is *owing* as a result, then perhaps it is not really a favour at all, but an investment.

According to Ross, that we have the prima facie duties he mentions is simply *self-evident* to any rational human being who thinks seriously about the requirements of morality. The existence of these duties, and the validity of the principles which describe them, are known through *moral intuition*. To say that a principle is self-evident and known through intuition is to say that its truth is evident to an attentive mind, that it neither needs supporting evidence nor needs to be deduced from other propositions. It stands alone as something obviously true. In this instance, it stands alone as something whose truth is known directly through *moral* intuition.

This feature of Ross's theory is very controversial among philosophers, who are generally suspicious of "self-evident principles" and "intuition." In the case of morality, the apparent obviousness of some principles, and the certainty with which many believe them, seem better explained by such things as uniform moral upbringing and common experiences. And then there is the problem of disagreement. If a principle truly is self-evident, then should not everyone agree on its validity? Yet this is seldom, if ever, the case with moral principles, including those on Ross's list.

This is not the place to discuss further the reasons behind the philosopher's suspicions concerning self-evidence and moral intuition, except to add the following. One who claims self-evidence for his views has little to say to those holding conflicting self-evident claims. He can ask that we think again, but he cannot undertake to prove his claims to us. If his claims truly are self-evident and known through intuition, they are in need of no proof. Perhaps more importantly, none can be given. So if, after careful reflection, you continue to disagree with some of the principles on Ross's list, he has little recourse but to accuse you of moral blindness. He must view you as equivalent to a person who cannot see the difference between red and blue; your moral blindness is on a par with his colour blindness. One might ask whether this is a satisfactory response to serious moral disagreements among reasonable people of good will and integrity.

Ross believes that his self-evident principles articulate prima facie moral obligations. These are obligations which hold unless overridden in individual cases by a more stringent or weightier duty. As for how we are to determine which of two or more prima facie duties has greater weight in a given case, Ross simply says that we must use our best judgment. This is of little help because it fails to tell us the considerations upon which our judgments are to be based. Ross is fully aware that in most cases of conflicting obligations it is far from clear which duty is more stringent. Reasonable people of moral integrity will disagree. We therefore seem left with a serious gap in the theory and must either accept that in cases of conflict there is no one right thing to do, that the best we can do is fulfil one of our conflicting duties and violate the other; or we must continue to look for a *criterion* in terms of which conflicts can be resolved.

It is at this point that the utilitarian will be more than happy to offer assistance. In his view, Ross has isolated the basis for a set of rules which are indeed important in everyday moral thinking. According to the defender of AU, these Rossian rules are useful guidelines or rules of thumb which we are well advised in most cases to follow. If we follow them regularly, our actions will in the long run end up maximizing utility. The act of promising usually does maximize utility, as does a display of gratitude. But in those cases in which a conflict in the rules arises, or where an applicable rule seems inappropriate for good utilitarian reasons, we must resort directly to the AU criterion and decide which action will maximize utility. As for the proponent of RU, he will likely claim that Ross's rules will almost certainly figure in the set of rules general observance of which, within a modern society, will maximize utility. He too is likely to claim that in cases in which the rules conflict direct recourse must be made to the principle of utility. We must follow the rule which in the circumstances will lead to the maximization of utility. Of course Ross must reject the utilitarian's offer of rescue. Were he to follow the utilitarian's lead he would in effect be adopting the principle of utility as defining a single, ultimate obligation, and this would be to deny Ross's central claim that each of his prima facie duties is ultimate and irreducible. But then it is far from clear how this plurality of irreducible duties is to be dealt with in cases of conflict. We seem truly left with a serious gap. Without a means of adjudicating among conflicting prima facie duties, we are left short just where we need guidance the most.

(d) Virtue Ethics: Aristotle

(i) What should we be? versus What ought we to do? Despite their many differences, the theories of Kant, Ross, and the utilitarians had at least one thing in common: they were all designed to answer directly the question "What ought I to do?" In other words, these theories were designed to help us determine what action(s) we should perform in particular circumstances. The concern, in short, was with the rightness of actions, with determining wherein our duty lies. According to Kant, the question "What ought I to do?" is answered by determining whether the maxim of one's action can be universalized. For rule utilitarians the answer lies in whether the rule(s) under which one acts maximize(s) overall utility. Although act utilitarians believe that rules have no role in our moral reasoning, except as rules of thumb, the question remains: "What is the right thing for me to do in these circumstances?" According to act utilitarians, we answer this question by determining which of the actions open to us would maximize utility. Ross too was concerned to help us determine what we should do in particular circumstances, with determining the course of (right) action wherein our moral duty lies. Modern theories sometimes transform the questions of Mill, Ross, and Kant into questions about our rights, but still the emphasis is on the evaluation of actions, on determining what we have or do not have rights to *do*.

Much earlier in the history of moral philosophy, the Greek philosopher Aristotle sought to cast ethics in an entirely different mould. This is a mould which some contemporary moral philosophers find highly appealing partly because it allows us to avoid many of the difficulties encountered by the traditional deontological and utilitarian theories, but also because it is thought to provide a much better understanding of our moral lives, what it is we strive to be in pursuing the moral life and why the moral life is important to us. The fundamental ethical question for Aristotle is not "What should I *do*?" but "What should I *be*?" As one similarly minded theorist put it,

> ... morality is internal. The moral law ... has to be expressed in the form, "be this," not in the form "do this." ... the true moral law says "hate not," instead of "kill not." ... the only mode of stating the moral law must be as a rule of character.[19]

For Aristotle, moral behaviour expresses *virtues* or qualities of *character*. There is a much greater emphasis on "character traits" and "types of persons," than on rules, obligations, duties, and rights. Aristotle is interested in questions such as these: Should we *be* stingy or generous? Hateful or benevolent? Cowardly or courageous? Over-indulgent or temperate? In what do these traits consist? How are they cultivated? And how do they figure in a life well lived? In discussing these questions about the character traits integral to moral life, Aristotle offered exemplars of virtue to emulate and vices to avoid rather than rules or principles to be obeyed or disobeyed. In short, for Aristotle, morality is *character-oriented* rather than *rule-driven*. Aristotle would no doubt have frowned on modern ethical theories which divorce actions and questions about them from the character of moral (or immoral) agents who perform them. Praiseworthy and blameworthy actions are not those which match up to a particular template of rules or principles, but rather ones which flow from and reveal a certain type of character. Moral agency is not merely a matter of which rules to follow; it flows from a whole way of life which requires a unity of thought and feeling characteristic of what Aristotle called "virtue."

(ii) Theoretical and practical reason

Aristotle divided knowledge into the theoretical and the practical. *Episteme* is concerned with speculative or theoretical inquiries, and its object is knowledge of the truth. This he contrasted with *phronesis* or practical knowledge which focuses on what is *"doable"* rather than on what is *knowable* for its own sake. Without *phronesis,* particular virtues of character (e.g., courage, moderation, and generosity) would not be achievable by human beings, and the conduct which flows from and expresses these virtues would not be likely. It is central to Aristotle's view of human knowledge and moral excellence that whereas the intellectual virtues associated with *episteme* can be acquired through teaching, the virtues of character achievable via phronesis require practice until they become "second nature." Moral virtue can not just be taught; it requires "training" and "habituation," the doing of virtuous actions. In order to be a virtuous person one must develop the disposition to be virtuous; and this requires training and the doing of virtuous actions till this becomes a settled disposition.

(iii) Human good

Aristotle's ethical theory is teleological. "Every art and every inquiry, every action and choice, seems to aim at some good; whence the good has rightly been defined as that at which all things aim."[20] There are different goods corresponding to the various arts and modes of inquiry. Navigation aims at safe voyages, the musical arts at the creation of beautiful music, and the medical arts aim at health. Is there, Aristotle asks, a good for human beings as such? If so, then perhaps we can begin to understand what we might call the art of living well by considering what is necessary to the achievement of that end? Just as we can understand proper medical practice in relation to the good which medicine strives to achieve, perhaps we can also understand moral life in relation to the good for humans which moral life strives to achieve. So Aristotle is interested in action in so far as it contributes to the good for human beings. The right thing to do is best understood in relation to what is conducive to the good for human beings, just as a "proper prescription" is best understood in relation to what is conducive to the patient's health.

In his classic work, the *Nicomachean Ethics,* Aristotle confines his discussion of the good, that at which all things aim, to human good. The good aimed at by human beings is *eudaemonia,* usually translated as "happiness" or "well-being."[21] Some people identify human good with such things as wealth, pleasure, and honour, but Aristotle quickly shows that these people cannot be right. Wealth, for example, is at best a (very unreliable) means to happiness, not happiness itself. Pleasure is not the good for human beings even though it is true, as Aristotle's teacher Plato argued, that the good person takes pleasure in virtuous activity. Pleasure is not itself the good, but only an external sign of the presence of goodness. One will experience pleasure when one does things well; doing well does not consist of the achievement of pleasure. In Aristotle's sense of the term, happiness or well-being is something enjoyed over a lifetime in the exercise of virtues such as courage, moderation, and generosity of spirit. In one sense the exercise of the virtues is a means to the achievement of happiness or well-being. In a deeper sense it is not. The exercise of virtue is integral to the achievement of happiness, constitutive of it, not merely a pre-payment of dues to insure happiness. In short, the virtuous life is not a means to the end of well-being; it *is* the life of well-being.

(iv) Virtue

Central to the Aristotelian conception of ethics and the good life is, as we have seen, the notion of "virtue." Aristotle's definition of this key notion is as follows. Virtue is "a state of character concerned with choice, lying in a mean, i.e. the mean relative to us, this being determined by rational principle, that principle by which the man [sic] of practical wisdom would determine it ..."[22] The key notions in this definition need to be clarified.

A central element in Aristotle's conception of virtue is "disposition." Virtue, as we will see, is a kind of disposition. William Frankena summarizes the nature of dispositions as follows:

> ... dispositions or traits ... are not wholly innate; they must all be acquired, at least in part, by teaching and practice, or, perhaps by grace. They are also traits of "character," rather than traits of "personality" like

charm or shyness, and they all involve a tendency to do certain kinds of action in certain kinds of situations, not just to think or feel in certain ways. They are not just abilities or skills, like intelligence or carpentry, which one may have without using.[23]

Linguistically, terms describing dispositions are often contrasted with "occurrence" terms. A dispositional term like "timid" tells us a good deal more about a person than the occurrence word "frightened." The former tells us something about the character of the individual, whereas the latter may tell us nothing more than that the person was in a particular state on some occasion or other. It is possible that the state we might call "Tom's being frightened" occurred on some occasion even though Tom has no disposition to be frightened. Very little future behaviour can be predicted from being told that someone is frightened or angry, even if we know the reasons why he is frightened or angry. On the other hand, if we are told that Sue is timid or irascible, then we can predict that she will tend to get frightened or angry in circumstances that would not frighten or anger other people with a more courageous or gentler disposition. Having such dispositions does not, of course, rule out the possibility of sometimes acting "out of character." There are provocations that would try even the patience of Job, some tasks so dangerous as to deter the most courageous and resolute persons, and some offers that even the most conscientious person cannot refuse. Dispositions, as tendencies, have an elasticity about them.

Aristotle's definition of virtue begins with virtue as a disposition, but it does not end there. Virtue is a disposition *to choose well*. Commenting on the etymology of the Greek word for choice, *prohairesis*, Aristotle writes: "the very term *prohairesis* ... denotes something chosen before other things."[24] Choosing something before other things requires (a) the presence of alternatives. Without alternatives there can be no choice. It also requires (b) deliberation about the relative merits of the alternatives open to the agent. Virtuous actions are principled and thoughtful. They are responses rather than reactions. Deliberation about the alternatives open to the agent requires (c) ranking of those alternatives. One alternative is preferred to another and chosen. Finally,

prohairesis presupposes (d) voluntarism. Virtue requires that we are responsible for our own actions. We are the begetters or efficient causes of our own actions, agents not patients. Our actions must be "self-caused," i.e., "in our power and voluntary."[25]

Aristotle emphasizes that primarily choice is restricted to means and not ends. The ultimate and remote end of our choosing, *eudaemonia* or happiness, is fixed by human nature.

(v) Human nature, essentialism, relativism
Just as all things within the universe have an essential nature (understood by Aristotle in terms of a unique function the thing serves) in relation to which their "good" can be understood, human nature provides a natural basis for understanding the good for human beings. This particular feature of Aristotle's view allows him to avoid arbitrariness in his ethics; ethics is not based on variable social norms or customs, or on the personal predilections of individuals or groups of individuals. Ethics is not "culturally relative" or "subjective" on this account; it is grounded in nature and to that extent "objective." Although the "objectivity" of the Aristotelian schema allows Aristotle to avoid relativism, it is a serious source of concern for some. Many critics see danger in the idea that there is a largely fixed, essential human nature in terms of which the moral life, and the requirements it places upon us, are to be understood. Some followers of Aristotle have argued that procreation is "natural" to human beings (as it is to all organisms) and that so-called "artificial" means of reproduction are therefore inherently suspicious and perhaps even immoral. Others take a similar line of argument in supporting the view that homosexuality is immoral. Whether such views follow from the Aristotelian system is highly questionable. But there is, nevertheless, cause to be concerned about a theory which seeks to define the moral in terms of what is "natural" for human beings. All too often what is thought to be "natural" is really only the conventional. And as feminists and other social critics point out, the conventional is often the result of bias, misunderstanding, and oppression.

If the ultimate end of our choosing is fixed by human nature, and the alternatives open to us when we seek to be virtuous are alternative ways of promoting this end, i.e., alternative ways of promoting *eudaemonia*, then the following question arises. Is Aristotle in fact advocating what we might call the *principle of eudaemonia*, as opposed to the principle of utility? And is this not a principle which can be applied, either directly or indirectly, to our actions in such a way that we have a means of determining morally right actions? For example, particular virtues like truth-telling, promise-keeping, and their ilk could be viewed as means toward achieving the ultimate end of *eudaemonia* or happiness. If this is so, then in actual fact there may be little to distinguish Aristotle's so-called "virtue ethics" from the action-centred "duty ethics" of Kant, Mill, and Ross.

(vi) The Aristotlean mean

Although there is some truth in this assessment of Aristotle's ethics, it would be a mistake to exaggerate it. This is because, for Aristotle, virtuous action is not action which accords with a principle, but rather action which springs from a disposition to choose a way which lies between two extremes, the one an excess and the other a deficiency. Virtuous action lies in choosing *the mean* between extremes of behaviour one of which is a vice through excess, the other of which is a vice through deficiency. And Aristotle is clear that there is no arithmetical formula which allows us to determine with precision what lies at the mean in a particular set of circumstances. This is one reason why he says that the mean must be determined "relatively to us," and as determined not by a rule universally applicable and established in advance, but by a rule "by which a practically wise man [sic] would determine it." On Aristotle's account, there is a kind of indeterminacy in moral judgments when it comes to deciding on particular courses of action. The variable contexts of moral life prevent us from fashioning hard-and-fast rules or procedures for settling what we ought to do. The best we can do is rely on *phronesis*, our virtuous dispositions, and the examples set by paragons of virtue. We must, in other words, try under the circumstances to act as "the man [sic] of practical reason would act." This is the best that we can do. Whether this is a weakness in Aristotle's account of moral life is a good question. Perhaps this inherent indeterminacy better reflects moral reality and the perplexing

dilemmas with which we are often faced, than theories which purport to provide ready-made answers which fail to emerge when we seek to apply the theories to concrete circumstances. Is it any more helpful to be told that one must maximize utility, or seek to treat humanity as an end in itself, than it is to be told that one must seek a mean between deficiency and excess? In explicitly acknowledging that moral theory can provide only a limited amount of help, Aristotle's theory may in fact be the more honest one.

Virtue lies at the mean between the vices of excess and deficiency. The virtues of courage and moderation (or temperance) are among those chosen by Aristotle to elucidate his doctrine of the mean. The accounts are perhaps dated, but they nevertheless serve to illustrate the main lines of Aristotle's thought. For Aristotle, courage is primarily a virtue of soldiers and his examples are culled entirely from the battlefield. Courage is located between the defect of fear and the excess of over-spiritedness or brashness. When the occasion arises, a courageous soldier can be counted on to subdue fear and enter bravely into the fray even in the face of death. Cowardice is the vice (defect) associated with fear. In more modern parlance, we may link it with the instinct of "flight" in the face of danger. But rashness is also a vice, in this case an excess associated with spiritedness. This vice we may link with the instinct of "fight" in the face of danger. But one can be too spirited. Soldiers emboldened by anger may rush impulsively into the fray, "blind to the dangers that await them."[26] "Right reason" moderates fear, and courage emerges as fear tempered by spirit.

The application of Aristotle's model of course need not be limited. One may as readily look for displays of courage in the more familiar domains of sickness and death. These domains are also "battlefields" of sorts, in which individuals face handicap, major surgery, debilitating illness, and prolonged and painful dying. Aristotle's ethics-of-virtue may prove helpful in such circumstances. While it may prove impossible to determine a hard-and-fast rule to answer our moral questions in such instances, it may be possible to answer the question: "What kind of people do we wish to *be* when we are faced with such circumstances?" Do we wish, for example, to be cowardly, cringing in fear in the face of death, demanding that everything conceivable be done to prolong our lives regardless of quality? Or is this an option which would not be pursued by the person of courage? Is this how the person "of practical wisdom" would act, lacking in regard for others, insensitive to the fact that the resources used to prop up his life might be of more benefit to others with a more favourable prognosis? Or do we want to be courageous, moderating our fear of death and insensitivity to the needs of others as much as it lies within us to do so? In another context the relevant question might be: What kind of people do we want to be in the face of severe handicap or disability? Cowardly, living each moment in fear; or brash—at the opposite extreme from fear—living in denial, masking our true feelings from others and conducting ourselves in an unwarranted display of over-confidence or *bravado* rather than bravery? Or will we try to avoid both extremes and be courageous, striving to temper fear of death or handicap with a more reasonably nuanced and spirited response, trying to live life to the full within our disability, even though such daring involves risk? To these questions we may find reasonable answers, even if there are no rules by which they can be determined, and even if we must in the end still choose for ourselves that course of action which best exemplifies the virtuous mean.

The second virtue upon which Aristotle focuses is temperance—the trait which moderates our appetites for food, drink, and sex. One can eat too little or too much food. Aristotle designates health as the goal of eating. Gluttons are guilty of excess. They live to eat rather than eat to live. They dig their graves with their teeth. They imperil rather than preserve their health by over-eating. This is a vice of excess. The vice of defect or deficiency involves eating insufficient food in circumstances where there is enough to go around. In time of scarcity and famine, failure to eat sufficient food is not morally blameworthy. Strictly speaking, in such circumstances eating insufficient food does not qualify as a voluntary activity. Although Aristotle does not mention it, malnutrition can be caused by eating the wrong foods, not just by failing to eat enough food. One can be malnourished on a diet of soda pop and chips, or with fad diets motivated by a perceived

need to be slim. In such cases, Aristotle would attribute malnutrition to vice rather than misfortune or famine.

To be clear on Aristotle's ordering of values in this context, it must be borne in mind that while health is an immediate end of eating, it is not good in itself. Rather it is a means to happiness or well-being, i.e. *eudaemonic*, and is properly conceived only in this way. Relative to moderation in partaking of food and drink, health is a proximate end, but relative to the final end, happiness, it is *usually* a necessary means. This last point must be kept clearly in mind in medical contexts where there is sometimes a tendency to confuse means with ends. Life and "health" are important ends of human action, including medical action, but only if and to the extent that they contribute to what really counts: *eudaemonia*. When they do not, the person of practical reason and virtue will no longer see them as worthy of pursuit. The implications of this point for decisions concerning the "saving" of people who judge their lives no longer worth living are apparent and profound. Life and "health" are goods which confer rightness on the means for their achievement, but only when these contribute to *eudaemonia*.

(e) Feminist Perspectives

Many contemporary women and not a few men find all the approaches to ethics outlined above to be in many respects unsatisfactory and alienating. These theories were all developed by men who, it is claimed, inadvertently brought to bear upon their theoretical positions a number of biases and ways of viewing the world which skew the results of their analyses. The resultant theories do little justice to the moral concerns and experiences of women. Indeed, in the view of most feminist ethicists, the traditional theories "do not constitute the objective, impartial theories that they are claimed to be; rather, most theories reflect and support explicitly gender-biased and often blatantly misogynist values."[27] It would be impossible to provide a complete and fully accurate account of the important, multi-faceted themes pursued by feminist ethicists. Instead, we will attempt, in what follows, to sketch two of the most common concerns of feminists regarding traditional ethical theories.

First, there is the issue of power relationships, for which the health care context provides an obvious set of examples. Built right into most medical situations is a power imbalance between, on the one hand, vulnerable patients in need of assistance, and on the other hand, health-care workers whose knowledge, skill, and special privileges often place them in a superior position. But for women the inherent power imbalance has traditionally been all the more difficult to overcome because of a further factor: gender imbalance. According to many theorists, evidence shows that male physicians (which is to say, until recently, the overwhelming majority of doctors) have tended to treat female patients with condescension or disdain—and that the medical system itself has been heavily biased towards taking male afflictions much more seriously than female ones. In similar fashion, the role of (primarily male) doctors was often the near-exclusive focus of attention, and the role of (primarily female) nurses was often ignored. Such systemic gender-based imbalances have been a major focus of feminist attention.

Many feminists share a broader concern with power imbalances—between men and women, certainly, but also between other advantaged and oppressed groups such as adults and children, the able and the disabled, and the rich and the poor. Many feminists have pointed out that the field of ethical theory (like most fields) has historically been dominated largely by men whose perspectives may have been biased against women. Some traditional ethicists, e.g. Kant and Aristotle, thought that women have a decidedly different character from men, and are to a much greater extent than men moved by emotion as opposed to reason. In the view of these theorists, this tendency towards the emotional serves as a barrier to the level of abstract reasoning required for satisfactory moral thought. Feminist ethicists are concerned to undermine these stereotypes and to assert the equal ability of women to engage in moral thought.

More widely, one strain of feminist thought is opposed to the search for abstract, universalizable principles and rules (or even virtues) with which to answer everyone's moral questions. The theories of Kant and Mill are often cited as illustrative of the insufficiency of traditional ethical theory. In the view of many feminist critics, Kant's theory rejects the emotional, personal component of moral life in favour of the rational universalizability of individual maxims. In seeking rationally to universalize our maxims, we are inescapably led to ignore or submerge our concern for all those complex factors which *individuate* our situations and the relationships in which we find ourselves. Most importantly perhaps, in seeking such abstractions, we are led to ignore or abstract away all that makes us individual persons enmeshed in inter-personal relationships involving caring and trust. Among the factors so eliminated are the emotional bonds between people and the special concerns they have for one another, as parents, friends, siblings, and colleagues. In seeking to universalize we are, it is claimed, led to forget that most of the time we approach one another—and believe ourselves right in doing so—not as strangers subject to the same set of universalized maxims or rights, but as unique individuals in highly personal, context-specific relationships in which we have much invested emotionally. These are relationships which, by their very nature, cannot be reduced to universalized rules and principles. According to Susan Sherwin, a leading feminist philosopher:

> Because women are usually charged with the responsibility of caring for children, the elderly, and the ill as well as the responsibility of physically and emotionally nurturing men, both at work and at home, most women experience the world as a complex web of interdependent relationships, where responsible caring for others is implicit in their moral lives. The abstract reasoning of morality that centres on the rights [and duties] of independent agents is inadequate for the moral reality in which they live. Most women find that a different model for ethics is necessary; the traditional ones are not persuasive.[28]

The feminist concern for the importance of context leads in another direction as well. Many feminist philosophers argue not only for the importance of appreciating the factors which individuate one case from the other, and tie us to one another in a variety of personal ways; they also stress the importance of appreciating the wider context of decision-making. This is a context which, more often than not, profoundly influences the options available, or the options thought available, to us. Feminists look beyond the individual situations in which decisions are made and question the social and political institutions, practices, and beliefs that create those situations and define the available options. Consider, for example, the case of reproductive technologies. Here a plethora of ethical questions arises whenever a woman requests reproductive assistance in the face of infertility. Should any woman who asks for such aid be accommodated? What if she is unmarried, a lesbian, or already has children of her own? Is it permissible to create multiple fertilized eggs when only a few will actually be implanted at any one time? If so, may some of the extra eggs be used for purposes of medical research? These questions, and many others like them, are ones which everyone agrees deserve attention.

But many feminist ethicists want to dig much deeper. They want to uncover for discussion the variety of social, political, and environmental factors which give rise to such questions and possibly frame the available answers. They wish to expose certain social factors which arguably lead many women to request treatment despite the negligible chance of success and the profound disappointment which often accompanies failure. Many argue that the conventionally accepted view of women's social role, as fundamentally involving the production and rearing of offspring, encourages infertile women to see themselves as defective and lacking in value. As a consequence, they are in effect "coerced" into seeking biomedical interventions to correct themselves. And they suffer great feelings of inadequacy and worthlessness if, as is all too common, such interventions fail to bring about the desired result. Similar points are made in relation to cosmetic surgery which, it is argued, is often pursued by women only because of the force of socially generated stereotypes of femininity which ground a woman's value in her good looks.

To sum up, many feminist approaches to ethics are marked by their rejection of traditional ethical theory as far too abstract and concerned with universalized rules and principles. As such, traditional ethical theory misses out on two fronts. First, it renders irrelevant a host of individuating factors which inform our moral lives and which most of us, women in particular, consider integral to moral assessment. These include the importance of personal relationships and the emotional bonds which exist between individuals who care for one another. Second, traditional ethical theory often ignores the wider social, political, and environmental contexts in which moral questions are shaped and the available options are defined.

For much of the 1980's and 1990's a great deal of attention was paid to a strain of feminist thought that we have not yet mentioned—care ethics. According to theories put forward by Carol Gilligan and others, women had particular claims to ethical insight as a result of their being (whether from nature or from nurture) predisposed to an ethic of caring and concern for their fellow creatures. While this theory has attracted a great deal of attention, it has attracted considerable criticism as well, not least of all from feminists of a different stamp, who have seen in care ethics unfortunate echoes of 19th-century views of women's "special role"—views that supported restrictions against women becoming involved in society outside the home or the "helping professions" of teacher, governess, nurse.

Care ethics may have helped to raise the level of esteem in which such professions are held. But it has proved to be only one current of feminist thought, and not the main stream. This last is an important point in that it illustrates that there are many feminisms rather than one. Within the discipline of philosophy it is now broadly recognized that there are many varieties of feminist thought—and that they provide a range of challenges to traditional moral theory.

THE LANGUAGE OF RIGHTS

An introduction to the basic theories and concepts of ethics would be radically incomplete without some mention of "rights." At one time it was quite natural to express moral requirements using concepts such as *ought, duty*, and *obligation*. It was in terms of the latter three concepts that the ethical theories just discussed were presented by their authors. Today, however, our moral vocabulary is dominated by the notion of rights. Instead of saying "You ought not to have done that," or "Your responsibility was to have done this rather than that," a modern person is more apt to remark "You had no *right* to do that." But rights come in a variety of different forms which are often confused with one another. In order to facilitate discussion of the moral issues raised in this book, a brief analysis of these differences follows. The conceptual map sketched is largely derivative from the theory proposed early in the twentieth century by the American legal scholar, Wesley Hohfeld and from the more recent account developed by the contemporary moral philosopher Joel Feinberg.[29]

(a) Claim-rights

What is a "right?" Where does it come from? On what does it rest? Strictly speaking, Hohfeld thought, a right is an enforceable claim to someone else's action or non-action. If one has a right to X, then one can demand X as one's due. It is not merely good, desirable, or preferable that one should have X: one is entitled to it and another person, or group of persons, has a correlative duty or obligation to respect your entitlement to X. For instance, I have a right not to be assaulted by you. This entails that you are under an obligation of non-action, that is, a duty *not* to assault me. This kind of right, a claim against other people, is what Hohfeld called a *claim-right*. A claim-right is always paired with a corresponding duty or obligation which applies to at least one other person. Violation of my claim-right is always the violation by someone else of his or her duty towards me.

Claim-rights come in a variety of different forms. In sorting these out, Joel Feinberg develops three important distinctions:

(i)   in personam versus in rem rights
(ii   positive versus negative rights
(iii) passive versus active rights.

In personam rights are said to hold against one or more determinate, specifiable persons. These are determinate persons who are under corresponding or correlative obligations. For example, if Bill owes Jean a weekend at Camp David, then there is a specific person, Bill, against whom Jean enjoys his claim-right. Other examples are rights under contract, rights of landlords to payment of rent from their tenants, the right against one's employer to a safe and healthy working environment, the right against one's doctor to her best professional judgment about one's medical care, and so on. Many of the duties on Ross's list of prima facie duties could easily be expressed in terms of the correlative claim-rights. Paired with a Rossian duty of fidelity, for example, will be a claim-right against a person with whom one has made an agreement to the honouring of that agreement. That person has a duty to perform his end of the deal; you have a correlative claim-right to his performance.

Not all claim-rights, however, are held against specifiable persons. Some hold against people generally. These kinds of rights, called *in rem rights*, are said to hold against "the world at large." For instance, my right not to be assaulted holds not against any particular person or group of persons, but against anyone and everyone who might be in a position to commit such an offence against me. This includes my neighbours, people at bus stops, and surgeons who might be tempted to operate on me in a non-emergency situation without first obtaining my consent. All such persons have a correlative duty not to assault me. This latter, correlative duty, would no doubt fall under Ross's duties of non-maleficence.

Positive and negative rights form another subclass of claim-rights. A positive right is a right to someone else's positive action. A negative right, on the other hand, is a right to another person's non-action or forbearance. If I have a positive right to something, this means that there is at least one other person who has an obligation actually to do something, usually something for my benefit. By contrast, I have a negative right when there is at least one other person who has a duty to refrain from doing something, usually something which would harm me. Depending on what it is that the other person(s) must refrain from doing, my negative right can be either passive or active.

Active rights are negative rights to go about one's own business free from the interference of others. Paired with active claim rights are duties of non-interference. Health-care professionals who complain that governments should allow them to practice medicine free from bureaucratic interference are usually asserting active claim-rights not to be interfered with or hindered in their medical pursuits. Corresponding to such rights would be a duty on the part of a government to allow health-care professionals a measure of freedom and autonomy—even when this involves such things as "extra-billing" patients over and above what is provided by a government-sponsored Medicare programme.

Passive negative rights are rights not to have certain things done to us. We might, for convenience, call them "security rights." Obvious examples are the right not to be killed or assaulted, and the right not to be inflicted with disease and injury by negligent or reckless medical staff. Health-care workers who assert a right not to be exposed to the AIDS virus also have in mind a negative, passive right. In this case it is the right not to be infected by AIDS victims. Passive rights are not rights against interference with one's own activities. Rather they are rights not to have certain unwanted or harmful things done to us.

It is worth noting that typically active rights of non-interference can be protected only at the expense of other people's passive security rights. The active right of a manufacturer to pursue a livelihood within the capitalist system often competes with the passive, in personam, security rights of workers. It also competes with the passive, in rem rights of the community or world at large not to have its environment fouled by industrial activities. In general, a key problem of moral, legal and political philosophy is how to balance active freedom rights against passive security rights. Different theories will place differing emphases on the competing rights. The resolution of such conflicts is as difficult as the resolution of conflicts among Ross's prima facie duties.

To sum up, claim rights can be either in personam or in rem, positive or negative, and if they are negative, they can be either passive or active. Correlated with any one of these rights is always a duty or obligation on the part of at least one other individual. Such rights are claims against others who are under duty to respect them.

(b) Liberties or Privileges
Sometimes the situations in which people assert rights do not involve claims against others who are under correlative obligations. Rather they involve

what Hohfeld called "privileges" or "liberties." My having a privilege does not entail that others are under obligation towards me. Rather it entails only the *absence* of an obligation on *my* part. If I enjoy the privilege of doing something, then I am free or at liberty to do it (or not do it) and I do no wrong should I exercise my privilege. In short, a privilege is "freedom from duty." An example from law may help to clarify the nature of privileges.

In most legal systems there is a standing duty to provide the court with whatever information it requests. One must provide that information even if one would prefer not to. However, many jurisdictions also recognize a special area in which this standing duty does not apply. They recognize a right—a privilege—against self-incrimination. What this means is that in this special area—i.e., evidence which may implicate them in a crime—citizens are at liberty to decline the court's request. Here they enjoy an absence of duty. If the testimony in question may incriminate them, they don't have to testify if they don't want to. But notice, if I have no *claim-right* against self-incrimination, but only a privilege, then if a sharp lawyer somehow gets me to incriminate myself, he has in no way violated my rights. This would be true only if my right were a claim-right against him. Were it a claim-right, then the lawyer would be under a corresponding duty or obligation to respect a claim I would then have against him. But with privileges there are no such corresponding duties—only the absence of duty on my part. I have a freedom to act (or not to act) but it is not a freedom which enjoys the protection afforded by corresponding duties on the part of other people to respect my freedom. There is no requirement on their part that they refrain from interfering with my action or non-action.

Situations in health care where the notion of a privilege or liberty arises are not entirely obvious at first glance. Examples can be found, however, in any situation in which some people are exempt from duties to which they would otherwise be held. Certain health-care professionals, for example, are privileged with respect to confidential information about your medical history. Access to such private, confidential information is something from which the general public is barred. The general public is under a duty to respect the confidentiality of your medical records. They have no right to these privileged items. Those who are privileged, however, enjoy a freedom from this duty. They are exempt from the general duty to keep away or to mind their own business which applies to the public at large.

Privileges also figure prominently in the therapeutic relationship. By providing consent to surgery, for example, a patient waives his claim-right not to be "touched" by the surgeon, thereby relieving or freeing the latter from his standing duty not to touch the patient. In short, he grants the surgeon a privilege without which any act of touching would amount to assault or battery.

It is perhaps worth stressing once again that privileges are *unprotected* freedoms. Contrast a situation in which a patient grants me the privilege of examining his confidential medical records with a situation involving the Medical Officer of Health. If the Medical Officer has a claim-right to examine the files, say for purposes of tracking an infectious disease, then the Hospital (and the patient) must respect that right. They have a duty to turn the files over and do wrong if they should fail to do so. If, on the other hand, the patient simply forgets to arrange for his records to reach my hands, he has in no way violated my rights. This is because I have been granted a mere privilege, not a claim-right with its corresponding duty.

(c) Powers

Sometimes the terminology of rights is used to describe neither a claim-right nor a privilege. In some situations we have the capacity to alter existing legal or moral relationships involving rights and duties. In such cases we enjoy what Hohfeld called a normative *power*. In law, for example, we find powers of attorney which enable an agent to bring about changes in the legal relationships of his client. An agent may, for instance, be empowered to sign a contract on behalf of his client. In exercising this power, the agent imposes on his client a duty to honour his part of the agreement with the third party. He also, of course, invests in his client a right that the third party do the same. In these ways, then, the agent alters the existing normative relationships between his client and the third party.

Powers also enter into the practice of medicine. A surrogate is one empowered to act on behalf of a patient. He is able, for example, to alter the legal/moral relationship between patient and physician by consenting to surgery. In so doing the surrogate grants the surgeon the privilege of operating, relieving her of her otherwise standing duty not to invade the patient's body. Put another way, the surrogate *waives* the patient's claim-right not to be "touched." Without the exercise of this power by the surrogate on the patient's behalf, the surgeon's actions would, strictly speaking, amount to assault or battery. Of course in most cases patients themselves exercise the power of consent. But when for some reason a patient is unable to do so, the power and its exercise may fall to the surrogate, who must act on the patient's behalf. The surrogate is empowered to alter certain of the patient's normative relationships, but only when this is in the best interests of the patient.

The power to waive claim-rights will serve as a focus of attention in many of the cases that follow. In some instances, the question of who has the legal or moral power to waive patients' rights arises. In others, the issue will be whether such a power exists at all. Does anyone, patient included, have the power to waive someone's right to life?

(d) Further Reflections on Rights

While, nowadays, the rights approach to morality and ethics is most prominent, it offers no panacea for resolving moral conflicts. Instead of presenting the abortion dispute as a conflict of obligations, the obligation to protect human life (of the fetus) versus the obligation to respect human freedom (of the woman), now the tension is located in a conflict between the fetus's right to life and the woman's right to exercise control over her own reproductive processes, as it arguably distorts the moral relationship between the woman and her fetus while failing to resolve this tension.

One should be careful when encountering talk of "rights." It is always important to ask whether the right being asserted is a claim-right or a privilege, or possibly even a power. These are different conceptually and have very different implications. If the right is a claim-right, then one should ask whether it is in rem or in personam. In particular it may be crucial to determine whether the right is negative or positive. Does it require only that others *refrain* from doing something, or does it require positive action(s)? This is an important difference which figures prominently in many public debates. One famous case in which the difference proved crucial was the United State Supreme Court's decision in *Roe v Wade*. The Court ruled that every woman has a right to abort a fetus within specified limits. This was interpreted by some to mean that the Court had recognized a positive right to abortion which entailed aid and financial assistance from the government. A 1977 ruling, however, made it clear that while it was unconstitutional to prevent a woman from having an elective abortion, within the prescribed limits, women did not have a right to aid or financial assistance. In other words, *Roe v Wade* had granted only a *negative*, not a *positive*, right to an abortion.

CONCLUDING THOUGHTS

We have now looked at numerous moral theories and different vocabularies with which to express them. How may the insights of ethical theory be applied to actual practice? The strategies one could adopt in linking moral theory to practice are numerous and varied. Nevertheless, it is possible to isolate three basic patterns of response.

(i) Make decisions on an ad hoc, case-by-case, basis, ignoring ethical theories altogether.
Despite the undeniable importance of individual context, this is neither a promising nor an inviting option. Although there is some measure of truth in the adage that "no two cases are ever alike," it would be a mistake to exaggerate it. Any two cases will necessarily be unlike one another in many respects, but it fails to follow that they will be unlike one another *in the relevant respects.* No two murders are completely similar, but they are alike in what is often the only relevant respect: an innocent human being has been killed. If cases can be classified as being similar to one another in a limited number of relevant respects, and these cases are familiar and recurring ones, then the possibility arises of discovering moral rules and principles to govern them. We are able to fashion workable legal rules governing mur-

der because there are a limited number of recurring, relevant aspects of murder cases which can be dealt with in simple, general rules. The same is often true with moral rules and principles. So while we must be sensitive to the importance of varying contexts, to what individuates us in our personal relationships with others, and to the dangers inherent in Aristotle's attempt to ground morality on a fixed human nature, we should also be sensitive to the importance of similarities. My relationship with my daughter is unique and special to me. It may also be very different from the relationship shared by fathers and daughters in other, more patriarchal cultures. But the relationship I share with my daughter may yet be in many ways relevantly similar to the unique, special relationships many fathers have with their daughters.

If the possibility of moral norms, and ethical theories to support and explain them, exists, then it would be counter-productive to ignore them entirely. We would have to "start from scratch" every time we had to make a difficult moral decision. This would be inefficient, to say the least, and would be a hindrance to moral understanding. Understanding the world involves recognizing similarities and differences among situations and people. Without moral rules, principles, values and virtues, and theories to generate them, we make it difficult, if not impossible, to gain moral understanding. So long as we do not claim too much for it, working with an admittedly limited theory is better than working with no theory at all.

(ii) Make a firm and irrevocable commitment to a particular ethical theory.
While this option promotes single-mindedness, and simplifies our moral deliberations, it has the serious disadvantage of ignoring the possible insights of other ethical theories and approaches. It compels one to resolve all moral quandaries within the boundaries of the theory chosen and this smacks of artificiality and arbitrariness. This will be so unless one is convinced that one "knows the truth" with absolute certainty, an unlikely possibility for someone willing to ascend to the reflective level of moral thinking (see Section 3 above). Blindly committing oneself to an ethical theory or approach is no better than blindly committing oneself to a conventional rule. It is to

descend to the pre-reflective level where blind acceptance replaces critical reflection and the possibility of moral progress.

(iii) Allow for both fixity and flexibility.
This is clearly the preferred option. The fixity is provided by acknowledging that moral conflicts need not, and perhaps should not, be resolved within a moral vacuum, and that the application of an ethical theory with which one is not entirely happy can nevertheless shed light on the issues in dispute. It may at the very least bring some of the important considerations into relief where they may be more easily examined and discussed reasonably. Flexibility arises in acknowledging that competing theories and approaches may well offer insight as well and that one's own favoured theory is always open to improvement or, at some point, rejection. Reasonable flexibility may even lead us judiciously to extract rules, principles, or values from competing systems as determined by their apparent relevance to the case in question. It may be true that sometimes Mill provides a better answer than Kant—and that the tables are reversed at other times. Sometimes feminist theorists may be right in stressing the individuating features of a moral situation, features which might in some instance render the relevant issue incapable of resolution by way of a universalizable moral principle. This is not necessarily a cause for dismay, as Ross seemed to appreciate. Consider an analogous case in physics. Sometimes the wave theory provides a better account of the properties and behavior of light than the particle theory does. At other times the reverse is true. A single, unified theory would no doubt be preferable. But till such time as one becomes available, it would be imprudent to ignore the existing theories altogether, or to subscribe to one and forget about the other(s). The same is true in moral philosophy. We must not let our failures to achieve completeness, or our failures to appreciate in all cases the full range of factors at play in particular contexts, blind us to the incremental gains in knowledge that have been made. Perhaps we would do well, in the end, to heed Aristotle's caution that "precision is not to be sought alike in all discussions. We must be content, in speaking of such subjects [as ethics and

politics], to indicate the truth roughly and in outline."[30]

Notes

1. John Stuart Mill, *On Liberty*, Shields edn. (Indianapolis: Bobbs-Merrill, 1956), 56.

2. See G.E. Moore, *Principia Ethica* (London: Cambridge University Press, 1903).

3. John Stuart Mill, *Utilitarianism* (New York: Bobbs Merrill, 1957) 10.

4. Utilitarianism, 22.

5. John Rawls, "Two Concepts of Rules," in *The Philosophical Review*, January 1955.

6. See J.J.C. Smart and Bernard Williams, *Utilitarianism: For and Against* (London: Cambridge University Press, 1973), 10.

7. See David Lyons, *The Forms and Limits of Utilitarianism* (Oxford: Oxford University Press, 1965) where it is argued that any version of RU faithful to the utilitarian credo collapses logically into AU.

8. Immanuel Kant, *Groundwork of the Metaphysics of Morals*, trans. H.J. Paton (New York: Harper and Row, 1964), 67-8.

9. Kant, 70.

10. Kant, 89.

11. Kant, 89-90.

12. Kant, 90.

13. Kant, 96.

14. See Lloyd Tataryn "From Dust to Dust," in D. Poff and W. Waluchow, eds., *Business Ethics in Canada*, eds. (Scarborough: Prentice Hall Canada, 1987), 122-25.

15. W.D. Ross, *The Right and the Good* (Oxford: Clarendon Press, 1930), 21.

16. Ross, 13.

17. Immanuel Kant, "On a Supposed Right to Lie from Altruistic Motives" in Lewis White Beck, ed. and trans., *Critique of Practical Reason and Other Writings in Moral Philosophy*, (Chicago: University of Chicago Press, 1949), 346-350.

18. Ross, 21.

19. Leslie Stephen, *The Science of Ethics* (New York: G.P. Putnam's Sons, 1882), 155, 158.

20. Aristotle, *Nicomachean Ethics*, translated by J.L. Ackrill (New York: Humanities Press, 1973), 1094.

21. Aristotle, 1095 a16-20.

22. Aristotle, 1106 b36-1107 a2.

23. William Frankena, *Ethics* 2nd ed. (Englewood Cliffs: Prentice-Hall, 1973), 63.

24. Aristotle, 1112a 16-17.

25. Aristotle, 1113b 20.

26. Aristotle, 1116 b37.

27. Susan Sherwin, "Ethics, 'Feminine Ethics,' and Feminist Ethics," in Debra Shogan, ed., *A Reader in Feminist Ethics* (Toronto: Canadian Scholar's Press, 1993), p. 10.

28. Sherwin, p. 14.

29. See W. Hohfeld, *Fundamental Legal Conceptions* (New Haven: Yale University Press, 1919) and Joel Feinberg, "Duties Rights and Claims," in *Rights, Justice and the Bounds of Liberty* (Princeton: Princeton University Press, 1980).

30. Aristotle, 1094 b12, 18.

CHAPTER TWO

RELATIONSHIPS
IN HEALTH CARE

1.
FOUR MODELS OF THE PHYSICIAN-PATIENT RELATIONSHIP

Ezekiel J. Emanuel and Linda L. Emanuel

During the last two decades or so, there has been a struggle over the patient's role in medical decision making that is often characterized as a conflict between autonomy and health, between the values of the patient and the values of the physician. Seeking to curtail physician dominance, many have advocated an ideal of greater patient control.[1] Others question this ideal because it fails to acknowledge the potentially imbalanced nature of this interaction when one party is sick and searching for security, and when judgments entail the interpretation of technical information.[2] Still others are trying to delineate a more mutual relationship.[3] This struggle shapes the expectation of physicians and patients as well as the ethical and legal standards for the physician's duties, informed consent, and medical malpractice. This struggle forces us to ask, What should be the ideal physician-patient relationship?

We shall outline four models of physician-patient interaction, emphasizing the different understanding of (1) the goals of the physician-patient interaction, (2) the physician's obligations, (3) the role of patient values, and (4) the conception of patient autonomy. To elaborate the abstract description of these four models, we shall indicate the types of response the models might suggest in a clinical situation. Third, we shall also indicate how these models inform the current debate about the ideal physician-patient relationship. Finally, we shall evaluate these models and recommend one as the preferred model.

As outlined, the models are Weberian ideal types. They may not describe any particular physician-patient interaction but highlight, free from complicating details, different visions of the essential characteristics of the physician-patient interaction.[4] Consequently, they do not embody minimum ethical or legal standards, but rather constitute relative ideals that are "higher than the law" but not "above the law."[5]

THE PATERNALISTIC MODEL

First is the *paternalistic* model, sometimes called the parental[6] or priestly[7] model. In this model, the physician-patient interaction ensures that patients receive the interventions that best promote their health and well-being. To this end, physicians use their skills to determine the patient's medical condition and his or her stage in the disease process and to identify the medical tests and treatments most likely to restore the patient's health or ameliorate pain. Then the physician presents the patient with selected information that will encourage the patient to consent to the intervention the physician considers best. At the extreme, the physician authoritatively informs the patient when the intervention will be initiated.

The paternalistic model assumes that there are shared objective criteria for determining what is best. Hence the physician can discern what is in the patient's best interest with limited patient participation. Ultimately, it is assumed that the patient will be thankful for decisions made by the physician even if he or she would not agree to them at the time.[8] In the tension between the patient's autonomy and well-being, between choice and health, the paternalistic physician's main emphasis is toward the latter.

In the paternalistic model, the physician acts as the patient's guardian articulating and implementing what is best for the patient. As such, the physician has obligations, including that of placing the patient's interest above his or her own and soliciting the views of others when lacking adequate knowledge. The conception of patient autonomy is patient assent, either at the time or later, to the physician's determinations of what is best.

THE INFORMATIVE MODEL

Second is the *informative* model, sometimes called the scientific,[9] engineering,[10] or consumer model. In this model, the objective of the physician-patient interaction is for the physician to provide the patient with all relevant information, for the patient to select the medical interventions he or she wants, and for the physician to execute the selected interventions. To this end, the physician informs the patient of his or her disease state, the nature of possible diagnostic and therapeutic interventions, the nature and probability of risks and benefits associated with the intervention, and any uncertainties of knowledge. At the extreme, patients could come to know all medical information relevant to their disease and available interventions and select the interventions that best realize their values.

The informative model assumes a fairly clear distinction between facts and values. The patient's values are well defined and known; what the patient lacks is facts. It is the physician's obligation to provide all the available facts, and the patient's values then determine what treatments are to be given. There is no role for the physician's values, the physician's understanding of the patient's values, or his or her judgment of the worth of the patient's values. In the informative mode, the physician is a purveyor of technical expertise, providing the patient with the means to exercise control. As technical experts, physicians have important obligations to provide truthful information, to maintain competence in their area of expertise, and to consult others when their knowledge or skills are lacking. The conception of patient autonomy is patient control over medical decision making.

THE INTERPRETIVE MODEL

The third model is the *interpretive* model. The aim of the physician-patient interaction is to elucidate the patient's values and what he or she actually wants, and to help the patient select the available medical interventions that realize these values. Like the informative physician, the interpretive physician provides the patient with information on the nature of the condition and the risks and benefits of possible interventions.

Beyond this, however, the interpretive physician assists the patient in elucidating and articulating his or her values and in determining what medical interventions best realize the specified values, thus helping to interpret the patient's values for the patient.

According to the interpretive model, the patient's values are not necessarily fixed and known to the patient. They are often inchoate, and the patient may only partially understand them; they may conflict when applied to specific situations. Consequently, the physician working with the patient must elucidate and make coherent these values. To do this, the physician works with the patient to reconstruct the patient's goals and aspirations, commitments and character. At the extreme, the physician must conceive the patient's life as a narrative whole, and from this specify the patient's values and their priority.[11] Then the physician determines which tests and treatments best realize these values. Importantly, the physician does not dictate to the patient; it is the patient who ultimately decides which values and course of action best fit who he or she is. Neither is the physician judging the patient's values; he or she helps the patient to understand and use them in the medical situation.

In the interpretive model, the physician is a counselor, analogous to a cabinet minister's advisory role to a head of state, supplying relevant information, helping to elucidate values and suggesting what medical interventions realize these values. Thus the physician's obligations include those enumerated in the informative model but also require engaging the patient in a joint process of understanding. Accordingly, the conception of patient autonomy is self-understanding; the patient comes to know more clearly who he or she is and how the various medical options bear on his or her identity.

THE DELIBERATIVE MODEL

Fourth is the *deliberative* model. The aim of the physician-patient interaction is to help the patient determine and choose the best health-related values that can be realized in the clinical situation. To this end, the physician must delineate information on the patient's clinical situation and then help elucidate the types of values embodied in the available options. The physician's objectives include suggesting why certain health-related values are more worthy and should be aspired to. At the extreme, the physician and patient engage in deliberation about what kind of health-related values

Table 5.1 Comparing the Four Models

	Informative	*Interpretive*	*Deliberative*	*Paternalistic*
Patient values	Defined, fixed, and known to the patient	Inchoate and conflicting, requiring elucidation	Open to development and revision through moral discussion	Objective and shared by physician and patient
Physician's obligation	Providing relevant factual information and implementing patient's selected intervention	Elucidating and interpreting relevant patient values as well as informing the patient and implementing the patient's selected intervention	Articulating and persuading the patient of the most admirable values as well as informing the patient and implementing the patient's selected intervention	Promoting the patient's well-being independent of the patient's current preferences
Conception of patient's autonomy	Choice of, and control over, medical care	Self-understanding relevant to medical care	Moral self-development relevant to medical care	Assenting to objective values
Conception of physician's role	Competent technical expert	Counselor or advisor	Friend or teacher	Guardian

the patient could and ultimately should pursue. The physician discusses only health-related values, that is, values that affect or are affected by the patient's disease and treatments; he or she recognizes that many elements of morality are unrelated to the patient's disease or treatment and beyond the scope of their professional relationship. Further, the physician aims at no more than moral persuasion; ultimately, coercion is avoided, and the patient must define his or her life and select the ordering of values to be espoused. By engaging in moral deliberation, the physician and patient judge the worthiness and importance of the health-related values.

In the deliberative model, the physician acts as a teacher or friend,[12] engaging the patient in dialogue on what course of action would be best. Not only does the physician indicate what the patient could do, but, knowing the patient and wishing what is best, the physician indicates what the patient should do, what decision regarding medical therapy would be admirable. The conception of patient autonomy is moral self-development; the patient is empowered not simply to follow unexamined preferences or examined values, but to consider, through dialogue, alternative health-related values, their worthiness, and their implications for treatment.

COMPARING THE FOUR MODELS

The Table compares the four models on essential points. Importantly, all models have a role for patient autonomy; a main factor that differentiates the models is their particular conception of patient autonomy. Therefore, no single model can be endorsed because it alone promotes patient autonomy. Instead the models must be compared and evaluated, at least in part, by evaluating the adequacy of their particular conceptions of patient autonomy.

The four models are not exhaustive. At a minimum there might be added a fifth: the *instrumental* model. In this model, the patient's values are irrelevant; the physician aims for some goal independent of the patient, such as the good of society or furtherance of scientific knowledge. The Tuskegee syphilis experiment[13] and the Willowbrook hepatitis study,[14] are examples of this model. As the moral condemnation of these cases reveals, this model is not an ideal but an aberration. Thus we have not elaborated it herein.

A CLINICAL CASE

To make tangible these abstract descriptions and to crystallize essential differences among the models, we will illustrate the responses they suggest in a clinical situation, that of a 43-year-old premenopausal woman who has recently discovered a breast mass. Surgery reveals a 3.5 cm ductal carcinoma with no lymph node involvement that is estrogen receptor positive. Chest roentgenogram, bone scan, and liver function tests reveal no evidence of metastatic disease. The patient was recently divorced and has gone back to work as a legal aide to support herself. What should the physician say to this patient?

In the paternalistic model a physician might say, "There are two alternative therapies to protect against recurrence of cancer in your breast: mastectomy or radiation. We now know that the survival with lumpectomy combined with radiation therapy is equal to that with mastectomy. Because lumpectomy and radiation offers the best survival and the best cosmetic result, it is to be preferred. I have asked the radiation therapist to come and discuss radiation treatment with you. We also need to protect you against the spread of cancer to other parts of your body. Even though the chance of recurrence is low, you are young, and we should not leave any therapeutic possibilities untried. Recent studies involving chemotherapy suggest improvements in survival without recurrence of breast cancer. Indeed, the National Cancer Institute recommends chemotherapy for women with your type of breast cancer. Chemotherapy has side effects. Nevertheless, a few months of hardship now are worth the potential added years of life without cancer."

In the informative model a physician might say, "With node-negative breast cancer there are two issues before you: local control and systemic control. For local control, the options are mastectomy or lumpectomy with or without radiation. From many studies we know that mastectomy and lumpectomy with radiation result in identical overall survival, about 80% 10-year survival. Lumpectomy without radiation results in a 30% to 40% chance of tumor recurrence in the breast. The second issue relates to systemic control. We know that chemotherapy prolongs survival for premenopausal women who have axillary nodes involved with tumor. The role for women with node-negative breast cancer is less clear. Individual studies suggest that chemotherapy is of no benefit in terms of improving overall survival, but a comprehensive review of all studies sug-

gests that there is a survival benefit. Several years ago, the NCI suggested that for women like yourself, chemotherapy can have a positive therapeutic impact. Finally, let me inform you that there are clinical trials, for which you are eligible, to evaluate the benefits of chemotherapy for patients with node-negative breast cancer. I can enroll you in a study if you want. I will be happy to give you any further information you feel you need."

The interpretive physician might outline much of the same information as the informative physician, then engage in discussion to elucidate the patient's wishes, and conclude, "It sounds to me as if you have conflicting wishes. Understandably, you seem uncertain how to balance the demands required for receiving additional treatment, rejuvenating your personal affairs, and maintaining your psychological equilibrium. Let me try to express a perspective that fits your position. Fighting your cancer is important, but it must leave you with a healthy self-image and quality time outside the hospital. This view seems compatible with undergoing radiation therapy but not chemotherapy. A lumpectomy with radiation maximizes your chance of surviving while preserving your breast. Radiotherapy fights your breast cancer without disfigurement. Conversely, chemotherapy would prolong the duration of therapy by many months. Further, the benefits of chemotherapy in terms of survival are smaller and more controversial. Given the recent changes in your life, you have too many preoccupations to undergo months of chemotherapy for a questionable benefit. Do I understand you? We can talk again in a few days."

The deliberative physician might begin by outlining the same factual information, engage in a conversation to elucidate the patient's values, but continue, "It seems clear that you should undergo radiation therapy. It offers maximal survival with minimal risk, disfigurement, and disruption of your life. The issue of chemotherapy is different, fraught with conflicting data. Balancing all the options, I think the best one for you is to enter a trial that is investigating the potential benefit of chemotherapy for women with node-negative breast cancer. First, it ensures that you receive excellent medical care. At this point, we do not know which therapy maximizes survival. In a clinical study the schedule of follow-up visits, tests, and decisions is specified by leading breast cancer experts to ensure that all the women receive care that is the best available anywhere. A second reason to participate in a trial is altruistic: it allows you to contribute something to women with breast cancer in the future who will face difficult choices. Over decades, thousands of women have participated in studies that inform our current treatment practices. Without those women, and the knowledge they made possible, we would probably still be giving you and all other women with breast cancer mastectomies. By enrolling in a trial you participate in a tradition in which women of one generation receive the highest standard of care available but also enhance the care of women in future generations because medicine has learned something about which interventions are better. I must tell you that I am not involved in the study; if you elect to enroll in this trial, you will initially see another breast cancer expert to plan your therapy. I have sought to explain our current knowledge and offer my recommendation so you can make the best possible decision."

Lacking the normal interchange with patients, these statements may seem contrived, even caricatures. Nevertheless, they highlight the essence of each model and suggest how the objectives and assumptions of each inform a physician's approach to his or her patients. Similar statements can be imagined for other clinical situations such as an obstetrician discussing prenatal testing or a cardiologist discussing cholesterol-reducing interventions.

THE CURRENT DEBATE AND THE FOUR MODELS
In recent decades there has been a call for greater patient autonomy or, as some have called it, "patient sovereignty,"[15] conceived as patient *choice* and *control* over medical decisions. This shift toward the informative model is embodied in the adoption of business terms for medicine, as when physicians are described as health care providers and patients as consumers. It can also be found in the propagation of patient rights statements,[16] in the promotion of living will laws, and in rules regarding human experimentation. For instance, the opening sentences of one law state: "The Rights of the Terminally Ill Act authorizes an adult person to *control* decisions

regarding administration of life-sustaining treatment.... The Act merely provides one way by which a terminally-ill patient's *desires* regarding the use of life-sustaining procedures can be legally implemented" (emphasis added).[17] Indeed, living will laws do not require or encourage patients to discuss the issue of terminating care with their physicians before signing such documents. Similarly, decisions in "right-to-die" cases emphasize patient control over medical decisions. As one court put it:[18]

> The right to refuse medical treatment is basic and fundamental.... Its exercise requires no one's approval.... *[T]he controlling decision belongs to a competent informed patient....* It is not a medical decision for her physicians to make.... *It is a moral and philosophical decision that, being a competent adult, is [the patient's] alone.* (emphasis added)

Probably the most forceful endorsement of the informative model as the ideal inheres in informed consent standards. Prior to the 1970s, the standard for informed consent was "physician based."[19] Since 1972 and the *Canterbury* case, however, the emphasis has been on a "patient-oriented" standard of informed consent in which the physician has a "duty" to provide appropriate medical facts to empower the patient to use his or her values to determine what interventions should be implemented.[20]

> True consent to what happens to one's self is the informed exercise of a choice, and that entails an opportunity to evaluate knowledgeably the options available and the risks attendant upon each.... *[I]t is the prerogative of the patient, not the physician, to determine for himself the direction in which his interests seem to lie.* To enable the patient to chart his course understandably, some familiarity with the therapeutic alternatives and their hazards become essential.[21] (emphasis added)

SHARED DECISION MAKING
Despite its dominance, many have found the informative mode "arid."[22] The President's Commission and others contend that the ideal relationship does not vest moral authority and medical decision-making power exclusively in the patient but must be a process of shared decision making constructed

around "mutual participation and respect."[23] The President's Commission argues that the physician's role is "to help the patient understand the medical situation and available courses of action, and the patient conveys his or her concerns and wishes."[24] Brock and Wartman[25] stress this fact-value "division of labor"—having the physician provide information while the patient makes value decisions—by describing "shared decision making" as a collaborative process

> in which both physicians and patients make active and essential contributions. Physicians bring their medical training, knowledge, and expertise—including an understanding of the available treatment alternatives—to the diagnosis and management of patients' condition. Patients bring knowledge of their own subjective aims and values, through which risks and benefits of various treatment options can be evaluated. With this approach, selecting the best treatment for a particular patient requires the contribution of both parties.

Similarly, in discussing ideal medical decision making, Eddy[26] argues for this fact-value division of labor between the physician and patient as the ideal:

> It is important to separate the decision process into these two steps.... The first step is a question of facts. The anchor is empirical evidence.... [T]he second step is a question not of facts but of personal values or preferences. The thought process is not analytic but personal and subjective.... [I]t is the patient's preferences that should determine the decision.... Ideally, you and I [the physicians] are not in the picture. What matters is what Mrs. Smith thinks.

This view of shared decision making seems to vest the medical decision-making authority with the patient while relegating physicians to technicians "transmitting medical information and using their technical skills as the patient directs."[27] Thus, while the advocates of "shared decision making" may aspire toward a mutual dialogue between physician and patient, the substantive view informing their ideal reembodies the informative model under a different label.

Other commentators have articulated more mutual models of the physician-patient interaction.[28] Prominent among these efforts is Katz[29] *The Silent World of the Doctor and Patient.* Relying on a Freudian view in which self-knowledge and self-determination are inherently limited because of unconscious influences, Katz views dialogue as a mechanism for greater self-understanding of one's values and objectives. According to Katz, this view places a duty on physicians and patients to reflect and communicate so that patients can gain a greater self-understanding and self-determination. Katz' insight is also available on grounds other than Freudian psychological theory and is consistent with the interpretive model.[30]

OBJECTIONS TO THE PATERNALISTIC MODEL
It is widely recognized that the paternalistic model is justified during emergencies when the time taken to obtain informed consent might irreversibly harm the patient.[31] Beyond such limited circumstances, however, it is no longer tenable to assume that the physician and patient espouse similar values and views of what constitutes a benefit. Consequently, even physicians rarely advocate the paternalistic model as an ideal for routine physician-patient interactions.[32]

OBJECTIONS TO THE INFORMATIVE MODEL
The informative model seems both descriptively and prescriptively inaccurate. First, this model seems to have no place for essential qualities of the ideal physician-patient relationship. The informative physician cares for the patient in the sense of competently implementing the patient's selected interventions. However, the informative physician lacks a caring approach that requires understanding what the patient values or should value and how his or her illness impinges on these values. Patients seem to expect their physician to have a caring approach; they deem a technically proficient but detached physician as deficient, and properly condemned. Further, the informative physician is proscribed from giving a recommendation for fear of imposing his or her will on the patient and thereby competing for the decision making control that has been given to the patient.[33] Yet, if one of the essential qualities of the ideal physician is the ability to assimilate medical

Four Models of the Physician-Patient Relationship   45

facts, prior experience of similar situations, and intimate knowledge of the patient's view into a recommendation designed for the patient's specific medical and personal condition,[34] then the informative physician cannot be ideal.

Second, in the informative model the ideal physician is a highly trained subspecialist who provides detailed factual information and competently implements the patient's preferred medical intervention. Hence, the informative model perpetuates and accentuates the trend toward specialization and impersonalization within the medical profession.

Most importantly, the informative model's conception of patient autonomy seems philosophically untenable. The informative model presupposes that persons possess known and fixed values, but this is inaccurate. People are often uncertain about what they actually want. Further, unlike animals, people have what philosophers call "second order desires," that is, the capacity to reflect on their wishes and to revise their own desire and preferences. In fact, freedom of the will and autonomy inhere in having "second order desires"[35] and being able to change our preferences and modify our identity. Self-reflection and the capacity to change what we want often require a "process" of moral deliberation in which we assess the value of what we want. And this is a process that occurs with other people who know us well and can articulate a vision of who we ought to be that we can assent to.[36] Even though changes in health or implementation of alternative interventions can have profound effects on what we desire and how we realize our desires, self-reflection and deliberation play no essential role in the informative physician-patient interaction. The informative model's conception of autonomy is incompatible with a vision of autonomy that incorporates second-order desires.

OBJECTIONS TO THE INTERPRETIVE MODEL
The interpretive model rectifies this deficiency by recognizing that persons have second-order desires and dynamic value structures and placing the elucidation of values in the context of the patient's medical condition at the center of the physician-patient interaction. Nevertheless, there are objections to the interpretive model.

Technical specialization militates against physicians cultivating the skills necessary to the interpretive model. With limited interpretive talents and limited time, physicians may unwittingly impose their own values under the guise of articulating the patient's values. And patients, overwhelmed by their medical condition and uncertain of their own views, may too easily accept this imposition. Such circumstances may push the interpretive model towards the paternalistic model in actual practice.

Further, autonomy viewed as self-understanding excludes evaluative judgment of the patient's values or attempts to persuade the patient to adopt other values. This constrains the guidance and recommendations the physician can offer. Yet in practice, especially in preventive medicine and risk-reduction interventions, physicians often attempt to persuade patients to adopt particularly health-related values. Physicians frequently urge patients with high cholesterol levels who smoke to change their dietary habits, quit smoking, and begin exercise programs before initiating drug therapy. The justification given for these changes is that patients should value their health more than they do. Similarly, physicians are encouraged to persuade their human immunodeficiency virus (HIV)-infected patients who might be engaging in unsafe sexual practices either to abstain or, realistically, to adopt "safer sex" practices. Such appeals are not made to promote the HIV-infected patients's own health, but are grounded on an appeal for the patient to assume responsibility for the good of others. Consequently, by excluding evaluative judgements, the interpretive model seems to characterize inaccurately ideal physician-patient interactions.

OBJECTION TO THE DELIBERATIVE MODEL
The fundamental objections to the deliberative model focus on whether it is proper for physicians to judge patients' values and promote particular health-related values. First, physicians do not possess privileged knowledge of the priority of health-related values relative to other values. Indeed, since ours is a pluralistic society in which people espouse incommensurable values, it is likely that a physician's values and view of which values are higher will conflict with those of other physicians and those of his or her patients.

Second, the nature of the moral deliberation between physician and patient, the physician's recommended interventions, and the actual treatments used will depend on the values of the particular physician treating the patient. However, recommendations and care provided to patients would not depend on the physician's judgment of the worthiness of the patient's values or on the physician's particular values. As one bioethicist put it:[37]

> The hand is broken, the physician can repair the hand; therefore the physician must repair the hand—as well as possible—without regard to personal values that might lead the physician to think ill of the patient or of the patient's values.... [A]t the level of clinical practice, medicine should be value-free in the sense that the personal values of the physician should not distort the making of medical decisions.

Third, it may be argued that the deliberative model misconstrues the purpose of the physician-patient interaction. Patients see their physicians to receive health care, not to engage in moral deliberation or to revise their values. Finally, like the interpretive model, the deliberative model may easily metamorphose into unintended paternalism, the very practice that generated the public debate over the proper physician-patient interaction.

THE PREFERRED MODEL AND THE PRACTICAL IMPLICATIONS

Clearly, under different clinical circumstances different models may be appropriate. Indeed, at different times all four models may justifiably guide physicians and patients. Nevertheless, it is important to specify one model as the shared, paradigmatic reference; exceptions to use other models would not be automatically condemned, but would require justification based on the circumstances of a particular situation. Thus, it is widely agreed that in an emergency where delays in treatment to obtain informed consent might irreversibly harm the patient, the paternalistic model correctly guides physician-patient interactions. Conversely, for patients who have clear but conflicting values, the interpretive model is probably justified. For instance, a 65-year-old woman who has been treated for acute leukemia may have clearly decided against reinduction chemotherapy if she relapses. Several months before the anticipated birth of her first grandchild, the patient relapses. The patient becomes torn about whether to endure the risks of reinduction chemotherapy in order to live to see her first grandchild or whether to refuse therapy, resigning herself to not seeing her grandchild. In such cases, the physician may justifiably adopt the interpretive approach. In other circumstances, where there is only a one-time physician-patient interaction without an ongoing relationship in which the patients's values can be elucidated and compared with ideals, such as in a walk-in center, the informative model may be justified.

Descriptively and prescriptively, we claim that the ideal physician-patient relationship is the deliberative model. We will adduce six points to justify this claim. First, the deliberative model more nearly embodies our ideal of autonomy. It is an oversimplification and distortion of the Western tradition to view respecting autonomy as simply permitting a person to select, unrestricted by coercion, ignorance, physical interference, and the like, his or her preferred course of action from a comprehensive list of available options.[38] Freedom and control over medical decisions alone do not constitute patient autonomy. Autonomy requires that individuals critically assess their own values and preferences; determine whether they are desirable; affirm, upon reflection, these values as ones that should justify their actions; and then be free to initiate action to realize the values. The process of deliberation integral to the deliberative model is essential for realizing patient autonomy understood in this way.

Second, our society's image of an ideal physician is not limited to one who knows and communicates to the patient relevant factual information and competently implements medical interventions. The ideal physician—often embodied in literature, art, and popular culture—is a caring physician who integrates the information and relevant values to make a recommendation and, through discussion, attempts to persuade the patient to accept this recommendation as the intervention that best promotes his or her overall well-being. Thus, we expect the best physicians to engage their patients in evaluating discussions of health issues and related values. The physician's discussion does not invoke values that are unrelated or tangentially related to the patient's illness and potential therapies. Importantly, these efforts are not restricted to situations in which patients might make "irrational and harmful" choices[39] but extend to all health care decisions.

Third, the deliberative model is not a disguised form of paternalism. Previously there may have been category mistakes in which instances of the deliberative model have been erroneously identified as physician paternalism. And no doubt, in practice, the deliberative physician may occasionally lapse into paternalism. However, like the ideal teacher, the deliberative physician attempts to persuade the patient of the worthiness of certain values, not to impose those values paternalistically; the physician's aim is not to subject the patient to his or her will, but to persuade the patient of a course of action as desirable. In the Laws, Plato[40] characterizes this fundamental distinction between persuasion and imposition for medical practice that distinguishes the deliberative from the paternalistic model:

A physician to slaves never gives his patients any account of his illness ... the physician offers some order gleaned from experience with an air of infallible knowledge, in the brusque fashion of a dictator.... The free physician, who usually cares for free men, treats their disease first by thoroughly discussing with the patient and his friends his ailment. This way he learns something from the sufferer and simultaneously instructs him. Then the physician does not give his medications until he has persuaded the patient; the physician aims at complete restoration of health by persuading the patient to comply with his therapy.

Fourth, physician values are relevant to patients and do inform their choice of a physician. When a pregnant woman chooses an obstetrician who does not routinely perform a battery of prenatal tests or, alternatively, one who strongly favors them; when a patient seeks an aggressive cardiologist who favors procedural interventions or one who concentrates therapy on dietary changes, stress reduction, and life-style modifications, they are, consciously or not, selecting a physician based on the values that guide his or her medical decisions. And, when disagreements between physicians and patients arise, there are discussions over which values are more important and should be realized in medical care. Occasionally, when such disagreements undermine the physician-patient relationship and a caring attitude, a patient's care is transferred to another physician. Indeed, in the informative model the grounds for transferring care to a new physician is either the physician's ignorance or incompetence. But patients seem to switch physicians because they do not "like" a particular physician or that physician's attitude or approach.

Fifth, we seem to believe that physicians should not only help fit therapies to the patients' elucidated values, but should also promote health-related values. As noted, we expect physicians to promote certain values, such as "safer sex" for patients with HIV or abstaining from or limiting alcohol use. Similarly, patients are willing to adjust their values and actions to be more compatible with health-promoting values.[41] This is in the nature of seeking a caring medical recommendation.

Finally, it may well be that many physicians currently lack the training and capacity to articulate the values underlying their recommendations and persuade patients that these values are worthy. But, in part, this deficiency is a consequence of the tendencies toward specialization and the avoidance of discussion of values by physicians that are perpetuated and justified by the dominant informative model. Therefore, if the deliberative model seems most appropriate, then we need to implement changes in medical care and education to encourage a more caring approach. We must stress understanding rather than mere provisions of factual information in keeping with the legal standards of informed consent and medical malpractice; we must educate physicians not just to spend more time in physician-patient communication but to elucidate and articulate the values underlying their medical care decisions, including routine ones; we must shift the publicly assumed conception of patient autonomy that shapes both the physician's and the patient's expectations from patient control to moral development. Most important, we must recognize that developing a deliberative physician-patient relationship requires a considerable amount of time. We must develop a health care financing system that properly reimburses—rather than penalizes—physicians for taking the time to discuss values with their patients.

CONCLUSION

Over the last few decades, the discourse regarding the physician-patient relationship has focused on two extremes: autonomy and paternalism. Many have attacked physicians as paternalistic, urging the empowerment of patients to control their own care. This view, the informative model, has become dominant in bioethics and legal standards. This model embodies a defective conception of patient autonomy, and it reduces the physician's role to that of a technologist. The essence of doctoring is a fabric of knowledge, understanding, teaching, and action, in which the caring physician integrates the patients's medical condition and health-related values, makes a recommendation on the appropriate course of action, and tries to persuade the patient of the worthiness of this approach and the values it realizes. The physician with a caring attitude is the ideal embodied in the deliberative model, the ideal that should inform laws and policies that regulate the physician-patient interaction.

Finally, it may be worth noting that the four models outlined herein are not limited to the medical realm: they may inform the public conception of other professional interactions as well. We suggest that the ideal relationships between lawyer and client,[42] religious mentor and laity, and educator and student are well described by the deliberative model, at least in some of their essential aspects.

Acknowledgements

We would like to thank Robert Mayer, MD, Craig Henderson, MD, Lynn Peterson, MD, And John Stoeckle, MD, as well as Dennis Thompson, PhD, Arthur Applebaum, PhD, and Dan Brock, PhD, for their critical reviews of the manuscript. We would also like to thank the "ethics and the professions" seminar participants, especially Robert Rosen, JD, Francis Kamm, PhD, David Wilkins, JD, and Oliver Avens, who enlightened us in discussions.

Notes

1. Veatch R.M. *A Theory of Medical Ethics*. New York, NY: Basic Books Inc Publishers; 1981; also Macklin R. *Mortal Choices*. New York, NY: Pantheon Books Inc., 1987.

2. Ingelfinger F.J. "Arrogance" *N Engl J Med*. 1980; 304:1507; also Marzuk P.M. "The right kind of paternalism" *N Engl J Med*. 1985; 313: 1474-76.

3. Siegler M. "The progression of medicine: from physician paternalism to patient autonomy to bureaucratic parsimony" *Arch Intern Med*. 1985;145:713-15; also Szasz T.S, Hollender M.H. "The basic models of the doctor-patient relationship" *Arch Intern Med*. 1956; 97:585-92.

4. Weber M., Parsons T. ed. *The Theory of Social and Economic Organization*. New York, NY: The Free Press, 1974.

5. Ballantine H.T. "Annual discourse—the crisis in ethics, anno domini 1979" *N Engl J Med*. 1979, 301:634-38.

6. Burke G. "Ethics and medical decision-making" *Prim Care*. 1980; 7:615-24.

7. Veatch R.M. "Models for ethical medicine in a revolutionary age" *Hastings Cent Rep*. 1975; 2:3-5.

8. Stone A.A. *Mental Health and Law: A System in Transition*. New York, NY: Jason Aronson Inc., 1976.

9. See note 6.

10. See note 7.

11. MacIntyre A. *After Virtue*. South Bend, Ind.: University of Notre Dame Press; 1981; Sandel M.J. *Liberalism and the Limits of Justice*. New York, NY: Cambridge University Press, 1982.

12. Fried C. "The lawyer as friend: the moral foundations of the lawyer client relationship" *Yale Law J*. 1976; 85:1060-89.

13. Jones J.H. *Bad Blood*. New York, NY: Free Press; 1981; *Final Report of the Tuskegee Syphilis Study Ad Hoc Advisory Panel*. Washington, DC: Public Health Service, 1973; Brandt A.M. "Racism and research: the case of the Tuskegee Syphilis Study" *Hastings Cent Rep*. 1978; 8:21-29.

14. Krugman S, Giles J.P. "Viral hepatitis: new light on an old disease" *JAMA*. 1970; 212:1019-29; also Ingelfinger F.J. "Ethics of experiments on children" *N Engl J Med*. 1973; 288:791-92.

15. President's Commission for the Study of Ethical Problems in Medicine and Biomedical and Behav-

ioral Research. *Making Health Care Decisions.* Washington, DC: US Government Printing Office, 1982.

16. *Statement of a Patient's Bill of Rights.* Chicago, Ill.: American Hospital Association; November 17, 1972.

17. "Uniform Rights of the Terminally Ill Act" in *Handbook of Living Will Laws.* New York, NY: Society for the Right to Die; 1987:135-47.

18. *Bouvia v Superior Court.* 225 Cal Rptr. 297 (1986).

19. *Natanson v Kline*, 350 P2d 1093 (Kan 1960); also Applebaum P.S, Lidz C.W, Meisel A. *Informed Consent: Legal Theory and Clinical Practice.* New York, NY: Oxford University Press, 1987: ch. 3; Faden R.R, Beauchamp T.L. *A History and Theory of Informed Consent*, New York, NY: Oxford University Press, 1986.

20. Applebaum P.S, Lidz C.W, Meisel A. *Informed Consent: Legal Theory and Clinical Practice.* New York, NY: Oxford University Press, 1987: ch. 3; also Faden R.R, Beauchamp T.L. *A History and Theory of Informed Consent*, New York, NY: Oxford University Press, 1986; *Canterbury v Spence*, 464 F2d 772 (DC Cir 1972).

21. *Canterbury v Spence*, 464 F2d 772 (DC Cir 1972).

22. See note 16.

23. "President's Commission for the Study of Ethical Problems in Medicine and Biomedical and Behavioral Research" *Making Health Care Decisions.* Washington, DC: US Government Printing Office, 1982; also Brock D. "The ideal of shared decision making between physicians and patients" *Kennedy Institute J Ethics.* 1991; 1:28-47.

24. See note 16.

25. Brock D.W, Wartman S.A. "When competent patients make irrational choices" *N Engl Med.* 1990; 322:1595-99.

26. Eddy D.M. "Anatomy of a decision" *JAMA.* 1990; 263:441-43.

27. See note 23.

28. Siegler M. "The progression of medicine: from physician paternalism to patient autonomy to bureaucratic parsimony" *Arch Intern Med.* 1985;145:713-15; also Szasz T.S, Hollender M.H. "The basic models of the doctor-patient relationship" *Arch Intern Med.* 1956; 97:585-92; Applebaum P.S, Lidz C.W, Meisel A. *Informed Consent: Legal Theory and Clinical Prac-*

tice. New York, NY: Oxford University Press, 1987: ch. 3.

29. Katz J. *The Silent World of Doctor and Patient.* New York, NY: Free Press, 1984.

30. Sandel M.J. *Liberalism and the Limits of Justice.* New York, NY: Cambridge University Press, 1982.

31. Veatch R.M. *A Theory of Medical Ethics.* New York, NY: Basic Books Inc Publishers, 1981; also Macklin R. *Mortal Choices.* New York, NY: Pantheon Books, 1987.

32. Tannock I.F, Boyer M. "When is a cancer treatment worthwhile?" *N Engl J Med.* 1990; 322:989-90.

33. Applebaum P.S, Lidz C.W, Meisel A. *Informed Consent: Legal Theory and Clinical Practice.* New York, NY: Oxford University Press, 1987: ch. 3.

34. Ingelfinger F.J. Arrogance. *N Engl J Med.* 1980; 304:1507; Marzuk P.M. "The right kind of paternalism" *N Engl J Med.* 1985; 33: 1474-76; Siegler M. "The progression of medicine: from physician paternalism to patient autonomy to bureaucratic parsimony" *Arch Intern Med.* 1985;145: 713-15.

35. Frankfurt H. "Freedom of the will and the concept of a person" *J Philosophy.* 1971; 68: 5-20; Taylor C. *Human Agency and Language.* New York, NY: Cambridge University Press, 1985: 15-44. Dworkin G. *The Theory and Practice of Autonomy.* New York, NY: Cambridge University Press, 1988: ch. 1.

36. Sandel M.J. *Liberalism and the Limits of Justice.* New York, NY: Cambridge University Press, 1982.

37. Gorovitz S. *Doctors' Dilemmas: Moral Conflict and Medical Care.* New York, NY: Oxford University Press, 1982: ch. 6.

38. Taylor C. *Human Agency and Language.* New York, NY: Cambridge University Press, 1985:15-44; also Dworkin G. *The Theory and practice of Autonomy.* New York, NY: Cambridge University Press, 1988: ch. 1.

39. See note 25.

40. Plato; Hamilton E, Cairns H, eds; Emanuel E.J, trans. *Plato: The Collected Dialogues.* Princeton, NJ: Princeton University Press, 1961: 720 c-e.

41. Walsh D.C., Hingson R.W., Merrigan D.M., *et al.* "The impact of a physician's warning on recovery after alcoholism treatment" *JAMA.* 1992: 267; 663-67.

42. See note 12.

2.
THE VIRTUOUS PHYSICIAN AND THE ETHICS OF MEDICINE

Edmund D. Pellegrino

Consider from what noble seed you spring: you were created not to live like beasts, but for pursuit of virtue and of knowledge.

Dante, *Inferno* 26, 118-120

THE VIRTUOUS PERSON, THE VIRTUOUS PHYSICIAN

Virtue implies a character trait, an internal disposition, habitually to seek moral perfection, to live one's life in accord with the moral law, and to attain a balance between noble intention and just action. Perhaps C.S. Lewis has captured the idea best by likening the virtuous man to the good tennis player: "What you mean by a good player is the man whose eyes and muscles and nerves have been so trained by making innumerable good shots that they can now be relied upon.... They have a certain tone or quality which is there even when he is not playing.... In the same way a man who perseveres in doing just actions gets in the end a certain quality of character. Now it is that quality rather than the particular actions that we mean when we talk of virtue."[1]

On almost any view, the virtuous person is someone we can trust to act habitually in a "good" way — courageously, honestly, justly, wisely, and temperately. He is committed to *being* a good person and to the pursuit of perfection in his private, professional and communal life. He is someone who will act well even when there is no one to applaud, simply because to act otherwise is a violation of what it is to be a good person. No civilized society could endure without a significant number of citizens committed to this concept of virtue. Without such persons no system of general ethics could succeed, and no system of professional ethics could transcend the dangers of self interest. That is why, even while rights, duties, obligations may be emphasized, the concept of virtue has "hovered" so persistently over every system of ethics.

Is the virtuous physician simply the virtuous person practicing medicine? Are there virtues peculiar to medicine as a practice? Are certain of the individual virtues more applicable to medicine than elsewhere in human activities? Is virtue more important in some branches of medicine than others? How do professional skills differ from virtue? These are pertinent questions propadeutic to the later questions of the place of virtue in professional medical ethics.

I believe these questions are best answered by drawing on the Aristotelian-Thomist notion of virtues and its relationship to the ends and purposes of human life. The virtuous physician on this view is defined in terms of the ends of medicine. To be sure, the physician, before he is anything else, must be a virtuous person. To be a virtuous physician he must also be the kind of person we can confidently expect will be disposed to the right and good intrinsic to the practice he professes. What are those dispositions?

To answer this question requires some exposition of what we mean by the good in medicine, or more specifically the good of the patient — for that is the end the patient and the physician ostensibly seek. Any theory of virtue must be linked with a theory of the good because virtue is a disposition habitually to do the good. Must we therefore know the nature of the good the virtuous man is disposed to do? As with the definition of virtue we are caught here in another perennial philosophical question — what is the nature of the Good? Is the good whatever we make it to be or does it have validity independent of our desires or interest? Is the good one, or many? Is it reducible to riches, honors, pleasures, glory, happiness, or something else?

I make no pretense to a discussion of a general theory of the good. But any attempt to define the virtuous physician or a virtue-based ethic for medicine must offer some definition of the good of the patient. The patient's good is the end of medicine, that which shapes the particular virtues required for its attainment. That end is central to any notion of the virtues peculiar to medicine as a practice.

I have argued elsewhere that the architectonic principle of medicine is the good of the patient as expressed in a particular right and good healing action.[2] This is the immediate good end of the clinical encounter. Health, healing, caring, coping are all good ends dependent upon the more immediate end of a right and good decision. On this view, the virtuous physician is one so habitually disposed to act in the patient's good, to place that good in ordinary instances above his own, that he can reliably be expected to do so.

But we must face the fact that the "patient's good" is itself a compound notion. Elsewhere I have examined four components of the patient's good: (1) clinical or biomedical good; (2) the good as perceived by the patient; (3) the good of the patient as a human person; and (4) the Good, or ultimate good. Each of these components of patient good must be served. They must also be placed in some hierarchical order when they conflict within the same person, or between persons involved in clinical decisions.[3]

Some would consider patient good, so far as the physician is concerned, as limited to what applied medical knowledge can achieve in *this* patient. On this view the virtues specific to medicine would be objectivity, scientific probity, and conscientiousness with regard to professional skill. One could perform the technical tasks of medicine well, be faithful to the skills of good technical medicine per se, but without being a virtuous person. Would one then be a virtuous physician? One would have to answer affirmatively if technical skill were all there is to medicine.

Some of the more expansionist models of medicine — like Engel's biopsychosocial model, or that of the World Health Organization (total well-being) would require compassion, empathy, advocacy, benevolence, and beneficence, i.e., an expanded sense of the affective responses to patient need.[4] Some might argue that what is required, therefore, is not virtue, but simply greater skill in the social and behavioral sciences applied to particular patients. On this view the physician's habitual dispositions might be incidental to his skills in communication or his empathy. He could

achieve the ends of medicine without necessarily being a virtuous person in the generic sense.

It is important at this juncture to distinguish the virtues from technical or professional skills, as MacIntyre and, more clearly, Von Wright do. The latter defines a skill as "technical goodness" — excellence in some particular activity — while virtues are not tied to any one activity but are necessary for "the good of man."[5] The virtues are not "characterized in terms of their results."[6] On this view, the technical skills of medicine are not virtues and could be practiced by a non virtuous person. Aristotle held *techne* (technical skills) to be one of the five intellectual virtues but not one of the moral virtues.

The virtues enable the physician to act with regard to things that are good for man, when man is in the specific existential state of illness. They are dispositions always to seek the good intent inherent in healing. Within medicine, the virtues do become in MacIntyre's sense acquired human qualities "... the possession and exercise of which tends to enable us to achieve those goods which are internal to practices and the lack of which effectively prevents us from achieving any such goods."[7]

We can come closer to the relationships of virtue to clinical actions if we look to the more immediate ends of medical encounters, to those moments of clinical truth when specific decisions and actions are chosen and carried out. The good the patient seeks is to be healed — to be restored to his prior, or to a better, state of function, to be made "whole" again. If this is not possible, the patient expects to be helped, to be assisted in coping with the pain, disability or dying that illness may entail. The immediate end of medicine is not simply a technically proficient performance but the use of that performance to attain a good end — the good of the patient — his medical or biomedical good to the extent possible but also his good as he the patient perceives it, his good as a human person who can make his own life plan, and his good as a person with a spiritual destiny if this is his belief.[8] It is the sensitive balancing of these senses of the patient's good which the virtuous physician pursues to perfection.

To achieve the end of medicine thus conceived, to practice medicine virtuously, requires certain dispositions: conscientious attention to technical knowledge and skill to be sure, but also compassion — a capacity to feel something of the patient's experience of illness and his perceptions of what is worthwhile; beneficence and benevolence — doing and wishing to do good for the patient; honesty, fidelity to promises, perhaps at times courage as well — the whole list of virtues spelled out by Aristotle: "... justice, courage, temperance, magnificence, magnanimity, liberality, placability, prudence, wisdom" (*Rhetoric*, 1, c, 13666, 1-3).

Not every one of these virtues is required in every decision. What we expect of the virtuous physician is that he will exhibit them when they are required and that he will be so habitually disposed to do so that we can depend upon it. He will place the good of the patient above his own and seek that good unless its pursuit imposes an injustice upon him, or his family, or requires a violation of his own conscience.

While the virtues are necessary to attain the good internal to medicine as a practice, they exist independently of medicine. They are necessary for the practice of a good life, no matter in what activities that life may express itself. Certain of the virtues may become duties in the Stoic sense, duties because of the nature of medicine as a practice. Medicine calls forth benevolence, beneficence, truth telling, honesty, fidelity, and justice more than physical courage, for example. Yet even physical courage may be necessary when caring for the wounded on battlefields, in plagues, earthquakes, or other disasters. On a more ordinary scale courage is necessary in treating contagious diseases, violent patients, or battlefield casualties. Doing the right and good thing in medicine calls for a more regular, intensive, and selective practice of the virtues than many other callings.

A person who is a virtuous person can cultivate the technical skills of medicine for reasons other than the good of the patient — his own pride, profit, prestige, power. Such a physician can make technically right decisions and perform skillfully. He could not be depended upon, however, to act against his own self-interest for the good of his patient.

In the virtuous physician, explicit fulfillment of rights and duties is an outward expression of an inner disposition to do the right and the good. He is virtuous not because he has conformed to the letter of the law, or his moral duties, but because that is what a good person does. He starts always with his commitment to be a certain kind of person, and he approaches clinical quandaries, conflicts of values, and his patient's interests as a good person should.

Some branches of medicine would seem to demand a stricter and broader adherence to virtue than others. Generalists, for example, who deal with the more sensitive facets and nuances of a patient's life and humanity must exercise the virtues more diligently than technique-oriented specialists. The narrower the specialty the more easily the patient's good can be safeguarded by rules, regulations, rights and duties; the broader the specialty the more significant are the physician's character traits. No branch of medicine, however, can be practiced without some dedication to some of the virtues.[9]

Unfortunately, physicians can compartmentalize their lives. Some practice medicine virtuously, yet are guilty of vice in their private lives. Examples are common of physicians who appear sincerely to seek the good of their patients and neglect obligations to family or friends. Some boast of being "married" to medicine and use this excuse to justify all sorts of failures in their own human relationships. We could not call such a person virtuous. Nor could we be secure in, or trust, his disposition to act in a right and good way even in medicine. After all, one of the essential virtues is balancing conflicting obligations judiciously.

As Socrates pointed out to Meno, one cannot really be virtuous in part:

Why did not I ask you to tell me the nature of virtue as a whole? And you are very far from telling me this; but declare every action to be virtue which is done with a part of virtue; as though you had told me and I must already know the whole of virtue, and this too when frittered away into little pieces. And therefore my dear Meno, I fear that I must begin again, and repeat the same question: what is virtue? For otherwise, I can only say that every action done with a part of virtue is virtue; what else is the meaning of saying that every action done with justice is virtue? Ought I not to ask the question over again; for can any one who does not know virtue know a part of virtue? (*Meno*, 79)

VIRTUES, RIGHTS AND DUTIES IN MEDICAL ETHICS

Frankena has neatly summarized the distinctions between virtue-based and rights — and duty-based ethics as follows:

> In an ED (ethics of duty) then, the basic concept is that a certain kind of external act (or doing) ought to be done in certain circumstances and that of a certain disposition being a virtue is a dependent one. In an EV (ethics of virtue) the basic concept is that of a disposition or way of being — something one has, or if not does — as a virtue, as morally good; and that of an action's being virtuous or good or even right, is a dependent one.[10]

There are some logical difficulties with a virtue-based ethic. For one thing, there must be some consensus on a definition of virtue. For another there is a circularity in the assertion that virtue is what the good man habitually does, and that at the same time one becomes virtuous by doing good. Virtue and good are defined in terms of each other and the definitions of both may vary among sincere people in actual practice when there is no consensus. A virtue-based ethic is difficult to defend as the sole basis for normative judgments.

But there is a deficiency in rights- and duty-ethics as well. They too must be linked to a theory of the good. In contemporary ethics, theories of good are rarely explicitly linked to theories of the right and good. Von Wright, commendably, is one of the few contemporary authorities who explicitly connects his theory of good with his theory of virtue....

In most professional ethical codes, virtue- and duty-based ethics are intermingled. The Hippocratic Oath, for example, imposes certain duties like protection of confidentiality, avoiding abortion, not harming the patient. But the Hippocratic physician also pledges: "... in purity and holiness I will guard my life and my art." This is an exhortation to be a good person and a virtuous physician, in order to serve patients in an ethically responsible way.

Likewise, in one of the most humanistic statements in medical literature, the first century A.D. writer, Scribonius Largus, made *humanitas* (compassion) an essential virtue. It is thus really a role-specific duty. In doing so he was applying the Stoic doctrine of virtue to medicine.[11]

The latest version (1980) of the AMA "Principles of Medical Ethics" similarly intermingles duties, rights, and exhortations to virtue. It speaks of "standards of behavior," "essentials of honorable behaviour," dealing "honestly" with patients and colleagues and exposing colleagues "deficient in character." The *Declaration of Geneva*, which must meet the challenge of the widest array of value systems, nonetheless calls for practice "with conscience and dignity" in keeping with "the honor and noble traditions of the profession." Though their first allegiance must be to the Communist ethos, even the Soviet physician is urged to preserve "the high title of physician," "to keep and develop the beneficial traditions of medicine" and to "dedicate" all his "knowledge and strength to the care of the sick."

Those who are cynical of any protestation of virtue on the part of physicians will interpret these excerpts as the last remnants of a dying tradition of altruistic benevolence. But at the very least, they attest to the recognition that the good of the patient cannot be fully protected by rights and duties alone. Some degree of supererogation is built into the nature of the relationship of those who are ill and those who profess to help them.

This too may be why many graduating classes, still idealistic about their calling, choose the Prayer of Maimonides (not by Maimonides at all) over the more deontological Oath of Hippocrates. In that "prayer" the physician asks: "... may neither avarice nor miserliness, nor thirst for glory or for a great reputation engage my mind; for the enemies of truth and philanthropy may easily deceive me and make me forgetful of my lofty aim of doing good to thy children." This is an unequivocal call to virtue and it is hard to imagine even the most cynical graduate failing to comprehend its message.

All professional medical codes, then, are built of a three-tiered system of obligations related to the special roles of physicians in society. In the ascending order of ethical sensitivity they are: observance of the laws of the land, then observance of rights and fulfillment of duties, and finally the practice of virtue.

A legally based ethic concentrates on the minimum requirements — the duties imposed by human laws which protect against the grosser aberrations of personal rights. Licensure, the laws of torts and contracts, prohibitions against discrimination, good Samaritan laws, definitions of death, and the protection of human subjects of experimentation are elements of a legalistic ethic.

At the next level is the ethics of rights and duties which spells out obligations beyond what law defines. Here, benevolence and beneficence take on more than their legal meaning. The ideal of service, of responsiveness to the special needs of those who are ill, some degree of compassion, kindliness, promise-keeping, truth-telling, and non-maleficence and specific obligations like confidentiality and autonomy, are included. How these principles are applied, and conflicts among them resolved in the patient's best interests, are subjects of widely varying interpretation. How sensitively these issues are confronted depends more on the physician's character than his capability at ethical discourse or moral casuistry.

Virtue-based ethics goes beyond these first two levels. We expect the virtuous person to do the right and the good even at the expense of personal sacrifice and legitimate self-interest. Virtue ethics expands the notions of benevolence, beneficence, conscientiousness, compassion, and fidelity well beyond what strict duty might require. It makes some degree of supererogation mandatory because it calls for standards of ethical performance that exceed those prevalent in the rest of society.[12]

At each of these three levels there are certain dangers from over-zealous or misguided observance. Legalistic ethical systems tend toward a justification for minimalistic ethics, a narrow definition of benevolence or beneficence, and a contract-minded physician-patient relationship. Duty- and rights-based ethics may be distorted by too strict adherence to the letter of ethical principles without the modulations and nuances the spirit of those principles implies. Virtue-based ethics, being the least specific, can more easily lapse into self-righteous paternalism or an unwelcome over-involvement in the personal life of the patient. Misapplication of any moral system even with good intent converts benevolence into maleficence. The virtuous person might be expected to be more sensitive to these aberrations than someone whose ethics is more deontologically or legally flavored.

The more we yearn for ethical sensitivity the less we lean on rights, duties, rules, and principles, and the more we lean on the character traits of the moral agent. Paradoxically, without rules, rights, and duties specifically spelled out, we cannot predict what form a particular person's expression of virtue will take. In a pluralistic society, we need laws, rules, and principles to assure a dependable minimum level of moral conduct. But that minimal level is insufficient in the complex and often unpredictable circumstances of decision-making, where technical and value desiderata intersect so inextricably.

The virtuous physician does not act from unreasoned, uncritical intuitions about what feels good. His dispositions are ordered in accord with that "right reason" which both Aristotle and Aquinas considered essential to virtue. Medicine is itself ultimately an exercise of practical wisdom — a right way of acting in difficult and uncertain circumstances for a specific end, i.e., the good of a particular person who is ill. It is when the choice of a right and good action becomes more difficult, when the temptations to self-interest are most insistent, when unexpected nuances of good and evil arise and no one is looking, that the differences between an ethics based in virtue and an ethics based in law and/or duty can most clearly be distinguished.

Virtue-based professional ethics distinguishes itself, therefore, less in the avoidance of overly immoral practices than in avoidance of those at the margin of moral responsibility. Physicians are confronted, in today's morally relaxed climate, with an increasing number of new practices that pit altruism against self-interest. Most are not illegal, or, strictly speaking, immoral in a rights- or duty-based ethic. But they are not consistent with the higher levels of moral sensitivity that a virtue-ethics demands. These practices usually involve opportunities for profit from the illness of others, narrowing the concept of service for personal convenience, taking a proprietary attitude with respect to medical knowledge, and placing loyalty to the profession above loyalty to patients.

Under the first heading, we might include such things as investment in and ownership of for-profit hospitals, hospital chains, nursing homes, dialysis units, tie-in arrangements with radiological or laboratory services, escalation of fees for repetitive, high-volume procedures, and lax indications for their use, especially when third party payers "allow" such charges.

The second heading might include the ever decreasing availability and accessibility of physicians, the diffusion of individual patient responsibility in group practice so that the patient never knows whom he will see or who is on call, the itinerant emergency room physician who works two days and skips three with little commitment to hospital or community, and the growing over-indulgence of physicians in vacations, recreation, and "self-development."

The third category might include such things as "selling one's services" for whatever the market will bear, providing what the market demands and not necessarily what the community needs, patenting new procedures or keeping them secret from potential competitor-colleagues, looking at the investment of time, effort, and capital in a medical education as justification for "making it back," or forgetting that medical knowledge is drawn from the cumulative experience of a multitude of patients, clinicians, and investigators.

Under the last category might be included referrals on the basis of friendship and reciprocity rather than skill, resisting consultations and second opinions as affronts to one's competence, placing the interest of the referring physician above those of the patients, looking the other way in the face of incompetence or even dishonesty in one's professional colleagues.

These and many other practices are defended today by sincere physicians and even encouraged in this era of competition, legalism, and self-indulgence. Some can be rationalized even in a deontological ethic. But it would be impossible to envision the physician committed to the virtues assenting to these practices. A virtue-based ethic simply does not fluctuate with what the dominant social mores will tolerate. It must interpret benevolence, beneficence, and responsibility in a way that reduces self-interest and enhances altruism. It is the only convincing answer the profession can give to the growing perception clearly manifest in the legal commentaries in the FTC ruling that medicine is nothing more than business and should be regulated as such.

A virtue-based ethic is inherently elitist, in the best sense, because its adherents demand more of themselves than the prevailing morality. It calls forth that extra measure of dedication that has made the best physicians in every era exemplars of what the human spirit can achieve. No matter to what depths a society may fall, virtuous persons will always be the beacons that light the way back to moral sensitivity; virtuous physicians are the beacons that show the way back to moral credibility for the whole profession.

Albert Jonsen, rightly I believe, diagnoses the central paradox in medicine as the tension between self-interest and altruism.[13] No amount of deft juggling of rights, duties, or principles will suffice to resolve that tension. We are all too good at rationalizing what we want to do so that personal gain can be converted from vice to virtue. Only a character formed by the virtues can feel the nausea of such intellectual hypocrisy.

To be sure, the twin themes of self-interest and altruism have been inextricably joined in the history of medicine. There have always been physicians who reject the virtues or, more often, claim them falsely. But, in addition, there have been physicians, more often than the critics of medicine would allow, who have been truly virtuous both in intent and act. They have been, and remain, the leaven of the profession and the hope of all who are ill. They form the seawall that will not be eroded even by the powerful forces of commercialization, bureaucratization, and mechanization inevitable in modern medicine.

We cannot, need not, and indeed must not, wait for a medical analogue of MacIntyre's "new St. Benedict" to show us the way. There is no new concept of virtue waiting to be discovered that is peculiarly suited to the dilemmas of our own dark age. We must recapture the courage to speak of character, virtue, and perfection in living a good life. We must encourage those who are willing to dedicate themselves to a "higher standard of self effacement."[14]

We need the courage, too, to accept the obvious split in the profession between those who see and feel the altruistic imperatives in medicine, and those who do not. Those who at heart believe that the pursuit of private self-interest serves the public good are very different from those who believe in the restraint of self-interest. We forget that physicians since the beginnings of the profession have subscribed to different values and virtues. We need only recall that the Hippocratic Oath was the Oath of physicians of the Pythagorean school at a time when most Greek physicians followed essentially a craft ethic.[15] A perusal of the Hippocratic Corpus itself, which intersperses ethics and etiquette, will show how differently its treatises deal with fees, the care of incurable patients, and the business aspects of the craft.

The illusion that all physicians share a common devotion to a high-flown set of ethical principles has done damage to medicine by raising expectations some members of the profession could not, or will not, fulfill. Today, we must be more forthright about the differences in value commitment among physicians. Professional codes must be more explicit about the relationships between duties, rights, and virtues. Such explicitness encourages a more honest relationship between physicians and patients and removes the hypocrisy of verbal assent to a general code, to which an individual physician may not really subscribe. Explicitness enables patients to choose among physicians on the basis of their ethical commitments as well as their reputations for technical expertise.

Conceptual clarity will not assure virtuous behavior. Indeed, virtues are usually distorted if they are the subject of too conscious a design. But conceptual clarity will distinguish between motives and provide criteria for judging the moral commitment one can expect from the profession and from its individual members. It can also inspire those whose virtuous inclinations need re-enforcement in the current climate of commercialization of the healing relationship.

To this end the current resurgence of interest in virtue-based ethics is altogether salubrious. Linked to a theory of patient good and a theory of rights and duties, it could provide the needed groundwork for a reconstruction of professional medical ethics as that work matures. Perhaps even more progress can be made if we take Shakespeare's advice in *Hamlet*: "Assume the virtue if you have it not.... For use almost can change the stamp of nature."

Notes

1. Lewis C. 1952. *Mere Christianity*, MacMillan Co., New York.

2. Pellegrino, E. 1983. "The Healing Relationship: The Architectonics of Clinical Medicine," in E. Shelp (ed.), *The Clinical Encounter*, D. Reidel, Dordrecht, Holland, pp. 153-72.

3. Pellegrino, E. 1983 "Moral Choice, The Good of the Patient and the Patient's Good," in J. Moskop and L. Kopelman (eds.), *Moral Choice and Medical Crisis,* D. Reidel, Dordrecht, Holland.

4. Engel, G. 1980. "The Clinical Application of the Biopsychosocial Model," *American Journal of Psychiatry* 137: 2, 535-44.

5. Von Wright, G. 1965. *The Varieties of Goodness,* The Humanities Press, New York, pp. 139-40.

6. Ibid, p. 141.

7. MacIntyre, A. 1981. *After Virtue*, University of Notre Dame Press, Notre Dame, Indiana, p. 178.

8. Pellegrino, E. 1979. "The Anatomy of Clinical Judgments: Some Notes on Right Reason and Right Action," in H.T. Engelhardt, Jr., *et al.*(eds.), *Clinical Judgment: A Critical Appraisal*, D. Reidel, Dordrecht, Holland, pp. 169-94; Pellegrino, E. 1979. "Toward a Reconstruction of Medical Morality: The Primacy of the Act of Profession and the Fact of Illness," *Journal of Medicine and Philosophy* 4: 1, 32-56.

9. May W. Personal communication, "Virtues in a Professional Setting," unpublished.

10. Frankena, W. 1982. "Beneficence in an Ethics of Virtue," in E. Shelp (ed.), *Beneficence and Health Care*, D. Reidel, Dordrecht, Holland, pp. 63-81.

11. Cicero, 1967. *Moral Obligations,* J. Higginbotham (trans.), University of California Press, Berkeley and Los Angeles; Pellegrino, E. 1983. *"Scribonius Largus* and the Origins of Medical Humanism," address to the American Osler Society.

12. Reeder, J. 1982. "Beneficence, Supererogation, and Role Duty," in E. Shelp (ed.), *Beneficence and Health Care,* D. Reidel, Dordrecht, Holland, pp. 83-108.

13. Jonsen, A. 1983. "Watching the Doctor," *New England Journal of Medicine* 308: 25, 1531-35.

14. Cushing, H. 1929. *Consecratio Medici and Other Papers*, Little, Brown and Co., Boston.

15. Edelstein, L. 1967. "The Professional Ethics of the Greek Physician," in O. Temkin (ed.), *Ancient Medicine: Selected Papers of Ludwig Edelstein,* Johns Hopkins University Press, Baltimore.

3.
SEPARATING CARE AND CURE: AN ANALYSIS OF HISTORICAL AND CONTEMPORARY IMAGES OF NURSING AND MEDICINE

Nancy S. Jecker and Donnie J. Self

Care as a central organizing concept is a relative newcomer to moral theory (Blum, 1988; Kittay and Meyers, 1987; Noddings, 1984, 1987, 1989; Pearsall, 1986) and moral development theory (Gilligan, 1982, 1986; Gilligan and Wiggins, 1987; Lyons, 1983). However, its roots in American nursing trace back to nursing's early history. In the late nineteenth century, Florence Nightingale thought medical therapeutics and "curing" were of less importance to patient outcome and willingly left this realm to the physician. Caring, the arena she considered of greatest importance, she assigned to the nurse (Reverby, 1987a, 1987b).[1]

Although nurses and physicians entertain a more sophisticated picture of their professions today, the image of caring as the exclusive province of nurses continues to influence public perceptions. Because patients exert influence over professionals' self-perceptions, patients' attitudes have the potential to strengthen and reinforce traditional stereotypes, obstruct efforts to re-define professional relationships and provide political fuel for traditional hierarchies. In this way, the idea that "doctors cure and nurses care" continues to exercise a pervasive influence on health professionals' self-images and inter-professional relationships. In addition to these practical consequences, the care-cure division easily can produce a lack of philosophical clarity regarding the concept of care itself. In particular, dissociating the labor of physicians from the realm of care narrows our understanding of care, while treating nursing work as an exclusive care paradigm encourages one-dimensional thinking about care.

This essay provides a philosophical critique of professional stereotypes in medicine. In the course of this critique, we also offer a detailed analysis of the concept of care in health care. More precisely, our aims are to (1) identify factors that contribute to viewing care as the exclusive province of nurses; (2) fine tune the concept of care by exploring alternative forms of care; and (3) illustrate, through the use of cases, diverse models of caring.

GENDER-BASED EXPLANATIONS OF PROFESSIONAL STEREOTYPES

In a popular text on nursing ethics, Andrew Jameton observes that "Physicians are ... said to focus on the *cure* function, while nurses focus on the *care* functions" (1984, p. 10). Jameton goes on to explain that nurses are expected to perform such functions as follow hospital procedures, report significant incidents and mishaps to supervisors, and organize work on wards and hospital departments. Presumably, physicians order procedures, make medical decisions and take charge of wards and departments. What are the origins of this apparent division of labor? Why does the perception that nurses, and only nurses, perform care functions remain with us? Since nursing and medicine are largely gender segregated professions, the answers to these questions may lie as much in gender-related tendencies as in the histories of nursing and medicine.

One explanation for this apparent division is suggested by Gilligan and Pollak (1989). They report that the association of danger with intimacy is a more salient feature in the fantasies of men than of women. In their study, men projected more danger into situations of close, personal affiliation than situations of impersonal achievement. For example, male subjects expressed "a fear of being caught in a smothering relationship or humiliated by rejection or deceit" (1989, p. 246). Females, by contrast, perceived more danger in situations of impersonal achievement than situations of personal affiliation. For instance, females "connected danger with the isolation that they associated with competitive success" (1989, p. 246). If male and female attitudes toward attachment and separation do cluster in the way this study suggests, this indicates one fairly obvious explanation for care and cure stereotypes in the health professions. Female nurses would tend to cultivate skill at caring activities, because these activities involve the intimacy and close personal affiliation that women, as a group, prefer. Curing activities would, on the whole, be shunned by nurses, because such activities involve forms of impersonal achievement that women, as a group, find threatening. The opposite tendency should occur in medicine, a male dominated profession, namely: physicians would be likely to stress scientific and technical achievement, while down playing patient contact and physician-patient relationships.

Consistent with the above line of reasoning is a second possible explanation. According to this second account, the detached objectivity of scientific fields generally, and medical science in particular, discourages many women from excelling at them. Keller maintains that the goal of post-enlightenment science has been a method of perception that affirms empirical reality, while denying subjectivity (1985). This method of knowing implies a purely mechanical view of persons and objects: "no longer filling the void with living form," scientists in the modern age "learned to fill it with dead form" (Keller, 1985, pp. 69-70). In our culture, such a view of self and world is, according to Keller, pervasively associated with masculinity (1985, p. 71).

If Keller is correct about both the association between science and objectivity and the association between objectivity and masculinity, her analysis sheds light on the alleged cure-care division. Following Keller's analysis, once scientific medicine became the dominant mode of medicine in this country, a method of perception that denied the significance of subjectivity took hold. Such an approach focused attention on patients' physical signs and symptoms, while down playing the significance of their subjective preferences, feelings and experiences. The masculine image this method portrayed in the culture induced males to practice medicine, but encouraged women to assume healing roles that fit better the culture's idea of femininity.

A third explanation of professional stereotypes in nursing and medicine also appeals to gender stereotypes. This explanation holds that our culture associates ethics and humanism with femininity rather than masculinity. For example, ethics and values frequently are referred to as being learned at mother's knee. Morantz-Sanchez (1985) traces this association between ethics and femininity to the early nineteenth century. She argues that during this time, the popular image of women shifted from the biblical and puritan idea of an innately sexual temptress to the idea of women as naturally passionless, spiritual and moral. When women were no longer seen as "the inheritors of Eve's questionable legacy" (Morantz-Sanchez, 1985, p. 22), their prudery confined the social roles they were qualified to fill. In particular, women were judged unqualified to enter the medical profession because, unlike men, they could not restrain their natural sympathies as a physician must. For example, women could not be brought into the dissecting room and undergo other rigors of medical training without destroying their innate moral sensibilities.

Referring to the modern tradition, Jameton makes the point that it is "women [not men who] have carried the humane tradition in modern western cultures: they educate children, soften the blows of the world, nurture others and humanize modern life. Nursing and medicine have reified this stereotype" (1987, p. 67). Jameton also notes the long standing tradition of ethics in the female dominated profession of nursing, and the comparatively weaker and more recent tradition of ethics in medicine. According to Jameton, since 1900 not a single decade has passed without publication of at least one basic text in nursing ethics. Moreover, in its very first volume (1901), *The American Journal of Nursing* published an article on ethics. In the 1920s and 1930s, the *Journal* carried a regular column of ethics cases. In addition to ethics publications, ethics courses have a long history in nursing: they were included in the first formal training programs for nurses. In medicine, by contrast, the tradition of ethics teaching in a sustained and consistent manner is much more recent. It was not until the 1970s that medicine incorporated a significant formal ethics curriculum into medical school classes, and even then "it resulted in large part from outside pressures" (Jameton, 1987, p. 67). Assuming Morantz-Sanchez's and Jameton's historical analyses are correct, they illuminate another possible source of professional stereotypes. If our culture associates ethical concern and response with femininity, one would expect females in general to gravitate toward roles that call upon these abilities. Men who wished to enter the health care profession would fill other roles.

It should be noted that all of the above explanations take for granted the idea that American nursing and medicine are gender segregated professions. This assumption is historically accurate, since a generation or more ago over ninety percent of medical students and physicians were white men (Relman, 1989), and nursing has long been dominated by women. Yet despite this historical precedence, today more men are becoming nurses and women are much more likely to enter the medical profession. In 1972, for example, 1,694 men graduated from American nursing schools, a fourfold increase over 1963, and in 1981 the number of men graduating from R. N. programs jumped to 3,492 (Rowland, 1984). Since women continue to dominate nursing, it is not surprising that overall they occupy more high-level administrative and supervisory positions than men. Yet, the percentage of male nurses who have reached administrative or supervisory positions is much larger than the percentage of female nurses who have reached administrative or supervisory positions (Rowland, 1984). Thus men who do enter nursing are more likely to be in positions where their presence and influence is felt.

Likewise, in the American medical profession, the percentage of female applicants and matriculants to medical school began to rise abruptly in 1970-1971. The number of applications from men, which had been rising steeply, reached a peak in 1974-1976 and has been falling ever since (Relman, 1989). Although few women serve on medical faculty (Eisenberg, 1989), and women are underrepresented in positions of power in academic institutions and as leaders in medical organizations (Levinson, Tolle, Lewis, 1989), their presence in medicine is growing and their influence in shaping medicine's professional identity is increasing.

For these reasons, the above explanations of professional stereotypes are incomplete as they stand. A more complete account would need to explain recent changes in the gender constitution of each profession, perhaps by appealing to shifts in the culture's gender ideas. For example, new gender ideals for men may lie behind changes currently underway in the medical profession. For example, the Association of American Medical Colleges has substantially revised its Medical College Admission Test (MCAT) to place greater emphasis on "humanistic" skills in selecting physicians; the American Board of Internal Medicine has requested directors of residency programs to assess compassion, respect for patients and integrity in candidates for board certification; and the American Medical Association recently embarked on a major quality assurance initiative which will include research into attributes of "interpersonal exchange" (Nelson, 1989). Alternatively, a fuller explanation might uncover ways in which traditional gender attitudes persist, despite greater integration of men in nursing and women in medicine. For example, despite greater numbers of male nurses, the American nursing profession is still overwhelmingly female: ninety seven percent of the total nurse population is female (American Nurses' Association, 1987). Moreover, the majority (56.3 percent) of men cite employment availability as their reason for entering nursing, while most women (62.1 percent) cite interest in people (Rowland, 1984). This suggests that practical economic considerations, rather than a desire to enter a caring role, are more frequent motives among men. Furthermore, the fact that more men are entering nursing may simply indicate that more men are willing to challenge prevailing stereotypes, rather than indicating that these stereotypes and the expectations associated with them no longer apply. Evidence for this is that males who become nurses are more likely than female nurses to be viewed as gay or asked why they do not become doctors (Rowland, 1984). Male nurses also report greater difficulty than female nurses in telling others of their occupational choice: in one study, only sixty-six percent felt comfortable doing so, as compared with eighty-three percent of women (Rowland, 1984). Finally, although more men are choosing nursing, gender segregation reportedly persists between nursing specialties. Men's highest priorities after graduation are jobs in critical or acute care settings, whereas women prefer pediatric and public health fields (Rowland, 1984). In one study of nursing students, male students preferred, in rank order: emergency nursing, then outpatient, intensive care, medical-surgical, psychiatric, and coronary care nursing, and lastly, anesthesia. By contrast, female students ranked pediatric nursing first, then public health, medical-surgical, obstetrics/maternity, and psychiatric nursing (Rowland, 1984).

HISTORICAL EXPLANATIONS OF PROFESSIONAL STEREOTYPES

Another kind of explanation for the cure-care division has less to do with hypothesized gender differences and more to do with the unique histories of the nursing and medical professions. First, the history of nursing, and its domestic roots in particular, may shed light on the association of nursing with care. Although historians sometimes ignore these roots and begin the history of nursing with the introduction of formal training programs for nurses in the 1870s, a growing number of revisionist historians reject this approach. For example, Reverby makes the point that American nursing "did not appear *de novo* at the end of the nineteenth century ... [instead,] nursing throughout the colonial era and most of the nineteenth century took place within the family" (1987a, p. 5). O'Brien also finds the roots of nursing "deep in the domestic world of the family" (1987). And Starr maintains that "care of the sick was part of the domestic economy for which the wife assumed responsibility. She would call on the networks of kin and community for advice and assistance when illness struck" (1982, p. 32, 1982).

According to these historians, the history of American nursing begins prior to the 1870s. During this earlier period, mothers, daughters and sisters nursed their families at home, sometimes aided by female neighbors who called themselves "professed" or "born" nurses and had previous experience caring for their own families (O'Brien, 1987, p. 13). So long as the locus of nursing remained domestic, its

primary task was the nurturing of loved ones through ongoing feeding, clothing, bathing and comforting.

Increasingly, the nurturing tasks in which home-based nurses engaged during the colonial era were set apart from the responsibility of their physicians counterparts. First, the medical manuals that domestic nurses consulted drew a sharp line between "what could be accomplished by a loving mother and nurse and what needed the skilled consultation of a physician" (O'Brien, 1987, p. 13). The popular 18th century book, *Domestic Medicine,* assured readers that physicians need be consulted rarely, and that most people underestimate their own abilities and knowledge (Buchanan, 1778). Second, the very fact that nurses lived with their patients and constantly were immersed in the practical activity of caring for them, meant that their job took on a distinctive character. In contrast to nurses, physicians made house calls or were visited by patients in offices. Patients were not primarily relatives, but neighbors and town's people. The physician's job was to offer expert advise or perform specific medical procedures, while nurses carried out physicians' instructions. Thus, physicians used their presumed expertise to direct the caring process, while nurses who lived with patients carried out the actual tasks of ongoing care.

According to this account, the association of American nursing with care traces back to the time when nurses' chief task was caring for sick offspring in the home. Later in the nineteenth century, when nurses left the domestic front to care for patients in hospitals and during wartime, and when they attended the first professional training schools, these early domestic roots continued to shape nursing's identity. In these new locations, nurses' roles continued to include traditional domestic tasks, such as bedmaking, feeding and hygiene. Thus, a significant emphasis of early training programs was on practical skills. Later educational reforms which sought to introduce scientific content into the nursing curriculum stirred heated debate, attesting to the continued influence of the domestic tradition on the nursing profession.

While American nursing was linked intimately with caregiving activities, American physicians achieved professional status and identity by fashioning a separate sphere. Given the association between caring and "women's work," physicians surely had little incentive to identify their own professional function as caring. As Benner and Wrubel note, "caring is devalued because caring is associated with women's work and women's work is devalued and most often unpaid" (1989, p. 368). During the colonial era, physicians had only part time medical practices. They earned a livelihood performing other tasks, such as clergy, teaching and farming (Conrad and Schnieder, 1990). Not until the nineteenth century did medicine become a full time vocation, but during this period its dangerous and often unsuccessful therapies undermined its prestige. According to Starr, "while some physicians were seeking to make themselves into an elite profession with a monopoly of practice, much of the public refused to grant them any such privileges" (1982, p. 31). In addition, physicians were fiercely competitive with homeopaths and other medical sects for a share of the medical market. Thus, much of American medicine's early history was characterized by repeated efforts to gain repute and professional standing. The first state licensing laws, which granted to physicians with special training and class sole authority to practice medicine, were repealed during the Jacksonian period (Starr, 1982). Later in the nineteenth century, with the formation of the American Medical Association, physicians were finally successful in their efforts to professionalize medicine and control medical markets. Medicine was credited with the decline in incidence and mortality of diseases, such as leprosy, malaria, small pox and cholera, thereby increasing the public's faith in its healing powers. During the latter part of the nineteenth century, the rise of scientific medicine ushered in significant progress and ensured the continued prestige and dominance of the medical profession.

The early history of American medicine suggests a possible explanation for the association of medicine with cure, rather than care. The presence of fierce competition and marginal status during its early years forged a mission for medicine that focused on achieving cultural authority and an elite status for its practitioners. Efforts to gain authority and status required physicians to stand apart from laypersons and develop exclusive modes of language, technique and theory. This put physicians at odds with activities, such as patient empathy and care, that call upon abilities of engagement and identification with others. The scientific paradigm that became the language and practice of medicine further reinforced a separation between physician and patient. This paradigm pictured the human being as a machine, and disease as an objective entity that interfered with the human being's mechanical functioning. Such a perspective implied that the "ghost in the machine" was superfluous to the healing process.

RETHINKING THE CONCEPT OF CARE

Having considered several possible explanations for the association of nursing with care, and medicine with cure, we need to consider next whether these common stereotypes are justified. To address this question, we now turn to a critical analysis of the concept of care. To begin with, it should be noted that the very idea of separating care from cure assumes that these ideas are distinct and non-overlapping. An alternative view sees caring as part of the very meaning of curing. According to this view, physicians who cure also care. Interestingly, the *Oxford English Dictionary* supports this interpretation of cure. Cure comes from the Latin word "curare" meaning "to care for, take care of." Cure refers to "care, heed, concern; to do one's (busy) care, to give one's care or attention to some piece of work; to apply one's self diligently." This definition renders the idea of a physician who cures without caring unintelligible. A person who heals a wound, or otherwise restores a patient to health, cures only if this outcome is the result of devoted caring.

On this reading, although curing entails applying one's care to some one or thing, caring does not imply curing. Thus, physicians can and often do *care* for patients, while suspending attempts to *cure* them. This occurs, for example, when physicians withdraw medical treatments they judge futile, while continuing palliative measures. Hauerwas notes the practical importance of acknowledging the possibility of caring *without* curing. Physicians who fail to recognize the possibility of caring without curing might attempt futile therapies, based on the false belief that efforts to cure patients are all they have to offer.

The *Oxford English Dictionary* distinguishes two distinct senses of care. First, care means "a burdened state of mind arising from ... concern about anything

... mental perturbation," and "serious or grave mental attention, the charging of the mind." In this first sense, to "have a care" or "keep a care" is to be in a subjective state of concern about something. Second, care refers to "oversight with view to protection, preservation, or guidance; hence to have the care of." In this second sense, care implies an activity of looking out for or safeguarding the interests of others.

We shall designate the first sense of care, "caring about." Caring about indicates an attitude, feeling, or state of mind directed toward a person or circumstance (Hauerwas, 1978, p. 145). To assert that "My nurse cares about me" or that "Everyone ought to care about the environment" refers to care in this first sense. The second sense of care involves the exercise of a skill, with or without a particular attitude or feeling toward the object upon which this skill is exercised. We shall refer to this as "caring for." For example, we use care in this sense when we say that "Nurse Jones is caring for your mother" or "The mechanic down the street offered to take care of my car." Caring in both senses is a relational term, referring to an attitude or skill directed to someone or something. One's concern about others may be more or less deep, and one's skill at caring for others may display more or less ability. Thus, we refer to the quality of caring to describe how deeply one feels, or how good or poor one is at caring for another. Whereas caring about can occur at a distance from its object, caring for usually requires direct contact with the one who is cared for. Excellence at caring for particular patients typically requires repeated contacts and skill in ascertaining each patient's particular needs. Thus, an expert caregiver learns "through repeated experience with patients ... to perceive the particular rather than the typical care, becomes individualized rather than standardized and planning becomes anticipatory of change rather than simply responsive to change" (Benner and Wrubel, 1989, p. 382).

Applying these definitions of cure and care to the medical setting enables us to say that a health professional who cares *about* a patient makes a cognitive or emotional decision that the welfare of the patient is of great importance. Caring about requires keeping the patient's best interest in the forefront of mind and heart. By contrast, a health professional who cares *for* a patient engages in a deliberate and ongoing activity of responding to the patient's needs. Caring for, executed in an exemplary or excellent way, involves deciphering the patient's particular condition and needs. This calls upon verbal skills of questioning and listening and requires attending to and translating non-verbal cues. Caring for thus requires cultivating a capacity to understand others' subjective experiences. Understood in this light, caring for draws upon and teaches a way of knowing that involves "awareness of the complexities of a particular situation" and "inner ... resources that have been garnered through experience in living" (Benoliel, 1987). The source of this knowledge tends to be participation in relationships with others and observation of others' actions, rather than verbal debate and conversation or the reading of texts (Benner, 1983). Knowledge in this form is practical and interpersonal (Schultz and Meleis, 1988). In the case of unconscious or mentally compromised patients and infants, caring for especially draws upon a person's skill at interpreting gestures, postures, sounds, grimaces, eye scans and bodily movements (Jecker, 1990a). For instance, through intimate engagement, a daughter who serves as a caretaker for a disoriented elderly parent may be able to decipher what counts as pain and comfort, or boredom and interest to the parent. Evidence is gleaned through partaking in daily rituals, such as bathing and feeding, and interpreting the parent's responses.

Caring *about* does not imply caring for. For example, a ward supervisor may care deeply about her patients, without being engaged in the activity of caring directly for them. Nor does caring *for* entail caring about. For instance, one who skillfully cares for patients may be meticulous in her efforts to interpret patients' needs, without actually caring about patients: she may regard them as just one more puzzle to be solved, excel at caring for its own sake, or simply seek to impress colleagues or a boss.

While it is fairly easy to tell who cares *for* a patient, it can be exceedingly difficult to construe who cares *about* a patient. Some professionals may prefer colleagues and supervisors to think they care about their patients, even if they in fact are preoccupied with other matters. Others may learn to cover up the fact that they do care about patients. For example, the idea of masculinity to which some aspire discourages outward expressions of care and concern for others. It would be difficult to gauge whether males who express masculinity in this way care about their patients. Still others may appear uncaring because they learn deference in conflict. For example, women or nurses who are taught to follow orders blindly may appear not to take a genuine interest in their patients. Historically, nurses were instructed to discharge medical orders in an obedient, unquestioning manner (Jameton, 1987), but this expectation does not necessarily entail the absence of caring about.

EXAMPLES OF CARE

In order to bring the concept of care into sharper focus, it is useful to review cases in which individuals exhibit care in different ways. In the course of this review, we shall consider in more detail the protective qualities associated with different kinds of care and the positive and negative forms these qualities can take.

1. Case One: Caring For and About a Patient

I was taking care of a 40-year old female who had been hospitalized for 3 months in another hospital and came to our hospital the day before to have her abdominal fistulas corrected. The night before I met her, the bag collecting her fistula drainage fell off three times and was reapplied the same way each time by her former nurse due to the patient's insistence that nothing else works. Her skin was very excoriated in spots and tender. When I removed the leaking bag I noticed that the problem was that she had a large crease between two recessed fistulas. I attempted to reapply it to avoid these. She was resistant to my suggestions, and protested my efforts to replace the bag. So I told her that she should trust me because I've had numerous similar situations with which I've had positive outcomes. I pointed out that if the bag was not replaced to avoid the fistulas it would continue to fall off and her pain and discomfort would only increase. She reconsidered. I told her that I was sure I could get a bag to stay on her for at least 24 hours, if not more. She said she'd love that to happen and told me I could do what I wanted (Benner, 1984, pp. 138-139).

In this first case, a nurse appears to care both for and about a patient. Each effort calls upon a distinct set of responses. Caring *for* manifests itself in the activities of removing the leaking bag, locating the problem in adhering it to the patient's skin and replacing the bag. Caring *about* is shown by the *manner* in which the nurse cares for the patient, a manner which expresses concern and involves efforts to reassure and gain the patient's confidence.

Notice too the nurse's response to her patient's initial resistance. This response exhibits the nurse's ability to persuade a recalcitrant patient that a certain procedure (replacing the bag) is in the patient's best interest and that she can execute this procedure successfully. A different response would have been simply to say, "you *must* let me do this." The difference between these two responses reveals alternative forms of parentalism (Taylor, 1985). In the medical setting, parentalism is an attempt to justify performing (or omitting) an action that is contrary to a patient's expressed wishes, yet judged to be in a patient's best interest. Were the nurse in this situation to respond to the refusal of treatment by saying "that's my final word," she would illustrate a kind of parentalism that justifies medical actions by presuming to abrogate a patient's *rights*. An alternative mode of parentalism invokes a morality of *responsibility*, rather than rights (Taylor, 1985; Ruddick, 1989). Here, one appeals to the patient's self-interest and personal responsibility, rather than invoking one's own authority to override the patient. For example, the nurse in case one displays this latter kind of parentalism by effectively laying out for the patient the consequences that attach to different alternatives: replacing the bag properly ensures that it will adhere; not doing so may result in the bag falling off and so heighten the patient's pain and discomfort. In this way, the patient is led to choose between taking responsibility for safeguarding her own interests, or behaving in a less responsible fashion.

Parentalism that is based on promoting the patient's sense of personal responsibility elicits our powers of practical persuasion, and it is often cultivated by those who care *for* others. This is because those charged with caring for others are more often in the position of having to gain other's cooperation. Those who care about, but not for, may need only to confirm in their *own* mind that a certain course of action is justified.

Both kinds of parentalism can be instantiated in positive and negative ways. For example, parentalism that fosters the patient's sense of responsibility can be a positive force. However, this kind of parentalism can also deteriorate into a manipulative tool, for example, when it is used merely to produce guilt in patients, block the expression of patient's feelings, or manipulate patients to acquiesce to decisions they do not prefer in order to gain petty conveniences for caregivers (Taylor, 1985).

The other form of parentalism, that appeals to the health professional's rights and authority over the patient, can represent both positive and negative approaches as well. Negative expressions include a doctor or nurse who knowingly assumes greater authority than she is morally entitled to claim. Or negative parentalism occurs when the justified exercise of authority is conjoined with callousness, e.g., bullying a patient or giving patients orders in an abrupt or cruel fashion. By contrast, an example of positive parentalism of this sort is overriding the rights of someone that one is close to in order to protect that person's interests. Hardwig, for example, notes that in the context of close personal relationships, parentalistic behavior is often warranted and failing to show parentalism can signal a failure to fulfill special responsibilities (Hardwig, 1984). Elsewhere (Jecker, 1989, 1990b, 1990c), it is argued that the responsibilities of individuals in close relationships are different and often greater than the responsibilities that exist between acquaintances or strangers. If this approach is correct, then whether or not abrogating others' rights is justified in the health care setting depends, in part, upon whether particular health professionals stand in close relationships with their patients. Between virtual strangers, interference with others for their own good is less often desirable and more apt to overstep moral boundaries between persons.

2. Case Two: Caring For, But Not About a Patient

A demented thirty year old man had AIDS for eight months. His final admission to our hospital was prompted by the development of large decubitus ulcers. On the ward his oral intake was minimal, and the attending physician instructed me to administer parenteral nutrition. I didn't like taking care of this patient. I kept thinking that he had brought this fate upon himself by his gay lifestyle. Gays repulsed me, and I was unable to feel any compassion for this fellow. I also found his medical problems disgusting and resented the fact that caring for him exposed me to life threatening risks. The patient had copious diarrhea; the decubiti were oozing fluids; and administering parenteral nutrition was complicated by high, spiking fevers that twice necessitated removal of the central line (Cooke, 1986).

In case two a nurse is involved in caring *for* a patient. Caring for is manifest in the activities of treating the patient's ulcers and administering parenteral nutrition. Although the nurse is engaged in the activity of caregiving, her negative feelings about the patient suggest that she lacks an attitude of caring *about* the patient. Mustering such an attitude would require the nurse to reject or subdue her negative responses to the patient. On the other hand, particular nurses will always dislike particular patients, and subduing negative feelings will not necessarily change or mitigate bad feelings. Attempting and failing to reduce negative feelings may simply compound a nurse's difficulties by festering guilt or lowering self-esteem. Where dislike for patients is likely to persist, it is important to keep separate the ideas of *dislike* and *disrespect*. A nurse who dislikes a particular patient may still express respect toward the patient as a fellow human being, for example, through her ongoing activity of caring *for* the patient. Thus, although the nurse may not care *about* the patient, she can still regard the patient in a positive manner and express this regard in action.

3. Case Three: Caring About, but Not For a Patient

A twenty-seven year old model was admitted to the emergency room after an automobile accident that caused multiple fractures and burns over sixty-five per cent of his body. Glass had penetrated both eyes so severely as to leave him blind, although a good chance for survival existed. In the emergency room, the patient was met by friends who candidly told him that his physician expects that his life can be saved. Later when

I, the physician, met with the patient to discuss treatment, the patient bluntly told me that he had enjoyed a life in which he had identified with his body and physical pleasure and abilities. He had few intellectual or other interests. On these grounds, he flatly refused treatment and asked me to keep him comfortable. My only concern was to promote this patient's welfare. I had seen many burn patients begin with a negative attitude toward treatment and then undergo a change of heart. Based on these experiences, I decided to order aggressive treatment and arranged for a psychiatric consult (Brody and Engelhardt, 1987, pp. 327-328).

The third case is about a physician who cares about a patient, but may not be engaged, in an ongoing way, in caring for the patient. For example, the physician orders burn treatments, but may not be the one who actually will provide these treatments to the patient. Unlike the nurse in case one, the physician in this case does not need to gain the patient's cooperation immediately. Moreover, the physician expresses parentalism by appealing to her authority and presumed superior knowledge to justify overriding the patient's wishes. The justification she gives for this is the silent refrain: "I know better; I've seen many burn patients in this situation change their mind." A different kind of parentalism would involve persuading the patient, as well as herself, of the wisdom of continued treatment. The alternative response intends to justify an action *to the patient* through iteration of the consequences of different choices. By contrast, the physician in case three seeks to justify the action mainly *to herself.* Thus her reasoning is "silent" and she does not attempt negotiation of a solution agreeable to the patient.

4. Case Four: Caring Neither For nor About a Patient

I supervise a ward of terminally ill cancer patients. I deliberately avoid getting emotionally involved with these patients because I realize it would be terribly depressing. Fortunately, most of my responsibilities involve management of nurses, paper work and general organization, so I by and large can steer clear of patients and families. Most of the time, I limit my contact with nursing staff while eschewing patient contact. This

enables me to direct my energy toward problems I can solve effectively and prevents me from feeling overwhelmed and powerless about dying patients.[2]

The nurse in this last case does not assume the responsibility of caring *for* patients. Nor does she display an attitude of caring *about* patients on her ward. Instead, she strives to maintain a neutral or indifferent stance. Presumably, such a stance affords her a sense of control in an otherwise emotionally charged environment.

FORMS OF CARE IN HEALTH CARE PROFESSIONS

The foregoing analysis of the concept of care places us in a better position to consider traditional stereotypes with a critical eye. In rethinking the idea that "doctors cure and nurses care," it is helpful to be aware of four possible models of caring. These models parallel the cases discussed above:

1. Health professionals who care for and about their patients,
2. Health professionals who care for, but not about their patients,
3. Health professionals who care about, but not for their patients,
4. Health professionals who care neither for nor about their patients.

In the first model, health professionals care for and about patients. Since caring for is an ongoing and deliberate activity, a health professional whose patient contact is limited to brief visits or to discrete medical interventions, such as taking vital signs, does not fit the first model. Rather, to care in the sense defined by the first model a health professional must both carry out the tasks required to provide health care to the patient and possess an attitude of being concerned about what happens to the patient.

The difference between the first and second models of caring is that in the second it does not ultimately matter much to the professional what happens to patients. Nonetheless, it would be misleading to say that the second professional "does not care." After all, the second kind of health professional cares *all the time*: he or she is an ongoing caregiver, even though she lacks an attitude of caring *about* patients. This lack may impede her ability to care for patients, but (as noted above), it need not.

Similarly, it would be misleading to state that health professionals whose caring exemplifies the third model "do not care." Such professionals (who care about but not for their patients) may think about patients with great frequency, pray for their recovery and be deeply moved to witness it. These kind of professionals do indeed care, but their care is more remote by virtue of being removed from the immediate context of the patient. This does not imply that caring *about* is "intellectual" or "cold," but it does represent a more abstract mode of caring.

The grounds for saying that a health professional "does not care" can only be that the professional cares neither for nor about patients. In the fourth model, health professionals do not care in either sense. An *uncaring* health professional is neither a caregiver nor concerned about the welfare of patients. Multiple factors may contribute to health professionals' lacking an attitude of caring about patients. In the cases discussed in the previous section, the absence of caring is prompted, in part, by feeling superior, being emotionally indifferent, needing control, blaming the patient for the disease and disliking the patient. Caring neither for nor about patients often will be an unacceptable role for health professionals. Yet it also may represent a legitimate coping tool, for example, when one's responsibilities are experienced as overwhelming and the need to distance oneself emotionally is felt forcefully.

It is now time to ask how the above models can serve to deepen our understanding of nurses' and physicians' professional roles. To begin with, it is never correct to hold that nurses who function as caregivers do not care. Caring, in the sense of *caring for*, is an inextricable part of their role. The history of nursing is *essentially* a history of caring in this sense. In the colonial era, home-based nurses always cared in the sense of caring *for* family members. Nursing also has a caring tradition in the sense of caring *about* patients. As noted earlier, the first training programs for nurses sought to cultivate moral virtues, including devotion to the welfare of patients.

Despite the historical tradition of care by nurses, there are, and always have been, nurses who do not care much *about* patients in general, or *about* particular patients they nurse. Moreover, as more and more nurses become engaged in administrative and supervisory roles, they may do less caring *for* patients. On these grounds, it is misleading to accept the traditional stereotype that "nurses care." This stereotype obscures the fact that over time nursing has changed in its stratification and fields of specialization. These changes have meant that in some areas nurses have less direct patient contact and are less engaged in caring *for* patients. In addition, the traditional stereotype obscures the fact that there always have been nurses who do not care *about* patients.

Turning to physicians, a similar cautionary note is in order. Although some physicians may be less likely to care for patients, and so less likely to exemplify the first two models of caring, many physicians obviously care profoundly *about* patients. Moreover, physicians are a diverse group. In a university hospital, medical students or residents-in-training may seek or be delegated a considerable amount of caring for responsibilities, while attendings or senior staff may assume very little. Likewise, in health maintenance organizations, physician assistants and nurse practitioners may be utilized to perform a majority of caring for activities. By contrast, in private practices, physicians may undertake most of the caring for responsibilities. Such physicians may establish ongoing relationships with each patient over several years, e.g., monitoring medications, performing regular check-ups and treating minor emergencies. However, regardless of whether physicians care directly *for* patients, they usually assume a stance of caring *about* patients. Attempting to *cure* a patient is ordinarily an expression of a physician's caring about the patient. It is unfortunate, as well as confusing, then, to assume that doctors cure, as *opposed* to care. Thus, to the extent that the care-cure distinction informs our present thinking, it wrongly denies to the medical profession a caring role and unfortunately clouds our conception of the complexities of nursing care.

CONCLUSION

In closing, this paper has intended to take a careful look at professional stereotypes in nursing and medicine. Doing so required clarifying the concept of care and articulating different models of caring. That the concept of care is multiform and the models of caring many should attune us to the dangers of buying into popular stereotypes. Holding tenaciously to traditional stereotypes can prevent us from seeing the evidence that both medicine and nursing are caring professions and both men and women care for and about their patients.

Appreciating the richness of the concept of care also should infuse new energy into research on care in health care and professional settings. The following are suggested research topics that merit further consideration. (1) How can cure and care be joined and integrated into the curriculum of both nursing and medical schools? (2) Is care a virtue? If so, under what circumstances might it deteriorate into a vice? Is care ever a duty or obligation? (3) Is caring a way of knowing? How do cure and care relate to both scientific and intuitive forms of knowledge? (4) What is the proper balance between cure and care in developing an ethic for specific patient groups, such as the elderly, the terminally ill and the chronically ill? Although answering these questions is a tall order, our analysis shows the importance and promise of further research in this area.

Authors' Notes

We wish to thank Sara T. Fry, Albert R. Jonsen and an anonymous reviewer of this journal for valuable comments. A version of this paper was presented at a University of Maryland School of Nursing conference on Ethics and Nursing Practice in May of 1990 and at a conference on The Politics of Caring held at the Emory University Institute for Women's Studies in October of 1990.

Notes

1. Throughout this paper, we will use the terms "care" and "caring" interchangeably. There may be important shades of meaning unique to each term, but exploring this is beyond the scope of the present inquiry.
2. Whereas the previous cases are drawn from the medical ethics literature, we could find no cases in the literature to illustrate the fourth model. We believe this is significant if it represents a lack of attention to the ethical problems of health care workers who exemplify this model.

References

American Nurses' Association: 1987, *Facts About Nurses,* American Nurses' Association, Kansas City, Missouri.

Benner, P.: 1983, "Recovering the knowledge embedded in clinical practice", *Image: Journal of Nursing Scholarship* 15, 30-41.

Benner, P.: 1984, *From Novice to Expert: Excellence and Power in Clinical Nursing Practice,* Addison-Wesley Publishing Company, Menlo Park, California.

Benner, P., and Wrubel, J.: 1989, *The Primacy of Caring,* Addison-Wesley Publishing Company, Menlo Park, California.

Benoliel, J.Q.: 1987, "Response to 'toward holistic inquiry in nursing: A proposal for synthesis of patterns and methods,'" *Scholarly Inquiry for Nursing Practice: An International Journal* 1, 147-152.

Blum, L.A.: 1988, "Gilligan and Kohlberg: Implications for moral theory," *Ethics* 98, 472-491.

Brody, B.A., and Engelhardt, H.T.: 1987, *Bioethics: Readings and Cases,* Prentice-Hall, Englewood Cliffs, New Jersey.

Buchanan, W.: 1778, *Domestic Medicine, The Third American Edition,* John Trumbull, Boston.

Conrad, P., and Schneider, J.W.: 1990, "Professionalization, monopoly, and the structure of medical practice," in P. Conrad and R. Kern (eds.), *The Sociology of Health and Illness: Critical Perspectives, Third Edition,* St. Martin's Press, New York, pp. 141-147.

Cooke, M.: 1986, "Ethical issues in the care of patients with AIDS," *Quality Review Bulletin,* October, 343-346.

Eisenberg, C.: 1989, "Medicine is no longer a man's profession," *New England Journal of Medicine* 321, 1542-1544.

Gilligan, C.: 1982, *In a Different Voice: Psychological Theory and Women's Development,* Harvard University Press, Cambridge, Massachusetts.

Gilligan, C.: 1986, "Remapping the moral domain: New Images of the self in relationship," in T.C. Heller, M. Sosna, and D.E. Wellbery (eds.), *Reconstructing Individualism: Autonomy, Individuality, and the Self in Western Thought,* Stanford University Press, Stanford, California, pp. 237-252.

Gilligan, C., and Wiggins, G.: 1987, "The origins of morality in early childhood," in J.Kagan and S. Lamb (eds.), *The Emergence of Morality in Young Children,* University of Chicago Press, Chicago, pp. 277-305.

Gilligan, C., and Pollak, S.: 1989, "The vulnerable and invulnerable physician," in C. Gilligan, J.V. Ward, and J.M. Taylor (eds.), *Mapping the Moral Domain,* Harvard University Press, Cambridge, Massachusetts, pp. 245-262.

Hardwig, J.: 1984, "Should women think in terms of rights?" *Ethics* 94, 441-455.

Hauerwas, S.: 1978, "Care," in W.T. Reich (ed.), *The Encyclopedia of Bioethics,* Free Press, New York, Vol. 1, 145-150.

Levinson, W., Tolle, S., and Lewis, C.: 1989, "Women in academic medicine," *New England Journal of Medicine* 321, 1511-1517.

Jameton, A.: 1984, *Nursing Practice: The Ethical Issues,* Prentice-Hall, Englewood Cliffs, New Jersey.

Jameton, A.: 1987, "Physicians and nurses: A historical perspective," in B.A. Brody and H.T. Engelhardt, *Bioethics, Readings and Cases,* Prentice-Hall, Englewood Cliffs, New Jersey, pp. 66-73.

Jecker, N.S.: 1989, "Are filial duties unfounded?" *American Philosophical Quarterly* 26, 73-80.

Jecker, N.S.: 1990a, "The role of intimate others in medical decision making," *The Gerontologist* 30, 65-71.

Jecker, N.S.: 1990b, "Conceiving a child to save a child: Reproductive and filial ethics," *The Journal of Clinical Ethics* 1, 99-103.

Jecker, N.S.: 1990c, "Anencephalic infants and special relationships," *Theoretical Medicine* 11, 333-342.

Keller, E.F.: 1985, *Reflections on Gender and Science,* Yale University Press, New Haven, Connecticut.

Kittay, E.F., and Meyers, D.T. (eds.): 1987, *Women and Moral Theory,* Rowman and Littlefield, Totowa, New Jersey.

Lyons, N.P.: 1983, "Two perspectives: On self, relationships, and morality," *Harvard Educational Review* 53, 125-145.

MacIntyre, A.: 1987, "How virtues become vices," in B.A. Brody and H.T. Engelhardt (eds.), *Bioethics: Readings and Cases,* Prentice-Hall, Englewood Cliffs, New Jersey, pp. 100-101.

Morantz-Sanchez, R.M.: 1985, *Sympathy and Science: Women Physicians in American Medicine,* Oxford University Press, New York.

Nelson, A.R.: 1989, "Humanism and the art of medicine: Our commitment to care," *Journal of the American Medical Association* 262, 1228-1230.

Noddings, N.: 1984, *Caring: A Feminine Approach to Ethics and Moral Education,* University of California Press, Berkeley.

Noddings, N.: 1987, "Do we really want to produce good people?," *Journal of Moral Education* 16, 177-188.

Noddings, N.: 1989, *Women and Evil,* University of California Press, Berkeley.

O'Brien, P.: 1987, "All a woman's life can bring: The domestic roots of nursing in Philadelphia, 1830-1885," *Nursing Research* 36, 12-17.

Pearsall, M. (ed.): 1986, *Women and Values,* Wadsworth Publishing Company, Belmont, California.

Relman, A.: 1989, "The changing demography of the medical profession," *New England Journal of Medicine* 321, 1540-1542.

Reverby, S.: 1987a, "A caring dilemma: Womanhood and nursing in historical perspective," *Nursing Research* 36, 5-11.

Reverby, S.: 1987b, *Ordered to Care: The Dilemma of American Nursing,* Cambridge University Press, New York.

Rowland, H.S.: 1984, *The Nurse's Almanac, 2nd edition,* Aspen Systems Corporation, Rockville, Maryland.

Ruddick, S.: 1989, *Maternal Thinking,* Beacon Press, Boston.

Schultz, P.R., and Meleis, A.I.: 1988, "Nursing epistemology: Traditions, insights, questions," *Image: Journal of Nursing Scholarship* 20, 217-221.

Star, P.: 1982, *The Social Transformation of American Medicine,* Basic Books, New York.

Taylor, S.G.: 1985, "Rights and responsibilities: Nurse-patient relationships," *Image: Journal of Nursing Scholarship* 17, 9-13.

4.
A RELATIONAL APPROACH TO AUTONOMY IN HEALTH CARE

Susan Sherwin

Respect for patient autonomy (or self-direction) is broadly understood as recognition that patients have the authority to make decisions about their own health care. The principle that insists on this recognition is pervasive in the bioethics literature: it is a central value within virtually all the leading approaches to health care ethics, feminist and other. It is not surprising, then, that discussions of autonomy constantly emerged within our own conversations in the Network; readers will recognize that autonomy is woven throughout the book in our various approaches to the issues we take up. It is, however, an ideal that we felt deeply ambivalent about, and, therefore, we judged it to be in need of a specifically feminist analysis.

In this chapter, I propose a feminist analysis of autonomy, making vivid both our attraction to and distrust of the dominant interpretation of this concept. I begin by reviewing some of the appeal of the autonomy ideal in order to make clear why it has achieved such prominence within bioethics and feminist health care discussions. I then identify some difficulties I find with the usual interpretations of the concept, focusing especially on difficulties that arise from a specifically feminist perspective. In response to these problems, I propose an alternative conception of autonomy that I label "relational" though the terms *socially situated* or *contextualized* would describe it equally well. To avoid confusion, I explicitly distinguish my use of the term *relational* from that of some other feminist authors, such as Carol Gilligan (1982), who reserve it to refer only to the narrower set of interpersonal relations. I apply the term to the full range of influential human relations, personal and public. Oppression permeates both personal and public relationships; hence, I prefer to politicize the understanding of the term *relational* as a way of emphasizing the political dimensions of the multiple relationships that structured an individual's

selfhood, rather than to reserve the term to protect a sphere of purely private relationships that may appear to be free of political influence.[1] I explain why I think the relational alternative is more successful than the familiar individualistic interpretation at addressing the concerns identified. Finally, I briefly indicate some of the implications of adopting a relational interpretation of autonomy with respect to some of the issues discussed elsewhere in this book, and I identify some of the changes that this notion of relational autonomy suggests for the delivery of health services.

THE VIRTUES OF A PRINCIPLE OF RESPECT FOR PATIENT AUTONOMY

It is not hard to explain the prominence of the principle of respect for patient autonomy within the field of health care ethics in North America: respect for personal autonomy is a dominant value in North American culture and it plays a central role in most of our social institutions. Yet, protection of autonomy is often at particular risk in health care settings because illness, by its very nature, tends to make patients dependent on the care and good will of others; in so doing, it reduces patients' power to exercise autonomy and it also makes them vulnerable to manipulation and even to outright coercion by those who provide them with needed health services. Many patients who are either ill or at risk of becoming ill are easily frightened into overriding their own preferences and following expert advice rather than risking abandonment by their caregivers by rejecting that advice. Even when their health is not immediately threatened, patients may find themselves compelled to comply with the demands of health care providers in order to obtain access to needed services from health professionals who are, frequently, the only ones licensed to provide those services (e.g., abortion, assistance in childbirth, legitimate excuses from work, physiotherapy).[2]

Without a strong principle of respect for patient autonomy, patients are vulnerable to abuse or exploitation, when their weak and dependent position makes them easy targets to serve the interests (e.g., financial, academic, or social influence) of others. Strong moral traditions of service within medicine and other health professions have provided patients with some measure of protection against such direct harms, though abuses nonetheless occur.[3] Most common is the tendency of health care providers to assume that by virtue of their technical expertise they are better able to judge what is in the patient's best interest than is the patient. For example, physicians may make assumptions about the advantages of using fetal heart monitors when women are in labor without considering the ways in which such instruments restrict laboring-women's movement and the quality of the birthing experience from their perspective. By privileging their own types of knowledge over that of their patients (including both experiential knowledge and understanding of their own value scheme), health care providers typically ignore patients' expressed or implicit values and engage in paternalism[4] (or the overriding of patient preferences for the presumed benefit of the patient) when prescribing treatment.

Until very recently, conscientious physicians were actually trained to act paternalistically toward their patients, to treat patients according to the physician's own judgment about what would be best for their patients, with little regard for each patient's own perspectives or preferences. The problem with this arrangement, however, is that health care may involve such intimate and central aspects of a patient's life—including, for example, matters such as health, illness, reproduction, death, dying, bodily integrity, nutrition, lifestyle, self-image, disability, sexuality, and psychological well-being—that it is difficult for anyone other than the patient to make choices that will be compatible with that patient's personal value system. Indeed, making such choices is often an act of self-discovery or self-definition and as such it requires the active involvement of the patient. Whenever possible, then, these types of choices should be made by the person whose life is central to the treatment considered. The principle of respect for patient autonomy is aimed at clarifying and protecting patients' ultimate right to make up their own minds about the specific health services they receive (so long as they are competent to do so). It also helps to ensure that patients have full access to relevant information about their health status so that they can make informed choices about related aspects of their lives. For example, information about a terminal condition may affect a person's decisions to reproduce, take a leave of absence from work, seek a reconciliation from estranged friends or relatives, or revise a will.

Although theorists disagree about the precise definition of *autonomy*,[5] there are some common features to its use within bioethics. In practice, the principle of respect for patient autonomy is usually interpreted as acknowledging and protecting competent patients' authority to accept or refuse whatever specific treatments the health care providers they consult find it appropriate to offer them (an event known as informed choice). Since everyone can imagine being in the position of patient, and most can recognize the dangers of fully surrendering this authority to near strangers, it is not surprising that the principle of respect for patient autonomy is widely endorsed by nearly all who consider it. Despite different theoretical explanations, the overwhelming majority of bioethicists insist on this principle as a fundamental moral precept for health care. Support is especially strong in North America, where it fits comfortably within a general cultural milieu in which attention to the individual and protection of individual rights are granted (at least rhetorical) dominance in nearly all areas of social and political policy.[6] Both Canadian and U.S. Courts have underlined the importance of protection of individual rights as a central tenet of patient-provider interactions, making it a matter of legal as well as moral concern.

Further, the principle requiring respect for patient autonomy helps to resolve problems that arise when health care providers are responsible for the care of patients who have quite different experiences, values, and world views from their own; under such circumstances, it is especially unlikely that care givers can accurately anticipate the particular needs and interests of their patients. This problem becomes acute when there are significant differences in power between patients and the health care professionals who care for them. In most cases, the relevant inter-actions are between patients and physicians, where, typically, patients have less social power than their physicians: doctors are well educated and they tend to be (relatively) healthy and affluent, while the patients they care for are often poor, and lacking in education and social authority. In fact, according to most of the standard dichotomies supporting domi-nance in our culture—gender, class, race, ability sta-tus—odds are that if there is a difference between the status of the physician and the patient, the physician is likely to fall on the dominant side of that distinc-tion and the patient on the subordinate side. The ten-dency of illness to undermine patients' autonomy is especially threatening when the patients in question face other powerful barriers to the exercise of their autonomy, as do members of groups subject to sys-temic discrimination on the basis of gender, race, class, disability, age, sexual preference, or any other such feature. A principle insisting on protection of patient autonomy can be an important corrective to such overwhelming power imbalances.

Moreover, physician privilege and power is not the only threat to patient autonomy. Increasingly, the treatment options available to both patients and physi-cians are circumscribed by the policies of govern-ments and other third-party payers. In the current eco-nomic climate, those who fund health care services are insisting on ever more stringent restrictions on access to specific treatment options; physicians find themselves asked to perform gate-keeping functions to keep costs under control. In such circumstances, where patient care may be decided by general guide-lines that tend to be insensitive to the particular cir-cumstances of specific patients, and where the finan-cial interests of the institution being billed for the patient's care may take priority over the patient's needs or preferences, the principle of respect for patient autonomy becomes more complicated to inter-pret even as it takes on added importance.

The principle of respect for patient autonomy can also be seen as an attractive ideal for feminists because of its promise to protect the rights and inter-ests of even the most socially disadvantaged patients. Feminist medical historians, anthropologists, and sociologists have documented many ways in which health care providers have repeatedly neglected and misperceived the needs and wishes of the women they treat.[7] The ideal of respect for patient autonomy seems a promising way to correct much that is objec-tionable in the abuses that feminist researchers have documented in the delivery of health services to women and minorities. Most feminists believe that the forces of systematic domination and oppression work together to limit the autonomy of women and members of other oppressed groups; many of their political efforts can be seen as aimed at disrupting those forces and promoting greater degrees of auton-omy (often represented as personal "choice") for individuals who fall victim to oppression. For exam-ple, many feminists appeal at least implicitly to the moral norm of autonomy in seeking to increase the scope of personal control for women in all areas of their reproductive lives (especially with respect to birth control, abortion, and childbirth, often dis-cussed under a general rubric of "reproductive free-dom" or "reproductive choice").

In a world where most cultures are plagued by sex-ism, which is usually compounded by other deeply entrenched oppressive patterns, fundamental respect for the humanity, dignity, and autonomy of members of disadvantaged groups, though extremely fragile, seems very important and in need of strong ethical imperatives. Feminists strive to be sensitive to the ways in which gender, race, class, age, disability, sex-ual orientation, and marital status can undermine a patient's authority and credibility in health care con-texts and most are aware of the long history of pow-erful medical control over women's lives. They have good reason, then, to oppose medical domination through paternalism. Promotion of patient autonomy appears to be a promising alternative.[8] Understood in its traditional sense as the alternative to heteronomy (governance by others), autonomy (self-governance) seems to be an essential feature of any feminist strat-egy for improving health services for women and achieving a nonoppressive society.

PROBLEMS WITH THE AUTONOMY IDEAL

Nonetheless, despite this broad consensus about the value of a principle of respect for patient autonomy in health care, there are many problems with the principle as it is usually interpreted and applied in health care ethics. As many health critics have observed, we need to question how much control individual patients really have over the determination of their treatment within the stressful world of health care services. Even a casual encounter with most modern hospitals reveals that wide agreement about the moral importance of respect for patient autonomy does not always translate into a set of practices that actually respect and foster patient autonomy in any meaningful sense. Ensuring that patients meet some measure of informed choice— or, more commonly, informed consent[9]—before receiving or declining treatment has become accepted as the most promising mechanism for insuring patient autonomy in health care settings, but, in practice, the effectiveness of the actual procedures used to obtain informed consent usually falls short of fully protecting patient autonomy. This gap is easy to understand: attention to patient autonomy can be a time-consuming business and the demands of identifying patient values and preferences are often sacrificed in the face of heavy patient loads and staff shortages. In addition, health care providers are often constrained from promoting and responding to patients' autonomy in health care because of pressures they experience to contain health care costs and to avoid making themselves liable to lawsuits. Moreover, most health care providers are generally not well trained in the communication skills necessary to ensure that patients have the requisite understanding to provide genuine informed consent. This problem is compounded within our increasingly diverse urban communities where differences in language and culture between health care providers and the patients they serve may create enormous practical barriers to informed choice.

There are yet deeper problems with the ideal of autonomy invoked in most bioethical discussions. The paradigm offered for informed consent is built on a model of articulate, intelligent patients who are accustomed to making decisions about the course of their lives and who possess the resources necessary to allow them a range of options to choose among. Decisions are constructed as a product of objective calculation on the basis of near perfect information. Clearly, not all patients meet these ideal conditions (perhaps none does), yet there are no satisfactory

guidelines available about how to proceed when dealing with patients who do not fit the paradigm.

Feminist analysis reveals several problems inherent in the very construction of the concept of autonomy that is at the heart of most bioethics discussions.[10] One problem is that autonomy provisions are sometimes interpreted as functioning independently of and outweighing all other moral values. More specifically, autonomy is often understood to exist in conflict with the demands of justice because the requirements of the latter may have to be imposed on unwilling citizens. Autonomy is frequently interpreted to mean freedom from interference; this analysis can be invoked (as it frequently is) to oppose taxation as coercive and, hence, a violation of personal autonomy. But coercive measures like taxation are essential if a society wants to reduce inequity and provide the disadvantaged with access to the means (e.g., basic necessities, social respect, education, and health care) that are necessary for meaningful exercise of their autonomy. In contrast to traditional accounts of autonomy that accept and indeed presume some sort of tension between autonomy and justice, feminism encourages us to see the connections between these two central moral ideals.

In fact, autonomy language is often used to hide the workings of privilege and to mask the barriers of oppression. For example, within North America it seems that people who were raised in an atmosphere of privilege and respect come rather easily to think of themselves as independent and self-governing; it feels natural to them to conceive of themselves as autonomous. Having been taught that they need only to apply themselves in order to take advantage of the opportunities available to them, most learn to think of their successes as self-created and deserved. Such thinking encourages them to be oblivious to the barriers that oppression and disadvantage create, and it allows them to see the failures of others as evidence of the latter's unwillingness to exercise their own presumed autonomy responsibly. This individualistic approach to autonomy makes it very easy for people of privilege to remain ignorant of the social arrangements that support their own sense of independence, such as the institutions that provide them with an exceptionally good education and a relatively high degree of personal safety. Encouraged to focus on their own sense of individual accomplishment, they are inclined to blame less well-situated people for their lack of comparable success rather than to appreciate the costs of oppression. This familiar sort of thinking tends to interfere with people's ability to see the importance of supportive social conditions for fostering autonomous action. By focusing instead on the injustice that is associated with oppression, feminism helps us to recognize that autonomy is best achieved where the social conditions that support it are in place. Hence, it provides us with an alternative perspective for understanding a socially grounded notion of autonomy.

Further, the standard conception of autonomy, especially as it is invoked in bioethics, tends to place the focus of concern quite narrowly on particular decisions of individuals; that is, it is common to speak of specific health care decisions as autonomous, or, at least, of the patient as autonomous with respect to the decision at hand. Such analyses discourage attention to the context in which decisions are actually made. Patient decisions are considered to be autonomous if the patient is (1) deemed to be sufficiently competent (rational) to make the decision at issue, (2) makes a (reasonable) choice from a set of available options, (3) has adequate information and understanding about the available choices, and (4) is free from explicit coercion toward (or away from) one of those options. It is assumed that these criteria can be evaluated in any particular case, simply by looking at the state of the patient and her deliberations in isolation from the social conditions that structure her options. Yet, each of these conditions is more problematic than is generally recognized.

The competency criterion threatens to exclude people who are oppressed from the scope of autonomy provisions altogether. This is because competency is often equated with being rational,[11] yet the rationality of women and members of other oppressed groups is frequently denied. In fact, as Genevieve Lloyd (1984) has shown, the very concept of rationality has been constructed in opposition to the traits that are stereotypically assigned to women (e.g., by requiring that agents demonstrate objectivity and emotional distance),[12] with the result that women are often seen as simply incapable of

rationality.[13] Similar problems arise with respect to stereotypical assumptions about members of racial minorities, indigenous peoples, persons with disabilities, welfare recipients, people from developing countries, those who are nonliterate, and so on. Minimally, then, health care providers must become sensitive to the ways in which oppressive stereotypes can undermine their ability to recognize some sorts of patients as being rational or competent.

Consider, also, the second condition, which has to do with making a (reasonable) choice from the set of available options. Here, the difficulty is that the set of available options is constructed in ways that may already seriously limit the patient's autonomy by prematurely excluding options the patient might have preferred. There is a whole series of complex decisions that together shape the set of options that health care providers are able to offer their patients: these can involve such factors as the forces that structure research programs, the types of results that journals are willing to publish, curriculum priorities in medical and other professional schools, and funding policies within the health care system.[14] While all patients will face limited choices by virtue of these sorts of institutional policy decisions, the consequences are especially significant for members of oppressed groups because they tend to be underrepresented on the bodies that make these earlier decisions, and therefore their interests are less likely to be reflected in each of the background decisions that are made. In general, the sorts of institutional decisions in question tend to reflect the biases of discriminatory values and practices.[15] Hence, the outcomes of these multiple earlier decisions can have a significant impact on an oppressed patient's ultimate autonomy by disproportionately and unfairly restricting the choices available to her. Nevertheless, such background conditions are seldom visible within discussions of patient autonomy in bioethics.

The third condition is also problematic in that the information made available to patients is, inevitably, the information that has been deemed worthy of study and that is considered relevant by the health care providers involved. Again, research, publication, and education policies largely determine what sorts of data are collected and, significantly, what questions are neglected; systemic bias unquestionably influences these policies. Further, the very large gap in life experience between physicians, who are, by virtue of their professional status, relatively privileged members of society, and some of their seriously disadvantaged patients makes the likelihood of the former anticipating the specific information needs of the latter questionable. While an open consent process will help reduce this gap by providing patients with the opportunity to raise questions, patients often feel too intimidated to ask or even formulate questions, especially when they feel socially and intellectually inferior to their physicians and when the physicians project an image of being busy with more important demands. Often, one needs some information in order to know what further questions to ask, and large gaps in perspective between patients and their health care providers may result in a breakdown in communication because of false assumptions by either participant.

The fourth condition, the one that demands freedom from coercion in exercising choice, is extremely difficult to evaluate when the individual in question is oppressed. The task becomes even trickier if the choice is in a sphere that is tied to her oppression. The condition of being oppressed can be so fundamentally restrictive that it is distorting to describe as autonomous some specific choices made under such conditions. For example, many women believe they have no real choice but to seek expensive, risky cosmetic surgery because they accurately perceive that their opportunities for success in work or love depend on their more closely approximating some externally defined standard of beauty. Similar sorts of questions arise with respect to some women's choice of dangerous, unproven experiments in new reproductive technologies because continued childlessness can be expected to have devastating consequences for their lives. In other cases, women sometimes choose to have abortions because they fear that giving birth will involve them in unwanted and lifelong relationships with abusive partners. Some women have little access to contraceptives and find themselves choosing sterilization as the most effective way of resisting immediate demands of their partners even if they might want more children in the future. Or, some women seek out prenatal diagnosis and selective abortion of cherished fetuses because

they realize that they cannot afford to raise a child born with a serious disability, though they would value such a child themselves. Many middle-class Western women choose hormone replacement therapy at menopause because they recognize that their social and economic lives may be threatened if they appear to be aging too quickly. When a woman's sense of herself and her range of opportunities have been oppressively constructed in ways that (seem to) leave her little choice but to pursue all available options in the pursuit of beauty or childbearing or when she is raised in a culture that ties her own sense of herself to external norms of physical appearance or fulfillment associated with childbearing or, conversely, when having a(nother) child will impose unjust and intolerable costs on her, it does not seem sufficient to restrict our analysis to the degree of autonomy associated with her immediate decision about a particular treatment offered. We need a way of acknowledging how oppressive circumstances can interfere with autonomy, but this is not easily captured in traditional accounts.

Finally, there are good reasons to be wary of the ways in which the appearance of choice is used to mask the normalizing powers of medicine and other health-related institutions. As Michel Foucault (1979, 1980b) suggests, in modern societies the illusion of choice can be part of the mechanism for controlling behavior. Indeed, it is possible that bioethical efforts to guarantee the exercise of individual informed choice may actually make the exercise of medical authority even more powerful and effective than it would be under more traditionally paternalistic models. In practice, the ideal of informed choice amounts to assuring patients of the opportunity to consent to one of a limited list of relatively similar, medically encouraged procedures. Thus, informed consent procedures aimed simply at protecting autonomy in the narrow sense of specific choice among preselected options may ultimately serve to secure the compliance of docile patients who operate under the illusion of autonomy by virtue of being invited to consent to procedures they are socially encouraged to choose. Unless we find a way of identifying a deeper sense of autonomy than that associated with the expression of individual preference in selecting among a limited set of similar options, we run the risk of struggling to protect not patient autonomy but the very mechanisms that insure compliant medical consumers, preoccupied with the task of selecting among a narrow range of treatments.

FOCUS ON THE INDIVIDUAL

A striking feature of most bioethical discussions about patient autonomy is their exclusive focus on individual patients; this pattern mirrors medicine's consistent tendency to approach illness as primarily a problem of particular patients.[16] Similar problems are associated with each discipline. Within the medical tradition, suffering is located and addressed in the individuals who experience it rather than in the social arrangements that may be responsible for causing the problem. Instead of exploring the cultural context that tolerates and even supports practices such as war, pollution, sexual violence, and systemic unemployment—practices that contribute to much of the illness that occupies modern medicine—physicians generally respond to the symptoms troubling particular patients in isolation from the context that produces these conditions. Apart from population-based epidemiological studies (which, typically, restrict their focus to a narrow range of patterns of illness and often exclude or distort important social dimensions), medicine is primarily oriented toward dealing with individuals who have become ill (or pregnant, [in] fertile, or menopausal). This orientation directs the vast majority of research money and expertise toward the things that can be done to change the individual, but it often ignores key elements at the source of the problems.

For example, physicians tend to respond to infertility either by trivializing the problem and telling women to go home and "relax," or by prescribing hormonal and surgical treatment of particular women, rather than by demanding that research and public health efforts be aimed at preventing pelvic inflammatory disease, which causes many cases of infertility, or by encouraging wide public debate (or private reflections) on the powerful social pressures to reproduce that are directed at women. In similar fashion, the mainstream scientific and medical communities respond to the growth of breast cancer rates by promoting individual responsibility for self-examination and by searching for the gene(s) that makes some women particularly susceptible to the disease; when it is found in a patient, the principal medical therapy available is to perform "prophylactic" double mastectomies. Few physicians demand examination of the potential contributory role played by the use of pesticides or chlorine, or the practice of feeding artificial hormones to agricultural animals. Or they deal with dramatically increased skin cancer rates by promoting the personal use of sunscreens while resigning themselves to the continued depletion of the ozone layer. In another area, health care professionals generally deal with the devastating effects of domestic violence by patching up its victims, providing them with medications to relieve depression and advice to move out of their homes, and devising pathological names for victims who stay in violent relationships ("battered woman syndrome" and "self-defeating personality disorder"), but few actively challenge the sexism that accepts male violence as a "natural" response to frustration and fears of abandonment.[17]

Some qualifications are in order. Clearly, these are crude and imprecise generalizations. They describe a general orientation of current health practices, but they certainly do not capture the work of all those involved in medical research and practice. Fortunately, there are practitioners and researchers engaged in the very sorts of investigation I call for, but they are exceptional, not typical. Moreover, I do not want to imply that medicine should simply abandon its concern with treating disease in individuals. I understand that prevention strategies will not eliminate all illness and I believe that personalized health care must continue to be made available to those who become ill. Further, I want to be clear that my critique does not imply that physicians or other direct care providers are necessarily the ones who ought to be assuming the task of identifying the social and environmental causes of disease. Health care training, and especially the training of physicians, is directed at developing the requisite skills for the extremely important work of caring for individuals who become ill. The responsibility for investigating the social causes of illness and for changing hazardous conditions is a social one that is probably best met by those who undertake different sorts of training and study. The problem is that medicine, despite the limits of its expertise and focus, is the primary agent of health care activity in our society and physicians are granted significant social authority to be the arbiters of health policy. Hence, when medicine makes the treatment of individuals its primary focus, we must understand that important gaps are created in our society's ability to understand and promote good health.

In parallel fashion, autonomy-focused bioethics concentrates its practitioners' attention on the preferences of particular patients, and it is, thereby, complicit in the individualistic orientation of medicine. It asks health care providers to ensure that individual patients have the information they need to make rational decisions about their health care, yet it does not ask the necessary questions about the circumstances in which such decisions are made. The emphasis most bioethicists place on traditional, individualistic understandings of autonomy reinforces the tendency of health care providers and ethicists to neglect exploration of the deep social causes and conditions that contribute to health and illness. Moreover, it encourages patients to see their own health care decisions in isolation from those of anyone else, thereby increasing their sense of vulnerability and dependence on medical authority.

The narrow individual focus that characterizes the central traditions within both medicine and bioethics obscures our need to consider questions of power, dominance, and privilege in our interpretations and responses to illness and other health-related matters as well as in our interpretations of the ideal of autonomy. These ways of structuring thought and practice make it difficult to see the political dimensions of illness, and, in a parallel way, they obscure the political dimensions of the conventional criteria for autonomous deliberation. As a result, they interfere with our ability to identify and pursue more effective health practices while helping to foster a special environment that ignores and tolerates oppression. In both cases, a broader political perspective is necessary if we are to avoid the problems created by restricting our focus to individuals apart from their location.

Feminism offers just such a broader perspective. In contrast to the standard approaches in bioethics, feminism raises questions about the social basis for decisions about health and health care at all levels. Here, as elsewhere, feminists are inclined to ask whose interests are served and whose are harmed by the traditional ways of structuring thought and practice. By asking these questions, we are able to see how assumptions of individual-based medicine help to preserve the social and political status quo. For example, the current taxonomy in Canada designates certain sorts of conditions (e.g., infertility, cancer, heart disease, anxiety) as appropriate for medical intervention, and it provides grounds for ensuring that such needs are met. At the same time, it views other sorts of conditions (e.g., malnutrition, fear of assault, low self-esteem) as falling beyond the purview of the health care system and, therefore, as ineligible to draw on the considerable resources allocated to the delivery of health services.[18] In this way, individualistic assumptions support a system that provides expert care for many of the health complaints of those with greatest financial privilege while dismissing as outside the scope of health care many of the sources of illness that primarily affect the disadvantaged. A more social vision of health would require us to investigate ways in which nonmedical strategies, such as improving social and material conditions for disadvantaged groups, can affect the health status of different segments of the community.[19]

None of the concerns I have identified argues against maintaining a strong commitment to autonomy in bioethical deliberations. In fact, I have no wish to abandon this ideal (just as I have no desire to abandon patient-centered medical care). I still believe that a principle of respect for patient autonomy is an important element of good patient care. Moreover, I believe that appeal to a principle of respect for autonomy can be an important instrument in challenging oppression and it can actually serve as the basis for many of the feminist criticisms I present with respect to our current health care system.[20]

What these criticisms do suggest, however, is that we must pursue a more careful and politically sensitive interpretation of the range of possible restrictions on autonomy than is found in most of the nonfeminist bioethics literature. We need to be able to look at specific decisions as well as the context that influences and sometimes limits such decisions. Many of the troublesome examples I review above are entirely compatible with traditional conceptions of autonomy, even though the patients in question may be facing unjust barriers to care or may be acting in response to oppressive circumstances; traditional conceptions are inadequate to the extent that they make invisible the oppression that structures such decisions. By focusing only on the moment of medical decision making, traditional views fail to examine how specific decisions are embedded within a complex set of relations and policies that constrain (or, ideally, promote) an individual's ability to exercise autonomy with respect to any particular choice.

To understand this puzzle it is necessary to distinguish between agency and autonomy. To exercise agency, one need only exercise reasonable choice.[21] The women who choose some of the controversial practices discussed (e.g., abortion to avoid contact with an abusive partner, cosmetic surgery to conform to artificial norms of beauty, use of dangerous forms of reproductive technology) are exercising agency; clearly they are making choices, and, often, those choices are rational under the circumstances.[22] They also meet the demands of conventional notions of autonomy that ask only that anyone contemplating such procedures be competent, or capable of choosing (wisely), have available information current practice deems relevant, and be free of direct coercion. But insofar as their behavior accepts and adapts to oppression, describing it as autonomous seems inadequate. Together, the habits of equating agency (the making of a choice) with autonomy (self-governance) and accepting as given the prevailing social arrangements have the effect of helping to perpetuate oppression: when we limit our analysis to the quality of an individual's choice under existing conditions (or when we fail to inquire why some people do not even seek health services), we ignore the significance of oppressive conditions. Minimally, autonomous persons should be able to resist oppression—not just act in compliance with it—and be able to refuse the choices oppression seems to make nearly irresistible. Ideally, they should be able to escape from the structures of oppression altogether and create new options that are not defined by these structures either positively or negatively.

In order to ensure that we recognize and address the restrictions that oppression places on people's health choices, then, we need a wider notion of autonomy that will allow us to distinguish genuinely autonomous behavior from acts of merely rational agency. This conception must provide room to challenge the quality of an agent's specific decision-making ability and the social norms that encourage agents to participate in practices that may be partially constitutive of their oppression.[23] A richer, more politically sensitive standard of autonomy should make visible the impact of oppression on a person's choices as well as on her very ability to exercise autonomy fully. Such a conception has the advantage of allowing us to avoid the trap of focusing on the supposed flaws of the individual who is choosing under oppressive circumstances (e.g., by dismissing her choices as "false consciousness"), for it is able to recognize that such choices can be reasonable for the agent. Instead, it directs our attention to the conditions that shape the agent's choice and it makes those conditions the basis of critical analysis.

The problems that I identify with the conventional interpretation of patient autonomy reveal a need to expand our understanding of the types of forces that interfere with a patient's autonomy. On nonfeminist accounts, these are irrationality, failure to recognize that a choice is called for, lack of necessary information, and coercion (including psychological compulsion). Since each of these conditions must be reinterpreted to allow for the ways in which oppression may be operating, we must add to this list recognition of the costs and effects of oppression and of the particular ways in which oppression is manifested. But we must do more than simply modify our interpretation of the four criteria reviewed above. We also need an understanding of the ways in which a person can be encouraged to develop (or discouraged from developing) the ability to exercise autonomy. For this task, we need to consider the presence or absence of meaningful opportunities to build the skills required to be able to exercise autonomy well (Meyers 1989), including the existence of appropriate material and social conditions. In addition, our account should reflect the fact that many decision makers, especially women, place the interests of others at the center of their deliberations. Such an analysis will allow us to ensure that autonomy standards reflect not only the quality of reasoning displayed by a patient at the moment of medical decision making but also the circumstances that surround this decision making.

A RELATIONAL ALTERNATIVE

A major reason for many of the problems identified with the autonomy ideal is that the term is commonly understood to represent freedom of action for agents who are paradigmatically regarded as independent, self-interested, and self-sufficient. As such, it is part of a larger North American cultural ideal of competitive individualism in which every citizen is to be left "free" to negotiate "his" way through the complex interactions of social, economic, and political life.[24] The feminist literature is filled with criticism of such models of agency and autonomy: for example, many feminists object that this ideal appeals to a model of personhood that is distorting because, in fact, no one is fully independent. As well, they observe that this model is exclusionary because those who are most obviously dependent on others (e.g., because of disability or financial need) seem to be disqualified from consideration in ways that others are not. Many feminists object that the view of individuals as isolated social units is not only false but impoverished: much of who we are and what we value is rooted in our relationships and affinities with others. Also, many feminists take issue with the common assumption that agents are single-mindedly self-interested, when so much of our experience is devoted to building or maintaining personal relationships and communities.[25]

If we are to effectively address these concerns, we need to move away from the familiar Western understanding of autonomy as self-defining, self-interested, and self-protecting, as if the self were simply some special kind of property to be preserved.[26] Under most popular interpretations, the structure of the autonomy-heteronomy framework (governance by self or by others) is predicated on a certain view of persons and society in which the individual is thought to be somehow separate from and to exist independently of the larger society; each person's major concern is to be protected from the demands and encroachment of others. This sort of conception fails to account for the complexity of the relations that exist between persons and their culture. It idealizes decisions that are free from outside influence without acknowledging that all persons are, to a significant degree, socially constructed, that their identities, values, concepts, and perceptions are, in large measure, products of their social environment.

Since notions of the self are at the heart of autonomy discussions, alternative interpretations of autonomy must begin with an alternative conception of the self. Curiously, despite its focus on individuals, standard interpretations of autonomy have tended to think of selves as generic rather than distinctive beings. In the traditional view, individuals tend to be treated as interchangeable in that no attention is paid to the details of personal experience. Hence, there is no space within standard conceptions to accommodate important differences among agents, especially the effects that oppression (or social privilege) has on a person's ability to exercise autonomy. In order to capture these kinds of social concerns, some feminists have proposed turning to a relational conception of personhood that recognizes the importance of social forces in shaping each person's identity, development, and aspirations.[27] Following this suggestion, I now explore a relational interpretation of autonomy that is built around a relational conception of the self that is explicitly feminist in its conception.

Under relational theory, selfhood is seen as an ongoing process, rather than as something static or fixed. Relational selves are inherently social beings that are significantly shaped and modified within a web of interconnected (and sometimes conflicting) relationships. Individuals engage in the activities that are constitutive of identity and autonomy (e.g., defining, questioning, revising, and pursuing projects) within a configuration of relationships, both interpersonal and political, by including attention to political relationships of power and powerlessness, this interpretation of relational theory provides room to recognize how the forces of oppression can interfere with an individual's ability to exercise autonomy by undermining her sense of herself as an autonomous agent and by depriving her of opportunities to exercise autonomy. Thus, it is able to provide us with insight into why it is that oppressed people often seem less autonomous than others even when offered a comparable range of choices. Under a relational view, autonomy is best understood to be a capacity or skill that is developed (and constrained) by social circumstances. It is exercised within relationships and social structures that jointly help to shape the individual while also affecting others' responses to her efforts at autonomy.[28]

Diana Meyers (1989) has developed one such theory of personal autonomy. She argues that autonomy involves a particular competency that requires the development of specific skills. As such, it can be either enhanced or diminished by the sort of socialization the agent experiences. Meyers shows how the specific gender socialization most (Western) women undergo trains them in social docility and rewards them for defining their interests in terms of others, thereby robbing them of the opportunity to develop the essential capacity of self-direction. Such training relegates most women to a category she labels "minimally autonomous" (as distinct from her more desirable categories of medially autonomous and fully autonomous). Relational theory allows us to appreciate how each relationship a person participates in plays a role in fostering or inhibiting that individual's capacity for autonomous action by encouraging or restricting her opportunities to understand herself as an autonomous agent and to practice exercising the requisite skills. Such a conception makes clear the importance of discovering the ways in which oppression often reduces a person's ability to develop and exercise the skills that are necessary for achieving a reasonable degree of autonomy.

For instance, relational theory allows us to see the damaging effects on autonomy of internalized oppression. Feminists have long understood that one of the most insidious features of oppression is its tendency to become internalized in the minds of its victims. This is because internalized oppression diminishes the capacity of its victims to develop self-respect, and, as several feminists have argued, reduced (or compromised) self-respect undermines autonomy by undermining the individual's sense of herself as capable of making independent judgments (Meyers 1989; Dillon 1992; Benson 1991, 1994). Moreover, as Susan Babbitt (1993, 1996) has argued, these oppression-induced barriers to auton-

omy cannot necessarily be rectified simply by providing those affected with more information or by removing explicit coercive forces (as the traditional view assumes). When the messages of reduced self-worth are internalized, agents tend to lose the ability even to know their own objective interests. According to Babbitt, in such cases transformative experiences can be far more important to autonomy than access to alternative information. Feminist theory suggests, then, that women and members of other oppressed groups can be helped to increase their autonomy skills by being offered more opportunities to exercise those skills and a supportive climate for practicing them (Meyers 1989), by being provided with the opportunity to develop stronger senses of self-esteem (Benson 1994; Dillon 1992; Meyers 1989), by having the opportunity for transformative experiences that make visible the forces of oppression (Babbitt 1993, 1996), and by having experiences of making choices that are not influenced by the wishes of those who dominate them (Babbitt 1993, 1996).

Autonomy requires more than the effective exercise of personal resources and skills, however; generally, it also demands that appropriate structural conditions be met. Relational theory reminds us that material restrictions, including very restricted economic resources, ongoing fear of assault, and lack of educational opportunity (i.e., the sorts of circumstances that are often part of the condition of being oppressed), constitute real limitations on the options available to the agent. Moreover, it helps us to see how socially constructed stereotypes can reduce both society's and the agent's sense of that person's ability to act autonomously. Relational theory allows us to recognize how such diminished expectations readily become translated into diminished capacities.

The relational interpretation I favor is feminist in that it takes into account the impact of social and political structures, especially sexism and other forms of oppression, on the lives and opportunities of individuals. It acknowledges that the presence or absence of a degree of autonomy is not just a matter of being offered a choice. It also requires that the person had the opportunity to develop the skills necessary for making the type of choice in question, the experience of being respected in her decisions, and encouragement to reflect on her own values. The society, not just the agent, is subject to critical scrutiny under the rubric of relational autonomy.

It is important, however, to avoid an account that denies any scope for autonomy on the part of those who are oppressed. Such a conclusion would be dangerous, since the widespread perception of limited autonomy can easily become a self-fulfilling prophecy. Moreover, such a conclusion would be false. Many members of oppressed groups do manage to develop autonomy skills and, thus, are able to act autonomously in a wide variety of situations, though the particular demands of acting autonomously under oppression are easily overlooked (Benson 1991). Some feminists, such as bell hooks (1990) and Sarah Hoagland (1992), have observed that the marginality associated with being oppressed can sometimes provide people with better opportunities than are available to more well-situated citizens for questioning social norms and devising their own patterns of resistance to social convention. Because those who are especially marginalized (e.g., those who are multiply oppressed or who are "deviant" with respect to important social norms) may have no significant social privilege to lose, they are, sometimes, freer than others to demand changes in the status quo. They may be far more likely to engage in resistance to the norms of oppression than are those who derive some personal benefits from oppressive structures (e.g., middle-class, able-bodied, married women).

Still, we must not make the mistake of romanticizing the opportunities available to the oppressed. An adequate conception of autonomy should afford individuals more than the opportunity to resist oppression; it should also ensure that they have opportunities to actively shape their world. A relational conception of autonomy seems better suited than the traditional models to handle the complexities of such paradoxes because it encourages us to attend to the complex ways in which the detailed circumstances of an individual's social and political circumstances can affect her ability to act in different kinds of contexts.

When relational autonomy reveals the disadvantage associated with oppression in terms of autonomy, the response should not be that others are there-

by licensed to make decisions for those who are oppressed; this response would only increase their powerlessness. Rather, it demands attention to ways in which oppressed people can be helped to develop the requisite autonomy skills. The best way of course to help oppressed people to develop autonomy skills is to remove the conditions of their oppression. Short of that, long-term social projects can help to provide educational opportunities to counter the psychological burdens of oppression. In the short term, it may be necessary to spend more time than usual in supporting patients in the deliberative process of decision making and providing them with access to relevant political as well as medical information when they contemplate controversial procedures (e.g., information about the social dimensions of hormone replacement therapy).

Relational autonomy is not only about changing the individual, however. It also demands attention to ways in which the range of choices before those who belong to oppressed groups can be modified to include more nonoppressive options, that is, options that will not further entrench their existing oppression (as often happens, for example, when women choose cosmetic surgery or the use of many reproductive technologies). Whereas in traditional autonomy theory only the mode and quality of specific decisions are evaluated, feminist relational autonomy regards the range and nature of available and acceptable options as being at least as important as the quality of specific decision making. Only when we understand the ways in which oppression can infect the background or baseline conditions under which choices are to be made will we be able to modify those conditions and work toward the possibility of greater autonomy by promoting nonoppressive alternatives.

As in health matters, it is important in relational discussions not to lose sight of the need to continue to maintain some focus on the individual. Relational autonomy redefines autonomy as the social project it is, but it does not deny that autonomy ultimately resides in individuals. Our attention to social and political contexts helps deepen and enrich the narrow and impoverished view of autonomy available under individualistic conceptions, but it does not support wholesale neglect of the needs and interests of individuals in favor of broader social and political interests. Rather, it can be seen as democratizing access to autonomy by helping to identify and remove the effects of barriers to autonomy that are created by oppression. A relational approach can help to move autonomy from the largely exclusive preserve of the socially privileged and see that it is combined with a commitment to social justice in order to ensure that oppression is not allowed to continue simply because its victims have been deprived of the resources necessary to exercise the autonomy required to challenge it.

IMPLICATIONS OF A RELATIONAL INTERPRETATION OF AUTONOMY FOR HEALTH CARE

Let us now consider what a relational interpretation of autonomy offers when we consider some of the subjects explored elsewhere in this book. Many of the concerns we raise in Chapter 10 regarding the ethics of research with human subjects stem from the fact that ordinary criteria of informed consent are often insufficient to ensure that proper attention is paid to all the morally relevant circumstances; we seek ethical norms that will be concerned with relational autonomy and not merely individual consent to some predetermined research project. Whereas traditional bioethics relies on the familiar individualistic understanding of autonomy, and, hence, focuses on the ability of potential research subjects to refuse to participate in a proposed project, our relational conception leads us to a variety of broader concerns. Rather than just asking whether research subjects truly understand all relevant details about their involvement (a question we still consider important), we argue that questions must also be asked about who is invited to participate and who is not and how the specific research questions were selected. Our recommendations that new research ethics guidelines provide members of oppressed groups a larger say in the planning, structure, and conduct of research are intended to counteract the ways in which existing power relations foster research that selectively serves the interests of those with privilege at the expense of those who are oppressed.

Margaret Lock's discussion of how women's aging bodies are culturally constructed in North American and Japanese societies (Chapter 8) helps to make vivid the limitations of traditional autonomy conceptions when evaluating women's personal choices regarding the use of hormone replacement therapy at menopause. She explains how different cultural expectations about women's aging bodies seem to produce important differences not only in medical practices but also in the experience of aging for women in these two cultures. Women in North America are far more likely than their Japanese counterparts to be offered hormone replacement therapy as either relief from menopausal symptoms or as prevention of heart disease or osteoporosis (or, perhaps, Alzheimer disease). Most women, however, find the decision extremely difficult to make. The problem is not merely one of insufficient data—there is an overwhelming amount of data available, but much of it is inconclusive or contradictory and, very frequently, the data come from studies sponsored by the pharmaceutical companies that market these products and do not address questions of significance to women. Nor is it a problem of coercion— even though some women feel quite strong pressure from their physicians, most doctors are themselves sufficiently ambivalent about the risks and benefits of long-term hormone use that they are happy to leave the decision to their patients. Rather, the problem women face is trying to weigh up their discomfort about the visible signs of aging in a culture that prefers its women young against the uncertain risks of long-term artificial hormone use, their lifelong training to avoid being a burden on others as background to their fears of becoming disabled, their lack of experience in evaluating competing and incommensurable risks, and the background condition of having their whole prior reproductive lives subject to medical surveillance and intervention. What makes hormone replacement therapy a difficult choice for the mostly middle-class, middle-aged Western women who are wrestling with this decision are the social expectations (both external and internal) that women confront as they approach menopause, combined with their own habits of deferring to medical expertise to monitor and regulate their bodies' changes.[29] Relational autonomy makes visible the importance of considering how such social factors affect women's decision making, and it invites us to consider how the burden of unjust social demands might be made explicit so that it can be separated out of the calculations. It allows us to help reshape the considerations that should be operative in this type of choice and to seek political changes that will challenge those influential factors that are discriminatory; at the same time, it warns us of the need to help ensure that women have the necessary autonomy skills before confronting such decisions. And it makes clear the need to ensure that if hormone replacement therapy is of benefit to some women, it be made available to all who can be expected to benefit from it and not simply to those who can afford it or who find themselves in a society that considers medical intervention an appropriate response to women's aging.

Wendy Mitchinson invites us to consider the complexity of the relationships between women and their doctors in Canada between 1850 and 1950 (Chapter 6). She reminds us that power is seldom a straightforward relation where one party holds it all and the other is fully subservient. In the past, as in the present, physicians enjoyed a great deal of social and personal power relative to most of their women patients. But they have never been in full control. Women patients always make choices and thereby exercise agency. Further, patients often make demands and pressure physicians into offering services (e.g., twilight sleep at childbirth) that the physicians might initially resist. Perhaps the modern equivalent is the tendency of many women to demand access to reproductive technologies in order to try to fulfill their reproductive aspirations. As patients, women demand as well as comply; when sufficient numbers make similar demands, they may well affect the course of medical practice. But, for the reasons reviewed above, it is not clear that we should count such influence as full autonomy as long as the conditions of choice are restricted and oppressive.

Both patients and physicians recognize that the options they may reasonably consider are limited by economic and legal restrictions and by the force of professional standards of acceptable practice. Evaluating autonomous decision making in medical encounters, then, requires us to attend to the circumstances of particular physicians and patients and to the nature of their interactions. Increasing autonomy for patients is a matter not just of increasing their power relative to their physicians but of increasing patients' social power more broadly and restructuring the health care system to ensure that it is responsive to an appropriate range of women's needs by removing discriminatory attitudes and barriers and by promoting the necessary knowledge base. It is necessary to avoid simplistic understandings of the patient-physician (or, more generically, the patient-health care worker) relationship as a contractual agreement between two fully independent parties (as is often suggested in the nonfeminist bioethics literature). We need to attend to ways in which those involved in delivering health care participate in social understandings of women, and of specific groups of women, when offering women a predefined set of treatment options. Relational autonomy invites us to appreciate that both physicians and patients are socially situated and the options each considers, like the choices each makes, are a reflection of social expectations that may well be oppressive.

Consider also what a relational ideal of autonomy might mean in some of the concrete circumstances of health care services. First, under relational as under individualistic conceptions of autonomy, it is important for health care workers to continue their efforts to explore the needs, interests, and concerns of their patients at all stages of treatment—to seek informed choice in the fullest sense possible. Under both relational and individualistic understandings, informed consent must be understood as an ongoing process; a relational interpretation can make it clearer that the pursuit of informed consent is also an interactive process in which both parties may be transformed. Also, both interpretations provide support for insisting that, apart from emergencies, health care providers should not presume to know what is best for their patients because they cannot have access to all of the relevant facts and values associated with the complexities of their patients' lives and interests.

A relational view helps us to understand how the specific social location of patients can affect their autonomy status. It explains why requiring health care providers to disclose relevant information and seek the permission of patients is a necessary, but not a sufficient, criterion for protecting patient autonomy. Because oppressive norms can undermine a patient's opportunities to develop the experience and skills necessary to practice autonomy, we need to explore ways of reversing such deficiencies and fostering greater autonomy skills. Clearly, this task extends far beyond the boundaries of health care and calls for social changes that will provide the oppressed with opportunities to develop autonomy skills that are comparable to the opportunities of the more privileged. Within health care, it is important to keep in mind that patients who have had little opportunity to exercise autonomy in other areas of their lives may need more time and more counseling than others before they are asked to give their decisions on health matters, in order to be sure that the patient understands that a choice is genuinely in her hands.

Moreover, a relational interpretation of autonomy should call into question health care orientations that view health-related services simply as consumer options, to be made available to anyone who chooses them. Policy questions about what health care procedures are developed and what services health professionals are trained to provide and encouraged to offer involve social and political values that should be subject to public debate and widespread ethical reflection. For example, each society needs to determine if it wants its medical researchers and practitioners occupied with the full range of emerging new reproductive technologies or if it wishes to set some restrictions;[30] each must also decide whether it supports massive genetic screening and testing efforts to reduce health problems associated with genetic variations, or whether it will focus its resources on other sorts of preventative initiatives and on strategies for relieving the burdens of genetic variations that now fall on individuals. It should not be the sole responsibility of physicians and researchers to determine whether to meet the demands of individuals who seek such procedures as assisted reproduction, cosmetic surgery, organ transplants, prenatal genetic testing, or diet aids.

The need for more sophisticated analyses and public policy is especially urgent when the services in question reflect and reinforce oppressive social norms that are difficult for those who are oppressed to resist.

Individualistic interpretations of autonomy seem to suggest that medical consumers should be provided with whatever services are voluntarily chosen (i.e., in the absence of explicit coercion), but a relational understanding of autonomy requires that we raise questions about the context of those choices. It encourages us to explore whether the growth of practices such as cosmetic surgery and prenatal diagnosis contribute to a climate in which these practices become so normalized that future patients may find themselves unable to refuse such services. Just as home births became virtually impossible to arrange once the majority of women in North America chose hospital births, there is a real risk that the current wide acceptance and popularity of prenatal genetic testing may soon make it nearly impossible for pregnant women to refuse. Because the autonomy of some may well be affected by the choices of others, we need to recognize the interpersonal implications of current practices on the autonomy of future patients.

In addition, because a relational conception highlights rather than obscures the roles played by social and material conditions, it helps us see the importance of ensuring that material constraints do not unduly restrict the options that are actually available to socially disadvantaged patients. This implies a duty on the part of each citizen to join the political fight to retain a commitment to the principles of universality and equal access in the Canadian health care system and other countries where these principles are now threatened and to seek to have such principles endorsed in the United States. It also suggests that we consider broadening the definition of health services to make certain that nonmedical services that improve health are also covered by public funding.

And, finally, a relational theory can show the importance of demanding that health care providers become sensitive to their own biases and assumptions so that they can better resist the common tendency to deny authority to patients with less social status. By disrupting norms that validate the experiences and perceptions of the powerful while dismissing those of the oppressed, relational ideals reveal the need for health care workers to listen carefully to the concerns and priorities of patients who belong to groups that are systematically oppressed. Health professionals must learn to stop assuming total expertise on health matters. They must broaden their understanding of their responsibilities; rather than seeing their task as simply one of educating and persuading patients to accept their learned advice, they need to develop the skills necessary to find out how the condition in question is experienced by the patient and what constraints on treatment options face the patient. Such a shift in orientation should lead to more effective, patient-centered health care. It may also help to transform the historical pattern in which health-related research and practice have focused on the specific needs and experiences of privileged members of society at the expense of less advantaged people whose distinctive health needs are largely neglected.

If we are truly to respect patient autonomy, we, as a society, need to develop a health care system that is more attentive to the actual needs of the diverse variety of citizens who depend on its services. That task will require that policy makers and providers learn to respond more appropriately to patients who are differently situated. A relational approach to autonomy allows us to maintain a central place for autonomy within bioethics, but it requires an interpretation that is both deeper and more complicated than the traditional conception acknowledges—one that sets standards that involve political as well as personal criteria of adequacy. It examines patient autonomy in the social and political dimensions within which it resides and provides us with theoretical resources that we need for restructuring health care practices in ways that will genuinely expand the autonomy of *all* patients.

Acknowledgments

This chapter has evolved over the course of the Network interactions and has benefited enormously from Network discussions. I am grateful to all Network members for careful readings of many earlier drafts and stimulating comments. In addition to input from Network members, I have also benefited from the generous attention paid by Keith Burgess-Jackson, Sue Campbell, Richmond Campbell, Carmel Forde, Jody Graham, Carl Matheson, Barbara Secker, and Eldon Soifer.

Notes

1. Some Network members prefer the terms "contextual" or "situated" as a way of avoiding all confusion with those feminists who reserve the term "relational" to refer exclusively to interpersonal relations. I feel that this usage perpetuates the misleading sense that interpersonal relations are themselves "apolitical." I have, therefore, chosen to insist on a thoroughly political reading of the term "relational" that applies to both interpersonal and more public sorts of relations.

2. While questions of patient autonomy arise in interactions with all health care providers, North American health care delivery is largely structured around provision of medical services; moreover, physicians control most of the decision making that determines provision of health care services. Hence, much of the subsequent discussion focuses explicitly on patient autonomy in relation to physician authority, even though many of the concerns raised also extend to other (nonmedical) types of health care practice.

3. The most vivid examples appear in distressing history of medical research with human subjects. See, for example, Katz 1972.

4. I deliberately retain the gendered term in this particular instance since it accurately reflects the connection to the traditional gendered role of patriarchal father who presumes authority to make decisions on behalf of all other family members. Traditional stereotypes of mothering and gender-neutral parenting do not retain this hierarchical flavor.

5. For a review of most of the common interpretations, see Dworkin 1988.

6. Interest in respect for patient autonomy is hardly unique to North America, however. See note 20.

7. See, for example, Corea 1985a; Ehrenreich and English 1979; Fisher 1986; Perales and Young 1988; and White 1990. This is not a straightforward history of constant abuse or one-sided power, however; as Wendy Mitchinson documents in Chapter 6, the relationship between women and their doctors has long been complex and ambiguous.

8. At the very least, we need a more complex analysis of the options for decision making than is provided by the familiar dichotomous structure of patient autonomy versus medical paternalism. See Mahowald 1993 for development of the idea of maternalism as an

alternative that is aimed at capturing both these aspects of medical responsibility; see also Sherwin 1992 for a brief proposal of "amicalism."

9. *Informed choice* suggests a wider scope for patient autonomy than *informed consent* in that it includes the possibility of patients' initiating treatment suggestions where *informed consent* implies that the role of the patient is merely to consent to the treatment proposed by the physician; further, *informed choice* makes more explicit that patients ought also to be free to refuse recommended treatments as well as to accept them.

10. Many of these concerns are not exclusive to feminists; several have also been raised by other sorts of critics. I call them feminist because I came to these concerns through a feminist analysis that attends to the role in society of systems of dominance and oppression, especially those connected with gender.

11. This reduction may be a result of a tendency to collapse the ideal of personal autonomy central to bioethics discussions with the concept of moral autonomy developed by Immanual Kant.

12. It is often taken as a truism in our culture that emotional involvement constitutes irrationality, that emotions are direct threats to rationality. It is hard to see, however, how decisions about important life decisions are improved if they are made without any emotional attachment to the outcomes.

13. Susan Babbitt (1996) argues that the traditional conception of rationality is defined in terms of propositional understanding in ways that obscure the experiences and needs of oppressed people.

14. For example, research priorities have led to the situation where birth control pills are available only for women and this increases the pressure on women seeking temporary protection against pregnancy to take the pill even when it endangers their health.

15. See chapter 10.

16. I focus primarily on medicine since it is the dominant health profession and is responsible for organization of most health services in developed countries. Most health professions involve a similar bias toward treatment of individuals, though some (e.g., social work) pride themselves on attending to social structures as well as individual need, and most health professions, including medicine, include subspecialties concerned with matters of public health.

17. See chapter 9.

18. Because health care is a provincial responsibility, there are differences in the precise services offered from province to province and from one administration to the next within provinces. The examples here are broad generalizations.

19. Such considerations do play a role in health care planning at a governmental level where the focus shifts from medical interventions to the idea of *health determinants,* but here, too, there is excessive attention paid to what the individual can and should be doing ("healthism") and insufficient concern about promoting egalitarian social conditions. See Chapters 3 and 4.

20. When I read an early version of this section of the paper to the Second World Congress of the International Association of Bioethics in Buenos Aires, Argentina, in November 1994, I was struck by how passionately committed local feminists were to retaining a version of the respect for autonomy principle. They felt that most women in their country had very little authority over decisions about their health care, and so they were struggling to reverse a strongly paternalistic bias on the part of physicians by appeal to the principle of respect for autonomy. While they acknowledged that this principle was not as well-entrenched in their society as it is in North America, they considered it very important to their own feminist health agenda. They see respect for patient autonomy as having profoundly liberatory potential in their own society; this perspective provides clear reason not to dismiss this principle lightly, flawed though it may be.

21. The language of agency and autonomy is quite varied within feminist (and other) discourse. For example, the term *agency* is used throughout the collection *Provoking Agents: Gender and Agency in Theory and Practice* (Gardiner 1995) in ways that sometimes appear to overlap with my usage of *relational autonomy.* Susan Babbitt (1996), on the other hand, seems to use the two terms in ways analogous to the use here.

22. The notion of agency is itself highly contested within current feminist theory. Postmodern accounts seem to deny the possibility of subjectivity in any familiar sense; since agency is traditionally assigned to a single subject, once the subject is eliminated, the possi-

bility of agency seems to disappear as well. I do not address this complex theoretical issue here but continue to rely on common sense understandings of both subjectivity and agency. Readers interested in understanding the feminist debates around agency may consult Gardiner 1995.

23. In addition, we need the conceptual space to be able to acknowledge that restrictive definitions of health sometimes preempt autonomy analysis by limiting the opportunity of some people even to enter the relatively well-funded health care system for assistance with problems (e.g., poverty) that affect their health.

24. The agent imagined in such cases is always stereotypically masculine.

25. Feminist discussion of these and other critiques can be found in Gilligan 1982; Baier 1985b; Code 1991; and Held 1993.

26. See Nedelsky 1989 for discussion of this view and its limitations.

27. For example, Baier 1985b; Code 1991; and Held 1993.

28. An alternative feminist conception of a relational view of autonomy is provided by Anne Donchin (1998). I see her account as complementary to, not competitive with, this one.

29. This cohort includes half of our research Network, so it is a question whose urgency we feel strongly.

30. For example, Canada funded the four-year Royal Commission on New Reproductive Technologies (1989-1993) to advise on public policy regarding these technologies. In June 1996, Bill C-47, which involves restrictions on commercialization of any aspects of human reproduction, including the buying or selling of gametes or embryos, prohibits human cloning and other sorts of technologies on the horizon and restricts the use of prenatal sex selection to medical conditions, was introduced to the House of Commons in Canada.

References

Babbitt, Susan. 1993. "Feminist and Objective Interests." In *Feminist Epistemologies*, ed. Linda Alcoff and Elizabeth Potter. New York: Routledge.

—. 1996. *Impossible Dreams: Rationality, Integrity, and Moral Indignation*. Boulder, Colo.: Westview Press.

Baier, Annette. 1985. "What do Women Want in a Moral Theory?" *Nous* 19(1): 53-63.

Benson, Paul. 1991. "Autonomy and Oppressive Socialization." *Social Theory and Practice* 17(3): 385-408.

—. 1994. "Free Agency and Self-Worth." *Journal of Philosophy* 91(12): 650-68.

Code, Lorraine. 1991. *What Can She Know? Feminist Theory and the Construction of Knowledge*. Ithaca, N.Y.: Cornell University Press.

Corea, Gena. 1985. *The Hidden Malpractice: How American Medicine Mistreats Women*. New York: Haper Colophon Books.

Dillon, Robin, 1992. "Toward a Feminist Conception of Self-Respect." *Hypatia* 7(1) 52-69.

Donchin, Anne. 1998. "Understanding Autonomy Relationally: Toward a Reconfiguration of Bioethical Principles." *Journal of Medicine and Philosophy* 23.

Dworkin, Gerald. 1988. *The Theory and Practice of Autonomy*. Cambridge: Cambridge University Press.

Ehrenreich, Barbara, and Deirdre English. 1972. *Wtiches, Midwives, and Nurses: A History of Women Healers*. Glass Mountain Pamphlet, no. 1. Old Westbury, N.Y.: The Feminist Press.

Fisher, Sue. 1986. *In the Patient's Best Interests: Women and the Politics of Medical Decisions*. New Brunswick, N.J.: Rutgers University Press.

Foucault, Michel. 1979. *Discipline and Punish*. New York: Vintage.

—. 1980. *Power/Knowledge*. Ed. Colin Gordon. Brighton, Eng.: Harvester.

Gardiner, Judith Kegan. 1995. *Provoking Agents: Gender and Agency in Theory and Practice*. Chicago: University of Illinois Press.

Gilligan, Carol. 1982. *In a Different Voice: Psychological Theory and Women's Moral Development*. Cambridge, Mass.: Harvard University Press.

Held, Virginia. 1993. *Feminist Morality: Transforming Culture, Society, and Politics*. Chicago: University of Chicago Press.

Hoagland, Sarah Lucia. 1992. "Lesbian Ethics and Female Agency." In *Explorations in Feminist Ethics: Theory and Practice*. Ed. Susan Browning Cole and Susan Coultrap-McQuin. Bloomington: Indiana University Press.

hooks, bell. 1990. *Yearning: Race, Gender, and Cultural Politics.* Toronto: Between The Lines.

Katz, Jay, ed. 1972. *Experimentation with Human Beings: The Authority of the Investigator, Subject, Professions, and State in the Human Experimentation Process.* New York: Russell Sage Foundation.

Lloyd, Genevieve. 1984. *The Man of Reason: "Male" and "Female" in Western Philosophy.* Minneapolis: University of Minnesota Press.

Mahowald, Mary Briody. 1993. *Women and Children in Health Care: An Unequal Majority.* New York: Oxford University Press.

Meyers, Diana. 1989. *Self, Society, and Personal Choice.* New York: Columbia University Press.

Nedelsky, Jennifer. 1989. "Reconceiving Autonomy." *Yale Journal of Law and Feminism* 1(1): 7-36.

Perales, Cesar A., and Lauren S. Young, eds. 1988. *Too Little, Too Late: Dealing with the Health Needs of Women in Poverty.* New York: Harrington Park Press.

Sherwin, Susan. 1992. *No Longer Patient: Feminist Ethics and Health Care.* Philadelphia: Temple University Press.

White, Evelyn C., ed. 1990. *The Black Women's Health Book: Speaking for Ourselves.* Seattle, Wash.: Seal Press.

5.
CARING FOR PATIENTS IN CROSS-CULTURAL SETTINGS

Nancy S. Jecker, Joseph A. Carrese, and Robert A. Pearlman

In our multicultural society, cross-cultural encounters are becoming increasingly common in the health care setting, often leading to distinct ethical and interpersonal tensions. Members of different cultures cannot take for granted a common catalog of recognized diseases; a shared understanding of their ascribed causes and usual treatments; or similar attitudes toward sickness, health, death, particular illnesses, and accidents. Although value differences also exist among different groups within a "shared" culture—across class, caste, gender, age, religious, and political lines—cross-cultural conflicts may be more deeply rooted, for such differences embody not just different opinions or beliefs, but different ways of everyday living and different systems of meaning.[1]

The difference between intra-and intercultural disagreements in health care may fall along a continuum, with intercultural tensions often appearing more striking and all encompassing. To illustrate this, consider the case of a Western patient diagnosed with carcinoma of the breast who disagrees with a Western physician's recommendation to undergo a mastectomy. The patient prefers instead to preserve the breast and treat the cancer with lumpectomy. In reaching her conclusion, the patient may stress the value she places on bodily integrity, physical wholeness, social attractiveness, and sexuality. Although the physician shares the patient's goal of preserving quality of life, the physician may place greater stress on curing disease. The physician may therefore reach a decision after consulting survival rates for the two procedures for patients at a similar stage of the disease. Despite the different concerns the patient and physician entertain, they are likely to share many of the same ethical concepts and principles. Thus they may articulate their differences in terms of a common moral vocabulary, for example, in terms of a tension between competing values of autonomy and beneficence. Or their discussion may refer to the relative priority of maximizing the quality versus the duration of the patient's life. This shared conceptual repertoire is likely to assist in reaching a treatment decision.

By contrast, intercultural disagreements in health care often involve the clash of different dominant social understandings. For example, consider the case of a Navajo patient who expresses to a Western physician a preference for a traditional healing ceremony to cure disease. Both the patient's and the physician's ideas about healing seem ordinary and "natural" within the context of their respective cultures. In attempting to communicate their respective orientations to each other, however, each will refer to practices and traditions, concepts and values, and systems and methods of knowledge that appear unusual from the other's perspective. Thus, cross-cultural debates often seem to introduce moral anarchy because people lack shared cultural standards or vantage points from which to communicate and resolve value differences.

There are at least two distinct ways in which cross-cultural differences may become especially striking in the clinical setting. First, a health provider may come from a dominant cultural group and the patient may be a representative of an immigrant or refugee group or of a historical ethnic minority. Alternatively, health professionals themselves may be members of immigrant, refugee, or ethnic minorities and patients may be from the mainstream of society. In this paper, we address the first sort of paradigm case.

BACKGROUND AND CONTEXT

Although individuals with culturally distinct identities exist across many different subgroups in society, cultural differences among dominant and minority ethnic groups have become especially pronounced in recent years. The influx of immigrant and refugee populations has meant that today physicians are more likely than ever before to encounter patients from diverse cultures in their daily practice, and the need for ethical analyses has increased.[2]

Despite the fact that the United States has long been "a nation of nations"—a mix of different cultural groups—American bioethicists have paid relatively little attention to the distinctive ethical challenges this poses. Some have charged that American bioethics "considers its principles, its style of reasoning, and its perceptions to be objective, unbiased, and reasonable to a degree that not only makes them socially and culturally neutral but also endows them with a kind of universality."[3] Others find bioethical analyses "entangled in asocial, acultural, and decontextualized philosophical, moral, and legal discourses" and therefore lacking tools to "investigate comprehensively the social and cultural realities that matter to diverse patient populaces."[4] Reflecting these concerns, standard bioethics textbooks often frame principles of ethics in health care to represent Western ethical traditions, while omitting discussion of pertinent and potentially conflicting values held by patients from non-Western cultures. When textbooks do address cross-cultural conflicts, they denounce ethical relativism and proceed to enumerate Western ethical standards,[5] or note cultural diversity on a case-by-case basis, without formulating general strategies for resolving differences.[6]

The dearth of coverage of cross-cultural issues in bioethics itself reflects the general paucity of scholarship in this area. Although a growing number of articles address specific cross-cultural problems,[7] only a few cover a full range of topics in a systematic fashion.[8] Reports of health care ethics in other countries have been forthcoming yet fail to touch upon the problems that arise when cultures collide.[9] Undoubtedly, such analyses can benefit from the contribution of diverse disciplines,[10] yet social science contributions to cross-cultural health care ethics have only recently begun to appear.[11]

A PRACTICAL ETHICAL APPROACH
We propose addressing the ethical predicaments cross-cultural medical encounters raise by means of an approach consisting of three distinct steps: identi-

fying goals; identifying mutually agreeable strategies; and meeting ethical constraints.

Identifying Goals
The first step in this process asks the health practitioner to identify the central aims that health professional and patient bring to the medical encounter. This requires the health professional to solicit information about the patient's ethical values and cultural orientation. Like an ethnographer, the clinician in a cross-cultural setting must try

> to get things right from the native's point of view ... he practices an intensive, systematic, and imaginative empathy with the experiences and modes of thought of persons who may be foreign to him but whose foreignness he comes to appreciate and to humanly engage.[12]

Like the ethnographer, providers in cross-cultural settings should function as observational scientists, attending carefully to particular details, gathering information not only by communicating directly with the patient, but also by speaking with important persons in the patient's life. In clarifying their own goals, health providers must be self-reflective, distinguishing the purpose they bring to a patient encounter from the practices typically employed to realize this purpose.

Identifying Mutually Agreeable Strategies
Once the provider in a cross-cultural encounter has clarified provider and patient goals, the provider should take the initiative in identifying alternative mutually agreeable strategies to meet these goals. For example, signing informed consent forms represents but one method, among others, of realizing health providers' goal of ensuring that patients receive the treatment they truly want. Other ways of realizing informed consent include communicating with family members who then speak directly with patients, or postponing discussion of treatment options until the patient begins to know and trust the provider. The general point is that the goals of the medical encounter serve only as general guideposts, indicating a direction without charting a specific course; providers should search for alternative paths to realize the aims that patient and provider hold.[13]

Ideally, health professionals caring for patients in cross-cultural settings have access to consultants familiar with the patient's cultural circumstances, fluent in the patient's native language, and trained in medical interpreting. Health care institutions that regularly serve non-Western patient groups have special responsibilities to make such resources available, and new tools have become available to hospitals in many areas. For example, the AT&T Language Line provides a twenty-four-hour service that guarantees access to interpreters who speak 147 different languages. Health care institutions also have developed "language banks" (that is, computerized lists of bilingual staff members), utilized flash cards containing common phrases written in different languages, and provided intensive language training to staff to assist them in interactions with clients from commonly served non-English-speaking populations.[14]

Meeting Ethical Constraints

The final step of our approach engages the health professional in ethical deliberation about the acceptability of alternative means of realizing goals. At an initial stage, the provider brings two central ethical criteria to bear. (Figure 1). First, the means chosen to achieve the goals of the medical encounter should be compatible with the health care provider's own conscientiously held values as well as with the ethics of the health care profession to which the provider belongs. As the American College of Physicians notes, "The physician [in a cross-cultural setting] cannot be required to violate fundamental personal values, standards of scientific or ethical practice, or the law."[15] A second criterion holds that the means employed should be compatible with the patient's values and the values of the culture with which the patient identifies. This constraint is necessary to ensure that relationships between providers and patients remain mutually respectful and to safeguard patients against abuses of power and authority by health professionals. Health professionals generally have greater authority and power than patients, and patients are frequently confused, upset, and compromised by their illness. When these power dynamics are compounded by cultural differences, with the health care provider representing the dominant culture and the patient coming from a "different" culture, the risk of unjustly coercing the patient is heightened.

Both constraints gain justification from the concept of ethical integrity. Integrity refers to the disposition to act in accordance with one's own moral beliefs and character.[16] It presupposes having the self-knowledge and moral commitment necessary to know and honor one's moral convictions. Understood in this light, integrity cannot be identified with any particular set of moral virtues or principles, but is instead compatible with diverse moral perspectives. For example, two persons with different positions on the morality of assisted suicide may show integrity by acting in opposite ways. Someone who believes that the sanctity of human life prohibits assisting with suicide may display integrity by refusing to meet a friend's request for aid in dying. By contrast, someone in the same situation who maintains that compassion for human suffering permits assisting with suicide may show integrity by assisting with suicide. Thus, if it can be called a virtue, integrity is a higher-order virtue. It does not presuppose any specific lower-order virtues to which a person's actions must conform.[17]

Within the limits set by integrity, alternative practical means for resolving culturally based conflicts may emerge, as people are frequently able to agree about particular cases without ever agreeing at all about the basic ethical tenets underlying them. A particularly impressive illustration of this phenomenon is the work of the National Commission for the Protection of Human Subjects of Biomedical and Behavioral Research. In describing the development of the commission's guidelines, one member notes that although the eleven commissioners had different ethical, religious, and professional orientations, "so long as the Commission stayed on the taxonomic or casuistical level, they usually agreed in their practical conclusions."[18]

When examination of more basic ethical goals is necessary, the health professional proceeds to a second stage of ethical analysis (figure 2). At this stage, integrity again furnishes guidance. Properly understood, integrity does not manifest itself merely as exceptional resoluteness. Rather, persons of true integrity make convictions and principles their own through critically examining and questioning them. By contrast, someone who acts blindly or stubbornly, holding fast to principles for their own sake, does not evince genuine integrity. Nor does the individual who accepts on faith whatever moral principles she or he receives from others. Instead, persons with integrity scrutinize their moral principles and commitments carefully to interpret and apply them to new situations. They regard their moral convictions as potentially mistaken and as continuously open to criticism and improvement in the wake of new circumstances and challenges. Whereas an ideologue claims "a monopoly of truth and justice," a person of integrity shows the qualities of a reasonable person, including "a disposition to find reasons for and against the possible lines of conduct ... open to him, ... to consider [viewpoints] ... in the light of further evidence and reasons which may be presented, ... [and] to know his own emotional, intellectual, and moral predilection."[19]

Understood in this light, integrity directs health professionals to examine critically the values they bring to the medical encounter. Similarly, the patient with integrity is "empowered not simply to follow unexamined preferences ... but to consider, through dialogue, alternative health-related values, their worthiness and their implications for treatment."[20] Providers and patients who show integrity may continue to assume that their own views are correct; however, they will also recognize that they could be mistaken. As Martin Benjamin notes, the give and take of conversation may lead thoughtful persons to alter their positions, replacing an initial viewpoint with a different viewpoint that comes to be regarded as superior.[21] This process of amending ethical beliefs does not necessarily show that persons have betrayed their principles; instead, it may show that ethical beliefs have been changed in light of new evidence and circumstances. Therefore, although the idea of integrity may conjure up images of people who hold tenaciously to principles in the face of enticements to give them up, many instances of integrity do not conform to this model. Persons manifest integrity by reexamining existing values and changing their course of action to conform to new or more fully enunciated values. Thus, integrity is able to survive changes in basic allegiances over time.[22]

Figure 1. First Level of Ethical Analysis.
Requirements
The means chosen should be
• consistent with the health care provider's conscientiously held beliefs
• compatible with the patient's values and the values of the culture with which the patient identifies
Justification
Integrity requires acting in accordance with ethical convictions and beliefs that are one's own

Figure 2. Second Level of Ethical Analysis.
Requirements
Reexamine personal values and consider reinterpreting, reordering, or changing them in light of the case
Justification
Integrity requires scrutinizing one's values and regarding them as open to criticism and improvement

The interpretation of integrity as nondogmatic is supported by the observation that context influences the weight ethical principles bring to bear. In the health care setting, for example, the force of ethical principles depends upon circumstances of context, such as the values of patients, family members, and relevant social groups; personal and professional values of health care providers; and the institutional setting in which ethical situations arise.[23] In addition, a nondogmatic reading of integrity is persuasive when one considers the myriad ways in which context shapes the actual meaning ethical principles hold.[24] Thus, in health care the very generality of bioethical principles to "do good" and "avoid harm" renders interpretation inescapable, and health professionals cannot get along on a diet of general principles alone.[25]

CASE ANALYSES
To illustrate the strategy outlined above we now turn to two cases drawn from the clinical setting. Each reveals ethical tensions that arise between Western

physicians and Navajo patients. The first case is relatively straightforward and is intended primarily to illustrate the approach we have described. It bears some resemblance to the intracultural example described at the outset of the paper, in which a patient and provider share common goals but place different emphases on curing disease versus preserving quality of life. Unlike the intracultural case, however, the Western physician and Navajo patient we describe below do not share a common moral vocabulary and framework, nor do they function with similar systems of meaning and modes of interacting. These cultural differences make the resolution of even a relatively straightforward ethical conflict more challenging. In the second cross-cultural encounter we describe, the provider and patient bring different goals to the medical encounter, and have different ethical frameworks, meaning systems, and ways of interacting.

Case 1

A fifty-five-year-old Navajo man, Mr. Begay, presented with hypertension for a routine clinic appointment. On this visit, as on previous visits, the patient's blood pressure was elevated. In the past, the physician had devoted considerable energy to educating Mr. Begay about high blood pressure: its etiology, natural history if untreated, and the benefits of controlling it. In addition, he had stressed the importance of non-pharmacologic measures, such as restricting salt, moderating alcohol use, exercising appropriately and losing weight. At the time of this visit Mr. Begay was being treated with two drugs. The physician considered adding a third drug; however, he was concerned that Mr. Begay would not adhere to a new medical regimen. Mr. Begay had not followed the physician's recommendations pertaining to diet and exercise in the past, and the physician suspected that he had not taken medication with prescribed frequency. Despite the physician's efforts, Mr. Begay's blood pressure was elevated and he was at risk for stroke, renal injury, and coronary artery disease.

Complicating the situation was the fact that the physician's ordinary manner of relating to patients involved disclosing negative possibilities and risks in order to inform and educate patients. In this situation, his inclination was to stress to Mr. Begay the negative risks asso-

ciated with his refusal to follow medical advice. Mr. Begay, however, was a traditional Navajo and his expectations reflected his culture's ideas about healing as a process of moving the patient from a negative state of illness or "imbalance" to a positive state of harmony and health. Hopefulness and positive thinking are perceived as integral to healing, while negative thinking is regarded as potentially deleterious. Thus, "Navajos emphasize that if one thinks of good things and good fortune, good things will happen. If one thinks of bad things, bad fortune will be one's lot."[26] According to traditional Navajos, people can acquire disease through a process of "witching." Witching involves manipulating agents that produce disease, and can occur through explicit discussion of potential morbid events.[27]

In view of how explicit disclosure of possible bad outcomes may adversely affect traditional Navajo patients, how should the physician proceed? The strategy proposed in the previous section instructs the physician to begin by identifying the underlying goals at stake in the situation for both Mr. Begay and himself. Through eliciting the patient's values and engaging others who know the patient well, the physician may learn that Mr. Begay's central goals include staying healthy, existing in harmony with nature, thinking in a positive and hopeful manner about the future, and living long enough to see his grandchildren's children. The physician may identify his own objectives to include minimizing Mr. Begay's risks of morbidity and mortality from hypertension and persuading Mr. Begay to adhere to treatment. These objectives of the physician are themselves instrumental to a more fundamental end, namely, keeping Mr. Begay healthy. The physician's aims also may include keeping Mr. Begay informed and educated about the purpose and importance of treatment.

Our second step directs the physician to determine mutually acceptable means to realize the goals patient and provider bring to the medical encounter. Stating goals explicitly helps to show that although the goal of achieving health is shared, there is not a shared conception of the appropriate means to achieve this goal. The physician's means of ensuring Mr. Begay's health are educating Mr. Begay; Mr. Begay's means of ensuring his health are avoiding witching by thinking only in positive and hopeful terms about the future. How can the physician accomplish both his and the patient's objectives and act in accordance with the values that both he and Mr. Begay hold? One approach that traditional Navajos use is to communicate information about possible bad outcomes by making reference to a hypothetical third party. This approach would avoid direct reference to Mr. Begay and avert his concern about being witched. Another option consists of reframing the interaction with the patient to focus on the positive benefits that Mr. Begay would gain if he abides by treatment. Thus, the physician might begin by affirming that he shares with Mr. Begay the goal that Mr. Begay stay healthy or "move to a state of harmony." The physician might then make the case that taking medication facilitates these positive ends. Similarly, the physician may explain to Mr. Begay that taking medication furthers his positive aim of seeing his grandchildren's children. This approach contrasts with the alternative, to which the physician was initially drawn, namely, focusing on his perception of the negative risks of non-adherence. The physician's goal of educating the patient is still achieved, but the means used accommodate the patient's concern not to be witched and to think affirmatively about the future.

Applying our approach to case 1 makes evident the central importance of integrity in cross-cultural conflicts. In the case resolutions we develop, the physician makes adjustments in his ordinary manner of communicating with patients, but does this without violating the standards he or the patient holds. In the actual resolution of the case, the physician caring for Mr. Begay had learned through experience with Navajo patients to devise innovative strategies that accomplish both his and the patient's goals. On previous occasions, however, the physician had taken the opposite tack and discussed explicit risks, thereby offending patients and discouraging them from returning to Western physicians.

Case 2

A sixty-five-year-old widowed Navajo woman, Mrs. Tsosie, presented to the hospital with her two adult daughters following nearly two months of lethargy, impaired memory, confusion, possible visual hallucinations, anorexia, and fever. These symptoms had progressed in the two weeks prior to admission, but the patient had refused to come to the hospital for treatment. She had instead sought a healing ceremony from a traditional Navajo medicine man, but the medicine man had refused to perform the ceremony, claiming that she was too sick to participate. When Mrs. Tsosie had become too weak and confused to protest going to the hospital, her daughters brought her there.

The patient had a history of rheumatic heart disease. Despite two admissions over the past three years for congestive heart failure, Mrs. Tsosie had refused an echo-cardiogram and cardiac catheterization to evaluate the severity of her disease. The patient, a weaver and shepherd, conceived of illness and healing in terms of the traditional Navajo worldview. Since childhood, cross-cultural tensions had rendered her relationship with Western physicians tentative.

Medical evaluation of Mrs. Tsosie's change in mental status included electroencephalogram, computerized axial tomography scan, and blood workup to rule out metabolic causes. When these tests were unrevealing, Mrs. Tsosie's daughters refused to consent to a lumbar puncture to rule out meningitis as a possible basis for delirium. The daughters explained that their mother had consistently refused surgical or invasive procedures. They believed this was due to their mother's skepticism about Western medicine. Especially when the perceived harm was great, Mrs. Tsosie was reluctant to put her trust in Western doctors.

Following one week in the hospital, the two daughters requested that their mother be discharged to participate in a healing ceremony. Mrs. Tsosie had apparently communicated to her daughters that she wished to have a healing ceremony performed. The patient's daughters insisted that they must honor their mother's wishes. As they perceived their mother's condition to be slightly improved, they hoped that the medicine man who had previously refused to perform a healing ceremony would now agree to do so.

In contrast to case 1, case 2 shows that sometimes there may seem to be no mutually agreeable means available to meet both the patient's and the health care provider's goals. How does the approach we endorse fare in light of this more challenging case? As before, the first step involves stating explicitly the goals of both physician and patient. The physician's primary goals might be diagnosing the patient and prescribing beneficial treatment. The alternative the physician sees is postponing diagnosis indefinitely with the expectation that the patient's status would deteriorate. Empirically based treatments for acute bacterial meningitis, such as broad spectrum antibiotics, had been tried without significant improvement in the patient's condition. Pursuing other treatment options was potentially hazardous without the more definitive diagnosis that the lumbar puncture would provide. Thus, the physician regarded the risks associated with acceding to the family's wishes as extremely high: an undiagnosed and inappropriately treated central nervous system infection was potentially fatal. The patient's goals, as conveyed by her daughters, included leaving the hospital to participate in a healing ceremony. The daughters' goals included abiding by their mother's wishes and returning her to an active and healthy state. The alternative for them was to violate their filial duties and perpetuate their mother in her current unhealthy state. There appeared to be no mutually acceptable means that respected the concerns of both sides. To the physician, performing the lumbar puncture seemed to be the only way to make an accurate diagnosis and identify appropriate treatments; to the patient and family, leaving the hospital to participate in a healing ceremony appeared to be the sole path to restoring harmony.

In applying our approach to case 2, the requirements of integrity indicate that the physician should engage in a critical process of examining, and possibly reconfiguring, her values. Earlier, we noted that altering one's values is possible without compromising personal integrity. How might the physician in case 2 weigh her values differently in view of the circumstances of the case? Although the physician perceives her primary responsibility to be minimizing Mrs. Tsosie's risks of morbidity and mortality, she also subscribes to values other than preservation of life and avoidance of harm. Among the physician's other values are respect for patient autonomy and self-determination. Thus, the contemporary Western ethics that this physician endorses pays homage to the idea that all persons possess a right to liberty and to freedom from interference by outside parties.

Evaluating these commitments in the context of the case, the physician might decide, on balance, to assign greater weight to the value of freedom from outside interference, represented by having the family pursue other (non-Western) modes of healing. This would entail assigning comparatively less weight to saving life and avoiding harm in situations where the patient or a valid surrogate prefers to incur risks. On this analysis, the physician does not sever her attachment to prior values. Instead, she casts these values in a different light by considering them in the context of other values that apply to the case. Needless to say, from the patient's perspective the Western ethics the physician endorses would appear unfamiliar, and perhaps unappealing. Yet despite disparate value frameworks, the physician and patient may be able to agree about how the medical encounter should proceed.

A different, and more demanding, strategy would be for the physician not only to reinterpret her present values but to make fundamental changes in them. Individuals compelled to reexamine their values in new situations generally resist making more than the minimal changes necessary to resolve the immediate problem. This avoids constant and disruptive upheavals in value frameworks. Had an examination of basic values been necessary in case 2, it might have taken the following form. The physician might have initially placed considerable emphasis on benefitting the patient, and interpreted benefitting her to mean performing the lumbar puncture. She might have reasoned at the outset that any disappointment resulting from omitting a healing ceremony was far outweighed by the benefit of accurately diagnosing and treating Mrs. Tsosie's illness. Yet the meaning the physician assigned to beneficence might have undergone a profound change had the physician exerted a genuine effort to understand Mrs. Tsosie's perspective. Mrs. Tsosie, like other traditional Navajos, viewed herself primarily in the context of her relationships with others and with the physical and spiritual universe. She held in high regard the values of connectedness and solidarity with others and with nature. In keeping with traditional Navajo practice, Mrs. Tsosie might have regularly included her family members in medical decisions, or deferred to them entirely. Thus, from her perspective it would be comforting and right to know that her daughters were looking out for her interests. Similarly, the healing ceremony is intended to establish in Mrs. Tsosie a state of harmony and balance. Whereas "in the hospital a Navajo is lonely and homesick, living by a strange routine and eating unfamiliar foods ... during the chant [of a traditional ceremony] the patient feels himself personally ... being succored and loved, for his relatives are ... rallying round to aid in the ceremonial."[28]

These considerations might have led the physician to think empathically about the meaning of benefit from the patient's perspective and the perspective of her traditional Navajo culture. For example, the physician might ask herself, Do the benefits of competent diagnosis and treatment fit into the broader view of what the patient conceives as the good life? This question may lead the physician to see the paradox of applying the word *benefit* to an outcome that the person in question does not appreciate. Although the physician does not subscribe to traditional Navajo medicine, she may come to appreciate that the patient would benefit by participating in a healing ceremony. Although the physician does not concur with the daughters' wish to refuse the lumbar puncture, she may nevertheless recognize that Mrs. Tsosie stands to benefit by placing matters in her daughters' hands. Understood in this light, the subject of medicine becomes the suffering patient, and the injunction to benefit the patient does not necessarily require producing certain physiological effects on the body, but requires instead caring for the patient and producing outcomes that patients themselves can appreciate.

In the actual resolution of the case, Mrs. Tsosie's daughters took her out of the hospital to participate in a healing ceremony. In reflecting on the case, the physician felt she had acted in accordance with her sense of professional integrity. The patient's daughters also felt a sense of closure about the case, as they had abided by their mother's wishes and met their filial duties toward her.

As our framework and case analyses attest, health professionals who treat patients from cultures different from their own should expect to devise alternative ways of interacting with patients. But this need not entail giving up the fundamental values the provider holds. Instead, our approach advises health professionals to step back from their ordinary manner of relating to patients to distill the underlying purposes and goals of the medical encounter. This enables the provider to find a manner of coping with differences that respects the integrity of both provider and patient. We acknowledge the likelihood that disparate values will at times require reexamination in light of the context and relationships at stake in the case. In such instances, no practical measure may be available that is consistent with the values espoused by both parties. Faced with an intractable conflict of values, health care providers must interpret and weigh their values with sensitivity to context. Reaching a resolution may not be possible unless one or more parties reshape their values in light of the circumstances of the case. We underscore the point that genuine integrity requires humility and openness to change.

Although we have pressed the idea of integrity throughout, we also recognize its potential limits. Hence, we recognize that on some occasions it may not be possible to preserve the integrity of both sides and reach a resolution to the case. There will be occasions where a provider or patient regards the other's values as not only different but wrong or extremely offensive and therefore is unable to accommodate them. Although we are not aware of Navajo medical practices that Westerners would view in this extreme manner, there are many examples from other non-Western cultures. For example, most Western providers find wrong and offensive the practice of clitoridectomy, or excision of the clitoris, that is practiced in parts of Africa, and would refuse to meet an African patient's request for this procedure.

We submit that under circumstances where Western eyes see non-Western health care decisions as wrong, preference should not automatically be given to Western medicine and its representatives. Instead, a "negotiated settlement" of conflict should occur (Figure 3).[29] This requires both sides to agree upon a fair procedure for resolving of differences. Although the specific details of such a procedure can be developed to address the concerns at hand, the core idea is that intercultural disagreement should be publicly argued and negotiated. Beyond

---

Figure 3. Third Level of Ethical Analysis.
Requirements
Adjudicate differences through a fair procedure
that reflects a nonjudgmental stance
Justification
Inequalities of power in the provider-patient
relationship must be recognized and patients
protected against abuses

---

agreement on procedural standards of adjudication, it may be exceedingly difficult in cross-cultural situations to resolve ethical disagreements by finding substantive cross-cultural ethical generalizations to apply to the situation. As others have noted,

> What has made objectifying representations and universalist claims [in ethics] particularly offensive ... are ... the asymmetries of power that have prevented [people from nondominant cultures] ... from participating in the conversation on equal footing.[30]

To avoid imposing foreign values on either patient or physician, both parties should refrain from assuming that their own ethical standards and cultural traditions represent universally valid truths. Rather, a fair adjudicative process will call initially for a nonjudgmental stance, in which both provider and patient are regarded as having equally important ethical concerns.

One basis for requiring an equal starting point is the presumption that diverse cultures possess worth and dignity. This presumption may be defended on the ground that

> it is reasonable to suppose that cultures that have provided the horizon of meaning for large numbers of human beings of diverse characters and temperaments, over a long period of time ... are almost certain to have something that deserves our admiration and respect ... it would take a supreme arrogance to discount this possibility *a priori*.[31]

Alternatively, requiring an equal starting point may be justified by appealing, not to the worth or truth of different cultural beliefs and practices, but to the assumption that both provider and patient are equally invested in their cultures. For example, when providers feel strongly that Western medical practices are valid, a nonjudgmental stance is called for because patients feel just as strongly that their cultural beliefs and practices are valid.

In light of these considerations, we propose that a fair procedure for resolving cultural differences reflects a presumption of the equal validity of both sides' views. This requires a process involving a balanced representation of individuals from both Western medicine and the patient's culture. Initially, adjudication might proceed through a process of discovery, analogous to what occurs in legal proceedings. In the cross-cultural setting, discovery entails gathering further information about the patient's culture and way of life as well as the professional and personal values of the health care worker. The specific details of the case can then guide the adjudicative process toward a resolution.

In response to our proposal it might be objected that in fact we have not avoided the errors of arrogance and cultural imperialism. Instead, we have proposed applying Western democratic standards of adjudication upon people from non-Western cultures. Worse, we have defended and elaborated this approach by appealing to concepts such as integrity and procedural justice as interpreted and developed by Western moral philosophers. Perhaps our model for resolving cross-cultural differences would persuade Western readers, but how might we rationally defend our position to persons who have no ethical concept corresponding to our idea of "integrity"?

Our reply to this objection can only be to admit that our ethical approach reflects Western meanings and values. Rather than presuming to "step outside" our own cultural traditions, or presuming to represent all cultural perspectives, we have sought to find within our own ethical traditions a meaningful way for Western providers to understand and help to resolve intercultural differences. We fully expect that members of non-Western cultures will appeal to concepts and ideas quite different from the ones we have developed. If diverse cultural justifications can be given for the kind of intercultural adjudication we propose, this only strengthens the practical usefulness of the approach.

In closing, although we have suggested a philosophical grounding for our proposal in the concept of ethical integrity, its ultimate validity turns on its practical usefulness. We therefore welcome the application of our approach to diverse cross-cultural settings, including those in which health care providers belong to a cultural minority and patients come from a dominant cultural group. The varied contexts and circumstances in which our approach is deployed should direct its further refinement.

Acknowledgments

The cases described in the paper are drawn from the experience of one of the authors (JC) who practiced medicine for four years on the Navajo Indian reservation in northeast Arizona. The authors express appreciation to members of the Navajo tribe whose stories inspired them to reflect more deeply about medicine and culture.

The authors also wish to thank Linda L. Emanuel, Albert R. Jonsen, Arthur Kleinman, and Gary Witherspoon for generous assistance with the paper.

NJ received financial support for this project from the Robert Wood Johnson Clinical Scholars Program, Seattle. JC was a V.A. fellow in the Robert Wood Johnson Clinical Scholars Program, Seattle, when this paper was written. The views expressed in this paper do not necessarily reflect the views of the Robert Wood Johnson Foundation or of any individuals who provided assistance with the paper.

Notes

1. Norma C. Ware and Arthur R. Kleinman, "Culture and Somatic Experience," *Psychosomatic Medicine* 54 (1992): 546-60.

2. Judith Barker, "Cultural Diversity—Changing the Context of Medical Practice," *Western Journal of Medicine* 157, no. 3, (1992): 248-54: Alan M. Kraut, "Healers and Strangers: Immigrant Attitudes toward the Physician in America—A Relationship in Historical Perspective," *JAMA* 263 (1990): 1807-11.

3. Renée C. Fox and Judith P. Swazey, "Medical Morality Is Not Bioethics—Medical Ethics in China and the United States," *Perspectives in Biology and Medicine 27,* no. 3 (1984): 336-60, at 356.

4. Barker, "Cultural Diversity," p. 251.

5. C. E. Harris, *Applying Moral Theories,* 2nd ed. (Belmont, Calif.: Wadsworth Publishing Company, 1992).

6. Howard Brody, *Ethical Decisions in Medicine*, 2nd ed. (Boston: Little, Brown and Company, 1981).

7. John F. Kilner, "Who Shall Be Saved: An African Answer," *Hastings Center Report* 14, no. 3 (1984): 19-22, Peter Lurie et al., "Ethical, Behavioral, and Social Aspects of HIV Vaccine Trials in Developing Countries," *JAMA* 271 (1994): 295-301; John Klessig, "The Effect of Values and Culture on Life Support Decisions" *Western Journal of Medicine* 157, no. 3 (1992): 316-21.

8. Peter Kunstadter, "Medical Ethics in Cross-Cultural Perspective," *Social Science and Medicine* 14B (1980): 289-96; Geri-Ann Galanti, *Caring for Patients from different Cultures* (Philadelphia: University of Pennsylvania Press, 1991); Robert Veatch, *Cross Cultural Perspectives in Medical Ethics* (Boston: Jones and Bartlett, 1989).

9. Azim A. Nanji, "Medical Ethics and the Islamic Tradition," *Journal of Medicine and Philosophy* 13 (1988): 257-75; Zbigniew Szawarski, "Poland: Biomedical Ethics in a Socialist State," Special Supplement, *Hastings Center Report* 17, no. 3 (1987): 27-29; Bertha Mo, "Modesty, Sexuality, and Breast Health in Chinese-American Women," *Western Journal of Medicine* 157, no. 3 (1992): 260-64.

10. D. F. Philip, "New Voices Ask to Be Heard in Bioethics," *Cambridge Quarterly of Healthcare Ethics* 2 (1992): 169-77.

11. Arthur R. Kleinman, "Anthropology of Bioethics," in *Encyclopedia of Bioethics*, 2nd ed., ed. Warren T. Reich (New York: Macmillian, forthcoming); George Weisz, ed., *Social Science Perspectives on Medical Ethics* (Philadelphia: University of Pennsylvania Press, 1990); Patricia A. Marshall, "Anthropology and Bioethics," *Medical Anthropology Quarterly* 6, no. 1 (1992): 49-73.

12. Arthur R. Kleinman, *The Illness Narratives* (New York: Basic Books, 1988).

13. Lawrence R. Churchill and J.J. Siman, "Principles and the Search for Moral Certainty," *Social Science and Medicine* 23 (1986): 461-68.

14. Lisa Belkin, "Patients Say 'Ah' in Many Languages," *New York Times,* 31 December 1992.

15. American College of Physicians, Ethics Committee, American College of Physicians Ethics Manual, 3rd

ed., *Annals of Internal Medicine* 117, no. 11 (1992): 947-60.

16. Gabriele Taylor and Raimond Gaita, "Integrity," *Proceedings of the Aristotelian Society Supplement* 55 (1981): 143-59; Lynn McFall, "Integrity," *Ethics* 98, no. 1 (1987): 5-20.

17. Bernard Williams, *Moral Luck* (Cambridge: Cambridge University Press, 1981), pp. 40-53.

18. Albert R. Jonsen and Stephen Toulmin, *The Abuse of Casuistry* (Berkeley and Los Angeles: University of California Press, 1988), p. 17.

19. John Rawls, "An Outline for a Decision Procedure for Ethics," *Philosophical Review* 60, no. 2 (1950): 177-97.

20. Linda L. Emanuel and Ezekiel J. Emanuel, "Four Models of the Physician-Patient Relationship," *JAMA* 267 (1992): 2221-26, at 2222.

21. Martin Benjamin, *Splitting the Difference: Compromise and Integrity in Ethics and Politics* (Lawrence: University Press of Kansas, 1990).

22. Jeffrey Blustein, *Care and Commitment* (New York: Oxford University Press, 1992).

23. David C. Thomasma, "The Context as a Moral Rule in Medicine," *Journal of Bioethics* 5, no. 1 (1984): 63-79.

24. Thomas H. Murray, "Medical Ethics, Moral Philosophy and Moral Tradition," *Social Science and Medicine* 25, no.6 (1987): 637-44.

25. Stephen Toulmin, "The Tyranny of Principles," *Hastings Center Report* 11, no. 6 (1981): 31-39.

26. Gary Witherspoon, *Language and Art in the Navajo Universe* (Ann Arbor: University of Michigan Press, 1977).

27. S.J. Kunitz and J.E. Levy, "Navajos," in *Ethnicity and Medical Care,* ed. Allen Hardwood (Cambridge: Harvard University Press, 1981), pp. 337-95.

28. Clyde Kluckhohn and D. Leighton, *The Navajo* (Cambridge, Mass.: Harvard University Press, 1974).

29. Nicholas A. Christakis and Morris J. Panner, "Existing International Guidelines for Human Subjects Research," *Law, Medicine & Health Care* 19, no. 3-4 (1991): 214-21.

30. Thomas McCarthy, "Doing the Right Thing in Cross-Cultural Representation," *Ethics* 102, no. 3 (1992): 635-49.

31. Charles Taylor, *Multiculturalism and the Politics of Recognition* (Princeton, N.J.:Princeton University Press, 1992), pp. 25-74, at 72-73.

6.
INTEGRITY IN CROSS-CULTURAL CLINICAL ENCOUNTERS

Elisabeth Boetzkes

INTRODUCTION

In this paper I examine the recent proposal by Jecker, Carrese and Pearlman (hereafter, the Jecker proposal) for preserving integrity in cross-cultural clinical encounters.[1] While the Jecker proposal rightly identifies some of the ethical hazards in such encounters (for instance, the imperialism of Western ethical views, and the asymmetries that jeopardize equality in clinical negotiation), its three-stage solution gives inadequate protection to the patient/client. A more consistent analysis of the notion of integrity, combined with a sensitivity to the social and cultural determinants of one's moral outlook, will serve clients better.

In her appeal for a specialty in ethnonursing, Madeleine Leininger catalogues the dangers of dismissing cultural differences between client/patient and clinician.[2] Ethnic differences, she claims, may discourage people from seeking medical help. If they do seek help, they are often afraid to reveal their own cultural perspectives and, fearing lack of understanding or dismissal, they consent to suggested procedures out of politeness only. A consequence of this, not surprisingly, is poor cooperation in treatment plans, with recovery rates negatively affected, and persons feeling uncared for, disenchanted, alienated, and sometimes even threatening to sue! Thus, cultural differences have significance for care. Furthermore, as Leininger points out, such differences are not superficial; systems of meaning and ways of life embed patient disclosure and treatment preferences. Current Western practices, such as comforting by touch, inviting fathers to bond with their newborns, or encouraging self-reliance in the elderly, may constitute a cross-cultural affront. Touching practices reflect notions of privacy, dignity, and bodily integrity; parental bonding reflects notions about gender roles; and attitudes towards older patients reflect notions of filial obligation, the division of labour, and communal self-understanding (that is,

individualistic versus communitarian models of social existence).

These examples highlight the way in which deeply-embedded culture-specific attitudes and practices might be mismatched, leading to misunderstanding or even harm. Sometimes such cultural differences challenge not just the overall clinical culture, but specific clinical judgments. What if the client's treatment preferences include home remedies, a prayer circle, or even exorcism, procedures viewed as ineffective or even dangerous by the clinician? How much may she diverge from what she views as sound clinical practice to accommodate such preferences and still preserve her integrity? How far may the client be swayed by the clinician's judgment, and yet maintain her own?

Preserving integrity is not just a matter of increasing cultural sensitivity. A satisfactory analysis of the requirements for integrity must take seriously the social and political context of multiculturalism and clinical practice.[3] For cultural mismatches are exacerbated by biases arising from ethnic and racial prejudice and residual medical authoritarianism. These social realities may considerably inhibit the capacity of clients to express their wishes and of clinicians to listen to them sympathetically. While the clinician is asking, "Can I reconcile the requested procedure with my notion of good patient care?," the client may be struggling to find the courage to reveal non-standard preferences or to challenge authority. Therefore, preserving integrity must be both bi-lateral and fully contextualised, with a realistic recognition of existing asymmetries.

INTEGRITY

Recent ethical discussions have not shed much light on the problem of integrity in cross-cultural clinical practice. For instance, Michael Bayles, in his comprehensive discussion of professional ethics,[4] adopts a neo-Rawlsian approach, which evaluates the actions of professionals in terms of what "a reasonable member of the society might approve," overlooking the lack of cultural homogeneity within many societies and thus rendering the "test" of acceptable professional behaviour unhelpful. Kluge, in his *Bioethics in a Canadian Context*, refers to cultural differences (for instance, in his discussion of disclosure) and encourages us to increase our sensitivity and understanding, but this reduces the problematic situation to an epistemic one.[5] No advice is given as to how to proceed with integrity where cultural differences over treatments emerge.

Feminists have deepened the debate by asking how we can justify ethical criticism of such culture-relative practices as cosmetic surgery, footbinding, and genital mutilation. Operating in the tension between the context-sensitivity of ethical relativism (which must approve or at least tolerate such practices) and the absolutism required to condemn gender oppression, some have proposed a theoretical option between the two. For instance, in *No Longer Patient*, Susan Sherwin argues that cultural ethical perspectives must be respected only when they have been reached by a process of fair representation.[6] Thus, cultural viewpoints determined in the absence of groups affected by them and required to live by them need not be viewed by others as authoritative. Applied to the present question of cross-cultural clinical encounters, Sherwin's view would require that the clinician evaluate the history of dialogical procedures in the community to which the client belongs in order to decide what weight to put on her wishes. However, such a recommendation is epistemically problematic (can a clinician perform such a feat, and is she qualified to do so?) and overlooks an important interest of the client/patient.

What would an adequate account of integrity in cross-cultural clinical encounters involve, and how does the Jecker proposal measure up?

The Jecker proposal suggests a three-stage approach to preserving integrity in cross-cultural settings. Sound practice, say the authors, involves identifying mutually acceptable goals and strategies, both of which must be compatible with the ethical integrity of client and caregiver. Nothing is said about impasses over goals; however, where means

are being sought, the three-stage approach to preserving integrity is described. First, if the suggested means are compatible with the "health care provider's conscientiously held beliefs" and "the patient's values and the values of the culture with which the patient identifies," then the integrity requirement has already been met, for, they say, "Integrity requires acting in accordance with ethical convictions and beliefs that are one's own."[7] When agreement is problematic, we must move to the second stage. Here client and clinician are to reexamine their values, to see whether there is flexibility from within the value structure to reorder, reinterpret or change values so as to arrive at the desired agreement. An example from Western ethics would be to prioritize autonomy over non-maleficence by reinterpreting harm as the contravention of client's wishes. Stage two passes the integrity test because, say the authors, "Integrity requires scrutinizing one's values and regarding them as open to criticism and improvement."[8] If the respective re-assessment of values fails, the parties must move to stage three, where public negotiation and adjudication take place within a starting framework of mutual respect for basic cultural differences and with correctives in place to protect the client's cultural representative from being overpowered by the dominant medical ethical culture. At this third stage, the integrity paradigm is abandoned in favour of something like procedural justice.

What is admirable about the Jecker proposal is that it acknowledges the importance of bilateral integrity, and the reality of power asymmetries in the clinical situation—asymmetries arising from both residual medical paternalism and the dominance of Western ethical thinking. Unlike Bayles's account, it acknowledges cultural heterogeneity; unlike Kluge's, it recognizes that sensitivity may not be enough—often negotiation is called for. However, I will argue that neither stage one nor stage three adequately protects the client or preserves integrity.

CRITIQUE OF THE JECKER PROPOSAL

Integrity is preserved in stage one, say Jecker *et al*, because integrity is a matter of acting in accordance with one's own personal convictions. By stage two, however, a very different model of integrity is being appealed to—one which identifies integrity with self-scrutiny. Are the authors being inconsistent? Do they realize they are appealing to two different views? Can one account of integrity be reduced to the other? Is one preferable to the other? While we could render the Jecker account consistent by viewing self-scrutiny as simply a means of arriving at personal convictions according to which one acts, (that is, seeing stage two integrity as reducing to stage one) other comments they make suggest they would resist this reduction. For example, they justify their self-scrutiny interpretation of integrity by saying that persons of integrity "regard their moral convictions as potentially mistaken and as continuously open to criticism and improvement in the wake of new circumstances and challenges."[9] This dynamic view is in stark contrast to the inherently conservative view of integrity supposed to be adequate for stage one.

I suggest that, when examined, two different notions of integrity are being appealed to in the Jecker proposal, and that the second, the dynamic view of integrity as self-scrutiny, is superior when applied to cross-cultural clinical encounters.

Why?

In a recent article, Victoria Davion challenges the "received view" of integrity and proposes a revision to it.[10] According to traditional moral thinking (and stage one of the Jecker proposal), integrity is a matter of making an unconditional commitment to certain principles and acting out of that commitment. Davion criticizes this view on feminist grounds, for it fails to acknowledge both the possibility of a radical change in moral viewpoint and the contingency of our view of the world. Feminist analysis shows that our interpretation of reality may be skewed by dominant social interests and that radical consciousness-raising is possible. Not wanting to deny that moral identity and integrity could be maintained through such a process, Davion suggests instead that integrity be viewed as a commitment to a process of self-scrutiny (stage two of the Jecker proposal), rather than commitment to a set of substantive principles.

Davion's view has intuitive appeal. We would hardly deny integrity to the Somali who calls into question her acceptance of genital mutilation, or the Sikh who questions his son's preference, or the Western white who challenges the social norms that encourage breast implants. Indeed, the absence of self-scrutiny over such matters would invite scepticism about integrity. Acting out of my deeply held, but unquestioned, convictions seems insufficient for preserving integrity; challenging my deeply held convictions seems insufficient for its being denied to me.

Integrity, then, is arguably not just a matter of acting out of deeply held convictions, but of consciously scrutinizing one's values and evaluating their adequacy. It follows, then, that when client and clinician agree about goals and means, at Jecker's stage one, they don't necessarily have integrity.

Are we to require that they scrutinize their goals and the values underlying them?

There are sound client-centred reasons for insisting on self-scrutiny, even where there seems to be agreement. Two arguments may be presented in favour of raising the standard of integrity at stage one. First, Jecker *et al* acknowledge that inequalities may exist in cross-cultural clinical settings; that is why, at stage three, they recommend that we employ correctives against the domination of the vulnerable. But surely asymmetries exist in the narrower clinical setting too; as we have seen, clients may assent out of deference or fear, and if so, a humble willingness on the part of clinicians to put accepted values on the table for assessment might be an effective corrective against client self-effacement (not to mention clinician complacency!). Second, since values are appropriated in social settings, and not always autonomously, self-scrutiny on the part of the client provides her with an opportunity to evaluate the scope of her identification with the values of her community, and of the possible coercive influences that have shaped her moral thinking. In a clinical setting, engaged in a mutual re-examination of moral viewpoints, the client may be protected from the immediacy of others' interests and influences and encouraged to assert her own. The clinical encounter may provide her with a welcome critical distance from the culture that has formed her moral outlook, a distance that might result either in a reinforced commitment to it or reasoned deviation from it. Either way, client interests are served. Therefore, I am suggesting that at stage one, even where there is agreement over goals and means, the self-scrutiny standard of integrity should be applied.

What of stage three? At stage three, a public hearing takes place, in which cultural differences are negotiated against a background presumption of cultural equality. Data on the respective cultures from which client and clinician have emerged is collected, and differences are adjudicated by procedures agreed upon as fair by both sides. The merit of stage three is not that it preserves integrity (this has been jettisoned at stage two) but that it meets the requirements of justice. Stage three is just because it offsets asymmetries of authority and because it acknowledges, "that both provider and patient are equally invested in their cultures."[11]

Once again, however, there are sound client-centred reasons for concern. First, as Sherwin has pointed out, if a culture has been oppressive, and we are appealing to a notion of justice in activating stage three, can we simultaneously adopt the *a priori* position that cultures are equally authoritative for their members on moral matters?

Perhaps a better justification of stage three is the respective identification of each party with her culture. But this position too is problematic. For, as our critique of stage one revealed, persons may be ambivalent towards some aspects of their cultural formation, while nevertheless identifying strongly with it. Furthermore, the cultural home of any given individual may not be so easy to identify.

When discussing the dynamic model of integrity, Davion refers to the phenomenon of "multiplicitous selves," individuals who identify simultaneously with a number of cultural groups, groups which represent opposing moral points of view on some issues. Davion cites Maria Lugones, a lesbian Hispana-American, who denies that her identity can be reduced to one cultural membership, notwithstanding the fundamental tension that such cross-cultural identification creates for her.[12] Identifying her true self with one group or the other—indeed, requiring her to have a unitary self—is a serious violation of her personhood, she maintains. Were we to privilege one group over the other as "the culture" of multiplicitous selves for the purposes of facilitating clinical decision-making, we would lose the very benefit we are trying so hard to gain—namely, cultural sensitivity adequate for the provision of care.

Elizabeth Spelman, too, has written of the difficulties of multiple group identification.[13] Spelman, discussing the various parameters of oppression such as gender, race, and ethnicity, condemns the tendency of some theorists to dismiss one's connection to a group on the grounds that the group has been a vehicle of oppression. Notwithstanding the experience of oppression, strong cultural ties with a group are often forged, ties which one may wish to reappropriate to strengthen sense of self. Since we cannot measure for one another the respective weight of various injustices against the personal value of cultural involvement, such judgments must be left to the individuals concerned. (This is not an abandonment of the feminist principle that individual benefit should not outweigh deleterious effects on women as a group—rather, it is an observation about how to gauge those effects. Nor is it an endorsement of the provision of services judged to be dangerous to women, on demand. Policy issues are differently decided.)

Recognizing that many selves, particularly in multicultural societies, must be multiplicitous, we must question whether any assumptions can be made about the nature of an individual's moral investment in her culture, assumptions that appear to be necessary in order to justify stage three of the Jecker proposal. To the extent that stage three assumes a questionable cultural individuation, it lacks the moral authority to displace the client as spokesperson in the clinical negotiation. While nobly motivated by a rejection of cultural imperialism and a commitment to equality, stage three effectively jeopardizes the moral identity and autonomy of the client at a time when both could be vital to her well-being.

CONCLUSION

Maintaining integrity in cross-cultural clinical encounters is a matter of a bi-lateral exercise in self-scrutiny (i.e., stage two of the Jecker proposal). Recognizing that bias and paternalism are recurrent dangers in such encounters, a willingness to reassess one's moral position is both a corrective to clinician complacency and a way of creating a needed critical distance for clients from their cultures. I have rejected stages one and three of the Jecker proposal, on the grounds that neither gives adequate protection to the client—stage one, because correctives against clinician and cultural domination are inadequate, stage three because third-party representation of the specifics of one's cultural identification is impossible. It remains only to consider what to do if an impasse cannot be resolved, and whether the high standard of integrity I have endorsed is a practical measure.

My argument does not propose a solution to cross-cultural impasse nor to disagreements about goals. It suggests only that stage three is not an adequate answer to a breakdown in cross-cultural negotiation. If thorough bilateral scrutiny cannot bring persons to an agreement about means, there is clearly no mandate for clinicians to simply comply with client demands; neither may they abandon clients. As has been argued in familiar cases, a caring relationship is compatible with drawing lines to preserve integrity. In some cases, adopting the revisionist view of integrity simply postpones the breakdown. A mutual recognition of the effort involved in self-scrutiny will surely generate mutual respect and help to offset feelings of client abandonment.

And its practicality? Although maintaining integrity through self-scrutiny is more time-consuming than acting on agreement alone, it has precedents and much to be said in its favour. Precedents in good clinical practice include reproductive counselling, where unilateral scrutiny at least is viewed as appropriate, even though it clearly takes longer than simply performing the respective procedures. Indeed, as disclosure standards are raised, client/clinician dialogue is something for which time must be budgeted, in the interests of both client autonomy and well-being. The present argument simply adds integrity to the list of benefits to be gained by such dialogue.

Notes

1. Nancy S. Jecker, Joseph A. Carrese, and Robert A. Pearlman, "Caring for Patients in Cross-Cultural Settings," *Hastings Center Report* (January-February, 1995): 6-14.
2. Madeleine Leininger, "Culture: The Conspicuous Missing Link to Understand Ethical and Moral Dimensions of Human Care," *Ethical and Moral Dimensions of Care,* ed. Madeleine Leininger (Detroit: Wayne State University Press, 1990).
3. S. Sherwin, "A Relational Approach to Autonomy in Health Care," *The Politics of Women's Health*, ed. Susan Sherwin (Philadelphia: Temple University Press, 1998), 19-47.
4. Michael Bayles, *Professional Ethics* (Belmont, CA: Wadsworth, 1989).
5. Eike-Henner Kluge, *Biomedical Ethics in a Canadian Context* (Scarborough, ON: Prentice-Hall, 1992).
6. Susan Sherwin, *No Longer Patient* (Philadelphia: Temple University Press, 1992).
7. Jecker *et al* 8.
8. Jecker *et al.*
9. Jecker *et al.*
10. Victoria Davion, "Integrity and Radical Change," *Feminist Ethics,* ed. Claudia Card (Lawrence, KS: University of Kansas Press, 1991).
11. Jecker *et al* 13.
12. Davion 187 ff.
13. Elizabeth Spelman, *Inessential Woman* (Boston: Beacon Press, 1988).

7.
WHAT ABOUT THE FAMILY?

John Hardwig

We are beginning to recognize that the prevalent ethic of patient autonomy simply will not do. Since demands for health care are virtually unlimited, giving autonomous patients the care they want will bankrupt our health care system. We can no longer simply buy our way out of difficult questions of justice by expanding the health care pie until there is enough to satisfy the wants and needs of everyone. The requirements of justice and the needs of other patients must temper the claims of autonomous patients.

But if the legitimate claims of other patients and other (non-medical) interests of society are beginning to be recognized, another question is still largely ignored: To what extent can the patient's family legitimately be asked or required to sacrifice their interests so that the patient can have the treatment he or she wants?

This question is not only almost universally ignored, it is generally implicitly dismissed, silenced before it can even be raised. This tacit dismissal results from a fundamental assumption of medical ethics: medical treatment ought always to serve the interests of the patient. This, of course, implies that the interests of family members should be irrelevant to medical treatment decisions or at least ought never to take precedence over the interests of the patient. All questions about fairness to the interests of family members are thus precluded, regardless of the merit or importance of the interests that will have to be sacrificed if the patient is to receive optimal treatment.

Yet there is a whole range of cases in which important interests of family members are dramatically affected by decisions about the patient's treatment; medical decisions often should be made with those interests in mind. Indeed, in many cases family members have a greater interest than the patient in which treatment option is exercised. In such cases, the interests of family members often ought to *override* those of the patient.

The problem of family interests cannot be resolved by considering other members of the family as "patients," thereby redefining the problem as one of conflicting interests among *patients*. Other members of the family are not always ill, and even if ill, they still may not be patients. Nor will it do to define the whole family as one patient. Granted, the slogan "the patient is the family" was coined partly to draw attention to precisely the issues I wish to raise, but the idea that the whole family is one patient is too monolithic. The conflicts of interests, beliefs, and values among family members are often too real and run too deep to treat all members as "the patient." Thus, if I am correct, it is sometimes the moral thing to do for a physician to sacrifice the interests of her patient to those of nonpatients—specifically, to those of the other members of the patient's family.

But what is the "family"? As I will use it here, it will mean roughly "those who are close to the patient." "Family" so defined will often include close friends and companions. It may also exclude some with blood or marriage ties to the patient. "Closeness" does not, however, always mean care and abiding affection, nor need it be a positive experience—one can hate, resent, fear, or despise a mother or brother with an intensity not often directed toward strangers, acquaintances, or associates. But there are cases where even a hateful or resentful family member's interests ought to be considered.

This use of "family" gives rise to very sensitive ethical—and legal—issues in the case of legal relatives with no emotional ties to the patient that I cannot pursue here. I can only say that I do not mean to suggest that the interests of legal relatives who are not emotionally close to the patient are always to be ignored. They will sometimes have an important financial interest in the treatment even if they are not emotionally close to the patient. But blood and marriage ties can become so thin that they become *merely* legal relationships. (Consider, for example, "couples" who have long since parted but who have never gotten a divorce, or cases in which the next of kin cannot be bothered with making proxy decisions.) Obviously, there are many important questions about just whose interests are to be considered in which treatment decisions and to what extent.

CONNECTED INTERESTS

There is no way to detach the lives of patients from the lives of those who are close to them. Indeed, the intertwining of lives is part of the very meaning of closeness. Consequently, there will be a broad spectrum of cases in which the treatment options will have dramatic and different impacts on the patient's family.

I believe there are many, many such cases. To save the life of a newborn with serious defects is often dramatically to affect the rest of the parents' lives and, if they have other children, may seriously compromise the quality of their lives, as well.... The husband of a woman with Alzheimer's disease may well have a life totally dominated for ten years or more by caring for an increasingly foreign and estranged wife.... The choice between aggressive and palliative care or, for that matter, the difference between either kind of care and suicide in the case of a father with terminal cancer or AIDS may have a dramatic emotional and financial impact on his wife and children.... Less dramatically, the choice between two medications, one of which has the side effect of impotence, may radically alter the life a couple has together.... The drug of choice for controlling high blood pressure may be too expensive (that is, requires too many sacrifices) for many families with incomes just above the ceiling for Medicaid....

Because the lives of those who are close are not separable, to be close is to no longer have a life entirely your own to live entirely as you choose. To be part of a family is to be morally required to make decisions on the basis of thinking about what is best for all concerned, not simply what is best for yourself. In healthy families, characterized by genuine care, one wants to make decisions on this basis, and many people do so quite naturally and automatically. My own grandfather committed suicide after his heart attack as a final gift to his wife—he had plenty of life insurance but not nearly enough health insurance, and he feared that she would be left homeless and destitute if he lingered on in an incapacitated state. Even if one is not so inclined, however, it is irresponsible and wrong to exclude or to fail to consider the interests of those who are close. Only when the lives of family members will not be importantly affected can one rightly make exclusively or even predominantly self-regarding decisions.

Although "what is best for all concerned" sounds utilitarian, my position does not imply that the right course of action results simply from a calculation of what is best for all. No, the seriously ill may have a right to special consideration, and the family of an ill person may have a duty to make sacrifices to respond to a members's illness. It is one thing to claim that the ill deserve special consideration; it is quite another to maintain that they deserve exclusive or even overriding consideration. Surely we must admit that there are limits to the right to special treatment by virtue of illness. Otherwise, everyone would be morally required to sacrifice all other goods to better care for the ill. We must also recognize that patients too have moral obligations, obligations to try to protect the lives of their families from destruction resulting from their illnesses.

Thus, unless serious illness excuses one from all moral responsibility—and I don't see how it could—it is an oversimplification to say of a patient who is part of a family that "it's his life" or "after all, it's his medical treatment," as if his life and his treatment could be successfully isolated from the lives of the other members of his family. It is more accurate to say "it's their lives" or "after all, they're all going to have to live with his treatment." Then the really serious moral questions are not *whether* the interests of family members are relevant to decisions about a patient's medical treatment or *whether* their interests should be included in his deliberations or in deliberations about him, but how far family and friends can be asked to support and sustain the patient. What sacrifices can they be morally required to make for his health care? How far can they reasonably be asked to compromise the quality of their lives so that he will receive the care that would improve the quality of his life? To what extent can he reasonably expect them to put their lives "on hold" to preoccupy themselves with his illness to the extent necessary to care for him?

THE ANOMALY OF MEDICAL DECISION MAKING

The way we analyze medical treatment decisions by or for patients is plainly anomalous to the way we think about other important decisions family members make. I am a husband, a father, and still a son, and no one would argue that I should or even responsibly could decide to take a sabbatical, another job, or even a weekend trip *solely* on the basis of what I want for myself. Why should decisions about my medical treatment be different? Why should we have even *thought* that medical treatment decisions might be different?

Is it because medical decisions, uniquely, involve life and death matters? Most medical decisions, however, are not matters of life and death, and we as a society risk or shorten the lives of other people— through our toxic waste disposal decisions, for example—quite apart from considerations of whether that is what they want for themselves.

Have we been misled by a preoccupation with the biophysical model of disease? Perhaps it has tempted us to think of illness and hence also of treatment as something that takes place *within* the body of the patient. What happens in my body does not—barring contagion—affect my wife's body, yet it usually does affect her.

Have we tacitly desired to simplify the practice and the ethics of medicine by considering only the *medical* or health-related consequences of treatment decisions? Perhaps, but it is obvious that we need a broader vision of and sensitivity to *all* the consequences of action, at least among those who are not simply technicians following orders from above. Generals need to consider more than military consequences, businessmen more than economic consequences, teachers more than educational consequences, lawyers more than legal consequences.

Does the weakness and vulnerability of serious illness imply that the ill need such protection that we should serve only their interests? Those who are sick may indeed need special protection, but this can only mean that we must take special care to see that the interests of the ill are duly considered. It does not

follow that their interests are to be served exclusively or even that their interests must always predominate. Moreover, we must remember that in terms of the dynamics of the family, the patient is not always the weakest member, the member most in need of protection.

Does it make *historical*, if not logical, sense to view the wishes and interests of the patient as always overriding? Historically, illnesses were generally of much shorter duration; patients got better quickly or died quickly. Moreover, the costs of the medical care available were small enough that rarely was one's future mortgaged to the costs of the care of family members. Although this was once truer than it is today, there have always been significant exceptions to these generalizations.

None of these considerations adequately explains why the interests of the patient's family have been thought to be appropriately excluded from consideration. At the very least, those who believe that medical treatment decisions are morally anomalous to other important decisions owe us a better account of how and why this is so.

LIMITS OF PUBLIC POLICY

It might be thought that the problem of family interests *is* a problem only because our society does not shelter families from the negative effects of medical decisions. If, for example, we adopted a comprehensive system of national health insurance and also a system of public insurance to guarantee the incomes of families, then my sons' chances at a college education and the quality of the rest of their lives might not have to be sacrificed were I to receive optimal medical care.

However, it is worth pointing out that we are still moving primarily in the *opposite* direction. Instead of designing policies that would increasingly shelter family members from the adverse impact of serious and prolonged illnesses, we are still attempting to shift the burden of care to family members in our efforts to contain medical costs. A social system that would safeguard families from the impact of serious illness is nowhere in sight in this country. And we must not do medical ethics as if it were.

It is perhaps even more important to recognize that the lives of family members could not be sheltered from all the important ramifications of medical treatment decisions by *any* set of public policies. In any society in which people get close to each other and care deeply for each other, treatment decisions about one will often and *irremediably* affect more than one. If a newborn has been saved by aggressive treatment but is severely handicapped, the parents may simply not be emotionally capable of abandoning the child to institutional care. A man whose wife is suffering from multiple sclerosis may simply not be willing or able to go on with his own life until he sees her through to the end. A woman whose husband is being maintained in a vegetative state may not feel free to marry or even to see other men again, regardless of what some revised law might say about her marital status.

Nor could we desire a society in which friends and family would quickly lose their concern as soon as continuing to care began to diminish the quality of their own lives. For we would then have alliances for better but not for worse, in health, but not in sickness, until death appears on the horizon. And we would all be poorer for that. A man who can leave his wife the day after she learns she has cancer, on the grounds that he has his own life to live, is to be deplored. The emotional inability or principled refusal to separate ourselves and our lives from the lives of ill or dying members of our families is *not* an unfortunate fact about the structure of our emotions. It is a desirable feature, not to be changed even if it could be; not to be changed even if the resulting intertwining of lives debars us from making exclusively self-regarding treatment decisions when we are ill.

Our present individualistic medical ethics is isolating and destructive. For by implicitly suggesting that patients make "their own" treatment decisions on a self-regarding basis and supporting those who do so, such an ethics encourages each of us to see our lives as simply our own. We may yet turn ourselves into beings who are ultimately alone.

FIDELITY OR FAIRNESS?

Fidelity to the interests of the patient has been a cornerstone of both traditional codes and contemporary theories of medical ethics. The two competing paradigms of medical ethics—the "benevolence" model and the "patient autonomy" model—are simply different ways of construing such fidelity. Both must be rejected or radically modified. The admission that treatment decisions often affect more than just the patient thus forces major changes on both the theoretical and the practical level. Obviously, I can only begin to explore the needed changes here.

Instead of starting with our usual assumption that physicians are to serve the interests of the patient, we must build our theories on a very different assumption: the medical and nonmedical interests of both the patient and other members of the patient's family are to be considered. It is only in the special case of patients without family that we can simply follow the patient's wishes or pursue the patient's interests. In fact, I would argue that we must build our theory of medical ethics on the presumption of equality: the interests of patients and family members are morally to be weighed equally; medical and nonmedical interests of the same magnitude deserve equal consideration in making treatment decisions. Like any other moral presumption, this one can, perhaps, be defeated in some cases. But the burden of proof will always be on those who would advocate special consideration for any family member's interests, including those of the ill.

Even where the presumption of equality is not defeated, life, health, and freedom from pain and handicapping conditions are extremely important goods for virtually everyone. They are thus very important considerations in all treatment decisions. In the majority of cases, the patient's interest in optimal health and longer life may well be strong enough to outweigh the conflicting interests of other members of the family. But even then, some departure from the treatment plan that would maximize the patient's interests may well be justified to harmonize best the interests of all concerned or to require significantly smaller sacrifices by other family members. That the patient's interests may often outweigh the conflicting interests of others in treatment decisions is no justification for failing to recognize that an attempt to balance or harmonize different, conflicting interests is often morally required. Nor does it justify overlooking the morally crucial cases in which the interests of other members of the family ought to override the interests of the patient.

Changing our basic assumption about how treatment decisions are to be made means reconceptualizing the ethical roles of both physician and patient, since our understanding of both has been built on the presumption of patient primacy, rather than fairness to all concerned. Recognizing the moral relevance of the interests of family members thus reveals a dilemma for our understanding of what it is to be a physician: Should we retain a fiduciary ethic in which the physician is to serve the interests of her patient? Or should the physician attempt to weigh and balance all the interests of all concerned? I do not yet know just how to resolve this dilemma. All I can do here is try to envision the options.

If we retain the traditional ethic of fidelity to the interests of the patient, the physician should excuse herself from making treatment decisions that will affect the lives of the family on grounds of a moral conflict of interest, for she is a one-sided advocate. A lawyer for one of the parties cannot also serve as judge in the case. Thus, it would be unfair if a physician conceived as having a fiduciary relationship to her patient were to make treatment decisions that would adversely affect the lives of the patient's family. Indeed, a physician conceived as a patient advocate should not even *advise* patients or family members about which course of treatment should be chosen. As advocate, she can speak only to what course of treatment would be best for the patient, and must remain silent about what's best for the rest of the family or what should be done in light of everyone's interests.

Physicians might instead renounce their fiduciary relationship with their patients. On this view, physicians would no longer be agents of their patients and would not strive to be advocates for their patients' interests. Instead, the physician would aspire to be an impartial advisor who would stand knowledgeably but sympathetically outside all the many conflicting interests of those affected by the treatment options, and who would strive to discern the treatment that would best harmonize or balance the interests of all concerned.

Although this second option contradicts the Hippocratic Oath and most other codes of medical ethics, it is not, perhaps, as foreign as it may at first seem. Traditionally, many family physicians—especially small-town physicians who knew patients and their families well—attempted to attend to both medical and nonmedical interests of all concerned. Many contemporary physicians still make decisions in this way. But we do not yet have an ethical theory that explains and justifies what they are doing.

Nevertheless, we may well question the physician's ability to act as an impartial ethical observer. Increasingly, physicians do not know their patients, much less their patients' families. Moreover, we may doubt physicians' abilities to weigh evenhandedly medical and nonmedical interests. Physicians are trained to be especially responsive to medical interests and we may well want them to remain that way. Physicians also tend to be deeply involved with the interests of their patients, and it may be impossible or undesirable to break this tie to enable physicians to be more impartial advisors. Finally, when someone retains the services of a physician, it seems reasonable that she be able to expect that physician to be *her* agent, pursuing *her* interests, not those of her family.

AUTONOMY AND ADVOCACY

We must also rethink our conception of the patient. On one hand, if we continue to stress patient autonomy, we must recognize that this implies that patients have moral responsibilities. If, on the other hand, we do not want to burden patients with weighty moral responsibilities, we must abandon the ethic of patient autonomy.

Recognizing that moral responsibilities come with patient autonomy will require basic changes in the accepted meanings of both "autonomy" and "advocacy." Because medical ethics has ignored patient responsibilities, we have come to interpret "autonomy" in a sense very different from [German philosopher Immanuel] Kant's original use of the term. It has come to mean simply the patient's freedom or right to choose the treatment he believes is best for himself. But as Kant knew well, there are many situations in which people can achieve autonomy and moral well-being only by sacrificing other important dimensions of their well-being, including health, happiness, even life itself. For autonomy is the *responsible* use of freedom and is therefore diminished whenever one ignores, evades, or slights one's responsibilities. Human dignity, Kant concluded, consists in our ability to refuse to compromise our autonomy to achieve the kinds of lives (or treatments) we want for ourselves.

If, then, I am morally empowered to make decisions about "my" medical treatment; I am also morally required to shoulder the responsibility of making very difficult moral decisions. The right course of action for me to take will not always be the one that promotes my own interests.

Some patients, motivated by a deep and abiding concern for the well-being of their families, will undoubtedly consider the interests of other family members. For these patients, the interests of their family are *part* of their interests. But not all patients will feel this way. And the interests of family members are not relevant *if* and *because* the patient wants to consider them; they are not relevant because they are *part* of the patient's interests. They are relevant *whether or not* the patient is inclined to consider them. Indeed, the *ethics* of patient decisions is most poignantly highlighted precisely when the patient is inclined to decide without considering the impact of his decision on the lives of the rest of his family.

Confronting patients with tough ethical choices may be part and parcel of treating them with respect as fully competent adults. We don't, after all, think it's right to stand silently by while other (healthy) adults ignore or shirk their moral responsibilities. If, however, we believe that most patients, gripped as they often are by the emotional crisis of serious illness, are not up to shouldering the responsibility of such decisions or should not be burdened with it, then I think we must simply abandon the ethic of patient autonomy. Patient autonomy would then be appropriate only when the various treatment options will affect only the patient's life.

The responsibilities of patients imply that there is often a conflict between patient autonomy and the patient's interests (even as those interests are defined by the patient). And we will have to rethink our understanding of patient advocacy in light of this conflict: Does the patient advocate try to promote the patient's (self-defined) *interests*? Or does she promote the patient's *autonomy* even at the expense of those interests? Responsible patient advocates can hardly encourage patients to shirk their moral

responsibilities. But can we really expect health care providers to promote patient autonomy when that means encouraging their patients to sacrifice health, happiness, sometimes even life itself?

If we could give an affirmative answer to this last question, we would obviously thereby create a third option for reinterpreting the role of the physician: The physician could maintain her traditional role as patient advocate without being morally required to refrain from making treatment decisions whenever interests of the patient's family are also at stake *if* patient advocacy were understood as promoting patient autonomy *and* patient autonomy were understood as the responsible use of freedom, not simply the right to choose the treatment one wants.

Much more attention needs to be paid to all of these issues. However, it should be clear that absolutely central features of our theories of medical ethics—our understanding of physician and patient, and thus of patient advocacy as well as patient dignity, and patient autonomy—have presupposed that the interests of family members should be irrelevant or should always take a back seat to the interests of the patient. Basic conceptual shifts are required once we acknowledge that this assumption is not warranted.

WHO SHOULD DECIDE?

Such basic conceptual shifts will necessarily have ramifications that will be felt throughout the field of medical ethics, for a host of new and very different issues are raised by the inclusion of family interests. Discussions of privacy and confidentiality, of withholding/withdrawing treatment, and of surrogate decisionmaking will all have to be reconsidered in the light of the interests of the family. Many individual treatment decisions will also be affected, becoming much more complicated than they already are. Here, I will only offer a few remarks about treatment decisions, organized around the central issue of who should decide.

There are at least five answers to the question of who should make treatment decisions in cases where important interests of other family members are also at stake: the patient, the family, the physician, an ethics committee, or the courts. The physician's role in treatment decisions has already been discussed. Resort to either the courts or to ethics committees for treatment decisions is too cumbersome and time-consuming for any but the most troubling cases. So I will focus here on the contrast between the patient and the family as appropriate decision-makers. It is worth noting, though, that we need not arrive at one, uniform answer to cover all cases. On the contrary, each of the five options will undoubtedly have its place, depending on the particulars of the case at hand.

Should we still think of a patient as having the right to make decisions about "his" treatment? As we have seen, patient autonomy implies patient responsibilities. What, then, if the patient seems to be ignoring the impact of his treatment on his family? At the very least, responsible physicians must caution such patients against simply opting for treatments because they want them. Instead, physicians must speak of responsibilities and obligations. They must raise considerations of the quality of many lives, not just that of the patient. They must explain the distinction between making a decision and making it in a self-regarding manner. Thus, it will often be appropriate to make plain to patients the consequences of treatment decisions for their families and to urge them to consider these consequences in reaching a decision. And sometimes, no doubt, it will be appropriate for family members to present their cases to the patient in the hope that his decisions would be shaped by their appeals.

Nonetheless, we sometimes permit people to make bad or irresponsible decisions and *excuse* those decisions because of various pressures they were under when they made their choices. Serious illness can undoubtedly be an extenuating circumstance, and perhaps we should allow some patients to make some self-regarding decisions, especially if they insist on doing so and the negative impact of their decisions on others is not too great.

Alternatively, if we doubt that most patients have the ability to make treatment decisions that are really fair to all concerned, or if we are not prepared to accept a policy that would assign patients the responsibility of doing so, we may conclude that they should not be empowered to make treatment decisions in which the lives of their family members will be dramatically affected. Indeed, even if the patient were completely fair in making the decision,

the autonomy of other family members would have been systematically undercut by the fact that the patient alone decided.

Thus, we need to consider the autonomy of all members of the family, not just the patient's autonomy. Considerations of fairness and, paradoxically, of autonomy therefore indicate that the *family* should make the treatment decision, with all competent family members whose lives will be affected participating. Many such family conferences undoubtedly already take place. On this view, however, family conferences would often be morally *required*. And these conferences would not be limited to cases involving incompetent patients; cases involving competent patients would also often require family conferences.

Obviously, it would be completely unworkable for a physician to convene a family conference every time a medical decision might have some ramifications on the lives of family members. However, such discussion need not always take place in the presence of the physician; we can recognize that formal family conferences become more important as the impact of treatment decisions on members of the patient's family grows larger. Family conferences may thus be morally *required* only when the lives of family members would be dramatically affected by treatment decisions.

Moreover, family discussion is often morally *desirable* even if not morally required. Desirable, sometimes, even for relatively minor treatment decisions: after the family has moved to a new town, should parents commit themselves to two-hour drives so that their teenage son can continue to be treated for his acne by the dermatologist he knows and whose results he trusts? Or should he seek treatment from a new dermatologist?

Some family conferences about treatment decisions would be characterized throughout by deep affection, mutual understanding, and abiding concern for the interests of others. Other conferences might begin in an atmosphere charged with antagonism, suspicion, and hostility but move toward greater understanding, reconciliation, and harmony within the family. Such conferences would be significant goods in themselves, as well as means to ethically better treatment decisions. They would leave all family members better able to go on with their lives.

Still, family conferences cannot be expected always to begin with or move toward affection, mutual understanding, and a concern for all. If we opt for joint treatment decisions when the lives of several are affected, we need to face the fact that family conferences will sometimes be bitter confrontations in which past hostilities, anger, and resentments will surface. Sometimes, too, the conflicts of interest between patient and family, and between one family member and another will be irresolvable, forcing families to invoke the harsh perspective of justice, divisive and antagonistic though that perspective may be. Those who favor family decisions when the whole family is affected will have to face the question of whether we really want to put the patient, already frightened and weakened by his illness, through the conflict and bitter confrontations that family conferences may sometimes precipitate.

We must also recognize that family members may be unable or unwilling to press or even state their own interests before a family member who is ill. Such refusal may be admirable, even heroic; it is sometimes evidence of willingness to go "above and beyond the call of duty," even at great personal cost. But not always. Refusal to press one's own interests can also be a sign of inappropriate guilt, of a crushing sense of responsibility for the well-being of others, of acceptance of an inferior or dominated role within the family, or lack of a sense of self-worth. All of these may well be mobilized by an illness in the family. Moreover, we must not minimize the power of the medical setting to subordinate nonmedical to medical interests and to emphasize the well-being of the patient at the expense of the well-being of others. Thus, it will often be not just the patient, but also other family members who will need an advocate if a family conference is to reach the decision that best balances the autonomy and interests of all concerned.

8.
NORBERG V. WYNRIB

Supreme Court of Canada

[1992] 2 S.C.R. 226

Laura Norberg became addicted to pain killers and maintained her supply by "double doctoring"—obtaining narcotic prescriptions from doctors without telling them that she already had other prescriptions. She eventually went to Dr. Morris Wynrib who confronted her about her addiction. But instead of recommending treatment, Dr. Wynrib made it clear that he would provide her with the drug in exchange for sexual intercourse. She gave in to his demands, and soon Dr. Wynrib was directly giving her the narcotic after each sexual encounter. Not long after, Norberg was charged criminally for double doctoring and went to a rehabilitation centre on her own initiative. Then she sued Dr. Wynrib.

The Supreme Court of Canada split three ways, not on the question of *whether* Dr. Wynrib had done something wrong and so was liable to Laura Norberg for damages, but on the issue of *what* duty he owed her and which he failed to live up to. Two of the justices sought to capture this duty in a highly innovative way, one which may signal a change in our understanding of the patient-physician and other professional relationships.

Madam Justices McLachlin and L'Heureux-Dubé:
The relationship of a physician and patient can be conceptualized in a variety of ways. It can be viewed as a creature of contract, with the physician's failure to fulfil his or her obligations giving rise to an action for breach of contract. It undoubtedly gives rise to a duty of care, the breach of which constitutes the tort of negligence. In common with all members of society, the doctor owes the patient a duty not to touch him or her without his or her consent; if the doctor breaches this duty he or she will have committed the tort of battery. But perhaps the most fundamental characteristic of the doctor-patient relationship is its

fiduciary nature. All the authorities agree that the relationship of physician to patient also falls into that special category of relationships which the law calls fiduciary....

... I think it is readily apparent that the doctor-patient relationship shares the peculiar hallmark of the fiduciary relationship—trust, the trust of a person with inferior power that another person who has assumed superior power and responsibility will exercise that power for his or her good and only for his or her good and in his or her best interests. Recognizing the fiduciary nature of the doctor-patient relationship provides the law with an analytic model by which physicians can be held to the high standards of dealing with their patient which the trust accorded them requires.

The foundation and ambit of the fiduciary obligation are conceptually distinct from the foundation and ambit of contract and tort. Sometimes the doctrines may overlap in their application, but that does not destroy their conceptual and functional uniqueness. In negligence and contract the parties are taken to be independent and equal actors, concerned primarily with their own self-interest. Consequently, the law seeks a balance between enforcing obligations by awarding compensation when those obligations are breached, and preserving optimum freedom for those involved in the relationship in question. The essence of a fiduciary relationship, by contrast, is that one party exercises power on behalf of another and pledges himself or herself to act in the best interests of the other....

The fiduciary relationship has trust, not self-interest, at its core, and when breach occurs, the balance favours the person wronged. The freedom of the fiduciary is limited by the obligation he or she has undertaken—an obligation which "betokens loyalty, good faith and avoidance of a conflict of duty and self-interest": *Canadian Aero Service*

Ltd. v. O'Malley (1973). To cast a fiduciary relationship in terms of contract or tort (whether negligence or battery) is to diminish this obligation. If a fiduciary relationship is shown to exist, then the proper legal analysis is one based squarely on the full and fair consequences of a breach of that relationship.

As La Forest J. went on to note in *McInerney v. MacDonald* (1992), characterizing the doctor-patient relationship as fiduciary is not the end of the analysis: "not all fiduciary relationships and not all fiduciary obligations are the same; these are shaped by the demands of the situation. A relationship may properly be described as 'fiduciary' for some purposes, but not for others." So the question must be asked, did a fiduciary relationship exist between Dr. Wynrib and Ms. Norberg? And assuming that such a relationship did exist, is it properly described as fiduciary for the purposes relevant to this appeal?

[Several previous Supreme Court of Canada decisions have] attributed the following characteristics to a fiduciary relationship: "(1) the fiduciary has scope for the exercise of some discretion or power; (2) the fiduciary can unilaterally exercise that power or discretion so as to affect the beneficiary's legal or practical interests; (3) the beneficiary is peculiarly vulnerable or at the mercy of the fiduciary holding the discretion or power."

Dr. Wynrib was in a position of power vis-á-vis the plaintiff; he had scope for the exercise of power and discretion with respect to her. He had the power to advise her, to treat her, to give her the drug or to refuse her the drug. He could unilaterally exercise that power or discretion in a way that affected her interests. And her status as a patient rendered her vulnerable and at his mercy, particularly in light of her addiction.... All of the classic characteristics of a fiduciary relationship were present. Dr. Wynrib and Ms. Norberg were on an unequal footing. He pledged himself—by the act of hanging out his shingle as a medical doctor and accepting her as his patient—to act in her best interests and not permit any conflict between his duty to act only in her best interests and his own interests—including his interest in sexual gratification—to arise. As a physician, he owed her the classic duties associated with a fiduciary relationship—the duties of "loyalty, good faith, and avoidance of a conflict of duty and self-interest."

Closer examination of the principles enunciated by Wilson, J. In *Frame v. Smith* (1987) confirms the applicability of the fiduciary analysis in this case. The possession of power or discretion needs little elaboration. That one party in a fiduciary relationship holds such power over the other is not in and of itself wrong; on the contrary, "the fiduciary must be entrusted with power in order to perform his function." What will be a wrong is if the risk inherent in entrusting the fiduciary with such power is realized and the fiduciary abuses the power which has been entrusted to him or her. As Wilson J. noted in *Frame*, in the absence of such a discretion or power and the possibility of abuse of power which it entails, "there is no need for a superadded obligation to restrict the damaging use of the discretion or power."

As to the second characteristic, it is, as Wilson J. put it, "the fact that the power or discretion may be used to affect the beneficiary in a damaging way that makes the imposition of a fiduciary duty necessary." Wilson J. went on to state that fiduciary duties are not confined to the exercise of power which can affect the legal interests of the beneficiary, but extend to the beneficiary's "vital non-legal or 'practical' interests." This negates the suggestion inherent in some of the other judgments which this case has engendered that the fiduciary obligation should be confined to legal rights such as confidentiality and conflict of interests and undue influence in the business sphere....

The case at bar is not concerned with the protection of what has traditionally been regarded as a legal interest. It is, however, concerned with the protection of interests, both social and personal, of the highest importance. Society has an abiding interest in ensuring that the power entrusted to physicians by us, both collectively and individually, not be used in corrupt ways. On the other side of the coin, the plaintiff, as indeed does every one of us when we put ourselves in the hands of a physician, has a striking personal interest in obtaining professional medical care free of exploitation for the physician's private purposes. These are not collateral duties and rights created at the whim of an aggrieved patient. They are duties universally recognized as essential to the physician-patient relationship. The Hippocratic Oath reflects this universal concern that physicians not exploit their patients for their own ends, and in particular, not for their own sexual ends....

To the extent that the law requires that physicians who breach them be disciplined, these duties have legal force. The interest which the enforcement of these duties project are, to be sure, different from the legal and economic interests which the law of fiduciary relationships has traditionally been used to safeguard. But as Wilson J. said in *Frame* "[t]o deny relief because of the nature of the interest involved, to afford protection to material interests but not to human or personal interests would, it seems to me, be arbitrary in the extreme." At the very least, the societal and personal interests at issue here constitute "a vital and substantial 'practical' interest" within the meaning of the second characteristic of a fiduciary duty set out in *Frame v. Smith*.

The third requirement is that of vulnerability. This is the other side of the differential power equation which is fundamental to all fiduciary relationships. In order to be the beneficiary of a fiduciary relationship a person need not be *per se* vulnerable.... It is only where there is a material discrepancy, in the circumstances of the relationship in question, between the power of one person and the vulnerability of the other that the fiduciary relationship is recognized by the law. Where the parties are on a relatively equal footing, contract and tort provide the appropriate analysis....

At the case at bar, this requirement too is fulfilled. A physician holds great power over the patient. The recent decision of the Ontario Court (General Division) in *College of Physicians & Surgeons of Ontario v. Gillen* (1990), contains a reminder that a patient's vulnerability may be as much physical as emotional, given the fact that a doctor "has the right to examine the patient in any state of dress or undress and to administer drugs to render the patient unconscious." Visits to doctors occur in private; the door is closed; there is rarely a third party present; everything possible is done to encourage the patient to feel that the patient's privacy will be respected. This is essential to the meeting of the patient's medical and emotional needs; the unfortunate concomitant is that it also creates the conditions under which the patient may be abused without fear of outside intervention. Whether physically vulnerable or not,

however, the patient, by reason of lesser expertise, the "submission" which is essential to the relationship, and sometimes, as in this case, by reason of the nature of the illness itself; is typically in a position of comparative powerlessness. The fact that society encourages us to trust our doctors to believe that they will be persons worthy of our trust, cannot be ignored as a factor inducing a heightened degree of vulnerability....

Women, who can so easily be exploited by physicians for sexual purposes, may find themselves particularly vulnerable. That female patients are disproportionately the targets of sexual exploitation by physicians is borne out by the [College of Physicians and Surgeons of Ontario, *Final Report of the Task Force on Sexual Abuse of Patients*]. Of the 303 reports they received of sexual exploitation at the hands of those in a position of trust (the vast majority of whom were physicians), 287 were by female patients, 16 by males....

The principles outlined by Wilson J. in *Frame v. Smith* may apply with varying force depending on the nature of the particular doctor-patient relationship. For example, the uniquely intimate nature of the psychotherapist-patient relationship, the potential for transference, and the emotional fragility of many psychotherapy patients make the argument for a fiduciary obligation resting on psychotherapists, and in particular an obligation to refrain from any sexualizing of the relationship, especially strong in that context. American courts have, as a result, imposed higher duties on psychiatrists than they have on other physicians. The Task Force of the Ontario College of Physicians and Surgeons has in its report also recognized the greater danger of breach of trust inherent in psychotherapeutic relationships, and has as a consequence recommended even more stringent guidelines for appropriate psychotherapist behaviour than it has for physicians practising in other areas. While the medial relationship between Dr. Wynrib and Ms. Norberg was not psychotherapeutic in orientation, the treatment of a patient dependent on drugs would seem to me to share many of the same characteristics, thereby rendering the addicted patient even more vulnerable and in need of the protection which the law of fiduciary obligations can afford than other patients might be....

But, it is said, there are a number of reasons why the doctrine of breach of fiduciary relationship cannot apply in this case. I turn then to these alleged conditions of defeasibility.

The first factor which is said to prevent application of the doctrine of breach of fiduciary duty is Ms. Norberg's conduct. Two terms have been used to raise this consideration to the status of a legal or equitable bar—the equitable maxim that he who comes into equity must come with clean hands and the tort doctrine of *ex turpi causa non orbitur actio*. For our purposes, one may think of the two respectively as the equitable and legal formulations of the same type of bar to recovery. The trial judge found that although Dr. Wynrib was under a trust obligation to Ms. Norberg, she was barred from claiming damages against him because of her "immoral" and "illegal" conduct. While he referred to the doctrine of *ex turpi*, there seems to be little doubt that in equity the appropriate term is "clean hands" and consequently that is the expression I will use.

The short answer to the arguments based on wrongful conduct of the plaintiff is that she did nothing wrong in the context of this relationship. She was not a sinner, but a sick person, suffering from an addiction which proved to be uncontrollable in the absence of a professional drug rehabilitation program. She went to Dr. Wynrib for relief from that condition. She hoped he would give her relief by giving her the drug; "hustling" doctors for drugs is a recognized symptom of her illness. Such behaviour is commonly seen by family physicians. Patients may, as did Ms. Norberg, feign physical problems which, if bona fide, would require analgesic relief. They may, as Ms. Norberg also did, specify the drug they wish to receive. Once a physician has diagnosed a patient as an addict who is "hustling" him for drugs, the recommended response is to "(1) maintain control of the doctor-patient relationship, (2) remain professional in the face of ploys for sympathy or guilt and (3) regard the drug seeker as a patient with a serious illness"....

The law might accuse Ms. Norberg of "double doctoring" and moralists might accuse her of licentiousness; but she did no wrong because not she but the doctor was responsible for this conduct. He had the power to cure her of her addiction, as her suc-

cessful treatment after leaving his "care" demonstrated; instead he chose to use his power to keep her in her addicted state and to use her for his own sexual purposes.

It is difficult not to see the attempt to bar Ms. Norberg from obtaining redress for the wrong she has suffered through the application of the clean hands maxim as anything other than "blaming the victim"....

A[nother] objection raised to viewing the relationship between Dr. Wynrib and Ms. Norberg as fiduciary is that it will open the floodgates to unfounded claims based on the abuse of real or perceived inequality of power. The spectre has conjured up a host of actions based on exploitation—children suing parents, wives suing husbands, mistresses suing lovers, all for abuse of superior power. The answer to this objection lies in defining the ambit of the fiduciary obligation in a way that encompasses meritorious claims while excluding those without merit. The prospect of the law's recognizing meritorious claims by the powerless and exploited against the powerful and exploitive should not alone serve as a reason for denying just claim. This Court has an honourable tradition of recognizing new claims of the disempowered against the exploitive.

The criteria for the imposition of a fiduciary duty already enunciated by this court ... provide a good starting point for the task of defining the general principles which determine whether such a relationship exists. As we have seen, an imbalance of power is not enough to establish a fiduciary relationship. It is a necessary but not sufficient condition. There must also be the potential for interference with a legal interest or a non-legal interest of "vital and substantial 'practical' interest." And I would add this. Inherent in the notion of fiduciary duty ... is the requirement that the fiduciary have assumed or undertaken to "look after" the interest of the beneficiary.... It is not easy to bring relationships within this rubric. Generally people are deemed by the law to be motivated in their relationships by mutual self-interest. The duties of trust are special, confined to the exceptional case where one person assumes the power which would normally reside with the other and undertakes to exercise that power solely for the other's benefit. It is as though the fiduciary has taken the power which rightfully belongs to the beneficiary on the condition that the fiduciary exercise the power entrusted exclusively for the good of the beneficiary. Thus, the trustee of an estate takes the financial power that would normally reside with the beneficiaries and must exercise those powers in their stead and for their exclusive benefit. Similarly, a physician takes the power which a patient normally has over her body, and which she cedes to him for the purposes of treatment. The physician is pledged by the nature of his calling to use the power the patient cedes to him exclusively for her benefit. If he breaks that pledge, he is liable.

In summary, the constraints inherent in the principles governing fiduciary relationships belie the contention that the recognition of a fiduciary obligation in this case will open the floodgates to unmeritorious claims. Taking the case at its narrowest, it is concerned with a relationship which has long been recognized as fiduciary—the physician-patient relationship; it represents no extension of the law. Taking the case more broadly, with reference to the general principles governing fiduciary obligations, it is seen to fall within principles previously recognized by this court, and again represents no innovation. In so far as application of those principles in this case might be argued to give encouragement to new categories of claims, the governing principles offer assurance against unlimited liability while at the same time promising a great measure of justice for the exploited.

9.
REIBL V. HUGHES

Supreme Court of Canada, Laskin, C.J.C., Martland, Dickson, Beetz, Estey, McIntyre and Chouinard J.J. October 7, 1980.

LASKIN, C.J.C.:—The plaintiff appellant, then 44 years of age, underwent serious surgery on March 18, 1970, for the removal of an occlusion in the left internal carotid artery, which had prevented more than a 15% flow of blood through the vessel. The operation was competently performed by the defendant respondent, a qualified neurosurgeon. However, during or immediately following the surgery the plaintiff suffered a massive stroke which left him paralyzed on the right side of his body and also impotent. The plaintiff had, of course, formally consented to the operation. Alleging, however, that his was not an "informed consent," he sued for damages and recovered on this ground in both battery and negligence. The trial Judge, Haines J., awarded a global sum of $225,000 [78 D.L.R. (3d) 35, 16 O.R. (2d) 306].

A majority of the Ontario Court of Appeal ordered a new trial on both liability and damages [89 D.L.R. (3d) 112, 21 O.R. (2d) 14, 6 C.C.L.T. 227]. Speaking through Brooke J.A. (Blair J.A. concurring) the Court ruled out battery as a possible ground of liability on the facts of the case. Jessup J.A., dissenting in part, would have ordered a new trial on damages alone, accepting the judgment at trial on liability.

On the hearing of the appeal by this Court, leave to come here having been obtained by the plaintiff, counsel for the defendant respondent agreed to accept the award of damages and limited his contestation to liability, seeking not only to hold the judgment in appeal but a "variation" thereof by way of dismissal of the action. Although, strictly speaking, the claim for a variation should have been made the subject of a cross-appeal, counsel for the appellant took no objection and I see no reason why I should not regularize the claim for dismissal *nunc pro tunc*. Indeed, neither counsel wished to have a new trial,

an understandable position when the physical damage suffered took place more than ten years ago. Unless, therefore, there are good reasons to support the order for a new trial or liability alone, the proper course is to determine whether to restore the judgment at trial on either or both grounds upon which it proceeded or whether the defendant should be relieved of liability.

It is now undoubted that the relationship between surgeon and patient gives rise to a duty of the surgeon to make disclosure to the patient of what I would call all material risks attending the surgery which is recommended. The scope of the duty of disclosure was considered in *Hopp v. Lepp*, a judgment of this Court, delivered on May 20, 1980, ... [112 D.L.R. (3d) 67, 22 A.R. 361, [1980] 4 W.W.R. 645], where it was generalized as follows [at p. 81]:

> In summary, the decided cases appear to indicate that, in obtaining the consent of a patient for the performance upon him of a surgical operation, a surgeon, generally, should answer any specific questions posed by the patient as to the risks involved and should, without being questioned, disclose to him the nature of the proposed operation, its gravity, any material risks and any special or unusual risks attendant upon the performance of the operation. However, having said that, it should be added that the scope of the duty of disclosure and whether or not it has been breached are matters which must be decided in relation to the circumstances of each particular case.

The Court in *Hopp v. Lepp* also pointed out that even if a certain risk is a mere possibility which ordinarily need not be disclosed, yet if its occurrence carries serious consequences, as for example, paralysis or even death, it should be regarded as a material risk requiring disclosure.

In the present case, the risk attending the surgery or its immediate aftermath was the risk of a stroke, of paralysis and indeed, of death. This was, without question, a material risk. At the same time, the evidence made it clear that there was also a risk of a stroke and of resulting death if surgery for the removal of the occlusion was refused by the patient. The delicacy of the surgery is beyond question, and its execution is no longer in any way faulted. (I would note here that in this Court no issue was raised as to the adequacy of post-operative care.) How specific, therefore, must the information to the patient be, in a case such as this, to enable him to make an "informed" choice between surgery and no surgery? One of the considerations weighing upon the plaintiff was the fact that he was about a year and a half away from earning a life-time retirement pension as a Ford Motor Company employee. The trial Judge noted (to use his words) ... that "Due to this tragedy befalling him at the time it did, he was not eligible for certain extended disability benefits available under the collective agreement between the Ford Motor Company of Canada Limited and its hourly employees of 10 years' standing." At the time of the operation, the plaintiff had 8.4 years' service with his employer. He stated in his evidence that if he had been properly informed of the magnitude of the risk involved in the surgery he would have elected to forego it, at least until his pension had vested and, further, he would have opted for a shorter normal life than a longer one as a cripple because of the surgery. Although elective surgery was indicated for the condition from which the plaintiff suffered, there was (as the trial Judge found) no emergency in the sense that immediate surgical treatment was imperative.

This brings me back to the question of the nature of the information provided by the respondent surgeon to the plaintiff and its adequacy in the circumstances. I will deal, in turn, with: (1) the findings and conclusion of the trial Judge on this issue; (2) whether, even on his findings, there was a basis for imposing liability for battery; (3) the assessment made by the Court of Appeal in ordering a new trial; (4) the evidence in the case, which consisted, in support of the plaintiff's case, mainly of the testimony of the plaintiff and of two neurosurgeons, Dr. Irving Schacter and Dr. Robert Elgie, and portions of the examination for discovery of the defendant and, in support of the defendant's case, the testimony of the defendant and of a neurosurgeon, Dr. William Lougheed, who were the only two witnesses called for the defendant; (5) the duty of disclosure and review of the findings below; and (6) whether causation was established.

... The well-known statement of Cardozo J. In *Schloendorff v. Society of New York Hospital* (1914), 211 N.Y. 125 at p. 129, 105 N.E. 92 at p. 93, that "every human being of adult years and sound mind has a right to determine what shall be done with his own body; and a surgeon who performs an operation without his patient's consent commits an assault, for which he is liable in damages" cannot be taken beyond the compass of its words to support an action of battery where there has been consent to the very surgical procedure carried out upon a patient but there has been a breach of the duty of disclosure of attendant risks. In my opinion, actions of battery in respect of surgical or other medical treatment should be confined to cases where surgery or treatment has been performed or given to which there has been consent at all or where, emergency situations aside, surgery or treatment has been performed or given beyond that to which there was consent.

This standard would comprehend cases where there was misrepresentation of the surgery or treatment for which consent was elicited and a different surgical procedure or treatment was carried out. See, for example, *Marshall v. Curry,* [1933] 3 D.L.R. 260, 60 C.C.C. 136 (consent given to operation to cure hernia; doctor removes patient's testicle; action in battery); *Murray v. McMurchy*, [1949] 2 D.L.R. 442, [1949] 1 W.W.R. 989 (consent given to a caesarian operation; doctor goes on and sterilizes the patient; doctor liable for trespass to the person); *Mulloy v. Hop Sang,* [1935] 1 W.W.R. 714 (doctor told to repair hand and not to amputate; performs amputation; held liable in trespass); *Winn et al. V. Alexander et al.,* [1940] 3 D.L.R. 778, [1940] O.W.N. 238 (consent given to caesarian; doctor goes further and sterilizes the patient); *Schweizer v. Central Hospital et al.* (1974), 53 D.L.R. (3d) 494, 6 O.R. (2d) 606 (patient consented to operation on his toe; doctor operated on back instead [spinal fusion]; doctor liable for trespass to the person).

In situations where the allegation is that attendant risks which should have been disclosed were not communicated to the patient and yet the surgery or other medical treatment carried out was that to which the plaintiff consented (there being no negligence basis of liability for the recommended surgery or treatment to deal with the patient's condition), I do not understand how it can be said that the consent was vitiated by the failure of disclosure so as to make the surgery or other treatment an unprivileged, inconsented to and intentional invasion of the patient's bodily integrity. I can appreciate the temptation to say that the genuineness of consent to medical treatment depends on proper disclosure of the risks which it entails in my view, unless there has been misrepresentation or fraud to secure consent to the treatment, a failure to disclose the attendant risks, however serious, should go to negligence rather than to battery. Although such a failure relates to an informed choice of submitting to or refusing recommended and appropriate treatment, it arises as the breach of an anterior duty of due care, comparable in legal obligation to the duty of due care in carrying out the particular treatment to which the patient has consented. It is not a test of the validity of the consent.

3. The Assessment of the Court of Appeal

Brooke J.A., speaking for the majority of the Court of Appeal, noted, ... quite properly, that:

> The duty [of disclosure] to the patient is determined by the Court and the evidence of the expert witnesses, if accepted, is relevant to determining whether or not the defendant has discharged that duty. To be actionable [in negligence] the defendant's failure in his duty of care must cause the plaintiff loss and damage.

He went on to examine the reasons of Haines J. and made the following observations upon that trial Judge's determination:....

> In finding that the plaintiff was left with the impression that the surgery carried no risk of consequence other than those in any surgical procedure I think it must be assumed that the learned trial Judge has rejected the defendant's explanation that the plaintiff was aware of the risk of a stroke as a risk of the surgery. Of some

importance, the learned trial Judge makes no specific finding of credibility and indeed does not disbelieve the defendant's evidence that he thought the plaintiff understood the risk. However, the learned trial Judge did not put his judgment simply on the failure to warn, but also on the failure to take sufficient care to discuss the degree of risk. He relied upon the evidence of Dr. Elgie and Dr. Schacter and it is my respectful view that, having regard for the emphasis which the learned trial Judge places upon the statistical details, he has misunderstood the real significance of the evidence of these two doctors. Drs. Schacter and Elgie appear to have taken a similar approach to the question of explaining the risks of the surgery, but the emphasis is not on statistical detail. Dr. Elgie alone made reference to statistics in discussing the manner in which he would advise his patient when seeking a consent to perform this operation and in this respect his answer was different from that of Dr. Schacter.

Brooke J.A. was highly critical of the use of unexplained statistics which appeared to be directed to the degree of risk involved in the particular surgery. This is what he said in that respect....

> One need only look at the contrast in the evidence of the statistics quoted by Dr. Hughes and Dr. Elgie to demonstrate the confusion that could arise from their use. When asked in cross-examination, Dr. Hughes' figure as to the incidence of death because of surgery was 4%, which was equal to Dr. Elgie's highest figure where he put the range between 2% and 4%, and with respect to the incidence of stroke causing paralysis or transient weakness, Dr. Hughes put the figure at 10% which was five times Dr. Elgie's lowest figure and almost two and one-half times his highest figure. Taken cumulatively, Dr. Hughes' figure at 14% is more than three times Dr. Elgie's lowest estimate and almost twice his highest. They were really very different. The reason for the difference went unexplained. No one asked the doctors. And yet the trial Judge referred principally in his reasons, and particularly in testing the defendant's conduct, to the statistics recounted by Dr. Hughes, which there was no suggestion the doctor attempted to use. If the difference is based solely or partly on the personal

experience of the surgeons, and there is in the evidence some reason suggested that this may be so, then perhaps the explanation lies in the nature of the cases that each has dealt with and that the chance of survivorship of those undertaken by one was less than the other. If this is so, there may have been good reason not to mention statistics to the patient, but rather to simply contrast his position if he undertakes the surgery with that of not undertaking it and urge him to proceed because of his youth and strength giving some assurance of survivorship. I do not think the evidence justifies the statement made by the learned trial Judge and I would hesitate to lay down any such requirements, for in my view, statistics can be very misleading. The manner in which the nature and degree of risk is explained to a particular patient is better left to the judgment of the doctor in dealing with the man before him. Its adequacy can be simply tested.

I think the Ontario Court of Appeal went too far, when dealing with the standard of disclosure of risks, in saying, as it did in the passage of its reasons just quoted, that "the manner in which the nature and degree of risk is explained to a particular patient is better left to the judgment of the doctor in dealing with the man before him." Of course, it can be tested by expert medical evidence but that too is not determinative. The patient may have expressed certain concerns to the doctor and the latter is obliged to meet them in a reasonable way. What the doctor knows or should know that the particular patient deems relevant to a decision whether to undergo prescribed treatment goes equally to his duty of disclosure as do the material risks recognized as a matter of required medical knowledge.

It is important to examine this issue in greater detail. The Ontario Court of Appeal appears to have adopted a professional medical standard, not only for determining what are the material risks that should be disclosed but also, and concurrently, for determining whether there has been a breach of the duty of disclosure. This was also the approach of the trial Judge, notwithstanding that on the facts he found against the defendant. (Indeed, the trial Judge seems also to have overstated the duty of disclosure.

The Court of Appeal, in contrast, seems to have understated it. Generally, the failure to mention statistics should not affect the duty to inform nor be a factor in deciding whether the duty has been breached.) To allow expert medical evidence to determine what risks are material and, hence, should be disclosed and, correlatively, what risks are not material is to hand over to the medical profession the entire question of the scope of the duty of disclosure, including the question whether there has been a breach of that duty. Expert medical evidence is, of course, relevant to findings as to the risks that reside in or are a result of recommended surgery or other treatment. It will also have a bearing on their materiality but this is not a question that is to be concluded on the basis of the expert medical evidence alone. The issue under consideration is a different issue from that involved where the question is whether the doctor carried out his professional activities by applicable professional standards. What is under consideration here is the patient's right to know what risks are involved in undergoing or foregoing certain surgery or other treatment.

The materiality of non-disclosure of certain risks to an informed decision is a matter for the trier of fact, a matter on which there would, in all likelihood, be medical evidence but also other evidence, including evidence from the patient or from members of his family. It is, of course, possible that a particular patient may waive aside any question of risks and be quite prepared to submit to the surgery or treatment, whatever they be. Such a situation presents no difficulty. Again, it may be the case that a particular patient may, because of emotional factors, be unable to cope with facts relevant to recommended surgery or treatment and the doctor may, in such a case, be justified in withholding or generalizing information as to which he would otherwise be required to be more specific.

If Canadian case law has so far proceeded on a subjective test of causation, it is in Courts other than this one that such an approach has been taken: see *Koehler v. Cook* (1975), 65 D.L.R. (3d) 766 at p. 767, [1976] W.W.D. 71, and *Kelly v. Hazlett* (1976), 75 D.L.R. (3d) 536 at pp.565-6, 15 O.R. (2d) 290 at p. 320. The matter is *res integra* here. An alternative to the subjective test is an objective one, that is, what would a reasonable person in the patient's position have done if there had been proper disclosure of attendant risks. The case for the objective standard has been tersely put in the following passage from a comment in 48 N.Y.U.L. Rev. 548 (1973), at p. 550, entitled "Informed Consent—A Proposed Standard for Medical Disclosure":

> Since proximate causation exists only if disclosure would have resulted in the patient's foregoing the proposed treatment, a standard must be developed to determine whether the patient would have decided against the treatment had he been informed of its risks. Two possible standards exist: whether, if informed, the particular patient would have foregone treatment (subjective view); or whether the average prudent person in plaintiff's position, informed of all material risks, would have foregone treatment (objective view). The objective standard is preferable, since the subjective standard has a gross defect: it depends on the plaintiff's testimony as to his state of mind, thereby exposing the physician to the patient's hindsight and bitterness.

However, a vexing problem raised by the objective standard is whether causation could ever be established if the surgeon has recommended surgery which is warranted by the patient's condition. Can it be said that a reasonable person in the patient's position, to whom proper disclosure of attendant risks has been made, would decide against the surgery, that is, against the surgeon's recommendation that it be undergone? The objective standard of what a reasonable person in the patient's position would do would seem to put a premium on the surgeon's assessment of the relative need for the surgery and on supporting medical evidence of that need. Could it be reasonably refused? Brooke J.A. appeared to be sensitive to this problem by suggesting a combined objective-subjective test.

I doubt that this will solve the problem. It could hardly be expected that the patient who is suing would admit that he would have agreed to have the surgery, even knowing all the accompanying risks. His suit would indicate that, having suffered serious disablement because of the surgery, he is convinced that he would not have permitted it if there had been proper disclosure of the risks, balanced by the risks of refusing the surgery. Yet, to apply a subjective test

to causation would, correlatively, put a premium on hindsight, even more of a premium than would be put on medical evidence in assessing causation by an objective standard.

I think it is the safer course on the issue of causation to consider objectively how far the balance in the risks of surgery or no surgery is in favour of undergoing surgery. The failure of proper disclosure pro and con becomes therefore very material. And so too are any special considerations affecting the particular patient. For example, the patient may have asked specific questions which were either brushed aside or were not fully answered or were answered wrongly. In the present case, the anticipation of a full pension would be a special consideration, and, while it would have to be viewed objectively, it emerges from the patient's particular circumstances. So too, other aspects of the objective standard would have to be geared to what the average prudent person, the reasonable person in the patient's particular position, would agree to or not agree to, if all material and special risks of going ahead with the surgery or foregoing it were made known to him. Far from making the patient's own testimony irrelevant, it is essential to his case that he put his own position forward.

The adoption of an objective standard does not mean that the issue of causation is completely in the hands of the surgeon. Merely because medical evidence establishes the reasonableness of a recommended operation does not mean that a reasonable person in the patient's position would necessarily agree to it, if proper disclosure had been made of the risks attendant upon it, balanced by those against it. The patient's particular situation and the degree to which the risks of surgery or no surgery are balanced would reduce the force, on an objective appraisal, of the surgeon's recommendation. Admittedly, if the risk of foregoing the surgery would be considerably graver to a patient than the risks attendant upon it, the objective standard would favour exoneration of the surgeon who has not made the required disclosure. Since liability rests only in negligence, in a failure to disclose material risks, the issue of causation would be in the patient's hands on a subjective test, and would, if his evidence was accepted, result inevitably in liability unless, of course, there was a finding that there was no breach of the duty of disclosure. In my view, therefore, the objective standard is the preferable one on the issue of causation.

In saying that the test is based on the decision that a reasonable person in the patient's position would have made, I should make it clear that the patient's particular concerns must also be reasonably based; otherwise, there would be more subjectivity than would be warranted under an objective test. Thus, for example, fears which are not related to the material risks which should have been but were not disclosed would not be causative factors. However, economic considerations could reasonably go to causation where, for example, the loss of an eye as a result of nondisclosure of a material risk brings about the loss of a job for which good eyesight is required. In short, although account must be taken of a patient's particular position, a position which will vary with the patient, it must be objectively assessed in terms of reasonableness.

5. BREACH OF DUTY OF DISCLOSURE: THE FINDINGS BELOW REVIEWED

In my opinion, the record of evidence amply justifies the trial Judge's findings that the plaintiff was told no more or understood no more than that he would be better off to have the operation than not to have it. This was not an adequate, not a sufficient disclosure of the risk attendant upon the operation itself, a risk well appreciated by the defendant in view of his own experience that of the 60 to 70 such operations that he had previously performed, 8 to 10 resulted in the death of the patients. Although the mortality rate was falling by 1970, the morbidity (the sickness or disease) rate, according to Dr. Hughes, was still about 10%. The trial Judge was also justified in finding that the plaintiff, who was concerned about his continuing headaches and who was found to be suffering from hypertension, had the impression that the surgery would alleviate his headaches and hypertension so that he could carry on with his job. Dr. Hughes made it plain in his evidence that the surgery would not cure the headaches but did not, as the trial Judge found, make this plain to the plaintiff.

The foregoing findings have a basis in the evidence independent of any reliance on so-called statistics which was criticized by the majority of the Court of Appeal. Although Brooke J.A., speaking for the majority, appeared to discount the trial Judge's determinations because the latter made no specific finding on credibility, it is patent to me that the trial Judge's conclusions involved a weighing of the evidence and, hence, a measuring of its relative worth on the issues that he had to decide. There were inconsistencies in the defendant's evidence, as the trial Judge noted in his reasons, and it was for him to reconcile them in arriving at his findings. For example, the defendant said in-chief that he had told the plaintiff of the risk of a stroke during surgery and then said on cross-examination that the risks of the surgery were quite minimal. Again, on cross-examination, he said that he did not tell the patient that there was a risk of a stroke as a result of the surgery at any specific time thereafter, and he returned to an oft repeated statement that the chances of paralysis were greater without an operation than with it. (This was also the only reference by Dr. Lougheed, who testified for the defence, as to the risk involved in submitting to or foregoing the surgery. His evidence was almost exclusively related to post-operative care and whether a re-operation was feasible. He said it was not. However, as I noted earlier, post-operative care was not an issue in this Court.) Moreover, the defendant placed this risk as one within a few years and not within any immediate time. Indeed, when asked in cross-examination whether he told the patient that the surgery carried the risk of a stroke, he answered, "I didn't say that specifically." This was certainly a case in which a trial Judge, here an experienced Judge, was in a better position than an appellate Court or this Court to determine what evidence to accept and what conclusions to draw from it.

In the ... reasons of Brooke J.A., speaking for the majority of the Court of Appeal, there are two approaches on the crucial issue whether the defendant apprised the plaintiff of the risk of a stroke from the very operation. In the first ... passage, the learned Justice of Appeal appears to have viewed the trial Judge's finding on this question as a finding that the plaintiff was not made aware of that risk. This is clearly a correct assessment of the trial Judge's conclusion. However, Brooke J.A. went on to deal with the case and with the evidence as if there was a partial albeit not a sufficient disclosure of the particular risk, and he proceeded from there into an appraisal of the statistics to which the trial Judge referred and found fault in their use. In the second ... passage ... Brooke J.A. ... ignores the finding of the trial Judge that there was no disclosure of the risks inherent in the surgery itself. In my opinion, there was a failure by the Court of Appeal to address this point directly. In the light of the defendant's own evidence that there was a failure on his part to disclose the risk, even though the plaintiff himself raised the question of the risks he faced on the operating table, I do not see how there could be any doubt of a breach in this respect of the duty of disclosure.

Indeed, the reasons of the Court of Appeal ... appear to support the trial Judge's finding that there was no proper disclosure by the defendant of the risk of the surgery itself. Brooke J.A. said this on the question [at p. 119]:

He [the defendant] did not specifically discuss the questions of death or paralysis as risks of the surgery, his explanation being that he believed the patient was aware of the risk because of questions that he asked when the surgery was being discussed. It was his view that no further detail was necessary.

In this respect then, there would seem to be concurrent findings of fact against the defendant on a central point in case.

There were a number of relevant considerations informing the findings of the trial Judge, about which there was no dispute. First, there was no emergency making surgery imperative. There was no noticeable neurological deficit. The defendant himself placed the risk of a stroke as one off in the future, four to five years. Any immediate risk would be from the surgery and not from foregoing it. Moreover, it must have been obvious to the defendant that the plaintiff had some difficulty with the English language and that he should, therefore, have made certain that he was understood. Finally, there was no evidence that the plaintiff was emotionally taut or unable to accept disclosure of the grave risk to which he would be exposed by submitting to surgery. I do not see in the reasons of the majority of the Court of

Appeal any evidentiary basis for challenging the findings of the trial Judge on the defendant's breach of the duty of disclosure. Of course, the medical evidence was relevant to what that duty entailed but, that said, it was for the trier of fact to determine the scope of the duty and to decide whether there had been a breach of the duty. As I have already said, the so-called statistical data used by the trial Judge did not affect the grounds upon which he made his critical findings. The Court of Appeal held, however, that the trial Judge did not examine the issue of causation with the necessary care that this issue required. He did not ignore it, even if he might have gone into it at greater length. The question that remains, therefore, is whether this was a sufficient basis upon which to direct a new trial.

6. CAUSATION

Relevant in this case to the issue whether a reasonable person in the plaintiff's position would have declined surgery at the particular time is the fact that he was within about one and one-half years of earning pension benefits if he continued at his job; that there was no neurological deficit then apparent; that there was no immediate emergency making the surgery imperative; that there was a grave risk of a stroke or worse during or as a result of the operation, while the risk of a stroke without it was in the future, with no precise time fixed or which could be fixed except as a guess of three or more years ahead. Since, on the trial Judge's finding, the plaintiff was under the mistaken impression, as a result of the defendant's breach of the duty of disclosure, that the surgery would relieve his continuing headaches, this would in the opinion of a reasonable person in the plaintiff's position, also weigh against submitting to the surgery at the particular time.

In my opinion, a reasonable person in the plaintiff's position would, on a balance of probabilities, have opted against the surgery rather than undergoing it at the particular time.

CONCLUSION

I would, accordingly, allow the appeal, set aside the order of the Court of Appeal and restore the judgment at trial. The appellant is entitled to costs throughout.

CHAPTER THREE

CONSENT

10.
A MORAL THEORY OF CONSENT

Benjamin Freedman

Most medical codes of ethics, and most physicians, agree that the physician ought to obtain the "free and informed consent" of his subject or patient before attempting any serious medical procedures, experimental or therapeutic in nature. They agree, moreover, that a proxy consent ought to be obtained on behalf of the incompetent subject. And informed consent is seen as not merely a legal requirement, and not merely a formality: it is a substantial requirement of morality.

Acceptance of this doctrine, however, requires the solution of a number of problems. How much information need be imparted? At what age is a person mature enough to consent on his own behalf? Can prisoners give a "free, and informed consent" to be experimented upon? Lurking behind these and similar questions there are more fundamental difficulties. What are the functions of consent for the competent and the incompetent? What is the sense in which the patient/subject must be "free," "informed," and "competent"? It is by way of an approach to these latter questions that I shall attempt to respond to the more specific questions.[1]

I. CONSENT AND THE COMPETENT

The negative aspects of the doctrine of informed consent have ordinarily been the focus of attention; difficulties in obtaining the informed consent of the subject/patient render the ethics of experimentation and therapeutic measures questionable. Our common view of informed consent is that, when at all relevant, it represents a minimum condition which ethics imposes upon the physician. It is seen as a necessary condition for medical manipulation, but hardly as a sufficient condition.

The reasons why this is so—why it is not sufficient that an experimenter, for instance, have received informed consent from his subject before proceeding—are quite obvious. The scarcity of medical resources (which includes a scarcity of qualified physician-investigators) forbids us from wasting time upon poorly-designed experiments, or upon experiments which merely replicate well-established conclusions. There seems to be, as well, a limit to the dangers which we (ordinarily) allow subjects to face. We do not, as a matter of policy, think it wise to allow would-be suicides to accomplish their end with the aid of a scientific investigator. Many other reasons could be given for the proposition that a person does not have a right to be experimented upon, even when he has given valid consent to the procedure.

The Right to Consent

But there does seem to exist a positive right of informed consent, which exists in both therapeutic and experimental settings. A person who has the capacity to give valid consent, and who has in fact consented to the procedure in question, has a right to have that fact recognized by us. We all have a duty to recognize a valid consent when confronted with it.

From whence derives this right? It arises from the right which each of us possesses to be treated as a person, and in the duty which all of us have, to have respect for persons, to treat a person as such, and not as an object. For this entails that our capacities for personhood ought to be recognized by all—these capacities including the capacity for rational decision, and for action consequent upon rational decision. Perhaps the worst which we may do to a man is to deny him his humanity, for example, by classifying him as mentally incompetent when he is, in fact, sane. It is a terrible thing to be hated or persecuted; it is far worse to be ignored, to be notified that you "don't count."

If an individual is capable of and has given valid consent, I would argue that he has a right, as against the world but more particularly as against his physician, to have it recognized that valid consent has been given. (The same applies, of course, with still greater force, with regard to *refusals* to consent to medical procedures.) The limited force of this claim must be emphasized: it does not entail a right to be treated, or to be experimented upon. It is a most innocuous right, one which most of us would have little hesitation about granting.

It is, therefore, curious that the literature on informed consent has failed to recognize this right—has, in fact, tacitly denied this right, at least as regards experimentation. In writings on informed consent it seems to have been assumed that if, under certain conditions, it is *doubtful* that valid consent to an experiment has been granted, it is best to "play it safe" ethically. In cases of doubt, we prefer not to take chances: in this case, we will not take a chance upon violating the canons of ethics by experimenting without being certain that the subject has validly consented to the experiment. Since we do not at present know whether a prisoner can give a valid consent, let us not take chances: we call for a moratorium on prison experimentation. Since we do not know at what age a person has the capacity to give a valid consent, we avoid the problem by setting the age of majority at a point where it is beyond doubt that maturity has been attained. If we must err, we shall ensure that we err in being overly ethical.

The establishment of the innocuous right to have valid consent recognized as such eliminates this expedient. Other writers have conceptualized the conflict as one between a right and, at best, a mere liberty. From the patient's point of view, he has a right to have his health protected by the physician, and a mere liberty to be experimented upon. From the physician-investigator's point of view, he has a duty to protect the subject's health, and a mere liberty to experiment upon the subject (contingent, of course, upon obtaining the subject's consent). A recognition of the claims of personhood and autonomy, however, reveals this to be a conflict between rights and duties. The physician-investigator has a duty to recognize consent when validly offered. When the consent is of doubtful validity, therefore, the physician experiences a conflict between two duties. He will not be ethically well-protected by choosing not to experiment, for there exists the pos-

sibility—which, as cases are multiplied, becomes a probability—that he is violating a duty in so choosing. Problems in informed consent present us with a dilemma. It is no longer the case that the burden of proof devolves upon the would-be experimenter. The would-be abstainer-from-experiments may have to prove his case as well.

These considerations give us a new point of departure in investigating problems of informed consent. They show us that there is no "fail-safe" procedure which we can fall back upon in cases of doubt. Rather, what is required is an exhaustive examination of each case and issue, to see whether or not a valid consent has in fact been obtained.

When we fail to recognize a valid consent, of course, more is involved than a denial of personhood. Other benefits may be denied as well. Dr. Vernon Mark, for example, maintains that psychosurgery should not be done on prisoners with epilepsy because of the problem in obtaining a voluntary consent from prisoners.[2] But a resolution of this problem has not been shown to be impossible. Surely, the proper thing to do here would be to see whether prisoners can or cannot give valid consent to such a procedure. To remain satisfied with doubts, to fail to investigate this question, complex though it be, results in a denial of medical treatment for the prisoner, as well as representing a negation of the prisoner's human capacities. In depriving prisoners of the opportunity to serve as subjects in medical experiments, there are losses other than those of human respect.[3] Not the least of these is the loss of an opportunity to be of altruistic service to mankind.[4] Even a child feels at times a need to be useful; in promoting a moratorium on prison experimentation we deny prisoners the satisfaction of this psychic need. We should not need a reminder from John Stuart Mill that there are "higher" as well as "lower" pleasures and needs.

The right to have valid consent recognized as such does not indicate that we must experiment on prisoners. What it does indicate is that we have a moral responsibility to investigate in detail the question of whether prisoners can, under certain conditions, validly consent to experimentation. It also requires that we not prevent a researcher from experimenting on the basis of over-scrupulousness. If prisoners can give valid consent, we wrong not only the researcher but the prisoner as well by forbidding prison experimentation.

The Requirement of Information

The most common locution for the requirement which I am discussing is "informed consent"—we require "informed consent" to protect a doctor from legal liability resultant from his therapeutic endeavors, or to ensure the "ethicacy" of an experiment. But I believe "informed consent" to be a serious misnomer for what we do, in fact, want medical practice to conform to.

No lengthy rehearsal of the absurdities consequent upon taking the term "informed consent" at face value is necessary. The claim has been made, and repeated with approval, that "fully informed consent" is a goal which we can never achieve, but toward which we must strive. In order to ensure that fully informed consent has been given, it has seriously been suggested that only medical students or graduate students in the life sciences ought to be accepted as subjects for experimentation. *Reductio ad absurdum* examples of "fully informed consent" have been elaborated, in forms which list all the minutiae of the proposed medical procedure, together with all of its conceivable sequelae. With such a view of "informed consent" and its requirements, it is not surprising to find doctors who claim that since they cannot fully inform patients, they will tell them nothing, but instead will personally assume the responsibility for assuring the subject's safety.

In truth, a *reductio ad absurdum* of this view of "informed consent" need not be constructed; it serves as its own *reductio ad absurdum*. For there is no end to "fully informing" patients. When the doctor wishes to insert a catheter, must he commend to the subject's attention a textbook of anatomy? Although this, of course, would not suffice: he must ensure that the patient understand the text as well. Must he tell the patient the story of Dr. X, that bogey of first-year medical students, who, in a state of inebriation, inserted ("by mistake") his pen refill instead of the catheter? With, of course, the assurance that *this* physician never gets drunk ("Well,

rarely, anyway"). Must the patient be informed of the chemical formula of the catheter? Its melting point?

The basic mistake which is committed by those who harp upon the difficulties in obtaining informed consent (and by critics of the doctrine) is in believing that we can talk about information in the abstract, without reference to any human purpose. It is very likely impossible to talk about "information" in this way; but impossible or not, when we do in fact talk about, or request, information, we do not mean "information in the abstract." If I ask someone to "tell me about those clouds" he will, ordinarily, know what I mean; and he will answer me, in the spirit in which he was asked, by virtue of his professional expertise as an artist, meteorologist, astronomer, soothsayer, or what-have-you. The meteorologist will not object that he cannot tell you the optical refraction index of the clouds, and therefore that he cannot "fully answer" your question. He knows that you are asking him with a given end in mind, and that much information about the cloud is irrelevant *relative to that purpose.*

That this "abstract information" requirement is not in question in obtaining valid consent is hardly an original point, but it is worth repeating. One of the leading court opinions on human experimentation puts it like this: "... the patient's interest in information does not extend to a lengthy polysyllabic discourse on all possible complications. A minicourse in medical science is not required...."[5]

The proper question to ask, then, is not "What information must be given?" That would be premature: we must first know for what purpose information is needed. *Why* must the patient be informed? Put that way, the answer is immediately forthcoming. The patient must be informed so that he will know what he is getting into, what he may expect from the procedure, what his likely alternatives are—in short what the procedure (and forbearance from it) will mean, so that a responsible decision on the matter may be made. This is the legal stance, as well as, I think, a "common sensical" stance; as Alexander Capron writes, the information component in valid consent derives in law from the recognition that information is "necessary to make meaningful the power to decide."[6] The proper test of whether a given piece of information needs to be given is, then, whether the physician, knowing what he does about the patient/subject, feels that the patient/subject would want to know this before making up his mind. Outré, improbable consequences would not ordinarily, therefore, be relevant information. Exceptionally, they will be: for example, when there is a small risk of impotence consequent upon the procedure which the physician proposes to perform upon a man with a great stake in his sexual prowess. This is only sensible.

Our main conclusion, then, is that valid consent entails only the imparting of that information which the patient/subject requires in order to make a responsible decision. This entails, I think, the possibility of a valid yet ignorant consent.

Consider, first, the therapeutic context. It is, I believe, not unusual for a patient to give his doctor *carte blanche* to perform any medical procedure which the physician deems proper in order to effect a cure. He is telling the doctor to act as his agent in choosing which procedure to follow. This decision is neither unwise nor (in any serious sense) an abdication of responsibility and an unwarranted burden upon the physician. We each of us choose to delegate our power of choice in this way in dealing with our auto mechanic or stockbroker.

It may be harder to accept an ignorant consent as valid in the purely experimental context. I think, however, that much of this difficulty is due to our paucity of imagination, our failure to imagine circumstances in which a person might choose to proceed in this way. We might approach such a case, for example, by imagining a Quaker who chooses to serve society by acting as a research subject, but who has a morbid fear of knives and pointed instruments. The Quaker might say to the physician-investigator that he wants to serve science but is afraid that his phobia would overcome his better judgment. He might consequently request that any experiment which would involve use of scalpels, hypodermic needles, and such, be performed without informing him: while, say, he is asleep or unconscious. He might further ask the doctor not to proceed should the experiment involve considerable risk. In such a case, or one similar, we would find an instance of a valid yet ignorant consent to experimentation.

The ostensible differences between the therapeutic and experimental contexts may be resolved into two components: in the therapeutic context it is supposed that the physician knows what the sequelae to treatment will be, which information, by definition, is not available in the experimental situation; and in the therapeutic context the doctor may be said to be seeking his patient's good, in contrast to the experimental context where some other good is being sought. On the basis of these differences it may be claimed that a valid yet ignorant consent is enough permission for therapy, but not for experimentation.

Closer examination, however, reveals that these differences do not necessarily obtain. First, because I believe it would be granted that a valid yet ignorant consent can be given in the "therapeutic-experimental" situation, where a new drug or procedure is being attempted to aid the patient (in the absence of any traditional available therapy). In the therapeutic-experimental situation, as in the purely experimental situation, the sequelae are not known (although of course in both cases some definite result is expected or anticipated). If a valid yet ignorant consent is acceptable in the one, therefore, it must be acceptable in the other.

Secondly, because it is patently not the case that we can expect there to be no good accruing to the subject of an experiment by reason of his participation. There are, commonly, financial and other "tangible" benefits forthcoming (laboratory training, and so on). And it must once again be said that the pleasures of altruism are not negligible. The proposed differences between experimentation and therapy do not stand up, and so we must say that if a valid yet ignorant consent is acceptable in the one it must be acceptable in the other. It must be remembered that this statement only concerns itself with one part of the consent doctrine, which is, itself, only one of the requirements which the ethical experiment must satisfy.

To mention—without claiming totally to resolve—two problems which may be raised at this point: First, it is said that a doctor often does not know what will happen as a consequence of a recommended procedure, and so cannot tell the patient what the patient wants to know. The obvious response to this seems to be right: the physician should, in that case, tell the patient/subject that he does not know what will happen (which does not exclude an explanation of what the doctor expects to happen, and on what he bases this expectation).

Second, it will be objected that the adoption of a requirement such as I propose would forbid the use of placebos and blind experiments. I am not sure that this is so; sometimes it must be the case that the subjects in an experiment may be asked (without introducing artifacts into the results) to consent to an experiment knowing that some will, and some will not, be receiving placebos. Another alternative would be to inform the subjects that the experiment may or may not involve some subjects receiving placebos.[7] I am aware, however, that these remarks are less than adequate responses to these problems.

Our conclusion, then, is that the informing of the patient/subject is not a fundamental requirement of valid consent. It is, rather, derivative from the requirement that the consent be the expression of a responsible choice. The two requirements which I do see as fundamental in this doctrine are that the choice be responsible and that it be voluntary.

The Requirement of Responsibility

What is meant by saying that the choice must be "responsible"? Does this entail that the physician may at any time override a patient's judgment on the basis that, in the physician's view, the patient has not chosen responsibly? Surely not; to adopt such a criterion would defeat the purpose embodied in the doctrine of consent. It would mean that a person's exercise of autonomy is always subject to review.

Still, some such requirement would appear to be necessary. A small child can certainly make choices.[8] Small children can also be intelligent enough to understand the necessary information. Yet surely we would not want to say that a small child can give valid consent to a serious medical procedure.[9] The reason for this is that the child cannot choose *responsibly.*

We are faced with a dilemma. On the one hand, it appears that we must require that the choice be responsible. To require only that the choice be free would yield counter-intuitive results. On the other hand, if we do require that the choice made be a responsible one, we seem to presuppose some body which shall judge the reasonableness of choices; this represents a paternalism which is antithetical to the

doctrine of consent. An elderly patient chooses to forgo further life-saving measures. How are we to judge whether or not this choice is a responsible one?

The path between the horns of this dilemma involves saying that the "responsibility" which we require is to be predicated not on the nature of the particular choice, but on the nature of the patient/subject. What we need to know is whether *he* is a responsible man ("in general," so to speak), not whether the choice which has been made is responsible. In this way, we avoid the danger of upholding as "responsible" only those choices which we ourselves feel are good choices. We can and do admit into the community of responsible persons individuals who make choices with which we do not agree.

In this sense, responsibility is a dispositional characteristic. To say that someone is a responsible individual means that he makes choices, typically on the basis of reasons, arguments, or beliefs—and that he remains open to the claims of reason, so that further rational argument might lead him to change his mind. It is to say that a person is capable of making and carrying through a life-plan—that he is prepared to act on the basis of his choices. It is to say that a person is capable of living with his life-plan; he can live with the consequences of his choices, he *takes responsibility* for his choices.[10] Of course, none of these are absolutes: all responsible people are at times pigheaded, at times shortsighted, at times flighty. That is to say, all responsible men at times act irresponsibly. Should the lack of responsibility persist, of course, to an extreme degree, we may say that the person has left the community of responsible folk.

Voluntarism and Reward

The other requirement of valid consent is that it be given voluntarily. The choice which the consent expresses must be freely made.

We all know some conditions which, if satisfied, make us say that a consent has been given involuntarily. The case which immediately springs to mind occurs when an individual succumbs under a threat: we call this duress or coercion. But the threat need not be overt; and perhaps there need not be a threat at all to render consent involuntary.

Hence, the major problem currently engendered by the requirement of voluntariness. It is typified by the prisoner who "volunteers" for an experiment in the hope or expectation of a reward: significantly higher wages, an opportunity for job training, better health care while involved in the experiment, a favorable report to his parole board. Is the consent which the prisoner offers a voluntary consent? The problem may be stated more generally thus: At what point does reward render consent involuntary?

The problem of reward is particularly difficult, since it involves questions of degree. Is a prisoner's consent involuntary if the reward for his participation in the experiment is a three-month reduction of sentence? Is it relevant here that the prisoner is serving a twenty-year sentence, rather than a one-to-five-year sentence? Does a possible increase in the wages from twenty-five cents per hour to one dollar per hour constitute duress? Should we consider the percentage increase, or the increase in absolute value, or the increase in actual value which the seventy-five cent disparity represents in the prison environment?

To some, of course, questions like these have little meaning. They have little meaning to those who are indifferent to the demands of justice and autonomy which the consent doctrine represents, to those who are willing to buy guinea pigs, rather than to reward human beings. And they have little meaning for those who are convinced that prisoners are inherently unfree, and who thus would call for a total cessation of prison experimentation. Each of these positions denies, in *a priori* fashion, freedom to prisoners; each must be rejected. A recognition of the fact that decisions about consent may be over- as well as under-protective forces us to deal with this sort of question, complex though it may be.

As is so often the case, posing the question in a different way may facilitate response. We have been considering the question of how much reward nullifies the validity of consent, how much reward renders the subject unfree. But is it in fact the case that *reward* is the disruptive factor here?

This problem may be clarified by the following examples. Imagine an upper-middle-class individual, who can provide for his family all of their needs and most of the amenities of civilized life. Let us say

that this person is offered one hundred dollars to cross the street—if you like, make it one thousand or ten thousand dollars? He chooses to cross the street, is his choice *involuntary*? Despite the substantial reward, I think most of us would agree that the consent was freely offered (and would that we should have such problems!).

Consider a person who deeply wants to be an astronaut. He is told that as part of the program he must participate in experiments to determine resistance to high-G conditions. Is his consent to this invalid, involuntary? I think not. We would say, this is part of his job; he should have expected it; and if he can't stand the heat, he should get out of the kitchen. In this vein, consider Evel Knievel, a financially prosperous man, who is offered millions of dollars to perform daredevil stunts. His choice may be bizarre, even crazy; but has his reward rendered it unfree?

Finally, consider a man who is informed by this doctor that he will most likely die unless he has open-heart surgery. His "reward" for consenting is his life; the penalty for not consenting is death. Does this mean this man cannot give the doctor valid consent—morally valid consent—to proceed?

There are two distinctions which, I think, go a long way towards dispelling these problems. First, I think it must be granted that natural contingencies ("acts of God," things which come to pass naturally, those contingencies which we cannot hold anyone responsible for) do not render a person unfree, nor do they render unfree the choices which a person makes in light of those contingencies.[11]

That natural contingencies do not render a man unfree is a point which is apt to be forgotten in the present context. I am not—in the morally relevant sense—lacking in freedom because I cannot, unaided, fly through the air, or live on grass. Nor am I unfree because my heart is about to give out. Nor am I unfree when, recognizing that my heart may give out, I choose to undergo surgery. I may, of course, be so crazed by knowing that I am near death's door that I am in a state of general impotence, and hence must have the choice made for me; but general incompetence is not in question here. The distinction between choices forced by man, and choices forced by nature, is, then, of importance.

The second distinction is between those pressures which are, and those which are not, in Daube's words, "consonant with the dignity and responsibility of free life."[12] I would explain this as follows: there are certain basic freedoms and rights which we possess which *entitle* us (morally) to certain things (or states of affairs). We would all, no doubt, draw up different lists of these rights and freedoms; but included in them would be safety of person, freedom of conscience and religion, a right to a certain level of education, and, for some of us, a right to some level of health care. When the "reward" is such as only to give us the necessary conditions of these rights and freedoms—when all that the reward does is to bring us up to a level of living to which we are entitled, and of which we have been deprived by man—then the "reward," I think, constitutes duress. A reward which accrues to one who has achieved this level, or who can easily achieve it (other than by taking the reward-option), and which hence serves only to grant us "luxury" items, does not constitute duress, and hence does not render choice unfree, no matter how great this reward may be.

The rewards above the moral subsistence level are true rewards. In contrast, we may say (with some touch of metaphor) that the "rewards" which only bring us up to the level to which we were in any event entitled are properly viewed as functioning as *threats*: "Do this, or stay where you are"—when you should not have been "where you are" in the first place.

The astronaut, Evel Knievel, and the upper-middle-class street-crosser are being granted "luxury" items, and hence are capable of giving free consent. But consider a man who will not be admitted to the hospital for treatment unless he agrees to be a subject in an experiment (unrelated to his treatment). Those who feel, as I do, that we are, here and now, morally entitled to medical treatment would agree, I trust, that this illegitimate option coerces the man into agreeing. Or consider a man who has religious scruples against donating blood, who takes his daughter to a hospital for treatment. He is told that the doctors will not treat her unless the family donates a certain amount of blood. His freedom has been nullified: his "consent" to donating blood is morally invalid. Similarly, the college student whose

grade is contingent upon his participation in the instructor's psychological experiments is not validly consenting to serve. He is entitled to have his grade based upon his classroom work.

It yet remains to apply this distinction to our original problem, prison experimentation. The application will not be attempted here, for we would first need to be clear in our minds what rights and freedoms a prisoner is entitled to. I would not hesitate to say, though, that when a situation is created whereby a prisoner can only receive decent health care by participating in an experiment, he is being coerced into that experiment. I would have little hesitation in claiming that if subjecting himself to experimentation is the only way in which a prisoner could learn a trade which may be used "outside," then that prisoner is being coerced, his consent is not free. When we take into account the condition of our society, these would seem to be reasonable entitlements for the prisoner. Other rewards—for example, higher pay—may or may not constitute rewards above the moral subsistence level; if they are, then consent in light of these rewards could be freely offered. Perhaps too much has been said already; judgments like these must be made in an individualized fashion, one which is sensitive to the realities of prison life.

II. CONSENT AND THE INCOMPETENT

In this section will be discussed, first, the question of how the age of majority and minority with reference to valid consent ought to be set; and secondly, the problems associated with the concept of proxy consent.

The Age of Consent

It has been argued that the requirements for obtaining valid consent are that the patient/subject must have consented freely and that he must be a responsible individual. The requirement of voluntariness does not raise any novel problems when applied to minors. Rather, what we usually have in mind when restricting the power of the minor to consent is that he is not, in the sense required, a responsible individual.

I have claimed that to be a responsible individual one must be capable of rationally adopting, following through, and accepting the consequences of a life-plan. The age, therefore, at which society indicates a presumption that individuals can satisfy these conditions can be said to be the age at which society ought to grant the right to give valid consent to serious medical procedures. The examples which spring to mind are the age of conscription and the age of marriageability. At these ages society has indicated that one is capable of acting, in a complex society, as an individual.

This is not an argument like that which says "If you are old enough to fight, then you are old enough to vote." The requirements necessary for being a soldier may be wholly unrelated to the requirements necessary before the franchise may be properly exercised. In contrast, the responsibility which we assume to be possessed by those capable of soldiering and contracting marriage is the same responsibility which is required to make consent valid: the ability to work through and with a life-plan.

The first thing which needs to be said, then, is that the age of consent should be lowered from 21 to 18 in those jurisdictions which have not yet done so. This should not entail merely that an 18- year-old may consent in the absence of parental disapproval; it should be a full power to consent, irrespective of what others might say.

But the setting of an age of consent indicates only a presumption and nothing more. The fact that someone has passed the age of consent is not conclusive proof that he is responsible (in the sense required); the fact that someone is below the age of consent is not conclusive proof of irresponsibility. The presumption may be defeated in either direction.

It is clear, for example, that an adult is not, *ipso facto*, responsible. The adult may be insane.

It is equally clear that a minor need not be irresponsible. People mature at different rates. If evidence of responsibility may be supplied on behalf of one below the age of consent, the presumption of irresponsibility should be defeated. The sort of evidence which would be necessary is that which indicates that the person can work through a life-plan. It may be said that this notion is being approached by the law in the special provisions sometimes made for the "emancipated minor." Marriage or economic self-sufficiency are among the common requirements for being considered an emancipated minor. One of the special prerogatives of the emancipated minor is that he may consent on his own behalf to medical care. I would argue that this should be extended to cover participation in experimentation as well.

Proxy Consent

Proxy consent is consent given on behalf of an individual who is himself incapable of granting consent. The major category of those who require proxy consent are minors, but proxy consent may need to be obtained for the insane or the unconscious as well. My comments will nevertheless be restricted to the case of minors, leaving the other cases to be dealt with by implication. In minors, proxy consent is ordinarily granted by the child's parent or guardian; exceptionally, it may be given by another close relative or by an individual appointed by the court for the specific purpose of granting consent to some procedure.

I have argued that the function of informed consent is to respect the autonomy and dignity of the individual. This cannot be the function of proxy consent. The minor patient/subject cannot fully express autonomy and dignity through choices. It may be said that the function of proxy consent is to protect the right of the parents to raise their child as they see fit, to do with the child as they like. But the child is not the property of the parents; parents do not have an absolute right of disposal over the child. In law we recognize constraints upon the parental power, and common morality affirms the justice in this. What then is the function of proxy consent?

I think it would be best to turn this question on its head. By virtue of what right which the child possesses do we require the granting of proxy consent before a medical procedure may be initiated? What *could* be the source of such an obligation? We ordinarily recognize that there is only one fundamental right possessed by minors, a right to be protected and aided in development. "... A child, unlike an adult, has a right 'not to liberty but to custody.'"[13] All other rights which a child possesses, all other duties which we have towards children, are derivative from this single right, and are void when inconsistent with it. Broadly speaking, in consequence of this right, we must do what we may to promote the welfare of the child; we must abstain from doing what will injure the child, physically or otherwise; and, as far as this right goes, we are at liberty to deal with the child in ways which neither help nor hurt.

That proxy consent is ordinarily to be obtained from the parent or guardian of the child is understandable. We feel that the parent has the best interests of the child at heart, and knows how best to seek the child's welfare. It also follows from this right, however, that, when the parent does not have the best interests of the child in mind, the power of proxy consent should be transferred to another. It is on such a basis that society feels justified in removing a child from his parent's custody, and in appointing another to act *in parens patriae*. If this system is to be effective, society must, by and large, act on the basis of shared common views about what the welfare of the child consists of. We cannot allow anything which a parent considers to be a benefit to the child—being boiled in oil to save his eternal soul—to count as action in the child's best interests. This does not preclude a certain amount of leeway in a liberal society as to permitted views of welfare: if most feel that it is better, when the money is available, to send the child to a private school, we yet will not fault an affluent parent who decides to send his child to a public school.

The consequences of these propositions for cases when proxy consent is being sought for the purpose of giving therapy to a child accord well with the way the law handles this subject. The problem situation which arises concerns parents who, because of religious scruples, refuse to consent to needed medical treatment for their child. Jehovah's Witnesses, for example, who believe that blood transfusions are forbidden by the law of God, will not consent on behalf of their child to blood transfusions. Society feels that the benefit of the child is to be found in allowing the procedure. Because of this, the hospital will often turn to a judge, who appoints someone to act *in parens patriae* for the purpose of consenting to the specific procedure. I suggest that if it were clearly the view of society that it is to the mongoloid infant's benefit to survive, should a parent refuse to consent to a life-saving procedure for that infant, a similar course would be followed: the consent of a court-appointed guardian would be substituted.

Proxy consent to experimentation on children is a more complicated matter. In law, there are two kinds of intervention in the person of another which are actionable in the absence of consent: those interventions where harm does, and where harm does not, result. The latter are termed "wrongful" or "harmful touchings" (though no harm has occurred). In other words, the mere *doing* of something to a person without his consent is, in itself, an actionable wrong.

We may say that, corresponding to this division, there are two sorts of experiments: those which do, and those which do not, injure the subject appreciably. Beecher has noted, for example, that "Many thousands of psychomotor tests and sociological studies have been carried out in children during the child's development and have revealed much information of value.... Sound nutritional studies without risk have been carried out. So have certain blood studies."[14] It must be added that many studies of value cannot, due to metabolic and other differences, be carried out in adults with results which will be valid for children.

It is clear, on the basis of the principle of benefit, that proxy consent to dangerous or harmful experiments on children cannot be valid. What about those experiments which carry no appreciable risk—the "wrongful touchings" sort? In an adult, it would seem, the right to autonomy, the right "to be let alone," is sufficient basis for the action of wrongful touching. But the child does not have a right to autonomy, except insofar as some measure of autonomy is necessary to promote the child's development and well-being.

Harmless experiments on children, therefore, which satisfy the other canons of medical ethics—good design, well-trained experimenters, and so forth—could be performed. Parents would not be derelict in their duty should they consent, on behalf of their child, to experiments of this sort. Participation in these experiments does not infringe the child's right to welfare, unless they would result in a *harmful* (and not just any) restriction of autonomy.

As I see it, the fundamental problem with those who would forbid *all* experimentation upon children[15] is that they confuse consent in adults with proxy consent for children. These two are fundamentally different requirements. Children are not small adults; our relations with children must not be made to approach as nearly as possible to our relations with adults. There are things which you ought to grant to children which need not be granted to adults: if a child is thirsty you provide him with a drink. And there are things which may licitly be done to children which could not be done with adults: if my parents annoy me I may not send them to their room. A child is (morally) a different sort of thing than is an adult; we must adjust our relations with them according to their claims upon us.

CONCLUSION

This paper represents an attempt of formulate what I call a "moral theory" of the requirement of consent to serious medical procedures. The method used involves an interplay between cases and principles, such that each influences the other. Well-established moral intuitions about cases suggested some principles and called for the rejection of others. These principles in turn, once established, enabled the clarification of a proper approach to other, borderline cases.

Under the influence of situation ethics, much of the work on medical ethics has stressed the respects in which cases differ. This has resulted in the development of an *ad hoc* literature on cases which pose difficulty for the doctrine of informed consent. As the cases accumulated, the doctrine began to seem more and more amorphous.

In contrast, this paper has sought to unify the doctrine of consent. Principles which are developed through considering the problems raised by prison experimentation in turn suggested solutions to other situations; rather than stressing the differences between the experimental and the therapeutic contexts, their similarities were emphasized. There is, I think, a need for such efforts at unification, as there is a need for a literature which is committed to the unique aspects of different cases.

Author's Note

The research for this paper was begun during an internship at the Institute of Society, Ethics and the Life Sciences in the month of June, I gratefully acknowledge the help of Drs. Daniel Callahan, Marc Lappé, Peter Steinfels, and Robert Veatch, of the Institute, who helped make my internship profitable and enjoyable. My wife Barbara read the manuscript and suggested a number of needed changes.

Notes

1. For examples of a similar method applied to different problems, see Thomas I. Emerson, *Toward a General Theory of the First Amendment* (New York: Vintage Books, 1967).

2. "Brain Surgery in Aggressive Epileptics," in *Hastings Center Report,* February 1973.

3. See the insert to Alexander M. Capron's call for a moratorium on prison experimentation, "Medical Research in Prisons," *Hastings Center Report,* June 1973. The insert is a report from the *New York Times.* April 15, 1973, and reads in part: "Ninety-six of the 175 inmates at Lancaster County prison have written to a newspaper here protesting a recent decision by the state to halt all medical experiments on state prisoners. In their letter to the *Lancaster New Era,* they urged that state to allow the research [which] did not harm them and enabled them to pay off their fines and court costs."

4. See Henry K. Beecher, *Research and the Individual: Human Studies* (Boston: Little, Brown, 1970), p. 56. Professor Beecher notes a study of prison inmates, who, for participation in an experiment involving malaria, received pay but no reduction of sentence. Half of the volunteers cited "altruism" rather than money as their motive for volunteering. Those inmates who did not volunteer "expressed or implied respect for those who did volunteer."

5. *Cobbs* v. *Grant,* 502P. 2d1, 11.

6. Alexander M. Capron, "Legal Rights and Moral Rights," in Hilton, *et al.,* eds., *Ethical Issues in Human Genetics* (Plenum Press, 1973), 228.

7. If this sort of explanation were given as a matter of course in *all* experiments, this might still further reduce the problem of artifacts. The remarks, it should be noted, are directed towards medical experiments. By and large, they are inapplicable to, say, experiments in social psychology.

8. The counter-suggestion may be made that children cannot *really* make choices. This would, I think, put too great a weight upon the requirement of voluntarism. We would be recruiting the concepts of choice and volition to do a job which they have not been designed for.

9. I am speaking of course in the moral, not the legal, context. It may be that in an emergency a child may, in the absence of his parents, give legally valid consent.

10. This gives us the link between "responsible" in the dispositional sense explained here, and "responsible" in the blame-sense of the word ("I'll hold you responsible for that").

11. The *caveat* must be added: natural contingencies do not have, as their *sole* result, the rendering of a person unfree, in the sense which vitiates consent: a man's brain tumor can make the man an idiot, schizophrenia can make a man insane, but these do not so much affect a person's volition as they do disturb his entire psychic structure.

12. David Daube, quoted in Beecher, p. 146.

13. *In re Gault,* U. S. 1 (1967).

14. Beecher, p. 67.

15. See, for example, Paul Ramsey, "Consent as a Canon of Loyalty with Special Reference to Children in Medical Investigations," in *The Patient as Person* (New Haven: Yale University Press, 1970).

11.
COMPETENCY TO GIVE AN INFORMED CONSENT: A MODEL FOR MAKING CLINICAL ASSESSMENTS

James F. Drane

In January 1980, as one more indication of the growing importance of medical ethics, a presidential commission was formed and began work on the moral questions posed by the practice of contemporary medicine. After three years of intense work, the commission published a separate volume on 11 different ethical problems in the hope of stimulating thoughtful discussion. Some broad principles were uncovered that apply to any and every bioethical issue, such as the principle of patient respect and its concrete application in the right of informed consent. But there were also recurring perplexities, one of which was competency or, in the language preferred by the commission, the patient's capacity to choose.[1]

Respect for patients means ensuring their participation in decisions affecting their lives. Such participation is a basic form of freedom and stands at the core of Western values. But freedom, participation, and self-determination suppose a capacity for such acts. No one, for example, assumes that an infant has such a capacity and, time and again, doubts arise about the capacity of some older patients. Not to respect a patient's freedom is undoubtedly wrong. But to respect what may be an expression of freedom only in appearance would be a violation of another basic principle of ethical medicine: promotion of the patient's well-being.

Although the commission's report referred many times to competency or capacity to choose, commissioners and staff members privately expressed frustration and disappointment about their conclusions. The commission reports spelled out what are considered to be the components of competency: the possession of a set of values and goals, the ability to communicate and understand information, and the ability to reason and deliberate. In addition, the commission criticized some standards for determining

competency that either were too lenient and did not protect a patient sufficiently or were too strict and in effect transferred decision making to the physician. But the commission did not come up with its own standard and left unsettled the question of how to decide whether a particular patient's decision should be respected or overridden because of incompetency. Incompetency is not the only reason for overriding a patient's refusal or setting aside a consent, but it is the most common reason for doing so. Defining incompetency or establishing standards of competency is a complex problem because it involves law, ethics, and psychiatry.

COMPETENCY ASSESSMENT

Competency assessments focus on the patient's mental capacities, specifically, the mental capacities to make an informed medical decision. Does the patient understand what is being proposed? Can the patient come to a decision about treatment based on an adequate understanding? How much understanding and rational decision making capacity are sufficient for this particular patient to be considered competent? Conversely how deficient must this patient's decision-making capacity be before he is declared incompetent? A properly performed competency assessment should eliminate two types of error: (1) preventing a competent person from participating in treatment decisions and (2) failing to protect an incompetent person from the harmful effects of a bad decision.

MODEL FOR MAKING THE ASSESSMENT

The President's commission did not recommend a single standard for determining competency because any one standard is inappropriate for the many different types of medical decisions that people face. What is proposed here is a sliding standard, i.e., the more dangerous the medical decision, the more stringent the standards of competency. The basic idea, following a suggestion of Mark Siegler,[2] is to connect determination of competency to different medical situations (acute or chronic, critical or noncritical), and next to take this idea a step further by specifying three different standards or definitions of what it means to be competent. These standards are then correlated with three different medical situations, each more dangerous than the other. Finally, the sliding standards and different medical situations are correlated with the types of psychiatric abnormalities that ordinarily undermine competency. The interrelationship of all these entities creates a model that can aid the physician faced with a question about a patient's capacity to choose. This model brings together disparate academic disciplines, but its goal is thoroughly pragmatic: to provide a workable guide for clinical decision making.

STANDARD 1

The first and least stringent standard of competency to give a valid consent applies to those medical decisions that are not dangerous and objectively are in the patient's best interest. If the patient is critically ill because of an acute illness that is life threatening, if there is an effective treatment available that is low in risk, and if few or no alternatives are available, then consent to the treatment is prima facie rational. Even though patients are seriously ill and thereby impaired in both cognitive and conative functioning, they are usually competent to consent to a needed treatment.

The act of consent to such a treatment is considered to be an informed consent as long as the patient is aware of what is going on. *Awareness* in the sense of orientation or being conscious of the general situation satisfies the cognitive requirement of informed consent. *Assent* alone to what is the rational expectation in this medical context satisfies the decisional component. When adult patients go along with needed medical treatment, then a legal presumption of competency holds even though the patients are obviously impaired. To insist on higher standards for capacity to give a valid consent in such a medical setting would amount to requiring surplus mental capacities for a simple task and would result in millions of acutely ill patients being considered incom-

petent. Such an absurd requirement would produce absurd consequences. Altogether rational and appropriate decisions would be set aside as invalid, and surrogate decision makers would have to be selected to make the same decision. For what purpose? To accomplish what objective? To protect what value? None of the values and objectives meant to be safeguarded by the competency requirement is disregarded or set aside by a lenient standard for this type of decision.

Considering as competent seriously ill patients, even the mentally ill, who are aware and assent to treatment, eliminates the ambiguity and confusion associated with terms such as *virtually competent*, *marginally competent*, and *competent for practical purposes* that are used to excuse the commonsense practice of respecting the decisions of patients who would be judged incompetent by a more demanding single standard of decision-making capacity. Refusal by a patient dying of a chronic illness of treatments that are useless and only prolong the dying requires the same modest standard of competency.

Infants, unconscious persons, and the severely retarded would obviously fall short even of this least demanding standard. These persons, and patients who use psychotic defenses that severely compromise reality testing, are the only ones who fail to meet this first definition of decision-making capacity. Children who have reached the age of reason (6 years or older), on the other hand, as well as the senile, the mildly retarded, and the intoxicated, are considered competent.

The law considers 21 and sometimes 18 years to be the age below which persons are presumed incompetent to make binding contracts, including health care decisions. The President's commission, however, endorses a lower age of competency, and so do many authors who write about children and mental retardation. In this model, we are discussing ethical standards, but the physician cannot ignore the law and must obtain consent from the child's legal guardian.

STANDARD 2

If the illness is chronic rather than acute, or if the treatment is more dangerous or of less definite benefit (or if there are real alternatives to one or another course of action, e.g., death rather than lingering ill-ness), then the risk-benefit balance is tipped differ-ently than in the situation described in the previous section. Consequently, a different standard of com-petency to consent is required. The patient must be able to *understand* the risks and outcomes of the dif-ferent options and then be able to *choose* a decision based on this understanding. At this point, compe-tency means capacity to understand the real options and to make an understanding decision, a higher standard than that required for the first type of treat-ment choice.

Ability to understand is not the same as being able to articulate conceptual or verbal understanding. Some ethicists assume a rationalist epistemology and reduce all understanding to a conceptual or ver-bal type. Many, in fact, require that patients literally remember what they have been told as a proof of competence. Understanding, however, may be more affective than conceptual. Following an explanation, a patient may grasp what is best for him with strong feelings and convictions, and yet be hard pressed to articulate his understanding/conviction in words.

Competency as capacity for an understanding choice is also reconcilable with a decision to let a trusted physician decide what is the best treatment. Such a choice (waiver) may be made for good rea-sons and represent a decision in favor of one set of values (safety or anxiety reduction) over another (independence and personal initiative). As such, it can be considered as informed consent and creates no suspicion of incompetency.

Ignorance or inability to understand, however, undermines competency. The same is true of a severe mood disorder or severe shock, which may either impair thought processes or undermine capacity to make an understanding choice. Short-term memory loss, delusion, dementia, and delirium would also render a patient incompetent. On the other hand, mature adolescents, the mildly retarded, and persons with some personality disorders would be competent to make this type of decision.

STANDARD 3

The most stringent and demanding standard of com-petency is reserved for those decisions that are very dangerous and fly in the face of both professional and public rationality. When diagnostic uncertainty is minimal, the available treatment is effective, and death is likely to result from treatment refusal, a pre-sumption is established against refusal of consent to treatment. The medical decision now is not a balanc-ing of what are widely recognized as reasonable alternatives. Any decision other than the one to be treated seems to violate basic reasonableness. A decision to refuse treatment, then, is apparently irra-tional, besides being harmful. Yet, according to this model, such decisions can be respected as long as the patients satisfy the most demanding standard of competency.

Competency in this context requires a capacity to appreciate the nature and consequences of the deci-sion being made. *Appreciation* is a term used to refer to the highest degree of understanding, one that grasps more than just the medical details of the ill-ness and treatment. To be competent to make appar-ently irrational and very dangerous choices, the patient must be able to come to a decision based on the medical information and to appreciate the impli-cations of this decision for his life. Competency of this type requires a capacity that is both technical and personal, both cognitive and affective.

Since the patient's decision flies in the face of objective standards of rationality, it must at least be subjectively critical and *rational*. A patient need not conform to what most rational people do to be con-sidered competent, but the competent patient must be able to give reasons for his decision. The patient must be able to show that he has thought through the med-ical issues and related this information to his person-al value system. The patient's personal reasons need not be medically or publicly accepted, but neither can they be purely private, idiosyncratic, or incoherent. Their intelligibility may derive from a set of religious beliefs or from a philosophical view that is shared by only a small minority. This toughest standard of com-petency does, however, demand a more rationalistic type understanding: one that includes verbalization, argumentation, and consistency.

The higher-level mental capacities required for competency to make this type of decision are impaired by less severe psychiatric abnormality. In fact, much less serious mental affliction suffices to create an assumption of incompetency to refuse a needed and effective treatment. On the other hand, however, not any mental or emotional disturbance would constitute an impairment of decisional capacity. A certain amount of anxiety, for example, goes with any serious decision and cannot make a patient incompetent. Some mild pain would not impair decisional capacity, but severe pain might do so. Even a slight reactive depression may not render a patient incompetent for this type of decision. But intense anxiety associated with mild or severe shock, and/or a mild endogenous depression, would be considered incapacitating. In fact, any mental or emotional disorder that compromises appreciation and rational decision making would make a patient incompetent. For example, persons who are incapable of making the effort required to control destructive behavior (substance abusers and sociopaths), as well as neurotic persons, hysterical persons, and persons who are ambivalent about their choice, would all be incompetent to refuse life saving treatment. The same standard applies to consent to experiments not related to one's own illness.

CONCLUSION
Radical advocates of patient rights and doctrinaire libertarians will worry that this model shifts power back toward physicians who make competency determinations and away from patients whose choices ought to be respected. But only in situation 3 does the physician's power increase, and then only for the patient's welfare. Moreover, this loss in the patient's power never reaches the point where patients' self-determination is set aside. Patients can insist on their decision to refuse a treatment even when the physician knows that the outcome will be certain death, as long as every precaution is taken to ensure that such a decision is not the product of a pathological state.

A balancing of values is the cornerstone of a good competency assessment. Rationality is given its place throughout this model. Maximum autonomy is guaranteed for patients because they can choose to do what is not at all beneficial (a non-therapeutic experiment) or refuse to do what is most beneficial. Maximum benefit is also guaranteed because patients are protected against harmful choices that are more the product of abnormality than of their self-determination. All the values, in fact, on which competency requirements were originally based are guaranteed in this model.

No one proposal will settle the question of which standard or standards of competency are appropriate for medical decisions. More empirical research is required on the issue, and more physicians who have valuable practical experience with complex cases need to be heard from. After much more study and discussion, perhaps the medical profession itself, through its ethics committees, will take a stand on the issue. In the meantime, this proposal is meant to be a contribution to the discussion.

Author's Notes
This investigation was supported in part by grant ED 0652-78 from the National Endowment for the Humanities.

Notes
1. President's Commission for the Study of Ethical Problems in Medicine and Biomedical and Behavioral Research; *Deciding to Forego Life-Sustaining Treatment.* Washington, D.C., U.S. Government Printing Office, 1983.
2. Siegler, M., Goldblatt, A.D.: Clinical intuition: A procedure for balancing the rights of patients and the responsibilities of physicians, in Spicker, S. F., Healey, J.M., Engelhardt, H.T. (eds.): *The Law-Medicine Relation: A Philosophical Exploration.* Dordrecht, The Netherlands, D. Reidel Publishing Co., 1981, pp. 5-29; Also Jonsen, A.R., Siegler, M., Winslade, W.J.: *Clinical Ethics.* New York: Macmillan Publishing Co., Inc., 1982, pp. 56-85.

12.
THE PHYSICIAN AS THERAPIST AND INVESTIGATOR

John E. Thomas

Moral dilemmas posed by experimenting with human subjects cluster around a tension between the need for scientific investigation to improve the effectiveness of treatment and the patient's claim to care. Two values underlie this tension—scientific freedom and individual inviolability; the right of scientists to inquire and the rights of human beings to be respected as persons and not to be treated as experimental materials. Over a wide range of intricate interactions these values are compatible, even complementary. Sometimes, however, they are in conflict, and when that happens we need to be reassured that patients' rights will not be sacrificed to scientific inquiry.

Formerly the researcher's and the physician's roles seldom overlapped. In recent years, however, particularly in teaching and research centres, doctors increasingly sport two hats—that of investigator and that of physician. The differences between them can be brought out in three ways: by reference to

(i) the different models underpinning the roles of physician and experimenter;
(ii) the divergence of the avowed goals of physician and researcher; and
(iii) the disparity in the knowledge to which the physician and investigator respectively lay claim.

First, consider the different models underpinning the roles of the physician and researcher. In its simplest form the physician-patient relationship may be diagrammed as follows:

THE THERAPEUTIC MODEL

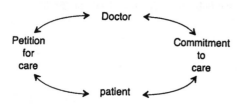

This contract or covenant is an agreement to which each party brings its own expectations. The primary thrust of the doctor-patient relationship, as the first model indicates, is *therapeutic*—the operative word is "care." In this relationship the doctor is the agent of the patient alone.

Contrast with this the different roles into which the doctor and patient are cast by the very nature of the experimental setting. Now the doctor confronts his subject as a scientist.

THE RESEARCH MODEL

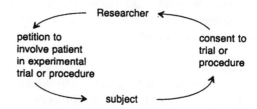

This contract is also an agreement to which each party brings its own expectations. Notice, in an experimental setting the doctor becomes a researcher and the patient a subject. The shift in the terms of the contract as well as in the roles of the parties to it are sufficiently radical to warrant disclosure to the patient. This is not to deny that the subject in the experimental situation will continue to receive care, perhaps even superior care to the recipients of standard or conventional treatment, but that fact in itself does not warrant withholding information about the change in the terms of the contract and the roles of the participants. Failure to keep these two models distinct may give rise to two serious misunderstandings. First, the patient is likely still to think of the researcher as a doctor (which, of course, he may be, but not in the sense relevant to this context). Second, the patient may mistake experiment for therapy.

Another undesirable consequence of the blurring of the distinction between physician and researcher is that the researcher may be tempted to claim for himself privileges that properly belong to the therapeutic model. This occurred in the notorious Brooklyn Jewish Hospital case. Ethically "the stone of stumbling and rock of offence" in the Brooklyn case was *not* that the procedure of injecting live cancer cells into geriatric patients was a particularly hazardous procedure (on the contrary, I have been assured it was a relatively harmless procedure). In court the researchers appealed to the physicians' right to withhold information from patients in certain circumstances. At this point in the trial the defence took a peculiar twist. The researchers defended their actions on the ground that the patients would *not* have agreed to the experiment if they had been told they were to be injected with live cancer cells—a curious justification for the waiver of the consent regulation that the court justifiably discounted.

In summing up their judgment of this case, the Board of Regents of the Brooklyn hospital put the whole matter in proper perspective:

> The physician when he is acting as an experimenter, has no claim to the doctor-patient relationship that, in a therapeutic situation would give him the generally acknowledged right to withhold information if he judged it in the best interest of the patient.[1]

So a shift in the roles of the parties to the contract radically affects the terms of the contract. Hence the investigator, even though also a physician, may not presume that the privileges accruing to the therapeutic model are automatically transferrable to the research model.

Second, not only do we witness a radical shift in the roles of the parties to the doctor-patient relationship as one moves from therapy to experimentation, there is also a *divergence in the goals* of the doctor and researcher. Primarily, the doctor is concerned to restore the patient to health, or where that proves impossible, to ameliorate his/her condition. These things the physician attempts to do as quickly and as efficiently as possible. By contrast the goal of the researcher is different. His objective is medical reconnaissance in which the emphasis now shifts from cure or amelioration of the subject's condition to a focus on *learning* more about the disease. This objective is accomplished by testing for more effective forms of treatment, which in turn hold promise of benefitting future sufferers if the present subjects are beyond hope. Getting clear about our goals in these situations need not cripple *bona fide* research. What it promises to do is to facilitate more intelligent and informed participation in the experiment.

Third, consider the disparity in the knowledge to which the physician and investigator, respectively, lay claim. In the experimental context the labels "researcher" and "subject" signal that the "patient" is no longer in the standard situation in which "the doctor knows best." In the standard setting the physician offers the most effective treatment consistent with the current state of the medical art. The scientific investigator, by his own admission, does *not* know best. Rather he is unsure whether the conventional treatment for the patient's malady is effective. Indeed it is this uncertainty that inspires the project and furnishes the moral imperative to undertake the clinical testing calculated to resolve the doubt. Because of this uncertainty the researcher is unable to say "This is the more effective treatment form." Instead, having acquainted the "patient" of the change in the terms of the contract or covenant signalled by the shift from the therapeutic to the research model and having informed the patient of the risks and potential benefits, he issues the invitation "While we don't know which treatment form is effective will you consent to being a party to finding out?"

The observation was made earlier that acquainting the patient-subject with such facts as we have been considering need not cripple *bona fide* research. It must be acknowledged, however, that it may slow down the pace of research. This is so for the following reasons. First, once the patient has an understanding of these factors he/she may decline to participate in an experimental procedure. I accept this as one of the risks associated with disclosure. Secondly, because the patients' physician performs a dual role—that of colleague of the investigator and that of patient advocate—tensions may arise in situations where there is a conflict between the patients' wishes and the experimenter's advice. In such cases, since I view the advocate's role of the patient as primary, again some refusals to participate may be forthcoming.

Another consideration involves some potentially coercive elements in a nontherapeutic experimental situation, that is, in a situation where the subject and benefittee are not identical.

The following imaginary conversation is put by Professor Hans Jonas into the mouth of a researcher:

> There is nothing more I can do for you. But you can do something for me. Speaking no longer as your physician but on behalf of medical science, we could learn a great deal about future cases of this kind if you would permit me to perform certain experiments on you. It is understood that you yourself would not benefit from any knowledge we might gain: but future patients would.[2]

One interesting thing about Jonas' example is that even though the experimental procedures envisaged hold no promise of direct benefit to the patient, they are nevertheless related to his disease, that is, they are potentially therapeutic from the researcher's standpoint, but not from the standpoint of the subject. The invitation to participate in such activities, however, poses an interesting ethical problem. Do patients have an obligation to acquiesce to such requests? If patients do have an obligation to participate in experimental procedures what is the source of this obligation? Frequently there are actions we feel obliged to perform from motives of gratitude. Are experimental procedures among such actions? After all, couldn't it be argued that the patients in question have been recipients of the physician's efforts on their behalf? What could be more natural than to claim that the sufferer now owes medicine a debt of gratitude? All other things being equal such a claim has some force. But all things are not equal in such circumstances, for the patient is already in an extremely disadvantageous and vulnerable position. Can we add to his/her burden by imposing yet another burden—the repayment of a debt of gratitude that might well involve further risk, discomfort, inconvenience and suffering? I think not. The patient's plight nullifies the obligation in this case. At most, sufferers at this kind of disadvantage may be "allowed to volunteer for" as opposed to "be expected to endure" such additional discomfort and risks as these experimental procedures are likely to incur. But, and this point is crucial, if such participation falls into the

category of moral obligation, then it falls into the category of unenforceable rather than enforceable obligation. In the case of proposals where the interests of the investigator are strongly in favour of research, special consideration and sensitivity are essential lest the patient be made to feel guilty if he/she refuses to acquiesce to experiments geared to the worthy goal of possibly benefitting future sufferers from the same complaint. The investigator must resist exploiting the motive of gratitude for services rendered or the worthy objective of possibly benefitting others. Indeed, in conjunction, gratitude and service may serve as powerful clubs to coerce participation in experimental procedures against the patient's wishes and better judgment.

Pressures on the subject to participate in experimental procedures, while often subtle, are nevertheless relentless. We have focussed on the temptation to exploit the motive of gratitude and incentive for service. Yet other patients respond from fear—the fear that if they refuse to acquiesce in the researcher's request that they will not receive proper treatment. A groundless fear from the researcher's viewpoint, especially since "patients" who are in an experiment "are likely to be more carefully observed and cared for than if they were not research subjects." But as groundless as the fear is from the researcher's vantage point, it may be so real from the patient's perspective as to count as duress. Not infrequently "patients" respond affirmatively to the invitation of the researcher to participate in an experimental procedure out of sheer physical weakness. Rendered less than sovereign by suffering, consent is marred by lowered resistance.

Sometimes even subtler influences brought to bear on the patient necessitate vigilance. These are the pressures resulting from pressures. The compulsion to do research easily translates itself into recruiting subjects for the project. After all, this is the *researcher's*, not the *subject's* project and its successful outcome will have a profound effect on his career. Medical schools and university hospitals are dominated by scientific investigations. Every young researcher knows that his/her professional career is contingent upon his/her ability as investigator as measured by publications.[3] Ramsey makes the same point: "it is not only that medical benefits are attained by research, but also that a man rises to the top in medicine by the success and significance of his research."[4] So, both the potential medical benefits to society as well as the investigator's promotion hinge upon conducting experiments that may place the patient at risk.

Earlier I referred to the conflict of values and obligations in the experimental situation—scientific freedom versus patient inviolability, the moral imperative to provide more effective treatment and the obligation to care for the patient. As delicate as the task of ranking values may be, it appears to be required in the present context. We have drawn attention to pressures to which the patient may be subjected in an experimental context—the exploitation of motives of gratitude, incentives for service, fear, the pressures born of pressures—all of which contribute to a powerfully coercive context for decision making. Given these pressures, as a compensatory move, it is necessary to give greater weight to the patient's rights than to the potential good to be achieved by the research project in which he/she is "invited" to participate. I am claiming with Hans Jonas, that ethically some justification is needed if an infringement of the primary inviolability of the human person is to be permitted. Such justification "must be by values and needs of a dignity commensurate with those sacrificed."[5]

But not only must we rank the individual's rights above the researcher's freedom to seek more effective remedies, we must also assert the patient's rights against the claims of society on behalf of future sufferers. Since the patient is in the potentially coercive situation outlined earlier it is necessary to give greater weight to his/her rights than to generosity of spirit, compassion for future sufferers, "zeal for humanity, reverence for the Golden Rule, enthusiasm for progress, homage to the call of knowledge ..."[6] Only by ranking the patient's rights above The call to sacrifice himself/herself for the common good can we hope to neutralize the combined effect of the convergence of a plurality of powerfully coercive factors in many experimental situations.

It may be objected that the main thrust of this part of the paper has been too negative. The emphasis has been on what is not required of the patient-subject rather than what is required. The subject is not required to act from motives of gratitude, not required

to act out of incentives for service, and not to yield to pressures born of pressures. But the question arises: "Is there no positive obligation on the subject's part to participate in experimental procedures?" "If so, in what moral principle or principles is such an obligation grounded?" Two such principles are referred to in the literature—beneficence and justice.

It may be claimed that the patient-subject has a *prima facie* obligation to engage in experimental procedures calculated to benefit others from a motive of beneficence. There are sufferers whose condition may be improved, whether in terms of reduced pain, or by the development of more effective treatment provided that the necessary experimental subjects exhibit a willingness to participate in research. Employed in isolation from other moral principles, however, appeals to beneficence function to predispose the patient to participate in research. Unless moderated by the principle of autonomy, beneficence lacks the necessary checks and balances either to facilitate refusal to participate in, or to withdraw from, an experiment. The respective weighting of beneficence and autonomy depends on an antecedent ranking of our priorities—patient inviolability versus social gain.

Likewise with grounding our obligation to participate in experimental procedures in the principle of justice. It may be claimed with a high degree of plausibility that the burdens as well as the benefits of medical research should be evenly distributed among the members of society. When, however, one recalls Mill's tortuous attempt to harmonize utility and justice, it is clear that justice was invoked to protect minority groups and individuals from undiluted applications of the principle of utility. By contrast, in the present context, the principle of justice is invoked not to moderate but to buttress the principle of utility. We are brought back again in a full circle to the question of weighting the individual against the social components in the context of research projects involving human subjects.

There is yet another constraint on the researcher, one that flows from the nature of the parties to the contract in the research model. The party I refer to is the subject. Herein lies a crucial problem, for human beings in experimental situations are not only subjects but the experimental materials. Because of this dual role it is easy to slip into treating persons as things, and treating ends as means. The difficulty, then, with medical research is that "research" carries overtones of impartiality that are inappropriate to human experimentation. This point may be brought out by contrasting the subject matter of the common-garden variety of scientific research with the subject matter of modern medicine. Originally, experimentation was housed within the domain of natural science, where it deals with inorganic matter. In science, particularly in physics, pure research is both permissible and laudable. A physicist, for example, may push "inert" matter around simply to discover what happens. One may not indulge one's curiosity about human subjects in the same way. The wide discrepancy between "inert" matter and human subjects demands a more conservative approach. "But as soon as animate, feeling beings become the subject of experiment, as they do in the life sciences, and especially in medical research, this innocence of the search for knowledge is lost, and questions of conscience arise."[7] Human subjects have rights which may not be violated simply "to see what happens." In pure science we may indulge ourselves, so far as research funding permits, to pursue knowledge *for its own sake*. Medicine as a profession cannot afford that luxury. Indeed, there are constraints on the profession of medicine lacking to the field of contemporary philosophical ethics. The professional ethicist may engage in a theoretical inquiry into the meanings of ethical terms, into the validity of ethical arguments, or may try to devise a system for the logic of ethical imperatives, or engage in a comparison of ethical systems noting the analogies and disanalogies between Kantianism and Utilitarianism. And he may do all of these things out of sheer intellectual curiosity.

Medicine as a profession can hardly devote all of its time and energies to such abstract pursuits. As a profession medicine is not concerned with experimental procedures *per se* but with procedures calculated to benefit human beings. There is a built-in practical bent to medicine lacking to pure science.[8] It has a built-in practical bent lacking to both normative and meta-ethics. Another way of putting this is that medicine as a profession is concerned with "the good for *humans*" not with "the good *itself*." If we couple this insight with the uniqueness of the human exper-

imental "material," constraints are imposed upon the medical researcher beyond the ken of the pure physicist or theoretical ethicist. Such constraints impose strict parameters within which guidelines governing human experimentation must be formulated.

In summary, I have no difficulty in acknowledging that experimentation with human subjects results in better medicine provided that the necessary proprieties are observed. As with other human enterprise so with human experimentation, the price of ethically acceptable research is perpetual vigilance. Only when we are sensitive to the implications of the shift in the doctor-patient relationships, alert ourselves to the potentially coercive elements in the experimental situation, and acknowledge the uniqueness of the humane experimental materials can we hope to treat subjects as persons rather than guinea pigs and in Bronowski's phrase, reconcile the welfare of man with the welfare of man.

Acknowledgment
A revised version of a paper presented at the 14th International Conference of Philosophy and Medicine, University of Tel Aviv, September, 1982.

Notes

1. As reported in Katz, Jay, *Experimentation with Human Beings*, New York, Russell Sage Foundation, 1972, 64.
2. Jonas, Hans, "Philosophical Reflections on Experimenting with Human Subjects," Beauchamp, Tom L., Walters, LeRoy, *Contemporary Issues in Bioethics*, California, Wadsworth, 1982, (2), 531.
3. Kieffer, George H., *Bioethics*, Addison-Wesley, 1978, 241; Beecher, Henry K., *Research and the Individual*, Boston, Little Brown, 1970, 16.
4. Ramsey, Paul, Consent as a Canon of Loyalty, Beauchamp, Walters, 534.
5. Jonas, *Ibid.*, 524.
6. *Ibid.*, 528.
7. *Ibid.*, 524.
8. For a variation on this theme see Thomas, John E., Medicine and Sociology: A Parting of the Ways, *The Journal of Medicine and Philosophy*, 1981, 6, 411-421.

13.
AFTER "EVE": WHITHER PROXY DECISION-MAKING?

Eike-Henner W. Kluge

One of the most difficult situations that physicians may face is one involving an incompetent patient. Normally, following what could be called a fiduciary model of the physician-patient relationship, physicians may feel that they have fulfilled their professional obligation when they have advised the patient of the various pertinent modalities of treatment, expressed an opinion and made a recommendation, and have done all this in language that the patient can and does understand. Whatever decision the patient then makes will be legally and ethically acceptable. If it should not accord with the physician's own better judgement, he or she may of course attempt to reason and persuade but not coerce; and all other things being equal, the physician may not overrule the patient's determination. *Reibl v. Hughes*[1] is very clear on that point. If all else fails and the physician cannot in good conscience accept the patient's decision, there is always the option of referring the patient to another physician and withdrawing from the case.[2] At no point, however, with the exceptions of emergency and therapeutic privilege, is the physician called on to assume the role of proxy decision-maker or to examine the ethical acceptability of the decision itself.

The case of the incompetent patient, however, is different. Here the physician must assume an evaluative role. As frontline workers, so to speak, physicians have to examine the way in which the proxy decision-makers—usually the next-of-kin—make the decision in order to assure themselves that it is the product of reflective consideration and not the offhand result of a hasty reaction. Furthermore, they must consider the criteria used by the proxy decision-makers in reaching the decision in order to make sure that they do not simply reflect the proxies' own standards, feelings or expectations but rather are ethically appropriate. When there is any doubt, the physician must engage the appropriate adminis-

trative or legal channels to prevent what may be an unacceptable exercise of proxy authority.[3]

To some degree, of course, this is a matter of subjective assessment on the part of the physician, but not entirely so. In cases in which the patient was once competent but is competent no longer, the physician will balance the quality of life expected from the various treatment options against the wishes and expectations expressed by the patient when competent in order to assess the reasonableness or acceptability of the particular proxy decision. The testimony of next-of-kin as well as formal and informal data to which the physician may have access will provide invaluable assistance. As to situations in which there is no evidence that the patient expressed preferences when competent, the physician will proceed on the basis of the quality-of-life standards that are currently accepted by the ordinary person, standards that are based not on the concept of social utility (whether defined within the ambit of the immediate family or social grouping or drawn more widely to include society as a whole) but rather on criteria that flow from the concept of the patient as a person. The physician will take into account the distinction between the continuation or sustaining of merely biologic life and support of the patient as a person who has (or retains the capacity for) sapient cognitive awareness and the possibility of meaningful social interaction.[4] Again, while this will involve a certain amount of subjectivity on the part of the physician, it need not and does not occur in complete isolation. Physicians can draw on the more or less standard perception of quality of life that prevails in society and are aided by their sensitivity to the cost of the various treatment options to the patient in purely human terms. Their professional knowledge of the nature and likelihood of the outcomes expected from the various modalities of treatment is invaluable, as is their awareness of what other, competent patients under similar circumstances have decided. Together, all this gives the physician a fairly good idea of what the ordinary reasonable person would decide under similar circumstances and provides a basis against which to measure the proxy decision. And although this sort of approach may present difficulties on occasion, it generally is workable and presents no serious ethical problems.

As to the case of the currently incompetent patient who never has been competent but in all likelihood will become competent in the future—i.e., an otherwise normal child—it, too, does not present the physician with fundamentally new issues. The physician will proceed on the assumption that, all other things being equal, the child's sensible experience and qualitative perception of the world is essentially like that of an adult and that the factor of incompetence involves the cognitive and judgemental plane. It is therefore entirely appropriate for the physician to take into account the child's subjective expressions (in so far as they are present or available) and balance them against the objective standard of what a reasonable person would decide when considering the proxy decision. The function of the proxy is to supply the cognitive and judgemental want of the child. Consequently, if the physician finds that the proxy decision-maker has introduced his or her own, nonstandard values in making the decision, the physician must challenge the decision. The situation becomes a little more complicated when the child has given assent in a particular direction, but even here it is not a matter of purely subjective evaluation. The assent must be seen as guiding, although not necessarily determining, depending on the facts of the cases.[5] Finally, in all cases of doubt, the courts must be the ultimate forum of appeal.

THE RADICALLY CONGENITALLY INCOMPETENT PATIENT

The case of the congenitally incompetent patient who, so far as medical science can tell, not only is barely at the limits of sapient cognitive awareness but also in all probability will never become competent is radically different. The sort of balancing of subjective expression against an objective standard that can at least be attempted in other cases seems inappropriate here. This is so not because the patient

is not reasonable—no incompetent patient is—but because the presumption on which such balancing is based may be false in such cases. The quality of life of the radically congenitally incompetent patient may be so fundamentally different from the norm that both the use of the objective standard of what a reasonable person would decide as a balance and the attempt to use the patient's own subjective expression would be untoward. The very significance of the latter may be fundamentally misconstrued because it would be based on the world experience of the physician, someone who fits the norm of the reasonable person. Consequently, there exists a danger that the use of the objective standard would violate the individuality of the patient and that the attempt to circumvent this by using subjective indicators from the patient would be so out of line with his or her actual experience that any treatment decision based on these criteria would be experienced as cruel and unusual treatment.[6]

If this is true, the physician who monitors proxy decisions made for radically congenitally incompetent patients is faced with a serious problem: What criteria—indeed, what evaluative approach—ought he or she to apply?

THE STEPHEN DAWSON DECISION

It was at least in part for this reason that the 1983 British Columbia Supreme Court decision *Re Stephen Dawson*[7] was welcomed by some members of the medical community. The case concerned a 7-year-old boy who had contracted meningitis shortly after birth, suffered severe brain damage and become hydrocephalic and as a consequence was exceedingly retarded, with no control over his faculties or limbs. At 5 months of age a shunt had been inserted and had been revised over the years, and at the time of application to the courts revision was again required. The reason for the court intervention was that the parents, as proxy decision-maker, had initially agreed to the revision, but after taking into account what they considered to be appropriate quality-of-life considerations from the perspective of the ordinary person—considerations involving the capacity for sapient cognitive awareness, the possibility of relatively pain-free and physically comfortable existence, and the potential for meaningful social interaction—and after consultation with a pediatric neurosurgeon they had withdrawn their permission. The superintendent of child welfare for the province intervened, and the matter came to trial in provincial court. The test used by the court to evaluate the parents' decision was whether, under the circumstances, the proposed revision constituted extraordinary treatment. The court decided in the affirmative and held in favour of the parents. On appeal to the British Columbia Supreme Court, the decision was reversed and an order for treatment was made. Stephen subsequently received treatment and continues to live.

It was the reasoning stated by the British Columbia Supreme Court that made the decision so important for the medical community. For the first time in Canadian medicolegal history the courts issued a ruling that explicitly addressed the question of what criteria and approach a proxy decision-maker and a physician should use when dealing with a congenitally incompetent person. Mr. Justice L. McKenzie, who decided the issue, ruled 1) that a congenitally incompetent person does not lose the rights to health care normally enjoyed by other persons simply in virtue of his or her incompetence, 2) that the duty of exercising this right normally rests in the parents as appropriate proxy decision-makers, 3) that their decision-making authority is appropriately challenged when it is not exercised in the best interests of the incompetent person, and 4) that what counts as being in the best interests of the incompetent person must not be determined from the point of view of the objective reasonable person. Rather, 5) it must be determined from the perspective of the incompetent person. As Judge McKenzie put it, "I do not think that it lies within the prerogative of any parent or of this court to look down upon a disadvantaged person and judge the quality of that person's life to be so low as not to be deserving of continuance." Quoting with approval Judge Asch in the US case *In the Matter of Eugene Weberlist* ("In this case, the court must decide what its ward would choose, if he were in a position to make a sound judgment.") he went on to say:

This last sentence puts it right. It is not appropriate for an external decision-maker to apply his standards of what constitutes a livable life and exercise the right to impose death if that standard is not met in his estimation. The decision can only be made in the context of the disabled person viewing the worthwhileness or otherwise of his life in its own context as a disabled person—and in that context he would not compare his life with that of a person enjoying normal advantages. He would know nothing of a normal person's life having never experienced it.

In adopting this position, Judge McKenzie was enunciating what had become known as a substituted-judgement approach to proxy decision-making for congenitally incompetent persons. As one US commentator put it, proxy decision-makers should try to put themselves as much as possible into the situation of the incompetent person and then decide in the way and from the perspective from which the latter would decide, where he or she able.[8]

The Stephen Dawson case injected an element of clarity into the Canadian context. The Canadian physician faced with the question of how to proceed in these sorts of cases now had definite guidelines on how to interpret "best interests" considerations and evaluate the appropriateness of a particular proxy decision. However, while definitive and clarifying, Judge McKenzie's decision was not without problems, some of which I pointed out at the time.[9] In the context of proxy decision-making the most important problem was the concept of a substituted-judgement approach itself. As I said then, the demand that the perspective of the congenitally incompetent person should constitute the basis of quality-of-life considerations by the proxy decision-maker and that any acceptance or rejection of medical treatment should be grounded on this basis is not only unworkable in practical terms but also and, indeed above all, logically incoherent. If the incompetent person lacks sapient cognitive awareness—or, less severely, if he or she lacks any standards or criteria—then, trivially, neither standards nor criteria can be ascribed to the person. That fact is definitive of the situation in which such people find themselves and characterizes their very nature. It is therefore logically impossible to determine what their wishes are or would be if they could make them known. To proceed otherwise is to do one of two things: to assume that despite this lack they have standards or criteria after all—a flat contradiction—or to project some other standards or criteria into the situation by substitution and thereby treat incompetent people as though they were not incompetent. In either case, however, the very concept of substituted judgement, of viewing the situation from the perspective of the incompetent person, "in its own context," is a fiction.

If this analysis was correct, the position of the physician faced with a congenitally incompetent patient was not improved but rather was worsened by the Stephen Dawson case: uncertainty over how to proceed had indeed been replaced by certainty, but at the price of logical impossibility.

THE CASE OF "EVE"

Then came *Eve v. Mrs. E.,*[10] which altered the whole picture. On the facts, the case was entirely different from that of Stephen Dawson. "Eve" was a 24-year-old moderately retarded woman suffering from extreme expressive aphasia. She was described to the courts as an extremely pleasant and affectionate person who, being physically adult, was capable of being attractive to and attracted by men. Her mother, of advancing years, feared that Eve might become pregnant, and since Eve was unable to take care of a child, the mother saw herself faced with the prospect of having to care for Eve's progeny. She found this unmanageable. She also felt that both pregnancy and childbirth would be incomprehensible to Eve. Consequently, acting as proxy decision-maker, she requested that Eve be sterilized.

The court of first instance rejected the request. It ruled that except for clinically therapeutic reasons, parents or other appropriate proxy decision-makers could not give valid proxy consent to such a procedure. On appeal to the Supreme Court of Prince Edward Island, the judgement was reversed and sterilization by hysterectomy was ordered. However, leave was granted to appeal the decision to the Supreme Court of Canada. On Oct. 23, 1986, that court handed down its ruling. It reinstated the trial court's order and rejected sterilization. Mr. Justice La Forest, writing the unanimous decision of the court, gave two reasons. One dealt with the historical nature of the *parens patriae* powers of the court. Here the thrust of Mr. Justice La Forest's deliberations was that these powers could be exercised only

in the best interests of the incompetent person, no matter what the position of society or next-of-kin. The second reason was an attempt to clarify the way in which such best interests could be determined. He here focused on the position advanced by the attorneys for Mrs. E. They had argued that as proxy decision-maker Mrs. E. had the duty to exercise Eve's rights for her and had argued further that, indeed, these rights ought to be exercised on the basis of what would be in Eve's best interests. However, they insisted that Eve's best interests could be determined only in a subjective fashion: by approximating as closely as possible the kind of situation in which Eve found herself and then making the kind of decision that she herself would make. In other words, they reasoned that a "substituted-judgement" approach to the determination of "best interests" would be appropriate "because it places a higher value on the individuality of the incompetent person."[11] Using such an approach, they argued, would result in a decision for sterilization.

For the purposes of this essay, it is irrelevant whether the logic of Mrs. E.'s position is valid. What is important is the court's reaction to the line of reasoning. While accepting the concept of best interests as appropriate, the court roundly rejected the contention that best interests could be appropriately determined with the substituted-judgement approach. In fact, the court brusquely rejected the concept of substituted judgement itself. Substituted judgement, it reasoned, is an attempt to determine what choice the incompetent person would make were he or she able. However, the court stated,[12]

> Choice presupposes that a person has the mental competence to make it. It may be a matter of debate whether a court should have the power to make the decision if that person lacks the mental capacities to do so. But it is obviously a fiction to suggest that a decision so made is that of the incompetent, however much the court may try to put itself in her place. What the incompetent would do if she or he could make a choice is simply a matter of speculation.

Mr. Justice La Forest went on to speak of "the sophistry embodied in the argument favouring substituted judgment" and quoted with approval from

Matter of Eberhardy (a US case), in which the court had stated:[13]

> We conclude that the question is not choice because it is sophistry to refer to it as such, but rather the question is whether there is a method by which others, acting on behalf of the person's best interests and in the interests, such as they may be, of the state, can exercise the decision.

Neither the US court nor the Supreme Court of Canada went on to detail such a method. They agreed in their focus on best interests considerations. One thing, however, was clear: by characterizing the substituted-judgement approach as legal "legerdemain," the Supreme Court effectively ruled out the very test enjoined by the Stephen Dawson case.

Of course, it could be argued that all this holds only for sterilization, that it leaves all other cases unaffected. That, however, is unlikely for three reasons. First, it would contradict the very *raison d'être* of Supreme Court decisions. They are, and are supposed to be, models for general types of cases. While *Eve v. Mrs. E.* is representative of sterilization cases, it is also and, indeed, above all representative of a type of case that deals with the problem of proxy decision-making for incompetent people. All cases of proxy decision for such people are thereby affected. The fact that the court itself saw it in this light is evidenced by the fact that the precedential cases it considered and cited in reaching its decision were drawn from a whole spectrum of cases proposing medical procedures for incompetent people, not only those advocating sterilization. Second, the fact that the Supreme Court intended its decision to have wider ambit is indicated by the fact that its rejection of substituted judgement is not explicitly directed to sterilization cases. It is couched independently of that issue in response to the argument that a substituted-judgement approach as such "is to be preferred to the best interests test because it places a higher value on the individuality of the mentally incompetent person."[14] In other words, it was a reply to the argument that because the substituted-judgement approach is the appropriate test for incompetent people in general, it should also be used in this case. It is to this general claim

that the court replied in the negative. Its rejection, therefore, has general implications. Finally, there is this to consider. Undoubtedly there are many strands intertwined in this case. However, to construe the rejection of substituted judgement in a limited fashion is to ascribe to the Supreme Court the position that different principles of law and of ethics hold for the very same problem—proxy decision-making—in different material cases. Not only would that undermine the very notion of the uniformity of legal and ethical principles, but also it lacks basis in any of the court's dicta.

I suggest, therefore, that *Eve v. Mrs. E.* ought to be seen as having general import. But if that is the case, it presents the Canadian physician with a problem: How to interpret best interests? The fact that the court recalled with approval Lord Eldon's remarks in *Wellesley v. Wellesley* ("It has always been the principle of this court, not to risk damage to children ... which it cannot repair")[15] may be considered guiding. However, that merely pushes the interpretational uncertainty onto the word "damage." Did the court intend this to apply to physiologic damage only, or did it intend to encompass psychologic, mental and emotional deficit as well as other repercussions? There are indications that it intended the wider construal; for example, it inveighed against a "grave intrusion on the physical and mental integrity of the person"[16] and included "health problems, religious upbringing and protection against harmful association."[17] But we do lack a really explicit statement. The physician is thus once again left in a domain of uncertainty. Only three—negative—guidelines are clear: physicians may not use a substituted-judgement approach to evaluate the appropriateness of proxy decisions, they may not accept a decision based on the proxy decision-maker's own idiosyncratic standards, and they may not use their own values, standards and expectations.

ATTEMPT AT A RESOLUTION

However, both the reasoning advanced in *Re Stephen Dawson* and that given in *Eve v. Mrs. E.* do point in the direction in which more positive criteria may be sought.[18] These stem not from the assumption of equality of life experience, which is the contentious concept, but from the assumption that whatever his or her handicap, the radically and congenitally incompetent patient is still a person. If this assumption is true—and here only incontrovertible evidence of the permanent lack of capability for sapient cognitive awareness can count as an indication to the contrary—that patient has the same panoply of rights as all other persons. More important, it follows that he or she must be treated as a person in all respects. This in turn means that the quality of life that the patient faces in the future as well as the quality at the present time, while it may be admitted to differ in degree of sophistication from that of the competent person, nevertheless cannot be held to differ in kind: no matter what the difference in degree, the quality itself, in its very nature, must be that of a person. This, however, immediately entails that the evaluative criteria that are appropriate in the case of all other persons must be applied here as well. Not, of course, in a straightforward fashion. That would be to ignore the difference in degree between the respective qualities of life. Rather, what it means is that the physician must use the quality of life of an otherwise heathy person with similar type and degree of incompetence as an evaluative baseline and consider the relative changes that would result in that quality under the various treatment options being considered. In this it is appropriate for the physician to take into account the incompetent person's subjective expressions of satisfaction with physical life, the psychologic affect and other attendant factors and balance these against the likelihood of retention of or improvement in sapient cognitive awareness, the possibility of meaningful social interaction at that level and the cost of the various options to the patient in purely human terms. Let us call this a comparative quality-of-life coefficient. The physician must then do a similar evaluation, with due alteration of detail, for an ordinary competent patient with a similar medical problem to determine what the comparative quality-of-life coefficient would be in his or her case. The physician must then compare the two coefficients. If, on balance, the comparative quality-of-life coefficient for the incompetent patient is the same as or higher than that for the competent patient, and if in the case of the latter the decision would normally be in favour of treatment (or of some specific form of treatment), the decision must be in favour of treatment for the incompetent patient as well. If the proxy decision-maker's decision is against treatment, the physician must oppose it, if necessary through administrative and judicial channels. In all other cases, he or she need not.

This way of approaching the problem provides a procedure that can be implemented in practice. At the same time, however—or perhaps precisely because of this—it allows us to reconcile *Eve v. Mrs. E.* with *Re Stephen Dawson*. For, in this way, Judge McKenzie's injunction to consider the situation of the radically congenitally incompetent person in the "context of the disabled person" can be given an interpretation that avoids the sophistry of substituted judgement while satisfying Mr. Justice La Forest's conclusion that the "best interests" of the person should be guiding.

A FINAL PROBLEM

At the same time, however, the case of Eve leaves the health care professional with a problem. The considerations that I have sketched are appropriate from the perspective of the incompetent person and under the *parens patriae* powers of the court. Ethically, however, they are insufficient. Medical decisions, after all, are not made in a vacuum, nor can health care decisions be reached in isolation from the overall context in which they must be implemented. The resources that will be involved in health care decisions and their distribution have ineluctable social implications. It is here the *Eve v. Mrs. E.* fails. By being focused narrowly within the *parens patriae* doctrine as traditionally understood, the decision paints an unrealistic picture. The rights of the incompetent person must never be less than those of the competent person solely by virtue of their incompetence, to be sure. However, justice and equality demand that they not be more either. It is ethically unacceptable to engage in reverse discrimination that accords a favoured ethical status to the incompetent person solely by virtue of his or her incompetence. That, however, would in fact occur if the powers of Eve's rights, as captured in the best-interests clause as expressed in the judgement, were to be given automatic precedence over the rights of others; if, in the words of Mr. Justice La Forest, we were to "sympathize with Mrs. E." but insist, as he did, that in cases such as these only the rights of the incompetent person are decisive.[19] The point of *Eve v. Mrs. E.* and analogous court actions surely is to insist that the rights of the incompetent person must be given due weight because incompetent people are persons. That, however, also means that with due alteration of detail their rights must be treated as subject to the same balancing process to which the rights of all other persons are subject under similar conditions. By rejecting the weight of the competing rights of Mrs. E. and the rest of society, Mr. Justice La Forest has created a special class of persons who are immune from the restrictive and balancing considerations that apply to everyone else. This seems to suggest that the physician who monitors proxy decisions for such people must refrain from taking into account the considerations of equity and justice that guide the allocation of resources in all other cases. Not only are the ethics of this highly questionable, but also it may lead to a distributive nightmare.

Notes

1. *Reibl v. Hughes,* 14 CCLT 1 (SCC 1980).
2. *Code of Ethics,* Can Med Assoc, Ottawa, 1978: 15.
3. Dickens, B.: The role of the family in surrogate medical consent. *Health Law Can* 1980; 1 (3): 49-52.
4. Keyserlingk, E.W.: Sanctity of life or quality of life. In *The Context of Ethics, Medicine and Law,* Law Reform Commission of Canada, Ottawa, 1979: 49-72.
5. McCormick, R.A.: Proxy consent in the experimentation situation. *Respect Biol Med* 1974; 18: 2-20; Ramsey, P.: *The Patient as Person,* Yale U Pr, New Haven, Conn, 1970: 1-58.
6. *Superintendent of Belchertown State School* v. *Saikewicz,* 370 NE (2d) 417 (Mass 1977); Annas, G.: Reconciling Quinlan and Saikewicz: decision making for the terminally ill incompetent. *AMJ Law Med* 1979; 4: 367-396.
7. *Re Stephen Dawson,* 3 WWR 618 (BC SC 1983) reversing 3 WWR 597 (BC Prov Ct 1983).
8. Annas, G.: The incompetent's right to die: the case of Joseph Saikewicz. *Hastings Cent Rep* 1978; 8 (1): 21-23.
9. Kluge, E.-H.W.: In the matter of Stephen Dawson: right v. duty of health care. *Can Med Assoc J* 1983; 129: 815-818.
10. *Eve v. Mrs. E.,* SCC, judgement handed down Oct 23, 1986, SCR 16654.
11. Ibid.
12. Ibid.
13. *Matter of Eberhardy,* 307 NW (2d) 881 (Wis 1981).
14. See note 10.
15. Ibid.
16. Ibid.
17. Ibid.
18. Magnet, J.E., Kluge, E.-H.W.: *Withholding Treatment From Defective Newborn Children,* Brown Legal Pubns, Cowansville, PQ, 1985: 3-306.
19. See note 10.

14.
PROXY CONSENT FOR RESEARCH ON THE INCOMPETENT ELDERLY

Barry F. Brown

In the past decade, the ethical issues of research with the elderly have become of increasing interest in gerontology, medicine, law, and biomedical ethics. In particular, the issue has been raised whether the elderly deserve special protection as a dependent group (Ratzan 1980). One of the most profound difficulties in this area of reflection is that of the justification of proxy consent for research on borderline or definitely incompetent patients.

Some diseases of the elderly, such as Alzheimer's disease, cause senile dementia: devastating for the patient and family and, in future, a considerable burden for society. This condition, in turn, renders a patient incapable of giving informed, voluntary consent to research procedures designed to learn about the natural history of the disease, to control it, and to find a cure. The research must be done on human subjects, since there is not as yet a suitable animal model; indeed some feel that there never can be such a model. A protection of the patient, rooted in concern for his best interests, from procedures to which he cannot give consent gives rise to a paradox: "If we can only perform senile dementia research using demented patients, but should not allow them to participate because they are incompetent, then we are left in a quandary. We cannot ethically conduct senile dementia research using demented patients because they are incompetent; but we cannot technically perform it using competent subjects because they are not demented" (Ratzan 1980: 36). Such a position seems to protect demented patients at the expense of their exposure, as a class, to prolonged misery or death.

If the patient cannot give consent, is the proxy consent of relatives ethically valid? That is, do the relatives have the moral right or capacity to give consent for procedures that may not offer much hope for the patient in that they may not offer a direct benefit to him?

Such procedures have by recent convention been called non-therapeutic. They might offer a possible benefit for other sufferers in the future, but little hope of benefit for *this* patient, here and now.

At present, an impasse has developed regarding such research. It appears that such procedures might be illegal under criminal laws on assault. If the research is strictly non-therapeutic, then no benefit is to be found for the patient-subject. If the requirement of therapeutic experimentation is that a direct, or fairly immediate, improvement in the patient's condition is the sole benefit that could count, then it is difficult to see how this could be discovered. For unlike the case of a curable disease or research on preventive measures for childhood diseases, such as polio, the Alzheimer's patients suffer from a presently terminal illness. Studies of the causation of this condition may hold little or no hope of alleviating the condition in them. There appears to be no present or future benefit directly accruing to them. Others may benefit, but they likely will not. Thus, it seems, there is no benefit in view.

If, in fact, such procedures, even relatively innocuous ones, are illegal, then such research cannot go ahead. If so, such persons will remain "therapeutic orphans" just as surely as infants and children unless proxy consent is valid. If proxy consent is also legally invalid, then the legal challenge to this impasse may be either legislative or judicial. In either case, ethical arguments must be offered as justification for the case that proxy consent is or ought to be legally valid. The following explorations are a contribution to that debate.

Can some kind of benefit for the demented be found in research that offers no immediate hope of improvement? I believe that it can, but the nature of that benefit will be unfamiliar or unacceptable to those who are sure that there are only two mutually exclusive alternatives: a utilitarian conception of the social good pitted against a deontological notion of the individual's rights.

Contemporary biomedical ethics routinely employs three principles in its effort to resolve such dilemmas (Reich 1970; Beauchamp & Childress 1983). These are the principle of beneficence, which demands that we do good and prevent harm; the principle of respect for persons (or the principle of autonomy), from which flows the requirement of informed consent; and the principle of justice, which demands the equitable distribution of the benefits and burdens of research. But the first two obviously conflict with each other in human experimentation: the principle of beneficence, which mandates research to save life and restore health, especially if this is seen as directed to the good of society, is in tension with the principle of respect for persons, which requires us to protect the autonomy of subjects. Moreover, the principle of beneficence requires us not only to benefit persons as patients through research, but also to avoid harming them as research subjects in the process. So there is an internal tension between moral demands created by the same principle. Finally, demented patients are no longer fully or sufficiently autonomous. Standard objections to paternalism do not apply. Consequently paternalism of the parental sort is not inappropriate, but rather necessary in order to protect the interest of the patient.

Simple application of these principles, therefore, will not provide a solution. Underlying the manner in which they are applied are radically different conceptions of the relationship of the individual good to the societal or common good.

In the present framework of philosophical opinion, there appear to be two major positions. On the one hand, some consequentialist arguments for non-therapeutic research justify non-consensual research procedures on the grounds that individual needs are subordinate to the general good conceived as an aggregate of individual goods. This good, that of the society as a whole, can easily be seen to take precedence over that of individuals. This is especially so if the disease being researched is conceptualized as an "enemy" of society. On the other hand, a deontological position argues that the rights of the individual take precedence over any such abstract general good as the advancement of science, the progress of medicine, or the societal good. In this view, to submit an individual incapable of giving or withholding consent to research procedures not for his own direct benefit is to treat him solely as a means, not as an end in himself. In this debate, one side characterizes the general good proposed by the other as much too broad and inimical to human liberty; the other sees the emphasis on individual rights as excessively individualistic or atomistic.

There are strengths and weaknesses in both approaches. The consequentialist rightly insists on a communal good, but justifies too much; the deontologist rightly protects individual interests, but justifies too little. I contend that if we are to resolve the dilemma concerning the incompetent "therapeutic orphan," it is necessary to go between these poles. In order to do so, I wish to draw upon and develop some recent explorations concerning non-therapeutic research with young children. In at least one important respect, that of incompetence, children and the demented are similar. We ought to treat similar cases similarly. I wish also to argue that research ethics requires: (1) a conception of the *common good* that is at once narrower than that of society as a whole and yet transcends immediate benefit to a single individual; and (2) a conception of the common good that sees it not in opposition to the individual good but including it, so that the good is seen as distributed to individuals.

THE LESSON OF RESEARCH WITH CHILDREN

As to the first, we may learn much from the discussions concerning research with children, particularly as they bear upon the distinction between therapeutic and non-therapeutic experimentation. In the 1970s a spirited debate took place between the noted ethicists Paul Ramsey and Richard McCormick on the morality of experimentation with children (Ramsey 1970, 1976, 1977; McCormick 1974, 1976). Ramsey presented a powerful deontological argument against non-therapeutic experimentation with children. Since infants and young children cannot give consent, an essential requirement of the canon of loyalty between researcher and subject, they cannot be subjected ethically to procedures not intended for their own benefit. To do so, he contended, is to treat children solely as means to an end (medical progress), not as ends in themselves (Ramsey 1970).

McCormick, arguing from a natural law position similar to that developed in the next section, argued that since life and health are fundamental natural goods, even children have an obligation to seek to preserve them. Medical research is a necessary condition of ensuring health, and this is a desirable social goal. Consequently children, as members of society, have a duty in social justice to wish to accept their share of the burdens of participating in research that promise benefit to society and is of minimal or no risk. Thus the parents' proxy consent is a reasonable presumption of the child's wishes if he were able to consent (McCormick 1974).

There are two major puzzles generated by this debate over non-therapeutic research in children. First, Ramsey stressed that the condition to which a child may be at risk need not reside within his skin, but could be an epidemic dread disease. Thus, testing of preventive measures such as polio vaccine on children is justified; indeed it counts for Ramsey as therapeutic. This is interesting for several reasons. First, the therapeutic benefit may be indirect or remote, not necessarily immediate. Second, it embodies the concept of a group or population at risk smaller than society as a whole. Third, it apparently allows for considerable risk. There was a risk of contracting polio from the vaccine. Although the risk might have been slight statistically, the potential damage was grave. By Ramsey's own account, a slight risk of grave damage is a grave risk. Thus, he was prepared to go beyond the limit of minimal or no risk on the grounds that the polio vaccine was *therapeutic,* while McCormick attempted to justify *non-therapeutic* research on children, but confined the risk to minimal or none. It is odd that in the subsequent protracted debate, this difference was not contested.

The second major puzzle arises from McCormick's view that fetuses, infants, and children ought to participate in low- or no-risk non-therapeutic research in order to share in the burden of social and medical progress in order that all may prosper. Note that only *burdens* are to be shared, not benefits. This is because the topic by definition was non-therapeutic experimentation. By putting it this way he seemed to many

to be subordinating the interests of such subjects to a very broadly construed societal good. But let us remember that the argument for such research in the first place was that without it, infants and children would be "therapeutic orphans." That is, without pediatric research, there could be fewer and slower advances in pediatric therapy.

Although not of direct benefit, such research is intended for the long-term benefit of children, and is thus indirectly or remotely therapeutic. It is not conducted for "the benefit of society" or for "the advancement of medical science"; it is for children in the future. Otherwise, it could be carried out on adults. Thus, such research should be construed as done not in view of broad social benefit but for the benefit of children as a group or a sub-set of society. Of course, if advances are made in medicine for the sake of children, society benefits as well, but this is incidental and unnecessary. The sole justification is provided by the benefits now and to come for *children.* At the same time, such benefits set one of the limits for such research: it should be confined to children's conditions, and it should not be directed at conditions for which the research may be done on competent persons.

THE COMMON GOOD OF A DISEASE COMMUNITY

Some of the hints arising from the foregoing debate can now be developed. It is indeed wrong to experiment on an incompetent person for "the benefit of society" if the research is unrelated to that person's disease and he is made a subject simply because he is accessible and unresistant. But is it necessarily unethical to conduct experiments on an incompetent person which attempt to discover the cause of the condition which causes the incompetence, and which may cure it or prevent it in others, even if he will not himself be cured?

In a "third way" of conceptualizing the relation between the individual and the group, the good in view is neither that of society as a whole nor that of a single individual. It involves the group of persons with a condition, such as Alzheimer's disease. Here I turn to a conception of the common good articulated by John Finnis of Oxford. Finnis defines the common good not as the "greatest good for the greatest number" but as "a set of conditions which enables the members of a community to attain for themselves reasonable objectives, or to realize reasonably for themselves the value(s) for the sake of which they have reason to collaborate with each other (positively and/or negatively) in a community" (Finnis 1980:155).

The community may be either the complete community or the political one, or it may be specialized, such as the medical community, the research community, or the community of children with leukemia, and so on. The common good is thus not the sum total of individual interests, but an ensemble of conditions which enable individuals to pursue their objectives or purposes, which enable them to flourish. The purposes are fundamental human goods: life, health, play, esthetic experience, knowledge, and others. Relevant to this discussion are life, health, especially mental integrity, and the consequent capacity for knowledge, all of which are threatened by diseases which cause dementia.

For my purposes, the community should be considered to be, at a minimum, those suffering from Alzheimer's disease. They have, even if they have never explicitly associated with each other, common values and dis-values: their lost health and the remaining health and vitality they possess. It could be said with McCormick that if they could do so, they would reasonably wish the good of preventing the condition in their relatives and friends.

But the community may be rightly construed more broadly than this. It naturally includes families with whom the patients most closely interact and which interact in voluntary agencies devoted to the condition, the physicians who treat them, the nurses, social workers, and occupational therapists who care for them, and the clinical and basic researchers who are working to understand, arrest, cure, and prevent the disease.

The participation of the patient, especially the demented patient, may be somewhat passive. He is a member of the specialized community by accident, not by choice, unless he has indicated his wish to become a research subject while still competent. Efforts to determine what a demented or retarded person would have wished for himself had he been competent have been made in American court decisions involving an incompetent patient's medical care. These "substituted judgment" approaches may have some worth, especially if the patient had expressed and recorded his wishes while still competent.

An individual might execute a document analogous to a human tissue gift—a sort of pre-dementia gift, in which he would officially and legally offer his person to medical research if and when he became demented. This might alleviate the problem of access to some extent, but it has its own difficulties. A pre-dementia volunteer cannot know in advance what types of research procedures will be developed in future, and so cannot give a truly informed consent except to either very specific procedures now known or to virtually anything. Such a pre-commitment may give some support to the decision to allow him to be a subject. But that decision, I contend, is justified by the claim, if valid, that it is for the common good of the dementia-care-research community, of which he is a member and to which, it is presumed, he would commit himself if he were capable of doing so at the time.

It is true, of course, that one might not ever have wished to participate in research procedures. In this case, the individual should be advised to register his or her objection in advance, along the lines that have been suggested for objection to organ donation in those countries that have a system of presumed consent for such donation. This can be achieved by carrying a card on which such an opt-out is recorded, or by placing one's name on a registry which might be maintained by support organizations. I suggest that unless one opt out in this manner, in the early stages of the disease, he or she be considered to have opted-in. That is, there should be a policy of presumed consent. In any event, as experience with organ retrieval has shown, in the final analysis it is the permission of relatives that is decisive in both those cases in which an individual has consented and those in which he or she has not made his or her wishes known.

The other members of the community may not all know each other. They do, however, have common values and, to a considerable degree, common objectives. There can be a high level of deliberate and active interaction, especially if there is close communication between the researchers, family, and volunteers in the voluntary health agencies.

What, then, is the ensemble of conditions which constitute the common good of the Alzheimer's community? Insofar as the purposes of collaboration include the effort to cure or to alleviate the disease, the common good would embrace, in addition to caring health professionals, a policy of promoting research, its ethical review, a sufficient number of committed clinical and scientific researchers, the requisite physical facilities and funding (some or all of which may be within other communities such as hospitals and medical schools), availability of volunteers for research, an atmosphere of mutual trust between research and subject, and finally ongoing research itself. This list is not exhaustive.

If access to the already demented is not allowed, and if this is essential for research on the disease to continue, it may well be impossible to find the answers to key questions about the disease. The common good of the Alzheimer's community would be damaged or insufficiently promoted. Since the goods of life and mental health are fundamental goods, this insufficiency would be profound.

One essential aspect of this common good is distributive justice. Each patient-subject shares not only in the burdens of research in order that all may prosper, but also the benefits. The benefits are not necessarily improved care or cure for the subject, but generally improved conditions for all such patient-subjects: a more aggressive approach to research, improved knowledge of the disease, increased probabilities for a cure, and others. Since the individual participates wholly in that good, he will be deprived of it in its entirety if it is not pursued. The common good is not so much a quantity of benefits as a quality of existence. It can therefore be distributed in its fullness to each member of the community. So, too, each can suffer its diminution.

Richard McCormick (1974) left his description of the common good unnecessarily broad and sweeping. According to some natural law theorists (Maritain 1947) the common good is always a distributed good, not simply the sum of parts. It is construed as flowing back upon the individual members of the community, who are not simply parts of a whole but persons, to whom the common good is distributed in

its entirety. Thus, not only can the common good of which McCormick speaks be narrowed to that of children as a group (equivalent to Ramsey's population at risk) but the benefits of such research can be seen as redistributed to the individuals of the group. The benefits are not to be taken in the sense of an immediately available therapy, but in the sense of improved general conditions under which a cure, amelioration, or prevention for all is more likely.

CONCLUSION

Some of these observations can now be applied to the case of the elderly demented. First, the debate showed the inadequacy of the simple distinction between therapeutic and non-therapeutic experimentation, which has been challenged on several grounds in past years. For example, May (1976: 83) includes diagnostic and preventive types of research under therapeutic experimentation, whereas Reich (1978: 327) observes that the terms "therapeutic" and "non-therapeutic" are inadequate because they do not seem to include research on diagnostic and preventive techniques. In the area of the development of experimental preventive measures such as vaccines for epidemic diseases, and in the area of diseases in which research is carried out on terminal patients with little or no expectation of immediate benefit for these patients, the distinction is somewhat blurred. In each case, there is a defined population at risk: one without the disease but at great risk of contracting it, the other with a disease but with little hope of benefiting from the research.

Such types of research seem to constitute an intermediate category: the "indirectly therapeutic," involving the hope of either prevention or alleviation or cure. This category as applied to dementia shows some characteristics of therapeutic experimentation in the accepted sense, since it is carried out on persons who are ill and it is directed to their own illness. But it also shares some properties of non-therapeutic research, since it is not for their immediate treatment and, therefore, benefit. The good to be achieved is more remote, both in time and in application, since it is less sharply located in the individual than is therapy as such.

It must be admitted that there is a difference between the testing of a vaccine for prevention of disease in young, healthy children and research on elderly, seriously ill patients. In the former, the child-subjects will benefit if the vaccine is successful, or at least be protected from harm. In the latter, the subjects will not benefit by way of prevention or cure of their disease, but rather simply by being part of a community in which those goals are being actively pursued. The identification of the demented patient's good with that common good is doubtless less concrete than the identification of the child's good with that of his peers. But it seems to me that underlying both these cases is a notion of the common good required to justify all cases of research that do not promise a hope of direct benefit to a person who is, here and now, ill.

Years ago, Hans Jonas (1969) noted that a physician-researcher might put the following question to a dying patient: "There is nothing more I can do for you. But there is something you can do for me. Speaking no longer as your physician but on behalf of medical science, we could learn a great deal about future cases of this kind if you would permit me to perform certain experiments on you. It is understood that you yourself would not benefit from any knowledge we might gain; but future patients would." Although greatly vulnerable and deserving of maximum protection, such a patient might be ethically approached to be a research subject, because the benefits to future patients are in a way a value to him: "At least that residue of identification is left him that it is his own affliction by which he can contribute to the conquest of that affliction, his own kind of suffering which he helps alleviate in others; and so *in a sense it is his own cause*" (Jonas 1969: 532, emphasis mine).

In this case, the individual apprehends a good greater than his personal good, less than that of society: that of his disease class, which is *his* good. Of course, the identification of which Jonas speaks is psychological; he would likely not agree with the approach herein outlined and might require that such participation be through a conscious, free choice of the patient. Nevertheless, it is a real, objective good which justifies his choice and prevents us from asking him to participate in research unrelated to his disease. Can a relative, a son or daughter perhaps, ethically make that decision for

an incompetent, demented Alzheimer's patient? If so, it is because, in a sense, it is the patient's cause, the patient's good as a member of a community which justifies that choice. It is not a matter of enforcing a social duty or minimal social obligation here, but seeking a good that lies in the relationship one has to others with the same disease. That same good, as noted above, limits the participation of the subject to research related precisely to his disease, not to anything else.

What is the implication of this for risk and the limits of risk? As has been seen, some wish to allow for exposure of subjects to greater than minimal risk provided only that it is classified as "therapeutic" (though the subjects are not ill). Others, in spite of the fact that the research is intended for the benefit of a group at risk, classify it as non-therapeutic and limit the acceptable risk to minimal levels. Are these the only alternatives? One advisory group has allowed, in the case of the mentally incompetent, for a "minor increase over minimal risk" in such circumstances (National Commission for the Protection of Human Subjects 1978:16). This is presumably permitted because the research is "of vital importance for the understanding or amelioration of the type of disorder or condition of the subjects" or "may reasonably be expected to benefit the subjects in future" (17). But what counts as minor increase in risk? Proposed research into Alzheimer's might involve invasive procedures such as brain biopsies, implantation of electrodes, spinal taps, and injections of experimental drugs. Are these of greater risk than that specified by the National Commission simply because they are invasive of the human brain? Or is there clear statistical risk of serious added damage to the brain? These are matters for empirical study. The invasiveness per se should not rule out a procedure. The major limitations should be whether the procedure is painful, causes anxiety, or adds to the already serious damage to the brain. If research involving procedures of greater risk than "minor increase over minimal" is ever to be justified, it must be so by the intent to avert the proportional evils of death or mental incapacity. If these are insufficient, than I fail to see what grounds might be available upon which to base a case for legislative change.

It is clear, then, that should such research be acceptable it also demands that stringent protective procedures be established in order to ensure that the demented are not drafted into research unrelated to their disease class. This is because the standard, being broader than that of "direct or fairly immediate benefit," is open to an accordionlike expansion, and therefore to abuse. Such safeguards could include: rigorous assurance that the proxy's consent (in reality, simply a permission) is informed and voluntary, the provision of a consent auditor, and various layers of administrative review and monitoring, from a local institutional review board up to a judicial review with a guardian appointed to represent the patient-subject's rights. These procedures may prove to be onerous. But we are on dangerous ground, and as we try to avoid overprotection, which may come at the expense of improved therapy for all, we must also avoid opening up a huge door to exploitation.

References

Beauchamp, T.L., & Childress, J.F. (1983). *Principles of Biomedical Ethics*. 2nd ed. New York: Oxford University Press.

Finnis, J. (1980). *Natural law and natural rights*. Oxford: Clarendon Press.

Jonas, H. (1969). Philosophical reflections on experimenting with human subjects. In T. Beauchamp and L. Walters (Eds.), *Contemporary issues in bioethics*. 2nd ed. Belmont, Ca: Wadsworth.

Maritain, J. (1974). *The person and the common good*. New York: Charles Scribner's Sons.

May, W. (1976). Proxy consent to human experimentation. *Linacre Quarterly, 43,* 73-84.

McCormick, R. (1974). Proxy consent in the experimentation situation. *Perspectives in Biology and Medicine, 18,* 2-20.

McCormick, R. (1976). "Experimentation in children: sharing in sociality. *Hastings Center Report, 6,* 41-46.

National Commission for the Protection of Human Subjects (1978). *Report and recommendations: Research involving those institutionalized as mentally infirm*. Washington, DC.

Ramsey, P. (1970). *The patient as person*. New Haven: Yale University Press.

Ramsey, P. (1976). The enforcement of morals: Non-Therapeutic research on children. *Hastings Center Report, 4,* 21-30.

Ramsey, P. (1977). Children as research subjects: a reply. *Hastings Center Report, 2,* 40-41.

Ratzan, R. (1980). "Being old makes you different": The ethics of research with elderly subjects. *Hastings Center Report, 5,* 32-42.

Reich, W. (1978). Ethical issues related to research involving elderly subjects. *Gerontologist, 18,* 326-37.

15.
BIOETHICS FOR CLINICIANS: INVOLVING CHILDREN IN MEDICAL DECISIONS

Christine Harrison, PhD; Nuala P. Kenny, MD; Mona Sidarous, LLB, LLM; Mary Rowell, MA, RN

Eleven-year-old Samantha is a bright, loving child who was treated for osteosarcoma in her left arm. The arm had to be amputated, and Samantha was given a course of chemotherapy. She has been cancer-free for 18 months and is doing well in school. She is self-conscious about her prosthesis and sad because she had to give away her cat, Snowy, to decrease her risk of infection. Recent tests indicate that the cancer has recurred and metastasized to her lungs. Her family is devastated by this news but do not want to give up hope. However, even with aggressive treatment Samantha's chances for recovery are less than 20%.

Samantha adamantly refuses further treatment. On earlier occasions she had acquiesced to treatment only to struggle violently when it was administered. She distrusts her health care providers and is angry with them and her parents. She protests, "You already made me give up Snowy and my arm. What more do you want?" Her parents insist that treatment must continue. At the request of her physician, a psychologist and psychiatrist conduct a capacity assessment. They agree that Samantha is probably incapable of making treatment decisions; her understanding of death is immature and her anxiety level very high. Nursing staff are reluctant to impose treatment; in the past Samantha's struggling and the need to restrain her upset them a great deal.

WHY IS IT IMPORTANT TO INCLUDE CHILDREN IN MEDICAL DECISION-MAKING?

Ethics

Traditionally, parents and physicians have made all medical decisions on behalf of children. However, just as the concept of informed consent has developed over the last 30 years with respect to competent adult patients, so new ways of thinking about the role of children in medical decision-making have evolved.

Ethical principles that provide guidance in the care of adults are insufficient in the context of caring for children.[1-3] Issues related to the voluntariness of consent, the disclosure of information, capacity assessment, treatment decisions and bereavement are more complex, as is the physician's relationship with the patient and the patient's family.[3,4] Adult models presume that the patient is autonomous and has a stable sense of self, established values and mature cognitive skills; these characteristics are undeveloped or underdeveloped in children.

Although it is important to understand and respect the developing autonomy of a child, and although the duty of beneficence provides a starting point for determining what is in the child's best interest, a family-centred ethic is the best model for understanding the interdependent relationships that bear upon the child's situation.[5] A family-centred approach considers the effects of a decision on all family members, their responsibilities toward one another and the burdens and benefits of a decision for each member, while acknowledging the special vulnerability of the child patient.

A family-centred approach presents special challenges for the health care team, particularly when there is disagreement between parent and child. Such a situation raises profound questions about the nature of the physician-patient relationship in pediatric practice. Integrity in this relationship is fundamental to the achievement of the goal of medicine,[6] which has been defined as "right and good healing action taken in the interest of a particular patient."[7] In the care of adults, the physician's primary relationship is with the particular capable patient. The patient's family may be involved in decision-making, but it is usually the patient who defines the bounds of such involvement.

The care of children, on the other hand, has been described in terms of a "triadic" relationship in which the child, his or her parents and the physician all have a necessary involvement (Dr. Abbyann Lynch, Director, Ethics in Health Care Associates, Toronto: personal communication, 1992). When there is disagreement between parent and child, the physician may experience some moral discomfort in having to deal separately with the child and parent.

The assumption that parents best understand what is in the interest of their child is usually sound. However, situations can arise in which the parents' distress prevents them from attending carefully to the child's concerns and wishes. Simply complying with the parents' wishes in such cases is inadequate. It is more helpful and respectful of the child to affirm the parents' responsibility for the care of their child while allowing the child to exercise choice in a measure appropriate to his or her level of development and experience of illness and treatment. This approach does not discount the parents' concerns and wishes, but recognizes the child as the particular patient to whom the physician has a primary duty of care. This approach seeks to harmonize the values of everyone involved in making the decision.[6,7]

Law

The legal right to refuse medical treatment is related to, but not identical with, the right to consent to treatment. The patient's right to refuse even life-saving medical treatment is recognized in Canadian law[8,9] and is premised on the patient's right to exercise control over his or her own body. Providing treatment despite a patient's valid refusal can constitute battery and, in some circumstances, negligence.

To be legally valid the refusal of medical treatment must be given by a person deemed capable of making health care choices, that is, capable of understanding the nature and consequences of the recommended treatment, alternative treatments and non-treatment. In common law the notion of the "mature minor" recognizes that some children are capable of making their own health care choices despite their age.[10] In common law and under the statutory law of some provinces patients are presumed capable regardless of age unless shown otherwise; in other provinces an age at which patients are presumed capable is specified.[11] When a child's capacity is in doubt an assessment is required.

In the case of children who are incapable of making their own health care decisions, parents or legal guardians generally have the legal authority to act as surrogate decision-makers. The surrogate decision-maker is obliged to make treatment decisions in the best interest of the child. Health care providers who believe that a surrogate's decisions are not in the child's best interest can appeal to provincial child welfare authorities. The courts have the authority to assume a *parens patriae* role in treatment decisions if the child is deemed to be in need of protection. This issue has arisen most commonly with respect to Jehovah's Witnesses who refuse blood transfusions for their children on religious grounds, and courts have authorized treatment in recognition of the state's interest in protecting the health and well-being of children.[12] Every province has child welfare legislation that sets out the general parameters of the "best interest" standard. Courts are reluctant to authorize the withholding or withdrawal of medical treatment, especially in the face of parental support for such treatment.

A special point to consider involves the use of patient restraints. The wrongful or excessive use of restraints could prompt an action of false imprisonment or battery. Restraint can involve the use of force, mechanical means or chemicals. The use of restraint compromises the dignity and liberty of the patient, including the child patient. Restraints should never be used solely to facilitate care but, rather, only when the patient is likely to cause serious bodily harm to himself or herself or to another. If restraint is required, the health care provider should use the least restrictive means possible, and the need for the restraint (as well as its effect on the patient) should be assessed on an ongoing basis.

Policy

The Canadian Paediatric Society has no policy regarding the role of the child patient in medical decision-making. The American Academy of Pediatrics statement on this question articulates the joint responsibility of physicians and parents to make decisions for very young patients in their best interest and states that "[p]arents and physicians should not exclude children and adolescents from decision-making without persuasive reasons."[13]

Empirical studies

As they grow, children develop decision-making skills, the ability to reason using complex concepts, an understanding of death[14] and the ability to imagine a future for themselves.[15] Children with a chronic or terminal illness may have experiences that endow them with insight and maturity beyond their years. Families often encourage children to participate in decision-making. Allowing even young children to make decisions about simple matters facilitates the development of skills that they will need to make more complex decisions later on.[16-18]

Because tools developed to assess the capacity of adults have not been tested with children, health care professionals working with children should be sensitive to the particular capacity of each child. Children are constantly developing their physical, intellectual, emotional and personal maturity. Although developmental milestones give us a general sense of capacities, two children of the same age will not necessarily have the same ability to make choices. Even when they are deemed capable of making health care choices, children need support for their decisions from family members and the health care team.

HOW SHOULD I DETERMINE THE APPROPRIATE ROLE OF A CHILD IN MEDICAL DECISION-MAKING?

Most children fall into one of three groups with respect to their appropriate involvement in decision-making.[19,20]

Infants and young children

Preschool children have no significant decision-making capacity and cannot provide their own consent. As surrogate decision-makers, parents should authorize (or refuse authorization) on their child's behalf, basing their decisions on what they believe to be in the child's best interest.

Primary-school children

Children of primary-school age may participate in medical decisions but do not have full decision-making capacity. They may indicate their assent or dissent without fully understanding its implications. Nonetheless they should be provided with information appropriate to their level of comprehension. Although the child's parents should authorize or refuse to authorize treatment, the child's assent should be sought and any strong and sustained dissent should be taken seriously.[21]

Adolescents

Many adolescents have the decision-making capacity of an adult.[22,23] This capacity will need to be determined for each patient in light of his or her

- ability to understand and communicate relevant information,
- ability to think and choose with some degree of independence,
- ability to assess the potential for benefit, risks or harms as well as to consider consequences and multiple options, and
- achievement of a fairly stable set of values.[24]

Many children and adolescents, particularly those who have been seriously ill, will need assistance in developing an understanding of the issues and in demonstrating their decision-making capacity. Age-appropriate discussion, perhaps with the assistance of teachers, chaplains, play therapists, nurses, psychologists or others skilled in communicating with children, are helpful. The child's participation may be facilitated by the use of art activities, stories, poems, role-playing and other techniques.[25,26]

Physicians should ensure that good decisions are made on behalf of their child patients. Although the interests of other family members are important and will influence decision-making, the child's interests are most important and are unlikely to be expressed or defended by the child himself or herself. Anxious, stressed or grieving family members may need assistance in focusing on what is best for the child. This may be especially difficult when a cure is no longer possible; in such cases a decision to stop treatment may seem like a decision to cause the child's death.

Whether or not the child participates, the following consideration should bear upon a treatment decision concerning that child:

- The potential benefits to the child
- The potential harmful consequences to the child, including physical suffering, psychological or spiritual distress and death
- The moral, spiritual and cultural values of the child's family

THE CASE

For Samantha, resuming aggressive treatment will have a serious negative effect on her quality of life. The chances of remission are small, yet a decision to discontinue treatment will likely result in her death. Because death is an irreversible harm, and decisions with serious consequences require a high level of competence in decision-making,[27] the capacity required would be very high. It has been determined that Samantha does not have this capacity.

Nevertheless, Samantha is included in discussions about her treatment options, and her reasons for refusing treatment are explored.[28] Members of the team work hard to re-establish trust. They and Samantha's parents come to agree that refusing treatment is not necessarily unreasonable; a decision by an adult patient in similar circumstances to discontinue treatment would certainly be honoured. Discussions address Samantha's and her parents' hopes and fears, their understanding of the possibility of cure, the meaning for them of the statistics provided by the physicians, Samantha's role in decision-making and her access to information. They are assisted by nurses, a child psychologist, a psychiatrist, a member of the clergy, a bioethicist, a social worker and a palliative care specialist.

Discussions focus on reaching a common understanding about the goals of treatment for Samantha. Her physician helps her to express her feelings and concerns about the likely effects of continued treatment. Consideration is given to the effects on her physical well-being, quality of life, self-esteem and dignity of imposing treatment against her wishes. Spiritual and psychological support for Samantha and her family is acknowledged to be an essential component of the treatment plan. Opportunities are provided for Samantha and her family to speak to others who have had similar experiences, and staff are given the opportunity to voice their concerns.

Ultimately, a decision is reached to discontinue chemotherapy and the goal of treatment shifts from "cure" to "care." Samantha's caregivers assure her and her family that they are not "giving up" but are directing their efforts toward Samantha's physical comfort and her spiritual and psychological needs. Samantha returns home, supported by a community palliative care program, and is allowed to have a new kitten. She dies peacefully.

Notes

1. Ruddick W. Parents and life prospects. In: O'Neill O, Ruddick W, editors. *Having children: philosophical and legal reflections on parenthood.* New York: Oxford University Press,; 1979:124.
2. Nelson J.L. Taking families seriously. *Hastings Cent Rep* 1992;22:6.
3. Hardwig J. What about the family? *Hastings Cent Rep* 1990; 20(2):5-10.
4. Leikin S. A proposal concerning decisions to forgo life-sustaining treatment for young people. *J Pediatre* 1989;115:17-22.
5. Mahowald M. *Women and children in health care.* New York: Oxford University Press; 1993:187,189.
6. Hellman J. In pursuit of harmonized values: patient/parent-pediatrician relationships. In: Lynch A, editor. *The "good" pediatrician: an ethics curriculum for use in Canadian pediatrics residency programs.* Toronto: Pediatric Ethics Network; 1996.
7. Pellegrino E.D. Toward a reconstruction of medical morality: the primacy of the act of profession and the fact of illness. *J Med Philos* 1979;4:47.
8. *Malett v. Shulman* [1990], 67 DLR (4th) (Ont CA).
9. Art. 11 CCQ.
10. Rozovsky L.E, Rozovsky F.A. *The Canadian law of consent to treatment.* Toronto: Butterworths; 1992:53-7.
11. Etchells E, Sharpe G, Elliott C, Singer P.A. Bioethics for clinicians 3: Capacity. *Can Med Assoc J* 1996; 155:657-61.
12. *R.B v. Children's Aid Society of Metropolitan Toronto,* [1995] 1 SCR 315 (SCC).

13. American Academy of Pediatrics. Informed consent, parental permission and assent in pediatric practice. *Pediatrics* 1995;95:314-7.

14. Matthews G.R. Children's conceptions of illness and death. In: Kopelman L.M, Moskop J.C, editors. *Children and health care: moral and social issues*. Dordrecht (Holland): Kluwer Academic Publishers; 1989:133-46.

15. Koocher G.P, DeMaso. Children's competence to consent to medical procedures. *Pediatrician* 1990;17:68-73.

16. King N.M.P., Cross A.W. Children as decision makers: guidelines for pediatricians. *J Pediatr* 1989;115:10-6.

17. Lewis M.A., Lewis C.E. Consequences of empowering children to care for themselves. *Pediatrician* 1990;17:63-7.

18. Yoos H.L. Children's illness concepts: old and new paradigms. *Pediatr Nurs* 1994;20:134-45.

19. Broome M.E., Stieglitz K.A. The consent process and children. *Res Nurs Health* 1992; 15:147-52.

20. Erlen J.A. The child's choice: an essential component in treatment decisions. *Child Health Care* 1987; 15:156-60.

21. Baylis F. *The moral weight of a child's dissent. Ethics Med Pract* 1993;3(1):2-3.

22. Weithorn L.A., Campbell S.B. The competency of children and adolescents to make informed treatment decisions. *Child Dev* 1982;53:1589-98.

23. Lewis C.C. How adolescents approach decisions; changes over grades seven to twelve and policy implications. *Child Dev* 1981;52:538-44.

24. Brock D.W. Children's competence for health care decisionmaking. In: Kopelman LM, Moskop JC, editors. *Children and health care: moral and social issues*. Dordrecht (Holland): Kluwer Academic Publishers; 1989:181-212.

25. Adams P.L., Fras I. *Beginning child psychiatry*. New York: Bruner/Mazel; 1988.

26. Kestenbaum C.J., Williams D., editors. *Handbook of clinical assessment of children and adolescents*. New York: University Press; 1988.

27. Dran J.F. The many faces of competency. *Hastings Cent Rep* 1985;15(2):17-21.

28. Freyer D.R. Children with cancer: special considerations in the discontinuation of life-sustaining treatment. *Med Pediatr Oncol* 1992;20:136-42.

CHAPTER FOUR

REPRODUCTION

16.
CLASS, FEMINIST, AND COMMUNITARIAN CRITIQUES OF PROCREATIVE LIBERTY

John A. Robertson

With procreative liberty as a beacon, this book[1] has visited the ethical, legal, and social conflicts presented by new reproductive technology. The journey has fleshed out the meaning of procreative liberty by arguing for presumptive moral and legal protection for reproductive technologies that expand procreative options. Those technologies that are not centrally connected to the values that underlie procreative liberty deserve less respect.

The resulting picture is a growing array of sophisticated technologies that can help individuals achieve their reproductive goals. As with many technologies, a bright, hopeful side coexists with dismay and distrust over how reproductive technologies might be used. For many people the technical ability to prevent or end pregnancy, to relieve infertility, to increase the chance of healthy offspring, or to obtain tissue for research and therapy is a great boon, and confirms one's faith in scientific progress.

Yet others feel profound discomfort with reproductive manipulations, and urge strict regulation or even prohibition. The source of their disquiet may be traced back to fears of manipulating nature and interfering with God's plans that have plagued science since its inception. Here the danger is even more ominous, because reproductive technologies manipulate the earliest stages of human life and potentially harm prenatal life, offspring, women, and the family.

In responding to this technology, individuals and society are both caught between autonomy and ambivalence—between the demands of personal choice and the disquiet that uses of autonomy causes them and society. One is damned either way—either overly technologizing the intimate, or losing the very real benefits that this technology provides.

The burden of this book has been to show the importance of procreative liberty in resolving these controversies. The lens of procreative liberty is essential because reproductive technologies are necessarily bound up with procreative choice. They are means to achieve or avoid the reproductive experiences that are central to personal conceptions of meaning and identity. To deny procreative choice is to deny or impose an all-encompassing reproductive experience on persons without their consent, thus denying them respect and dignity at the most basic level.

Although procreative liberty is a deeply held value, its scope and contours have never previously been fully elaborated. Past controversies have concerned contraception and abortion, and rarely, with the exception of eugenic sterilization and overpopulation in the Third World, dealt with limitations on procreation itself. The advent of new reproductive technologies has changed the landscape of conflict, and forced us to inquire into the meaning and scope of procreative liberty.

This book's discussion of seven controversial reproductive technologies has shown the intimate connection between procreative liberty and technology. Once this connection is made, the choice of individuals to use or not use these technologies should be presumptively respected because of the privileged position that procreative liberty occupies as a moral and legal right. Where only peripheral aspects of procreation are involved, the right to use those techniques must rest on some basis other than procreative liberty.

The invocation of procreative liberty as a dominant value is not intended to demolish opposition or end discussion. It is offered as a template to guide inquiry and evaluation, and to assure that moral inquiry and public policy do not ignore the importance of personal choice in these matters. No right is absolute. Even procreative liberty can be limited or restricted when adequate cause can be shown. Procreative choices that clearly harm the tangible interest of others are subject to regulation or even prohibition. Even if they cannot be prohibited, their use can be condemned as irresponsible or ill-advised, or not encouraged.

With this approach, however, we have seen that there are few instances in which the feared harms of the new technology are compelling enough to justify restrictive legal intervention (though the need for responsible use remains). Again and again the dire warnings of harm turn out to be baseless or speculative fears, or to reflect highly contested positions about fetal or embryo status, gestational motherhood, and the nature of families—positions that are usually insufficient to justify interference with procreation. In nearly every instance, public policy should keep the gateway to technology open, allowing individuals the freedom to enter as they will.

In the few instances in which choice could be limited, the core values of procreative liberty do not appear to be directly implicated, as with restrictions on pregnant women using drugs, Norplant for the retarded, and nontherapeutic genetic engineering. Even when a good case for restricting reproductive choice exists, the regulatory emphasis should be on counseling, education, notice, and noncoercive incentives, though criminal penalties or injunctions may in some cases be justified.

Some people, of course, will disagree with this analysis, either because they dispute the privileged position accorded procreative liberty or the assessment of harms from individual choice. For example, they may think that I have underestimated the impact of these technologies on women, children, and the family, or undervalued the moral status of embryos and fetuses. Or they may simply be more cautious. With technologies that have not yet been widely used, much less assimilated into the social fabric, it may be premature to pronounce them socially acceptable or even essential to procreative choice.

Yet even if one differs with the book's position in particular instances, the importance of procreative liberty in assessing other applications of technology should remain. For example, persons holding pro-life views will disagree with a biologically based, symbolic analysis of abortion and other prenatal conflicts. But this disagreement should affect only those situations in which embryos or fetuses are directly threatened, and not all other instances of procreative choice.

Even persons with pro-life beliefs might grant the importance of procreative liberty in deciding whether persons may or may not use technologies that do not destroy prenatal life. They may still recognize the right of infertile couples to use IVF, at least within certain limits, and may favor prenatal screening where therapeutic interventions are possible. They may also support uses of Norplant and other technologies when people are not equipped to raise children, as long as embryos and fetuses are not destroyed. Despite differences in some areas, considerable room remains for respecting procreative choice.

An additional advantage of a procreative liberty framework for assessing reproductive technology is the guidance that this approach provides in evaluating future innovations. The development of IVF, prenatal screening, contragestion, and other techniques marks a watershed in human reproduction from which there is no turning back. Future developments will push the envelope of technological control even further, as extracorporeal gestation, cloning, embryo splitting, genetic engineering, embryo tissue farms, posthumous birthing, and other variations come on line. Each of them will present the same dilemmas of individual choice and public policy that we now face.

Procreative liberty should provide a useful framework for evaluating those future developments as well. The effect of each new technology on procreative choice will have to be assessed. If procreative interests are centrally implicated, then only strong countervailing interests will justify limitation. As illustrated repeatedly throughout this book, many of the concerns and fears will, upon closer analysis, turn out to be speculative fears or symbolic perceptions that do not justify infringing core procreative interests. If we accept a strong version of procreative liberty, then public policy for those technologies, as for most of those surveyed in this book, may have to rely on education and persuasion rather than coercion.

THE PROBLEMS OF A RIGHTS-BASED APPROACH
The approach of this book has been explicitly and unswervingly rights based. Taking procreative liberty as a fundamental moral and legal right, it has

assumed that the individual's procreative liberty should rule unless there are compelling reasons to the contrary.

While such an approach characterizes many social issues in the United States, a right-based approach has been strongly criticized in recent years as overly individualistic and insufficiently sensitive to the needs of the community. In a recent book, for example, Professor Mary Ann Glendon has argued that rights talk is limiting because it is absolutist, individualist, and inimical to a sense of social responsibility.[2] Others have argued that rights talk is too private and individualistic, ignoring how public claims interpenetrate the private sphere.[3] It also exposes a social blindness to the claims of interdependence and mutual responsibility that are at the heart of social living.[4]

These criticisms of rights talk are especially applicable to reproduction. A rights-based perspective tends to view reproduction as an isolated, individual act without effects on others. The determinative consideration is whether an individual thinks that a particular technology will serve his or her personal reproductive goals. Except for the rare case of compelling harm, the effects of reproductive choices on offspring, on women, on family, on society and on the general tone and fabric of life are treated as irrelevant to moral analysis or public policy.[5]

Yet reproduction is the act that most clearly implicates community and other persons. Reproduction is never solipsistic. It always occurs with a partner, even if that partner is an anonymous egg or sperm donor, and usually requires the collaboration of physicians and nurses. Its occurrence also directly affects others by creating a new person who in turn affects them and society in various ways. Reproduction is never exclusively a private matter and cannot be completely accounted for in the language of individual rights. Emphasizing procreative rights thus risks denying the central, social dimensions of reproduction.

Critics of rights talk point particularly to the abortion debate, where the pro-choice claim ignores both the interests of fetuses and the interests of fathers and potential grandparents.[6] This criticism might also be leveled against other reproductive technologies, from IVF and collaborative reproduction to genetic screening and fetal tissue transplants. Emphasizing procreative rights necessarily deemphasizes the effects of these technologies on prenatal life, offspring, handicapped children, the family, women, and collaborators.

Although powerful and important, however, this critique of rights does not defeat the priority assigned to procreative rights anymore than it defeats the priority of free speech, due process, travel, and other important rights. To begin with, the critique does not always prove the ill effects that it claims. Glendon, for example, overlooks the fact that many rights "encourage precisely the form of deliberation and communal interaction" that Glendon herself favors.[7] This is true of political and social rights, which make communal deliberation and democracy possible.[8] It is also true of rights to use procreative technologies. Thus IVF encourages the formation of families and the cooperative, dependent relationships that inhere therein. The use of donors and surrogates requires a special kind of cooperation, often among strangers, that leads to new forms of community. Even aborting to get fetal tissue for a loved one can be a sacrifice that binds rather than divides.

Second, rights-based approaches to reproduction or other issues do not ignore other interests so much as judge them, after careful scrutiny, as inadequate to sustain interference with individual choice. If harmful effects are clearly established or the action in question does not implicate central features of fundamental liberty, public concerns may take priority over private choice. In many cases, however, the state is relegated to exhortation and noncoercive sanctions to protect communal interest because it cannot satisfy the burden of serious harm necessary to justify overriding fundamental rights.

A third problem with the critique of rights is that the alternative it offers is weak and thin, even less desirable than whatever excesses rights might breed. Without the protection of rights, important aspects of individual dignity and integrity have no protection from legislative majorities or policymakers. Elizabeth Kingdom's hope that getting beyond rights will enable public policy to make "a wider calculation of the proper distribution of social benefits" overlooks the need for rights to protect us from the policy calculations of zealous administrators.[9] Indeed, the emergence of rights is due to the failure of the community and public officials to give due regard to the needs of affected individuals.

This is especially clear in the case of abortion, which Glendon and Elizabeth Fox-Genovese claim shows the divisive, individualistic vices of a rights approach. The claim for a right to abortions comes out of a failed collective responsibility toward motherhood, which makes abortion an essential option. If pro-life groups were truly concerned with the weak and vulnerable, as their concern with the fetus claims, they would make greater efforts to rectify the social and economic conditions that make abortion a necessary option for women. Their failure in this regard suggests rather an interest in controlling "women's reproductive capacities ... (in order) ... to continue a system of discrimination that is based on sex."[10] Rights are essential precisely to guard against discriminatory agendas that deny dignity and integrity to women and men. They are responses to failures of social responsibility, not the causes of them.[11]

To be convincing, however, a right-based approach must acknowledge its defects even while proclaiming its strengths. It cannot ignore the social dimension, even if social claims are seldom sufficient to limit procreative choice. To assure that full credence is given to these dimensions, three specific criticisms of a rights-based approach are discussed. In each case we will see that procreative liberty, despite some qualifications, emerges alive and well.

MONEY AND CLASS

A major problem with a rights-based approach is that it ignores the social and economic context in which exercise of rights is embedded. Procreative rights are negative in protecting against private or state interference, but they give no positive assistance to someone who lacks the resources essential to exercise the right. A rights-based approach to reproductive choice thus has no way to take the effects of money and class into account. As Rhonda Copeland has noted:

The negative theory of privacy is ... profoundly inadequate as a basis for reproductive and sexual freedom because it perpetuates the myth that the ability to effectuate one's choices rests exclusively on the individual,

rather than acknowledging that choices are facilitated, hindered or entirely frustrated by social conditions. In doing so negative privacy theory exempts the state from responsibility for contributing to the material conditions and social relations that impede, and conversely, could encourage autonomous decision-making.[12]

The truth of this statement is evident in how the distribution of wealth operates as a prime determinant of who exercises reproductive rights. The most obvious wealth effect concerns access to reproductive technology. For example, women who lack the money to pay for Norplant or abortions are much less able to avoid reproduction than those who can pay. Yet the Supreme Court has held that the state's failure to fund abortions for indigent women does not violate their right to terminate pregnancy because it places no obstacle in their path that was not already there.[13] It is also the poor who feel the brunt of 24-hour waiting periods for abortions, and who would be most acutely affected if *Roe v. Wade* were ever reversed.

Lack of resources also affect one's ability to undergo IVF and related assisted reproductive techniques. At a cost of $7,000 per cycle, only middle- and upper-class couples can afford this treatment. Since several cycles may be needed to establish pregnancy, this is a technique that will clearly be wealth-based. Similarly, egg donation and surrogacy, which have equivalent or higher costs, will also be distributed according to wealth. Nor will prenatal screening and genetic manipulation be widely available to those who cannot pay for them.

There is irony in the financial disparities that determine differential access here. Poor and minorities have greater rates of infertility than middle and upper classes, yet only the latter can afford the high costs of IVF and other assisted reproductive treatment. Given the current crisis of access to health care for poor people, the idea of Medicaid payments for infertility treatments is politically unlikely, so these disparities are likely to continue.

Allocating reproductive technologies and other essential goods and services according to ability to pay raises profound questions of social justice. Because infertility impairs a basic aspect of species-typical functioning, a strong argument for including it in any basic health-care package can be made.[14] Yet it does not follow that society's failure to assure access to reproductive technologies for all who would benefit justifies denying access to those who have the means to pay. Such a principle has not been followed with other medical procedures, even life-saving procedures such as heart transplants. As troubled as we might be by differential access, the demands of equality should not bar access for those fortunate enough to have the means.

Class and money may also influence the roles individuals play in the collaborative reproductive process. Under the theory of procreative liberty proposed in this book, individuals have the right to hire or engage donors and surrogates, or to serve as donors and surrogates themselves.[15] Since donors and surrogates are usually paid for their contribution, the danger is that only the middle class and wealthy will have the resources to hire them, while only the lower classes will be inclined to assume these roles. If this is so, money and class will greatly skew the distribution of roles and services in collaborative reproduction.

The latter concern, however, may be most acute for surrogacy. Although lack of funds may prevent poor people from obtaining gamete donations, poverty has not been a determinant of who provides sperm and egg donations. Proximity, reliability, health, and fertility have been the main factors physicians have sought in gamete donors. While egg donations are paid as much as $1,500 to $2,000 per cycle, it is unlikely that only poor women in need of money will choose to be donors.

Class, however, may be a stronger factor in the selection of surrogate mothers. Again, poor people will not usually be able to buy surrogate services, if a willing family member is not available. However, they are more likely to be recruited as surrogates because of the $10,000 or more that they will be paid. It is not surprising that Mary Beth Whitehead, the surrogate in the *Baby M* case, was of a lower social class and less educated then the recipient couple. Similarly, in the *Anna C. v. Mark J.* gestational surrogate case, the surrogate was black, while the hiring couple was white/Asian.[16] Although many surrogates have gone to high school or college, there is a danger that class bias and financial need will

determine the supply of surrogates. Carried to extremes, a breeder class of poor, minority women whose reproductive capacity is exploited by wealthier people could emerge.

But what is to be done about this practice? Denying poorer women that opportunity by prohibiting payment or by allowing payment only to middle-class surrogates denies them a reproductive role which they find meaningful. Given that poorer women serve as nannies, babysitters, housekeepers, and factory workers, gestational services might also be sold, even though it will offend the respect that some persons have for maternal gestation. Should couples be denied access to surrogacy because of the risk of class bias, when the surrogate is freely and intelligently choosing that role? Whatever our qualms about such a practice, it may have to be tolerated because the procreative liberty of all the parties is so intimately involved.

A final area in which class and money will make itself felt is in state interventions to protect offspring from harmful prenatal conduct or to limit irresponsible reproduction by compulsory contraception. Punishing women for prenatal child abuse or ordering cesarean sections against their will appears to have a disproportionate racial and class impact. For example, a Florida study showed that while the same percentage of white and black women have signs of illegal drugs in their blood at birth, the state refers black women disproportionately to the criminal justice system or to child welfare agencies.[17] Other studies have shown that mandatory cesarean sections are most commonly sought for black and poor women, not for whites who also refuse the operation.[18] Similarly, compulsory contraception for child abusers or HIV women seems to target the poor and minorities more than other groups. Although an invidious discriminatory purpose has not been shown to underlie these disparities, the danger that wealth, class, and race will be factors in the state's coercive use of reproductive technology cannot be ignored.

These points about the role of money and class in distributing reproductive technologies and procreative choice show the limits of a negative rights-based approach to procreative liberty. It is another example of the disparities that differential distribution of wealth in a liberal society inevitably bring.

One can decry the disparities that exist and urge that society correct distributive inequities, however, without denying all persons the right to make these choices. In the end, the need for social justice is not a compelling reason for limiting the procreative choice of those who can pay.

THE FEMINIST CRITIQUE

A strong emphasis on procreative liberty has also been questioned by feminists who fear that technology will lessen women's control over reproduction and further oppression of women. Feminist critics have usually focused on the dangers to women in surrogate motherhood or objected to prenatal interventions for the sake of offspring. However, the feminist critique goes deeper than a challenge to these techniques, and calls into question all reproductive technologies that redound to the benefit of a male-dominated society at the expense of women.[19]

The feminist critique of a rights-based approach to reproductive technology has several strands. Sometimes the objections go to the very idea of subjecting the natural reproductive process to technological control, because such control is viewed as a male-driven violation of the natural order. The more central fear, however, is that because of men's greater access to wealth and power, they will use reproductive technologies to control and oppress women. Indeed, some feminists assert that men devised these techniques in order to control female reproduction just when women began gaining social and economic power. They fear that a rights-based approach to reproductive technology will further patriarchal domination of women by reinforcing the traditional identification of women with childbearing and child rearing. At the very least, it will result in women taking on additional reproductive burdens to serve male procreative agendas.

Given the long history of sexism in medicine, the feminist critique must be taken seriously. A long tradition exists of men controlling female reproduction. Male doctors wrested control of the birth process from female midwives in the eighteenth and nineteenth centuries. In the early twentieth century they developed techniques of twilight sleep and anesthesia to further that control, which the natural childbirth movement of the 1960s and 1970s fought hard to overcome.[20] Hysterectomy, involuntary sterilization, and mastectomy reflect further assaults on female sexuality and reproduction. Electronic fetal monitoring and high rates for cesarean births may also be seen as further examples of male control.[21]

Some developments in reproductive technology seem to be cut from the same cloth. Forced cesarean section or jail for drug use discovered by doctors during pregnancy strikes some people as a form of medical violence against women. Forced contraception to limit "irresponsible reproduction" could be viewed as a way to bring untrammeled female sexuality under control. Restrictions on abortion often seem more concerned with imposing sexual and reproductive orthodoxy than on protecting fetuses.

Noncoital treatments of infertility can also be seen in this light. Women undergo the burdensome roller-coaster ride of IVF treatment to please their husbands. IVF technologies assault the woman's body with powerful hormones to coax out eggs and make the uterus receptive to embryos. Women may also feel compelled to screen out defective embryos and fetuses to make sure that they deliver a "good baby."

Because women bear the brunt of reproductive work, injustice in the distribution of reproductive burdens and benefits is inescapable. However, the view that a rights-based view of reproductive technology places power increasingly in the hands of men to the detriment of women overlooks the many ways in which technology offers options that expand the freedom of women. It also overlooks how a rights-based approach, despite its contextual limitations, assures women a large measure of control over their reproductive lives.

Consider how several technologies discussed in this book help women to avoid unwanted pregnancy or to have healthy offspring. Norplant is a safe, effective, and reversible long-lasting contraception that many women will welcome. When RU486 becomes available in the United States, it will allow unwanted pregnancies to be terminated at early stages without surgery, and thus increase access to abortion. IVF and the other assisted reproductive techniques enable women to rear offspring when they previously would have had to remain childless or adopt. Earlier and less invasive prenatal diagnosis allows a woman to avoid giving birth to handicapped children. Tissue production techniques may eventually allow a woman to save the life of a child, a parent, or even herself. Given these possibilities, reproductive technologies would appear to advance the interests of women.

Although a rights-based approach to reproduction cannot eliminate the inherent inequalities in male and female procreation, it can provide substantial protection for women. It is the best guarantee of a woman's control over the options these technologies offer. Legal recognition of procreative liberty will protect women from public sector impositions on their procreative choice. Respecting this liberty will stop the state from outlawing early abortion. Respect of this right will also protect women against forced sterilization, forced abortion, or forced contraception to prevent harm to offspring or taxpayers. Some limits on reproductively related conduct, such as drug use during pregnancy, might still be possible, but the threat here is not to procreative liberty and neither men nor women have the right to harm offspring by egregious or irresponsible prenatal conduct. When everything is considered, a strong commitment to procreative liberty will protect more than it will harm the interests of women.

Of course this is not to deny the ways in which technology can be used to harm women, nor the barriers that stand in the way of women having the means and the situational power to exercise free choice in decisions about technology. However, the most common target of feminist attacks is the argument that procreative liberty leads to the enforcement of surrogate mother contracts against the wishes of the gestational mother. Although much less common than other assisted reproductive techniques, surrogacy has come to symbolize the struggle of women to gain control of pregnancy and reproduction.[22]

Many feminists always favor the gestational mother in these disputes, as do most of the courts and legislatures that have addressed the issue.[23] Yet which solution is most protective of women is debatable—the woman who provides the egg for gestational surrogacy also has important reproductive interests at stake as do women who wish to serve as surrogates who are denied the opportunity because

of the legal unenforceability of their preconception promise. Many liberal feminists now argue that the intentions of the contracting parties should control rearing.[24] In their view, such a solution puts women in ultimate control, even though it requires that they be bound by surrogacy contracts just as they are by their contracts in other settings. It also undercuts traditional notions of reproductive orthodoxy that identify women with gestation and child rearing.

In the private sphere, the main issue for women will be whether they will be free to use—to have access to—the technologies they desire. Pro-creative liberty will protect them against state restrictions that are based on speculative harms or particular moral views of proper reproductive behavior, a major threat in this area. They will thus be free to use or not use IVF, egg and embryo donation, gestational surrogacy, genetic screening, embryo biopsy, and fetal therapy to treat infertility or to have healthy children.

Of course, a right against the state to use these techniques will not overcome contextual constraints on a women's freedom. It does not help her if she lacks the funds to purchase the services in question. Nor will it remove the financial pressures that might lead her to choose to be an egg donor or a surrogate. It also does not protect her from her partner's, her family's, or her own internally generated demands— the product of socialization in a patriarchal society— to have children, despite the physical social, or psychological burdens to her of doing so. Yet these limitations do not diminish the importance of the negative protections that a recognition of procreative liberty establishes, even if women do end up carrying a heavier reproductive load than men.

Some philosophers argue that more reproductive choices are not always better for women because new options do not always leave all of a woman's previous alternatives unchanged.[25] As evidence they cite how the development of IVF lead to pressure on women to undergo several burdensome cycles of treatment, and how prenatal sex determination might lead to pressure to abort. They also point to how prenatal genetic testing now makes a woman responsible for having handicapped offspring if she rejects amniocentesis, when previously she would have been seen as a victim of the natural lottery.[26]

One cannot deny that reproductive choices will not increase self-determination for all women, because some will be pressured to make choices that they previously would not have had to face, or will lack the resources to take advantage of the opportunities presented. On balance, however, there is no reason to think that women do not end up with more rather than less reproductive freedom as a result of technological innovations. If so, procreative liberty is an important bulwark that helps women achieve the greater freedom that reproductive advances make possible. The more important lesson for social policy is the need to protect women from new forms of private sector coercion that arise because of these techniques, and to support their efforts to exercise procreative autonomy.

One need only imagine a world without procreative liberty to appreciate its contribution to the well-being of women. Although procreative liberty gives little protection from family or internal pressures to procreate or from lack of resources, it does prevent arbitrary, moralistic, or speculative governmental impositions on a woman's procreative choice. Even in a world without the technological options now available, recognition of negative procreative liberty would be an important achievement.

THE COMMUNITARIAN CRITIQUE: RIGHTS AND RESPONSIBILITY

Rights-based approaches are also criticized for their disregard of the needs of community. An emphasis on rights is necessarily individualist. It reflects a "do your own thing" mentality that ignores the impact of exercising rights on the shape, the tone, and the overall well-being of communities, and may obstruct the resolution of pressing economic and social problems[27] Responsibility in the exercise of rights is essential if communities are to survive and be vital, yet rights talk invariably slights one's responsibility to the community.

This criticism is especially applicable to reproductive rights. Procreative liberty emphasizes individual satisfaction and deemphasizes the social consequences of procreative choice. It respects individual desire but denigrates duty and responsibility in how desire is fulfilled. Yet responsibility in procreation is essential because of its effects on resulting offspring. Indeed, many persons would argue that no one should reproduce unless they are able and willing to care and nurture the children they produce. Yet this book except for the argument in chapter 8 for prenatal responsibility, largely rejects that conception of procreative liberty, as do feminists and others who want strict walls against any governmental intervention in reproductive choice.

Procreative liberty arguments for use of new reproductive technologies are vulnerable to the communitarian critique on several grounds. Many consumers of these techniques—and professionals who profit from offering them—rush to use them with little thought of their impact on off-spring, family, and society. One may ask whether it is socially responsible to spend a billion dollars a year on assisted reproduction when so many other health needs are unmet, and when so many children await in foster homes for adoption.[28] Couples who spend thousands of dollars on such treatments may be less concerned about their child's welfare than their own selfish desires. Cumulatively, such practices could undermine the bonds on which the welfare of children and the community depend.

The community also suffers from routinization of prenatal screening practices. Embryos and fetuses become objects to be discarded or destroyed if they do not meet standards of quality or convenience, thus diminishing respect for the first stages of human life and the well-being of children who are born simply ordinary or with minor handicaps. The willingness to employ gamete donors and surrogates as reproductive collaborators also undermines community. Infertile couples might view donors and surrogates not as equals in a mutually collaborative enterprise, but as depersonalized cogs in the production of children. Written contracts distance the infertile couple and surrogate from the emotional reality of their joint endeavor.[29] Disaggregation and recombination of reproductive components also undermine the traditional importance of genetic and gestation bonds in defining families, and may leave children and parents confused about their lineage and social responsibilities. Finally, couples who harvest the uterus for transplant and research material contribute, like slash-and burn farmers in the rain forest, to the increasing erosion of community conceptions of the sanctity of human life.

These concerns should be taken seriously, but the assumption that a rights-based approach to reproductive technology will inevitably diminish community greatly overstates the case. Procreative liberty does entitle women on welfare, convicted child abusers, and those with HIV to procreate, but as we saw in chapter 4, it is not clear that such reproduction is always irresponsible. We have also seen, in chapter 8, that procreative liberty does not give women or men the right to engage in prenatal conduct that will harm offspring. The expense and burdens of assisted reproduction is as likely to make the child loved and cherished as it is to commodify it as a product to satisfy parental selfishness. Prenatal genetic interventions to enhance the health of offspring may be more rooted in love than in narcissism.

Nor will the use of surrogates and donors necessarily be depersonalized and adversarial. Couples usually meet the surrogate, have frequent contact during pregnancy, and may correspond or meet in later years. Often egg donors are friends or family, and are increasingly sought out even when they are strangers. Written contracts; by providing certainty and understanding of mutual obligations, bring parties together more often than they divide. Contrary to rights critics, the use of donors and surrogates is as likely to be truly collaborative and cooperative as it is to be adversarial and antagonistic. Rather than undermine family, these practices present new variations of family and community that could help fill the void left by flux in the shape of the American family.

If this is so, an emphasis on reproductive rights is not inconsistent with reproductive responsibility and the needs of community, and is unlikely to damage individuals, families or larger social concerns more than it benefits them. The fears raised, however, do remind us of the possible reverberations of reproductive decisions on individuals and the community and thus the need for sensitivity and respect for others in their use.

Efforts to assure responsible use of reproductive technologies could take several forms. One is for both providers and consumers to resist the seductive urge to use a technology because it is there and might work. A technological solution of infertility is a powerful temptation, as the readiness of couples to try IVF and related procedures shows. Because the technology may be more onerous and less effective than at first appears, couples should be accurately informed of their prospects and counseled about the complications that could arise.[30]

A second approach is to ask potential users to think carefully about the social and psychological ramifications of collaborative reproduction for themselves, the children, and the donors and surrogates who assist them. Infertile couples, donors, and surrogates should explore the social and emotional uncertainties they face before embarking on such a weighty venture. They should be especially careful before undertaking truly novel procedures, such as splitting embryos to create twins born years apart, using related or intergenerational surrogates, creating embryos for tissue, and the like.[31]

A third approach is to develop guidelines or canons of ethical behavior. A legal right to use reproductive technologies does not necessarily entitle one to private-sector access. Health professionals are gatekeepers who ultimately determine who will use these technologies. They should use discretion in accepting patients and in acceding to their demands for technological help, yet not exclude persons on the basis of sexual preference, disability, or life-style alone. Above all, they should treat their patients with dignity and respect, and not mislead or exploit their desire to reproduce merely to make a profit. Regulatory measures to protect consumers from provider overreaching, as discussed in chapter 5, are clearly justified.

Finally, a rights approach to reproductive technology is not an imprimatur on all uses of the technology. It does not require that the state subsidize or otherwise encourage the use of all reproductive techniques, and provides no immunity from moral condemnation, persuasion, or noncoercive instruction in how that technology should be used. Thus not all forms of collaborative reproduction need be subsidized, even if health insurance should or does cover some infertility treatment. States may also refuse to enact laws that facilitate collaborative reproduction, though that approach might cause more problems than it presents.[32] In short, there is ample room for protecting the community while also respecting individual choice. How to encourage responsible use without infringing procreative liberty will remain a major challenge for public policy.

Conclusion: Autonomy and Ambivalence

Resort to technology is a powerful temptation to persons who wish to have or to avoid having offspring. Reliance on technology, however, has both a bright and a dark side. It can be used in a caring, supportive, and communal way, or it can be used to oppress, dominate, and alienate. The ultimate challenge is to use it well.

Despite the problems of a rights-based approach, I have argued that procreative liberty should be presumptively protected in moral analysis and in public policy determinations about new reproductive technology. Procreation is central to individual meaning and dignity, and respect for procreative liberty best resolves the many controversies surveyed. A commitment to autonomy, however, does not eliminate the ambivalence that use of these techniques creates at both the individual and societal level.

At the individual level, persons may be ambivalent about the manipulations and social uncertainties that technologized means of reproduction entail, yet feel that they have few alternatives if they are to overcome infertility, avoid handicapped children, or save a loved one. At the societal level, ambivalence arises from the unknown social effects of permitting individuals to engineer offspring and to alter traditional understandings of family. Yet restricting individual efforts to find reproductive meaning through technology engenders further ambivalence, for it violates procreative freedom and implicates the state in intimate decisions best left to personal choice.

As science produces more technologies to control reproduction, public response will oscillate between attraction and repulsion, between respect for autonomy and concern for how that freedom is used. In the end, the reception of individual reproductive technologies will depend on their efficacy, the goals they serve, and their real and symbolic effects. Ambivalence will dissipate only when a clear verdict on the desirability or undesirability of a particular technology is possible. Given normative differences and uncertain empirical effects, that will not quickly occur.

There is no stopping the desire for greater control of the reproductive process. Since this is so value-laden an area, ethical, legal, and social conflicts over reproductive technology are likely to continue for many years. In confronting those conflicts, we must not deny the importance of procreative liberty just to escape the discomfort that its use often engenders. There is no better alternative than leaving procreative decisions to the individuals whose procreative desires are most directly involved.

Notes

1. [John A. Robertson, *Children of Choice: Freedom and the New Reproductive Technologies* (Princeton University Press, 1994)–Ed.]
2. *Rights Talk: The Impoverishment of Political Discourse* (New York: Free Press, 1991).
3. Elizabeth Fox-Genovese, "Society's Child" (Review of *Life Itself: Abortion in the American Mind* by Roger Rosenblatt), *The New Republic*, 18 May 1992, 40-41.
4. This is one of Elizabeth Kingdom's criticisms of rights in *What's Wrong with Rights: Problems for Feminist Politics of Law* (Edinburgh U.K.: Edinburgh University Press 1991), 79-84.
5. I am grateful to Daniel and Sidney Callahan for first making me aware of this aspect of reproductive rights.
6. See Fox-Genovese, "Society's Child"; Daniel Callahan, "Bioethics and Fatherhood, " *Utah Law Review* 1992 (3): 735.
7. Cass Sunstein, "Righttalk," *The New Republic*, 2 September 1991, 34.
8. As Sunstein notes, rights of speech and association, jury trial and antidiscrimination, are basic preconditions for social involvement, thus enhancing rather than dividing community. In addition, rights and duties are correlative, thereby creating an implicit sense of social responsibility. Id. At 35.
9. Kingdom, *What's Wrong with Rights,* 83.
10. Sunstein, "Righttalk," 36. Sunstein further notes: "If one looks at the context in which restrictions on abortion take place, at their real purposes and real effects, then the abortion right is most plausibly rooted not in privacy but in the right to equality on the basis of sex. Current law nowhere compels men to devote their bodies to the protection of other people, even if life is at stake, and even if men are responsible for the very existence of those people.... Such restrictions are an

important means of reasserting traditional gender roles." Id. See also chapter 3 [of *Children of Choice* —Ed.].

11. If the social vision of reproduction is to claim our allegiance, then society's commitment to the sanctity of life must be reflected in a social commitment to support it at all stages, including in those pregnant women who desire an abortion because they lack the resources to care for a child.

12. "Losing the Negative Right of Privacy: Building Sexual and Reproductive Freedom," *New York University Review of Law and Social Change* 18 (1991): 46.

13. Maher v. Roe, 432 U.S. 464 (1977); Harris v. McCrae, 448 U.S. 297 (1980).

14. Norman Daniels, *Just Health Care* (New York: Cambridge University Press, 1985), 26-28.

15. Either directly or as a derivative right of the recipient. See chapters 2 and 6 [of *Children of Choice*—Ed.].

16. 822 p. 2d 1317, 4 Cal. Rptr. 2nd 170 (1992).

17. Ira J. Chasnoff, "The Prevalence of Illicit Drug Use during Pregnancy and Discrepancies in Mandatory Reporting in Pinellas County, Florida," *New England Journal of Medicine* 322 (1990): 1202. However, the differential treatment could be explained by the fact that the white women were more likely to have evidence of marijuana in their blood, while the black women had evidence of cocaine.

18. V.E. Kolder, J. Gallagher, and M.T. Parsons, "Court-Ordered Obstetrical Interventions," *New England Journal of Medicine* 316 (1987): 1192-1196.

19. Almost any issue of *Issues in Reproductive and Genetic Engineering: Journal of International Feminist Analysis* contains criticism of the dangers of new reproductive technologies, including IVF. See, for example, Bette Vanderwater, "Meanings and Strategies of Reproductive Control: Current Feminist Approaches to Reproductive technology," 5 (1992): 215.

Part of the feminist objection to the medicalization of pregnancy through ultrasound, amniocentesis, cesarean sections, and IFV, to name but a few examples, is that women lose control over their own pregnancies and childbirths. Martha Field, "Surrogacy Contracts—Gestational and Traditional: The Argument for Nonenforcement,"*Washburn Law Journal* 31 (1991): 1, 16. It is usually men who then control the process.

20. Judith Leavitt, "Birthing and Anesthesia: The Debate Over Twilight Sleep," *Signs* 6 (1980): 147.

21. Adrienne Rich, *Of Woman Born: Motherhood as Experience and Institution* (New York: W. W. Norton, 1976). 117-148; Bottoms, Rosen, and Sokol, "The Increase in the Cesarean Birth Rate," *New England Journal of Medicine* 302 (1980): 559; Banta, "Benefits and Risks of Electronic Fetal Monitoring," in *Birth Control and Controlling Birth,* ed., H. Holmes, B. Hoskins, and M. Gross (Atlantic Highlands, N. J.: Humanities Press, 1980), 147.

22. Martha Field notes: "A final thing about surrogacy is allocation of power between the sexes. Seen through one lens surrogacy concerns who will control pregnancy and reproduction. Surrogacy is one way for men to take control of reproduction, to have babies without being dependent upon women, or at least to be dependent only upon those women who are under contract.... The surrogacy debate is part of a range of hard-fought issues over who is going to make the greater part of the decision in this important facet of life." Field, "Surrogacy Contracts," 31.

23. See chapter 6 [of *Children of Choice*—Ed.].

24. M. Shultz, "Reproductive Technology and Intent-Based Patenthood: An Opportunity for Gender Neutrality," *Wisconsin Law Review* (1990: 298; L. Andrews, *New Conceptions* (New York: St. Martin's Press, 1984); L. Andrews, *Between Strangers: Surrogate Mothers, Expectant Fathers, and Brave New Babies* (New York: Harper and Row, 1989).

25. I am indebted to Dan Brock's "Reproductive Freedom: Its Nature, Bases, and Limits" (unpublished paper, 1992) for this particular formulation of the problem.

26. Barbara Katz Rothman, *The Tentative Pregnancy* (New York: Viking Press, 1986).

27. Sunstein notes that rights talk can sometimes "stop discussion in its tracks," leaving the impression that much more needs to be said but making it difficult to say it. Rights talk can also lead to "conclusions that masquerade as reasons." "Right talk," 34. Ideally, the claim of a right should not cut off the detailed argument about social consequences that recognition of rights often encapsulates.

28. Most of the money comes from persons buying reproductive services with their own funds, and thus would

not be available to satisfy other health needs of the community. For a discussion of IVF, surrogacy, and adoption, see Field, "Surrogacy Contracts," and Elizabeth Bartholet, *Family Bonds: Adoption and the Politics of Parenting* (Boston: Houghton Mifflin, 1993). Field and Bartholet never state why infertile couples alone and not all persons who reproduce have the obligation to adopt kids in need of parents.

29. See Maura Ryan, "The Argument for Unlimited Procreative Liberty: A Feminist Critique," *Hastings Center Report,* July/August 1990, 6.

30. See chapter 5 [of *Children of Choice*—Ed.].

31. Knowing when to proceed and when to stop is difficult precisely because so little is know about so many procedures.

32. See chapter 6 [of *Children of Choice*—Ed.] for elaboration of this point.

17.
REFLECTIONS ON REPRODUCTIVE RIGHTS IN CANADA

Christine Overall

The concept of "reproductive rights" plays a central role in discussions of issues relating to women's reproductive health. While the concept of rights in general does not by any means constitute all that is important in ethical discourse, and the concept of reproductive rights in particular does not exhaust all that is significant in the moral evaluation of reproductive issues, the idea of reproductive rights is, at this point at least, indispensable to a complete discussion of reproductive ethics and social policy.

Barbara Katz Rothman has expressed reservations about the use of the term "reproduction," arguing that we do not literally produce babies or reproduce ourselves.[1] While I agree with this observation, I shall continue to use the phrase "reproductive right" because I specifically want to explore the strengths and the ambiguities of that phrase. In particular, this chapter will analyse and evaluate the ways in which this notion of reproductive right has been given a unique legal and moral expression within Canadian society during the last two decades, manifesting itself within the struggle for abortion, the debates about midwifery and the place of birth, and the introduction of social practices relating to new reproductive technologies such as *in vitro* fertilization.

Originally, the concept of reproductive rights seemed to find a natural home within the abortion debate, but it is now being extended to discussions of new reproductive technologies. What is extraordinary is that the idea of reproductive rights is used not only by feminists concerned with promoting women's well-being and ending oppression, but also by non-feminists, whose agenda usually includes preservation of the traditional family, extension of male sexual and reproductive entitlements, and enforcement of a "pro-life" morality that sees women's bodies as instruments for the production of babies. In other words, while the idea of reproductive rights is both useful and central to the advance-ment of women's reproductive freedom, there are also ways in which it can be and is being used against women's best interests. For this reason feminists need to think carefully about what they mean when making claims for reproductive rights.

THE RIGHT NOT TO REPRODUCE

The term "reproductive right" has more than one meaning.[2] It is necessary, first, to distinguish between the right to reproduce and the right *not* to reproduce. The two are sometimes mistakenly conflated as, for example, when Justice Bertha Wilson referred in her Supreme Court decision on the Morgentaler case to "[t]he right to reproduce or not to reproduce which is in issue in this case."[3] The right not to reproduce is the entitlement not to be compelled to beget or bear children against one's will: the entitlement not to have to engage in forced reproductive labour. To say that women have a right not to reproduce implies that they have no obligation to reproduce. In its weak (liberty) sense it is the entitlement not to be compelled to donate gametes (eggs or sperm) or embryos against one's will. The right not to reproduce in the strong (welfare) sense is the right of access to services like abortion and contraception that enable women to avoid procreation. Women do not owe their reproductive products or labour to any person or institution, including male partners or the state.

Recognition of the right not to reproduce has been slower to develop in Canada than in the United States. Full exercise of such a right requires, among other protections, access to safe and effective contraception and abortion services. In other words, the moral entitlement to abortion access follows from the broader right not to reproduce. In 1969, stipulations were introduced into the Criminal Code that provided for the possibility, under certain carefully specified conditions, of therapeutic exceptions to the general law that using any means or permitting any means to be used for the purpose of procuring a miscarriage on a female person was an indictable offence. According to the then new Section 251 of the Code, such a therapeutic abortion had to be performed by a qualified medical practitioner who was not a member of a therapeutic abortion committee; in an accredited or approved hospital; and only after a decision by the hospital's therapeutic abortion committee, consisting of at least three members, each of them a qualified medical practitioner, that the continuation of the pregnancy would, or would be likely to, endanger the life or health of the pregnant woman.

In the ensuing years, variations in interpretation of and conformity to Section 251 gave rise in many cases to outright injustice. In some areas hospitals could not obtain accreditation or approval; in some hospitals there were not sufficient doctors to constitute a therapeutic abortion committee. Hospitals had no legal obligation to set up such a committee; and those committees that did exist had no obligation to meet. Some hospitals imposed quotas on the numbers of abortions performed, or limitations on patient eligibility based on place of residence. Women had no right to appear before the committees to present their case, and interpretation of the phrase "life or health" of the pregnant woman was left entirely to committee members. Interpretations varied enormously from one committee to another, and some even introduced extraneous considerations such as marital status of the applicant, consent of her spouse, or number of previous abortions.[4]

Section 251 of the Criminal Code placed severe constraints on Canadian women's right not to reproduce. In effect, it said that some women—directly, those whose abortion requests were rejected by therapeutic abortion committees, and indirectly, those who had no opportunity to bring their request to such a committee—had a legal obligation to procreate; it sentenced them to forced reproductive labour. This surely was a major violation of what the Charter of Rights and Freedoms now refers to as "security of the person." In the words of Supreme Court Judge Jean Beetz in the Morgentaler decision, "A pregnant woman's person cannot be said to be secure if, when her life or health is in danger, she is faced with a rule

of criminal law which precludes her from obtaining effective and timely medical treatment."[5]

The so-called "pro-life" movement in North America places heavy emphasis upon what is alleged to be the foetus's right to life. Even without specifically recognizing such a right, however—indeed, without making any direct references at all to the foetus or its physical condition—Section 251 implicitly attributed to the foetus a right to the use and occupancy of the woman's uterus. In effect, the woman's body was regarded simply as a container, with various utilities, that the foetus happened to need for nine months. Indeed, foetuses are the only group of entities that have been given entitlement under Canadian law to the medical use of the bodies of adult persons.

Section 251 also helped to perpetuate a right of access to women's reproductive labour that potentially benefited both individual men and the state. In the words of Justice Bertha Wilson, Section 251 of the Criminal Code "assert[ed] that the woman's capacity to reproduce is not to be subject to her own control. It is to be subject to the control of the state.... She is truly being treated as a means—a means to an end which she does not desire but over which she has no control."[6]

Fortunately, in January 1988 the Supreme Court removed these Criminal Code impediments to women's access to abortion.[7] No longer is a woman seeking an abortion required to obtain the approval of a therapeutic abortion committee. According to the judicial decision, "Forcing a woman, by threat of criminal sanction, to carry a foetus to term unless she meets certain criteria unrelated to her own priorities and aspirations, is a profound interference with a woman's body and thus a violation of security of the person."[8]

But this decision has by no means permanently removed a significant danger to women's right not to reproduce. Like women in the United States,[9] Canadian women cannot assume that access to abortion will remain indefinitely protected. Potential threats to abortion access can be found in at least three areas.

First, there is a danger that the recent expression of concerns about the reasons for abortion and abortion-related procedures may lead to renewed limitations on access to abortion. One example is the growing media discussion of abortion for the purpose of sex selection.[10] Another is the demand for regulation of and limitations on so-called selective termination in pregnancy (discussed in detail in Chapter 3 below). This procedure, performed in cases of multiple pregnancy in order to reduce the number of foetuses in the uterus, usually involves the injection of potassium chloride into the thorax of one or more of the foetuses to stop the heart. The "terminated" foetus is reabsorbed into the woman's body, without further need for surgery.[11] Recent media news reports have quoted Canadian ethicists and physicians as challenging the justification of the procedure and calling for limitations on the number of foetuses to be terminated.[12]

A second reason for concern about potential threats to the right not to reproduce is the persistence of the claim that there is a need for protection of foetal life and alleged foetal rights. In March 1989 the Supreme Court of Canada dismissed Joseph Borowski's argument that Section 251 of the Criminal Code contravened the life, security, and equality rights of the foetus, as a "person" protected by sections 7 and 15 of the Canadian Charter of Rights and Freedoms. In the absence of a law governing abortion, the Court found the appeal to be moot, and stated that the appellant no longer had standing to pursue the appeal. It added:

> In a legislative context any rights of the foetus could be considered or at least balanced against the rights of women guaranteed by s. 7.... A pronouncement in favour of the appellant's position that a foetus is protected by s. 7 from the date of conception would decide the issue out of its proper context. Doctors and hospitals would be left to speculate as to how to apply such a ruling consistently with a woman's rights under s. 7.[13]

Nevertheless, it is not impossible that a future government could use the decision in the Borowski case as part of the rationale for reintroducing a law to recriminalize some abortions. Indeed, even the 1988 decision striking down the existing abortion law left open the very real possibility that legal steps might be taken to protect so-called foetal rights. For example, Justice Wilson stated that "Section 1 of the Charter authorizes reasonable limits to be put upon the woman's right having regard to the fact of the developing foetus within her body." She added:

> A developmental view of the foetus ... supports a permissive approach to abortion in the early stages of pregnancy and a restrictive approach in the later stages.... [The woman's] reasons for having an abortion would ... be the proper subject of inquiry at the later stages of her pregnancy when the state's compelling interest in the protection of the foetus would justify it in prescribing conditions. The precise point in the development of the foetus at which the state's interest in its protection becomes "compelling" I leave to the informed judgment of the legislature which is in a position to receive guidance on the subject from all the relevant disciplines. It seems to me, however, that it might fall somewhere in the second trimester.[14]

Similarly, Chief Justice Brian Dickson said, "State protection of foetal interests may well be deserving of constitutional recognition under s. 1."[15] And Justice Beetz stated:

> [A] rule that would require a higher degree of danger to health in the latter months of pregnancy, as opposed to the early months, for an abortion to be lawful, could possibly achieve a proportionality which would be acceptable under s. 1 of the Charter.... Parliament is justified in requiring a reliable, independent and medically sound opinion in order to protect the state interest in the foetus.... [T]here would be a point in time at which the state interest in the foetus would become compelling. From this point in time, Parliament would be entitled to limit abortions to those required by therapeutic reasons and therefore require an independent opinion as to the health exception.... I am of the view that the protection of the foetus is and ... always has been, a valid objective in Canadian criminal law.... I think s. 1 of the Charter authorizes reasonable limits to be put on a woman's right having regard to the state interest in the protection of the foetus.[16]

More recently it has been claimed that without protection of foetal rights there is nothing to prevent abortion for purposes of sex selection, harm to foetuses by the use of dangerous drugs and by third-party attacks, and the buying and selling of foetuses and foetal parts.[17] The Law Reform Commission of Canada's Working Paper entitled "Crimes Against the Foetus" expresses serious concern about dangers to the foetus, and proposes a new category of criminal offence, "Foetal Destruction or Harm."[18] Thus the stage is set for a potential continuation of major conflict between women's right not to reproduce and the alleged rights of the foetus. Unfortunately, as the Working Paper makes clear, recognition of foetal rights would almost inevitably mean the judicial recognition, via the recriminalization of abortion,[19] of the foetus's alleged right to occupancy and use of a woman's body, and concomitant limitations on women's autonomy and self-determination.

A third reason for concern about threats to Canadian women's right not to reproduce is the growing use by anti-abortion groups of not only non-violent civil disobedience but also active interference in the operations of abortion clinics.[20] In addition, "pro-life" leaders such as Joseph Borowski have threatened the use of violence in defence of their cause:

The war goes on. There is no end to this fight, and certainly no compromise. They [pro-choice] are the enemy. It's a war. Our side has one advantage. We pray. They don't.... I'm glad I did not come to Ottawa for the [Morgentaler Supreme Court] decision. I probably would have gone into the court and punched the judges in the nose.... I'm a non-violent man, and I don't believe in violence but if the seven judges or whoever were here right now, I would have great difficulty restraining myself from punching them in the mouth.[21]

In the face of these potential threats to the right not to reproduce, feminist research and activism must insist that there is no need for the recriminalization of abortion, including late abortion. No woman deliberately sets out to kill a highly developed foetus, and abortion is not sought by women for its own sake. Rather, in the words of philosopher Caroline Whitbeck, it is often a "grim option."[22] While abortions late in pregnancy may seem particularly problematic, they are usually requested for one of the following reasons. In some instances it was impossible for the woman to obtain the abortion earlier, because convoluted legal procedures delayed

its approval. Cases such as these can be avoided by making very early abortions easily available and accessible. In other instances, a late abortion is sought either because prenatal testing reveals a foetal condition that is or is perceived as being severely disabling or even life-threatening, or because the woman's own life or health is endangered.[23] There is, therefore, insufficient justification for the introduction of legislation to protect the late-term foetus from the pregnant woman, or indeed for any new Criminal Code limitations on abortion.

Moreover, the entitlement to choose how many foetuses to gestate, and of what sort, should be seen as a part of the right not to reproduce. The protection of this choice is essential within a cultural context where mothering receives little social support, people with disabilities are subject to bias and stigmatization, and raising several infants simultaneously represents a personal and financial challenge of heroic dimensions. (It is also significant that the upsurge in the incidence of multiple pregnancies has been generated by the administration of fertility drugs and by the use of in vitro fertilization and the technology of gamete intrafallopian transfer, or GIFT.) There is no more reason to demand that a woman gestate a certain number of foetuses or type of foetus than there is to demand that she gestate a given foetus or foetuses. To set such requirements is to accord those foetuses an unjustified right of occupancy of the woman's uterus.

If protection of the foetus seems to be a worthwhile and neglected social goal, then what is needed is greater protection of the pregnant woman herself. Even, surely, on the basis of the non-feminist and implausible assumption of an adversarial relationship between pregnant woman and foetus, the reinstallation of physicians as "body police" enforcing foetal rights[24] is unlikely to improve the behaviour of pregnant women towards their foetuses. Furthermore, in order to prevent the commodification of foetuses and foetal parts, and other undesirable uses of the foetus, there is no more need to assign personhood or rights to the foetus than there is to assign personhood or rights to blood or body parts. Instead of using that blunt instrument the criminal law in post hoc fashion to attempt to manage undesirable reproductive practices, use can be made of existing regulations governing health care and the utilization of human tissues. Ultimately, of course, it will be necessary to minimize and finally eliminate the powerful underlying conditions of oppression that generate such practices as foetal commodification and sex selection.

THE RIGHT TO REPRODUCE

The right not to reproduce is distinct from the right to reproduce. In other words, it is independent, neither implying a right to reproduce nor following from such a right.

The right to reproduce has two senses, which may be called the weak (or liberty) sense and the strong (or welfare) sense. The weak sense of the right to reproduce is the entitlement not to be interfered with in reproduction, or prevented from reproducing. It would imply an obligation on the part of the state not to inhibit or limit reproductive liberty through, for example, racist marriage laws, forced sterilization,[25] or coercive birth-control programs.

In this weak sense, the right to reproduce is also compromised by restrictions on the place of birth and on birth attendants, and by court-ordered Caesarean sections for competent but unwilling pregnant women. Like the United States, Canada has a history of the gradual medicalization of birth. Midwives have been replaced by physicians, from general practitioners to obstetricians; hospitals have replaced the home; and medical innovations from foetal monitoring, amniotomy (the premature puncturing of the amniotic sac); and forceps deliveries to anaesthesia and Caesarean sections have made birthing into a health crisis. Without the genuine freedom to choose home birth, to be attended by midwives, and to avoid obstetrical technology, women's right to reproduce in the weak sense is seriously compromised.

In its strong sense, the right to reproduce would be the right to receive all necessary assistance to reproduce. It would imply entitlement to access to any and all available forms of reproductive products, technologies, and labour, including the gametes of other women and men, the gestational services of women, and the full range of procreative techniques including *in vitro* fertilization, gamete intrafallopian transfer, uterine lavage (a process in which one woman is inseminated with sperm, her uterus is flushed with fluid, and the embryo is retrieved for implantation in another woman's uterus), embryo freezing, and sex preselection.

Non-feminist writers such as American legal theorist John A. Robertson defend the right to reproduce in the strong sense by claiming that it is simply an extension of the right to reproduce in the weak sense. As he puts it, "the right of the married couple to reproduce noncoitally" and "the right to reproduce noncoitally with the assistance of donors and surrogates' both follow from 'constitutional acceptance of a married couple's right to reproduce coitally."[26] (Robertson's heterosexist bias is not much mitigated by his later concession that there is "a very strong argument for unmarried persons, either single or as couples, also having a positive right to reproduce.")[27] Robertson believes that these rights entitle married couples certainly, and perhaps single persons, to "create, store, transfer, donate and possibly even manipulate extra-corporeal embryos"; and "to contract for eggs, sperm, embryos, or surrogates." They would also, he thinks, justify compelling a contract mother to hand over a child to its purchasers, even against her will.[28]

In addition, American attorney Lori B. Andrews argues that the right to reproduce in the strong sense is probably founded upon the right to marital privacy, which, she claims, protects the full range of married people's choices about both sexual and reproductive behaviour.[29] Hence some feminists may want to claim the right to reproduce in the strong sense both because of arguments such as those of Robertson and Andrews, and because of a fear that otherwise access to reproductive technologies such as IVF may be treated by the state as a privilege— one to be gained only through possession of the requisite social criteria, such as being heterosexual and married.

Nevertheless, the legitimacy and justification of this right to reproduce are questionable. To recognize it would be to shift the burden of proof onto those who have doubts about the morality of technologies such as IVF and practices such as contract motherhood. For it suggests that a child is somehow owed to each of us, as individuals or as members of a couple, and that it is indefensible for society to fail to provide all possible means for obtaining one. Thus it might be used, as Robertson advocates, to imply an entitlement to hire contract mothers, to obtain other women's eggs, and to make use of donor insemination and uterine lavage of another woman, all in order to maximize the chances of reproducing.[30] In other words, recognition of the right to reproduce in the strong sense would create an active right of access to women's bodies and in particular to our reproductive labour and products. For example, it would condone the hiring of contract mothers, and force the latter to surrender their infants after birth. And it might be used to found a claim to certain kinds of children—for example, children of a desired sex, appearance, or intelligence.

Exercise of the alleged right to reproduce in this strong sense could potentially require violation of some women's right not to reproduce. There is already good evidence, in both the United States and Great Britain, that eggs and ovarian tissue have been taken from some women without their knowledge or informed consent.[31] It is not difficult to imagine that recognizing a strong right to reproduce could require either a similar theft of eggs or embryos from some women, if none can be found to offer them willingly, or a commercial inducement to sell these products. Such a right could be used as a basis for requiring fertile people to "donate" gametes and embryos. Even if some people would willingly donate gametes, there is no *right* on the part of the infertile that would entitle them to demand such donations.

The feminist language of reproductive rights is illegitimately co-opted when it is used to defend an alleged right to become or to hire a contract mother, to buy or to sell eggs, embryos, or babies, or to select or preselect the sex of one's offspring. There can be no genuine entitlement to women's reproductive labour, nor to buying or otherwise obtaining human infants. Contract motherhood entails a type of slave trade in infants, and it commits women to a modern form of indentured servitude.

It is to be hoped that Canada will choose neither the legalization of contract motherhood nor the criminalization of contract mothers. We should opt instead to reduce the potential motivation for such contracts by making them unenforceable and by rendering criminal both the operation of contract motherhood agencies and the actions of professionals who participate in such arrangements. It is important for Canadian social policy to resist the incursion of US-style commercialization of reproduction and reproductive entrepreneurialism, the most likely victims of which would be poor women and women of colour (see Chapter 7 below).

At the same time, there is no need to treat procedures like *in vitro* fertilization as privileges to which access may be limited on arbitrary and unfair grounds—grounds such as marital status, sexual orientation, putative stability or parenting potential, or economic level. While I cannot wholeheartedly support and endorse highly ineffective, costly, and painful procedures such as IVF, I also cannot endorse the call by some feminists for a total ban on the procedure. State provision and financing of IVF is different from state provision of contract motherhood. Many compelling reasons—primary among them being the sale of babies and the exploitation of women's reproductive labour—militate against state recognition of contract motherhood through legalization or financial support. These two reasons are not present, or not inevitably present, in the case of IVF.

Rather, without asserting a strong right to all possible reproductive assistance, we can critically examine the artificial barriers, such as marital status, sexual orientation, and ability to pay, that get in the way of women's fair access to reproductive technologies. We can also provide protections for women entering and participating in infertility treatment programs. This would require ensuring that applicants make a genuinely informed choice, in full knowledge of the short- and long-term risks, possible benefits, chances of success and failure, alternative approaches and treatments, and perhaps even the pronatalist social pressures to procreate. *If* IVF seems to be a valuable medical service (and that view is still debatable) then it deserves to be made available, like other medical services, through medicare, as is now the case in Ontario. It would also be important to ensure thorough screening of egg and sperm donors; to maintain adequate records that will make it possible to track the long-term effects of IVF on women and their offspring; and to ensure that any women who provide eggs for the program have genuinely chosen to do so. Finally, in the long run, feminists should be thinking about whether it is possible to incorporate high-tech infertility treatments such as IVF into women-centred and women-controlled reproductive health centres.

The approach sketched here avoids two tendencies that I believe are undesirable: on the one hand, treating access to reproductive technology as a privilege to be earned through the possession of certain personal, social, sexual, and/or financial characteristics; and on the other hand, a kind of feminist maternalism that seeks, in the best interests of women, to terminate IVF research and treatment.[32] While many feminists have stressed both the social construction of the desire for motherhood and the dangers and ineffectiveness of *in vitro* fertilization,[33] it is surely dangerous for feminists to claim to understand better than infertile women themselves the origins and significance of their desire for children. It is not the role of feminist research and action to protect women from what is interpreted as their own "false consciousness." Instead, we should assume that when women are provided with full information about the possibilities they will be empowered to make reproductive decisions that will genuinely benefit themselves and their children.[34]

CONCLUSION

The two themes that have structured the struggle over reproductive rights in Canada appear to have little in common: on the one hand, access to various reproductive services and technologies; on the other, the use and exploitation of women's bodies for reproductive purposes.

Nevertheless, the goals of access to reproductive technologies and access to women's bodies come together within conservative discourse on reproduction. Pronatalist, pro-family, and in favour of traditional roles for women, this discourse is also classist, racist, ableist, and heterosexist. The oppressive nature of this discourse is often disguised by the co-optation of feminist language and concepts. In recent lectures and papers, for example, members of the anti-abortion movement have claimed that there is "sexism" in the pro-choice movement,[35] which is alleged to favour the sexual agenda of men over the reproductive needs of women, and have depicted the foetus as a member of a maligned minority group. The same voices that want to ban abortion because women engage in sexual intercourse "by choice" also want to compel contract moth-

ers to sell their babies because they enter the contracts "by choice." Meanwhile, non-feminists are proclaiming that new reproductive technologies actually promote women's autonomy and reproductive choice.[36]

Paradoxically, however, both the non-existence and the existence of certain reproductive "choices" or alternatives can be coercive. While lack of access to contraception or abortion clearly violates reproductive choice by failing to respect the right not to reproduce, conversely practices such as contract motherhood and the sale of gametes and embryos have the potential to violate reproductive choice. In other words, respecting a right to reproduce in the strong sense for some may violate the right not to reproduce of others.

Feminists want to preserve and enhance access to the reproductive services and technologies that benefit women while preventing further encroachments on access to women's bodies, whether by the state or by individuals. The way to do this is by insisting upon both women's right not to reproduce and our right to reproduce in the weak sense, and also by developing a critical analysis of the ways in which the right to reproduce in the strong sense is now being exercised.

Notes

1. Barbara Katz Rothman, remarks at a conference on "Legal and Ethical Aspects of Human Reproduction," Canadian Institute of Law and Medicine, Toronto, Dec. 1989.

2. Christine Overall, *Ethics and Human Reproduction: A Feminist Analysis* (Boston: Allen and Unwin, 1987), Chapter 8.

3. R v. Morgentaler [1988] 1 SCR 30, 172.

4. Ibid., 56-61, 64-73.

5. Ibid., 90.

6. Ibid., 173.

7. Ignoring the Criminal Code provisions on abortion, community health clinics in Quebec had already been providing abortions for more than a decade before the Supreme Court decision.

8. R v. Morgentaler [1988] 1 SCR 32.

9. See George J. Annas, "Webster and the Politics of Abortion," *Hastings Center Report* 19 (March/April

1989): 36-8. In July 1989 the United States Supreme Court ruled that the state of Missouri had the right to ban the performance of abortions by public hospitals and public employees. It is anticipated that the court may in future uphold additional state-imposed restrictions on abortion services, seriously limiting access to abortion, particularly for poor women. See *Webster v. Reproductive Health Services*, 109 S. Ct. 3040 (1989).

10. For example, Brenda Large's editorial "If Sex-Based Abortions are Wrong, So Are All," *Kingston Whig-Standard* (11 Feb. 1989).

11. Mark I. Evans, John C. Fletcher, Evan E. Zador, Burritt W. Newton, Mary Helen Quigg, and Curtis D. Struyk, "Selective First-Trimester Termination in Octuplet and Quadruplet Pregnancies: Clinical and Ethical Issues," *Obstetrics and Gynecology* 71, 3, pt. 1 (March 1988): 291. For an extensive discussion of the ethics and social context of this procedure, see "Selective Termination in Pregnancy and Women's Reproductive Autonomy," chapter 3 below.

12. Dorothy Lipovenko, "Infertility Technology Forces People to Make Life and Death Choices," *The Globe and Mail* (21 Jan. 1989): A4; "Multiple Pregnancies Create Moral Dilemma," *Kingston Whig-Standard* (21 Jan. 1989): 3.

13. Borowski v. Canada (Attorney General) [1989] 1 SCR 342.

14. R. v. Morgentaler, 181, 183.

15. Ibid., 76.

16. Ibid., 82-3, 110, 113, 124.

17. Neil Reynolds, "Fetal Status Cannot Depend on Momentary Opinion," *Kingston Whig-Standard* (16 March 1989): 6.

18. Law Reform Commission of Canada, Working Paper 58, "Crimes Against the Foetus" (Ottawa, 1989), 64.

19. Ibid., 42, 56, and 64.

20. A Johnson, "Clinic Fights to Survive in B.C.," *Rites* (March 1989): 4; and Helen Armstrong, Debi Brock and Jennifer Stephen, "'Operation Rescue' Turns Into Fiasco," *Rites* (March 1989): 5.

21. Joseph Borowski, quoted in *The Toronto Star* and *The Globe and Mail*, 10 March 1989.

22. Caroline Whitbeck, "The Moral Implications of Regarding Women as People: New Perspectives on Pregnancy and Personhood," in William B. Bondeson, H. Tristram Engelhardt, Jr, Stuart F. Spicker, and Daniel H. Winship, eds., *Abortion and the Status of the Fetus* (Boston: Reidel, 1984), 251.

23. This is argued by Sanda Rodgers in "The Future of Abortion in Canada," in Christine Overall, ed., *The Future of Human Reproduction* (Toronto: Women's Press, 1989). This argument in no way endorses the use of abortion for supposed eugenic purposes. As disabled women and their allies have pointed out, feminists should be highly critical of the use of reproductive technologies to discriminate among human beings on the basis of their physical or mental condition, or to promote the notion of human perfectibility. See Marcia Saxton, "Prenatal Screening and Discriminatory Attitudes About Disability," in Elaine Hoffman Baruch, Amadeo F. D'Adamo, Jr, and Joni Seager, eds., *Embryos, Ethics, and Women's Rights: Exploring the New Reproductive Technologies* (New York: Haworth Press, 1988), 217-24, and Ruth Hubbard, "Eugenics: New Tools, Old Ideas," in ibid., 225-35.

24. In my view, this is the effect of the proposal of the Law Reform Commission of Canada's "Crimes Against the Foetus," which would require "medical authorization" of an abortion by one "qualified medical practitioner" before foetal viability, and by two such practitioners after the foetus is capable of independent survival (64).

25. "In North America there is a long history of the forced sterilization of native women and women of colour.

26. John A. Robertson, "Procreative Liberty, Embryos, and Collaborative Reproduction: A Legal Perspective," in Baruch et al., eds., *Embryos, Ethics and Women's Rights*, 180. Cf. Lori B. Andrews, "Alternative Modes of Reproduction," in Sherrill Cohen and Nadine Taub, eds., *Reproductive Laws for the 1990s* (Clifton, N.J.: Humana Press, 1989), 364.

27. Robertson, "Procreative Liberty," 181.

28. Ibid., 180, 186, and 190.

29. Lori B. Andrews, *New Conceptions: A Consumer's Guide to the Newest Infertility Treatments* (New York: Ballantyne Books, 1985), 138.

30. From this point of view, then, IVF with donor gametes is more problematic than IVF in which a woman and a man make use of their own eggs and sperm.

31. Genoveffa Corea, "Egg Snatchers," in Rita Arditti, Renate Duelli Klein, and Shelley Minden, eds., *Test-Tube Women: What Future for Motherhood* (London: Pandora Press, 1984), 37-51.

32. Renate Duelli Klein, quoted in Christine St. Peters, "Feminist Discourse, Infertility, and the New Reproductive Technologies," *National Women's Studies Association Journal* 1, 3 (Spring 1989): 358.

33. See, for example, Susan Sherwin, "Feminist Ethics and In Vitro Fertilization," in Marsha Hanen and Kai Nielsen, eds., *Science, Morality and Feminist Theory* (Calgary: University of Calgary Press, 1987), 265-84.

34. For a more detailed discussion of the fair provision of IVF, see "Access to *In Vitro* Fertilization: Costs, Care, and Consent," Chapter 8 [in *Human Reproduction*, Oxford University Press, 1993].

35. See, for example, Diane Marshall and Martha Crean, "The Human Face of a Woman's Agony," in Ian Gentles, ed., *A Time to Choose Life: Women, Abortion and Human Rights* (Toronto: Stoddart, 1990), 134-42, and Janet Ajzenstat, "The Sexism of Pro-Choice," Queen's University, Kingston, Ont., 14 March 1989. Ajzenstat is a member of the Department of Political Science, McMaster University.

36. John Robertson ("Procreative Liberty") claims that "'[e]xtra-corporeal conception seems to promote choice, to promote the autonomy of women (and men) in helping them overcome infertility, which for many women (and men) is a very serious problem" (192). It "makes possible new, partial reproductive roles for women" as "egg and embryo donors and surrogates" (193).

18.
FEMINIST ETHICS AND IN VITRO FERTILIZATION

Susan Sherwin

New technology in human reproduction has provoked wide ranging arguments about the desirability and moral justifiability of many of these efforts. Authors of biomedical ethics have ventured into the field to offer the insight of moral theory to these complex moral problems of contemporary life. I believe, however, that the moral theories most widely endorsed today are problematic and that a new approach to ethics is necessary if we are to address the concerns and perspectives identified by feminist theorists in our considerations of such topics. Hence, I propose to look at one particular technique in the growing repertoire of new reproductive technologies, in vitro fertilization (IVF), in order to consider the insight which the mainstream approaches to moral theory have offered to this debate, and to see the difference made by a feminist approach to ethics.

I have argued elsewhere that the most widely accepted moral theories of our time are inadequate for addressing many of the moral issues we encounter in our lives, since they focus entirely on such abstract qualities of moral agents as autonomy or quantities of happiness, and they are addressed to agents who are conceived of as independent, non-tuistic individuals. In contrast, I claimed, we need a theory which places the locus of ethical concerns in a complex social network of interrelated persons who are involved in special sorts of relations with one another. Such a theory, as I envision it, would be influenced by the insights and concerns of feminist theory, and hence, I have called it feminist ethics.[1]

In this paper, I propose to explore the differences between a feminist approach to ethics and other, more traditional approaches in examining the propriety of developing and implementing in vitro fertilization and related technologies. This is a complicated task, since each sort of ethical theory admits of a variety of interpretations and hence of a variety of conclusions on concrete ethical issues. Nonetheless, certain themes and trends can be seen to emerge. Feminist thinking is also ambivalent in application, for feminists are quite torn about their response to this sort of technology. It is my hope that a systematic theoretic evaluation of IVF from the point of view of a feminist ethical theory will help feminists like myself sort through our uncertainty on these matters.

Let me begin with a quick description of IVF for the uninitiated. In vitro fertilization is the technology responsible for what the media likes to call "test tube babies." It circumvents, rather than cures, a variety of barriers to conception, primarily those of blocked fallopian tubes and low sperm counts. In vitro fertilization involves removing ova from the woman's body, collecting sperm from the man's, combining them to achieve conception in the laboratory, and, a few days later, implanting some number of the newly fertilized eggs directly into the women's womb with the hope that pregnancy will continue normally from this point on. This process requires that a variety of hormones be administered to the women—which involve profound emotional and physical changes—that her blood and urine be monitored daily, and then at 3 hour intervals, that ultrasound be used to determine when ovulation occurs. In some clinics, implantation requires that she remain immobile for 48 hours (including 24 hours in the head down position). IVF is successful in about 10-15% of the cases selected as suitable, and commonly involves multiple efforts at implantation.

Let us turn now to the responses that philosophers working within the traditional approaches to ethics have offered on this subject. A review of the literature in bioethics identifies a variety of concerns with this technology. Philosophers who adopt a theological perspective tend to object that such technology is wrong because it is not "natural" and undermines God's plan for the family. Paul Ramsey, for instance, is concerned about the artificiality of IVF and other sorts of reproductive technology with which it is potentially associated, e.g. embryo transfer, ova as well as sperm donation or sale, increased eugenic control, etc.:

But there is as yet no discernable evidence that we are recovering a sense for man [sic] as a natural object ... toward whom a ... form of "natural piety" is appropriate ... parenthood is certainly one of those "courses of action" natural to man, which cannot without violation be disassembled and put together again.[2]

Leon Kass argues a similar line in "'Making Babies' Revisited."[3] He worries that our conception of humanness will not survive the technological permutations before us, and that we will treat these new artificially conceived embryos more as objects than as subjects; he also fears that we will be unable to track traditional human categories of parenthood and lineage, and that this loss would cause us to lose track of important aspects of our identity. The recent position paper of the Catholic Church on reproductive technology reflects related concerns:

> It is through the secure and recognized relationship to his [sic] own parents that the child can discover his own identity and achieve his own proper human development.... Heterologous artificial fertilization violates the rights of the child; it deprives him of his filial relationship with his parental origins and can hinder the maturing of his personal identity.[4]

Philosophers partial to utilitarianism prefer a more scientific approach; they treat these sorts of concerns as sheer superstition. They carefully explain to their theological colleagues that there is no clear sense of "natural" and certainly no sense that demands special moral status. All medical activity, and perhaps all human activity, can be seen in some sense as being "interference with nature," but that is hardly grounds for avoiding such action. "Humanness," too, is a concept that admits of many interpretations; generally, it does not provide satisfactory grounds for moral distinctions. Further, it is no longer thought appropriate to focus too strictly on questions of lineage and strict biological parentage, and, they note, most theories of personal identity do not rely on such matters.

Where some theologians object that "fertilization achieved outside the bodies of the couple remains by this very fact deprived of the meanings of the values which are expressed in the language of the body and in the union of human persons,"[5] utilitarians quickly dismiss the objection against reproduction without sexuality in a properly sanctified marriage. See, for instance, Michael Bayles in *Reproductive Ethics*: "... even if reproduction should occur only within a context of marital love, the point of that requirement is the nurturance of offspring. Such nurturance does not depend on the sexual act itself. The argument confuses the biological act with the familial context."[6]

Another area of disagreement between theological ethicists and their philosophical critics is the significance of the wedge argument to the debate about IVF. IVF is already a complex technology involving research on superovulation, "harvesting" of ova, fertilization, and embryo implants. It is readily adaptable to technology involving the transfer of ova and embryos, and hence their donation or sale, as well as to the "rental of womb space"; it also contributes to an increasing ability to foster fetal growth outside of the womb and, potentially, to the development of artificial wombs covering the whole period of gestation. It is already sometimes combined with artificial insemination and is frequently used to produce surplus fertilized eggs to be frozen for later use. Theological ethicists worry that such activity, and further reproductive developments we can anticipate (such as human cloning), violate God's plan for human reproduction. They worry about the cultural shift involved in viewing reproduction as a scientific enterprise, rather than the "miracle of love" which religious proponents prefer. "[He] cannot be desired or conceived as the product of an intervention of medical or biological techniques; that would be equivalent to reducing him to an object of scientific technology."[7] And, worse, they note, we cannot anticipate the ultimate outcome of this rapidly expanding technology.

The where-will-it-all-end hand-wringing that comes with this sort of religious futurology is rejected by most analytical philosophers; they urge us to realize that few slopes are as slippery as the pessimists would have us believe, that scientists are moral people and quite capable of evaluating each form of technology on its own merits, and that IVF must be judged by its own consequences and not the possible result of some future technology with which it may be linked. Samuel Gorovitz is typical:

> It is not enough to show that disaster awaits if the process is not controlled. A man walking East in Omaha will drown in the Atlantic—if he does not stop. The argument

must also rest on the evidence about the likelihood that judgment and control will be exercised responsibly.... Collectively we have significant capacity to exercise judgment and control ... our record has been rather good in regard to medical treatment and research.[8]

The question of the moral status of the fertilized eggs is more controversial. Since the superovulation involved in producing eggs for collection tends to produce several at once, and the process of collecting eggs is so difficult, and since the odds against conception on any given attempt are so slim, several eggs are usually collected and fertilized at once. A number of these fertilized eggs will be introduced to the womb with the hope that at least one will implant and gestation will begin, but there are frequently some "extras." Moral problems arise as to what should be done with these surplus eggs. They can be frozen for future use (since odds are against the first attempt "taking"), or they can be used as research material, or simply discarded. Canadian clinics get around the awkwardness of their ambivalence on the moral status of these cells by putting them all into the woman's womb. This poses the devastating threat of six or eight "successfully" implanting, and a woman being put into the position of carrying a litter; something, we might note, her body is not constructed to do.

Those who take a hard line against abortion and argue that the embryo is a person from the moment of conception object to all these procedures, and, hence, they argue, there is no morally acceptable means of conducting IVF. To this line, utilitarians offer the standard responses. Personhood involves moral, not biological categories. A being neither sentient nor conscious is not a person in any meaningful sense. For example, Gorovitz argues, "Surely the concept of person involves in some fundamental way the capacity for sentience, or an awareness of sensations at the very least."[9] Bayles says, "For fetuses to have moral status they must be capable of good or bad in their lives .... What happens to them must make a difference to them. Consequently some form of awareness is necessary for moral status."[10] (Apparently, clinicians in the field have been trying to avoid this whole issue by coining a new term in the hopes of identifying a new ontological category, that of the "pre-embryo.")[11]

Many bioethicists have agreed here, as they have in the abortion debate, that the principal moral question of IVF is the moral status and rights of the embryo. Once they resolve that question, they can, like Englehardt, conclude that since fetuses are not persons, and since reproductive processes occurring outside a human body pose no special moral problems, "there will be no sustainable moral arguments in principle ... against in vitro fertilization."[12] He argues:

in vitro fertilization and techniques that will allow us to study and control human reproduction are morally neutral instruments for the realization of profoundly important human goals, which are bound up with the realization of the good of others: children for infertile parents and greater health for the children that will be born.[13]

Moral theorists also express worries about the safety of the process, and by that they tend to mean the safety to fetuses that may result from this technique. Those fears have largely been put to rest in the years since the first IVF baby was born in 1978, for the couple of thousand infants reportedly produced by this technique to date seem no more prone to apparent birth defects than the population at large, and, in fact, there seems to be evidence that birth defects may be less common in this group—presumably because of better monitoring and pre and post natal care. (There is concern expressed, however, in some circles outside of the bioethical literature about the longterm effect of some of the hormones involved, in light of our belated discoveries of the effect of DES usage on offspring. This concern is aggravated by the chemical similarity of clomid, one of the hormones used in IVF, to DES.)[14]

Most of the literature tends to omit comment on the uncertainties associated with the effect of drugs inducing superovulation in the woman concerned, or with the dangers posed by the general anaesthetic required for the laparoscopy procedure; the emotional costs associated with this therapy are also overlooked, even though there is evidence that it is extremely stressful in the 85-90% of the attempts that fail, and that those who succeed have difficulty in dealing with common parental feelings of anger and frustration with a child they tried so hard to get. Nonetheless, utilitarian theory could readily accommodate such concerns, should the philosophers involved think to look for them. In principle, no new moral theory is yet called for, although a widening of perspective (to include the effects on the women involved) would certainly be appropriate.

The easiest solution to the IVF question seems to be available to ethicists of a deontological orientation who are keen on autonomy and rights and free of religious prejudice. For them, IVF is simply a private matter, to be decided by the couple concerned together with a medical specialist. The desire to have and raise children is a very common one and generally thought to be a paradigm case of a purely private matter. Couples seeking this technology face medical complications that require the assistance of a third party, and it is thought, "it would be unfair to make infertile couples pass up the joys of rearing infants or suffer the burdens of rearing handicapped children."[15] Certainly, meeting individuals' desires/needs is the most widely accepted argument in favour of the use of this technology.

What is left, then, in the more traditional ethical discussions, is usually some hand waving about costs. This is an extremely expensive procedure; estimates range from $1500 to $6000 per attempt. Gorovitz says, for instance, "there is the question of the distribution of costs, a question that has heightened impact if we consider the use of public funds to pay for medical treatment."[16] Debate tends to end here in the mystery of how to balance soaring medical costs of various sorts and a comment that no new ethical problems are posed.

Feminists share many of these concerns, but they find many other moral issues involved in the development and use of such technology and note the silence of the standard moral approaches in addressing these matters. Further, feminism does not identify the issues just cited as the primary areas of moral concern. Nonetheless, IVF is a difficult issue for feminists.

On the one hand, most feminists share the concern for autonomy held by most moral theorists, and they are interested in allowing women freedom of choice in reproductive matters. This freedom is most widely discussed in connection with access to safe and effective contraception and, when necessary, to abortion services. For women who are unable to conceive because of blocked fallopian tubes, or certain fertility problems of their partners, IVF provides the technology to permit pregnancy which is otherwise impossible. Certainly most of the women seeking IVF perceive it to be technology that increases their reproductive freedom of choice. So, it would seem that feminists should support this sort of technology as part of our general concern to foster the degree of reproductive control women may have over their own bodies. Some feminists have chosen this route. But feminists must also note that IVF as practiced does not altogether satisfy the motivation of fostering individual autonomy.

It is, after all, the sort of technology that requires medical intervention, and hence it is not really controlled by the women seeking it, but rather by the medical staff providing this "service." IVF is not available to every woman who is medically suitable, but only to those who are judged to be worthy by the medical specialists concerned. To be a candidate for this procedure, a woman must have a husband and an apparently stable marriage. She must satisfy those specialists that she and her husband have appropriate resources to support any children produced by this arrangement (in addition, of course, to the funds required to purchase the treatment in the first place), and that they generally "deserve" this support. IVF is not available to single women, lesbian women, or women not securely placed in the middle class or beyond. Nor is it available to women whom the controlling medical practitioners judge to be deviant with respect to their norms of who makes a good mother. The supposed freedom of choice, then, is provided only to selected women who have been screened by the personal values of those administering the technology.

Further, even for these women, the record on their degree of choice is unclear. Consider, for instance, that this treatment has always been very experimental: it was introduced without the prior primate studies which are required for most new forms of medical technology, and it continues to be carried our under constantly shifting protocols, with little empirical testing, as clinics try to raise their very poor success rates. Moreover, consent forms are perceived by patients to be quite restrictive procedures and women seeking this technology are not in a particularly strong position to bargain to revise the terms; there is no alternate clinic down the street to choose if a woman dislikes her treatment at some clinic, but there are usually many other women waiting for access to her place in the clinic should she choose to withdraw.

Some recent studies indicate that few of the women participating in current programs really know how low the success rates are.[17] And it is not apparent that participants are encouraged to ponder the medical unknowns associated with various aspects of the technique, such as the long term consequences of superovulation and the use of hormones chemically similar to DES. Nor is it the case that the consent procedure involves consultation on how to handle the disposal of "surplus" zygotes. It is doubtful that the women concerned have much real choice about which procedure is followed with the eggs they will not need. These policy decisions are usually made at the level of the clinic. It should be noted here that at least one feminist argues that neither the woman, nor the doctors have the right to choose to destroy these embryos: " ... because no one, not even its parents, owns the embryo/fetus, no one has the *right* to destroy it, even at a very early developmental stage ... to destroy an embryo is not an automatic entitlement held by anyone, including its genetic parents."[18]

Moreover, some participants reflect deep seated ambivalence on the part of many women about the procedure—they indicate that their marriage and status depends on a determination to do "whatever is possible" in pursuit of their "natural" childbearing function—and they are not helped to work through the seeming imponderables associated with their long term well-being. Thus, IVF as practiced involves significant limits on the degree of autonomy deontologists insist on in other medical contexts, though the nonfeminist literature is insensitive to this anomaly.

From the perspective of consequentialism, feminists take a long view and try to see IVF in the context of the burgeoning range of techniques in the area of human reproductive technology. While some of this technology seems to hold the potential of benefitting women generally—by leading to better understanding of conception and contraception, for instance—there is a wary suspicion that this research will help foster new techniques and products such as human cloning and the development of artificial wombs which can, in principle, make the majority of women superfluous. (This is not a wholly paranoid fear in a woman-hating culture: we can anticipate that there will be great pressure for such techniques in subsequent generations, since one of the "successes" of reproductive technology to date has been to allow parents to control the sex of their offspring; the "choice" now made possible clearly threatens to result in significant imbalances in the ratio of boy to girl infants. Thus, it appears, there will likely be significant shortages of women to bear children in the future, and we can anticipate pressures for further technological solutions to the "new" problem of reproduction that will follow.)

Many authors from all traditions consider it necessary to ask why it is that some couples seek this technology so desperately. Why is it so important to so many people to produce their "own" child? On this question, theorists in the analytic tradition seem to shift to previously rejected ground and suggest that this is a natural, or at least a proper, desire. Englehardt, for example, says, "The use of technology in the fashioning of children is integral to the goal of rendering the world congenial to persons."[19] Bayles more cautiously observes that "A desire to beget for its own sake ... is probably irrational"; nonetheless, he immediately concludes, "these techniques for fulfilling that desire have been found ethically permissible."[20] R.G. Edwards and David Sharpe state the case most strongly: "the desire to have children must be among the most basic of human instincts, and denying it can lead to considerable psychological and social difficulties."[21] Interestingly, although the recent pronouncement of the Catholic Church assumes that "the desire for a child is natural,"[22] it denies that a couple has a right to a child: "The child is not an object to which one has a right."[23]

Here, I believe, it becomes clear why we need a deeper sort of feminist analysis. We must look at the sort of social arrangements and cultural values that underlie the drive to assume such risks for the sake of biological parenthood. We find that the capitalism, racism, sexism, and elitism of our culture have combined to create a set of attitudes which views children as commodities whose value is derived from their possession of parental chromosomes. Children are valued as privatized commodities, reflecting the virility and heredity of their parents. They are also viewed as the responsibility of their parents and are not seen as the social treasure and burden that they are. Parents must tend their needs on pain of prosecution, and, in return, they get to keep complete control over them. Other adults are inhibited from having warm, stable interactions with the children of others—it is as suspect to try to hug and talk regularly with a child who is not one's own as it is to fondle and hang longingly about a car or a bicycle which belongs to someone else—so those who wish to know children well often find they must have their own.

Women are persuaded that their most important purpose in life is to bear and raise children; they are told repeatedly that their life is incomplete, that they are lacking in fulfillment if they do not have children. And, in fact, many women do face a barren existence without children. Few women have access to meaningful, satisfying jobs. Most do not find themselves in the centre of the romantic personal relationships which the culture pretends is the norm for heterosexual couples. And they have been socialized to be fearful of close friendships with others—they are taught to distrust other women, and to avoid the danger of friendship with men other than their husbands. Children remain the one hope for real intimacy and for the sense of accomplishment which comes from doing work one judges to be valuable.

To be sure, children can provide that sense of self worth, although for many women (and probably for all mothers at some times) motherhood is not the romanticized satisfaction they are led to expect. But there is something very wrong with a culture where childrearing is the only outlet available to most women in which to pursue fulfillment. Moreover, there is something wrong with the ownership theory of children that keeps other adults at a distance from children. There ought to be a variety of close relationships possible between children and adults so that we all recognize that we have a stake in the well-being of the young, and we all benefit from contact with their view of the world.

In such a world, it would not be necessary to spend the huge sums on designer children which IVF requires while millions of other children starve to death each year. Adults who enjoyed children could be involved in caring for them whether or not they produced them biologically. And, if the institution of marriage survives, women and men would marry because they wished to share their lives together not because the men needed someone to produce heirs for them and women needed financial support for their children. That would be a world in which we might have reproductive freedom of choice. The world we now live in has so limited women's options and self-esteem, it is legitimate to question the freedom behind women's demand for this technology, for it may well be largely a reflection of constraining social perspectives.

Nonetheless, I must acknowledge that some couples today genuinely mourn their incapacity to produce children without IVF and there are very significant and unique joys which can be found in producing and raising one's own children which are not accessible to persons in infertile relationships. We must sympathize with these people. None of us shall live to see the implementation of the ideal cultural values outlined above which would make the demand for IVF less severe. It is with real concern that some feminists suggest that the personal wishes of couples with fertility difficulties may not be compatible with the overall interests of women and children.

Feminist thought, then, helps us to focus on different dimensions of the problem than do others sorts of approaches. But, with this perspective, we still have difficulty in reaching a final conclusion on whether to encourage, tolerate, modify, or restrict this sort of reproductive technology. I suggest that we turn to the developing theories of feminist ethics for guidance in resolving this question.[24]

In my view, a feminist ethics is a moral theory that focusses on relations among persons as well as on individuals. It has as a model an inter-connected social fabric, rather than the familiar one of isolated, independent atoms; and it gives primacy to bonds among people rather than to rights to independence. It is a theory that focusses on concrete situations and persons and not on free-floating abstract actions.[25] Although many details have yet to be worked out, we can see some of its implications in particular problem areas such as this.

It is a theory that is explicitly conscious of the social, political, and economic relations that exist among persons; in particular, as a feminist theory, it attends to the implications of actions or policies on the status of women. Hence, it is necessary to ask questions from the perspective of feminist ethics in addition to those which are normally asked from the perspective of mainstream ethical theories. We must view issues such as this one in the context of the social and political realities in which they arise, and resist the attempt to evaluate actions or practices in isolation (as traditional responses in biomedical ethics often do). Thus, we cannot just address the question of IVF per se without asking how IVF contributes to general patterns of women's oppression. As Kathryn Payne Addelson has argued about abortion,[26] a feminist perspective raises questions that are inadmissible within the traditional ethical frameworks, and yet, for women in a patriarchal society, they are value questions of greater urgency. In particular, a feminist ethics, in contrast to other approaches in biomedical ethics, would take seriously the concerns just reviewed which are part of the debate in the feminist literature.

A feminist ethics would also include components of theories that have been developed as "feminine ethics," as sketched out by the empirical work of Carol Gilligan.[27] (The best example of such a theory is the work of Nel Noddings in her influential book *Caring*.)[28] In other words, it would be a theory that gives primacy to interpersonal relationships and woman-centred values such as nurturing, empathy, and co-operation. Hence, in the case of IVF, we must care for the women and men who are so despairing about their infertility as to want to spend the vast sums and risk the associated physical and emotional costs of the treatment, in pursuit of "their own children." That is, we should, in Noddings' terms, see their reality as our own and address their very real sense of loss. In so doing, however, we must also consider the implications of this sort of solution to their difficulty. While meeting the perceived desires of some women—desires which are problematic in themselves, since they are so compatible with the values of a culture deeply oppressive to women—this technology threatens to further entrench those values which are responsible for that oppression. A larger vision suggests that the technology offered may, in reality, reduce women's freedom and, if so, it should be avoided.

A feminist ethics will not support a wholly negative response, however, for that would not address our obligation to care for those suffering from infertility; it is the responsibility of those who oppose further implementation of this technology to work towards the changes in the social arrangements that will lead to a reduction of the sense of need for this sort of solution. On the medical front, research and treatment ought to be stepped up to reduce the rates of peral sepsis and gonorrhea which often result in tubal blockage, more attention should be directed at the causes and possible cures for male infertility, and we should pursue techniques that will permit safe reversible sterilization providing women with better alternatives to tubal ligation as a means of fertility control; these sorts of technology would increase the control of many women over their own fertility and would be compatible with feminist objectives. On the social front, we must continue the social pressure to change the status of women and children in our society from that of breeder and possession respectively; hence, we must develop a vision of society as community where all participants are valued members, regardless of age or gender. And we must challenge the notion that having one's wife produce a child with his own genes is sufficient cause for the wives of men with low sperm counts to be expected to undergo the physical and emotional assault such technology involves.

Further, a feminist ethics will attend to the nature of the relationships among those concerned. Annette Baier has eloquently argued for the importance of developing an ethics of trust,[29] and I believe a feminist ethics must address the question of the degree of trust appropriate to the relationships involved. Feminists have noted that women have little reason to trust the medical specialists who offer to respond to their reproductive desires, for, commonly women's interests have not come first from the medical point of view.[30] In fact, it is accurate to perceive feminist attacks on reproductive technology as expressions of the lack of trust feminists have in those who control the technology. Few feminists object to reproductive technology per se; rather they express concern about who controls it and how it can be used to further exploit women. The problem with reproductive technology is that it concentrates power in reproductive matters in the hands of those who are not directly involved in the actual bearing and rearing of the child; i.e., in men who relate to their clients in a technical, professional, authoritarian manner. It is a further step in the medicalization of pregnancy and birth which, in North America, is marked by relationships between pregnant women and their doctors which are very different from the traditional relationships between pregnant women and midwives. The latter relationships fostered an atmosphere of mutual trust which is impossible to replicate in hospital deliveries today. In fact, current approaches to pregnancy, labour, and birth tend to view the mother as a threat to the fetus who must be coerced to comply with medical procedures designed to ensure delivery of healthy babies at whatever cost necessary to the mother. Frequently, the fetus-mother relationship is medically characterized as adversarial and the physicians choose to foster a sense of alienation and passivity in the role they permit the mother. However well IVF may serve the interests of the few women with access to it, it more clearly serves the interests (be they commercial, professional, scholarly, or purely patriarchal) of those who control it.

Questions such as these are a puzzle to those engaged in the traditional approaches to ethics, for they always urge us to separate the question of evaluating the morality of various forms of reproductive technology in themselves, from questions about particular uses of that technology. From the perspective of a feminist ethics, however, no such distinction can be meaningfully made. Reproductive technology is not an abstract activity, it is an activity done in particular contexts and it is those contexts which must be addressed.

Feminist concerns cited earlier made clear the difficulties we have with some of our traditional ethical concepts; hence, feminist ethics directs us to rethink our basic ethical notions. Autonomy, or freedom of choice, is not a matter to be determined in isolated instances, as is commonly assumed in many approaches to applied ethics. Rather it is a matter that involves reflection on one's whole life situation. The freedom of choice feminists appeal to in the abortion situation is freedom to define one's status as childbearer, given the social, economic, and political significance of reproduction for women. A feminist perspective permits us to understand that reproductive freedom includes control of one's sexuality, protection against coerced sterilization (or iatrogenic sterilization, e.g. as caused by the Dalkon Shield), and the existence of a social and economic network of support for the children we may choose to bear. It is the freedom to redefine our roles in society according to our concerns and needs as women.

In contrast, the consumer freedom to purchase technology, allowed only to a few couples of the privileged classes (in traditionally approved relationships), seems to entrench further the patriarchal notions of women's role as childbearer and of heterosexual monogamy as the only acceptable intimate relationship. In other words, this sort of choice does not seem to foster autonomy for women on the broad scale. IVF is a practice which seems to reinforce sexist, classist, and often racist assumptions of our culture; therefore, on our revised understanding of freedom, the contribution of this technology to the general autonomy of women is largely negative.

We can now see the advantage of a feminist ethics over mainstream ethical theories, for a feminist analysis explicitly accepts the need for a political component to our understanding of ethical issues. In this, it differs from traditional ethical theories and it also differs from a simply feminine ethics approach, such as

the one Noddings offers, for Noddings seems to rely on individual relations exclusively and is deeply suspicious of political alliances as potential threats to the pure relation of caring. Yet, a full understanding of both the threat of IVF, and the alternative action necessary should we decide to reject IVF, is possible only if it includes a political dimension reflecting on the role of women in society.

From the point of view of feminist ethics, the primary question to consider is whether this and other forms of reproductive technology threaten to reinforce the lack of autonomy which women now experience in our culture—even as they appear, in the short run, to be increasing freedom. We must recognize that the interconnections among the social forces oppressive to women underlie feminists' mistrust of this technology which advertises itself as increasing women's autonomy.[31] The political perspective which directs us to look at how this technology fits in with general patterns of treatment for women is not readily accessible to traditional moral theories, for it involves categories of concern not accounted for in those theories—e.g. the complexity of issues which makes it inappropriate to study them in isolation from one another, the oppression in shaping individual desires, and potential differences in moral status which are connected with differences in treatment.

It is the set of connections constituting women's continued oppression in our society which inspires feminists to resurrect the old slippery slope arguments to warn against IVF. We must recognize that women's existing lack of control in reproductive matters begins the debate on a pretty steep incline. Technology with the potential to further remove control of reproduction from women makes the slope very slippery indeed. This new technology, though offered under the guise of increasing reproductive freedom, threatens to result, in fact, in a significant decrease in freedom, especially since it is a technology that will always include the active involvement of designated specialists and will not ever be a private matter for the couple or women concerned.

Ethics ought not to direct us to evaluate individual cases without also looking at the implications of our decisions from a wide perspective. My argument is that a theory of feminist ethics provides that wider perspective, for its different sort of methodology is sensitive to both the personal and the social dimensions of issues. For that reason, I believe it is the only ethical perspective suitable for evaluating issues of this sort.

_____

Author's Note

I appreciate the helpful criticism I have received from colleagues in the Dalhousie Department of Philosophy, the Canadian Society for Women in Philosophy, and the Women's Studies program of the University of Alberta where earlier versions of this paper were read. I am particularly grateful for the careful criticism it has received from Linda Williams and Christine Overall.

Notes

1. Susan Sherwin, "A Feminist Approach to Ethics," *Dalhousie Review* 64, 4 (Winter 1984-85) 704-13.
2. Paul Ramsey, "Shall We Reproduce?," *Journal of the American Medical Association* 220 (June 12, 1972), 1484.
3. Leon Kass, "'Making Babies' Revisited," *The Public Interest* 54 (Winter 1979), 32-60.
4. Joseph Card Ratzinger and Alberto Bovone, "Instruction on Respect for Human Life in its Origin and on the Dignity of Procreation: Replies to Certain Questions of the Day" (Vatican City: Vatican Polyglot Press 1987), 23-4.
5. Ibid., 28.
6. Michael Bayles, *Reproductive Ethics* (Englewood Cliffs, NJ: Prentice Hall 1984) 15.
7. Ratzinger and Bovone, 28.
8. Samuel Gorovitz, *Doctors' Dilemmas: Moral Conflict and Medical Care* (New York: Oxford University Press 1982), 168.
9. Ibid., 173.
10. Bayles, 66.
11. I owe this observation to Linda Williams.
12. H. Tristram Englehardt, *The Foundations of Bioethics* (Oxford: Oxford University Press 1986), 237.
13. Ibid., 241.
14. Anita Direcks, "Has the Lesson Been Learned?," *DES Action Voice* 28 (Spring 1986), 1-4; and Nikita A. Crook, "Clomid," DES Action/Toronto Factsheet # 442 (available from 60 Grosvenor St., Toronto, M5S 1B6).
15. Bayles, 32. Though Bayles is not a deontologist, he does concisely express a deontological concern here.
16. Gorovitz, 177.
17. Michael Soules, "The In Vitro Fertilization Pregnancy Rate: Let's Be Honest with One Another," *Fertility and Sterility* 43, 4 (1985) 511-13.
18. Christine Overall, *Ethics and Human Reproduction: A Feminist Analysis* (Allen and Unwin, forthcoming), 104 ms.
19. Englehardt, 239.
20. Bayles, 31.
21. Robert G. Edwards and David J. Sharpe, "Social Values and Research in Human Embryology," *Nature* 231 (May 14, 1971), 87.
22. Ratzinger and Bovone, 33.
23. Ibid., 34.
24. Many authors are now working on an understanding of what feminist ethics entail. Among the Canadian papers I am familiar with, are Kathryn Morgan's "Women and Moral Madness," Sheila Mullett's "Only Connect: The Place of Self-Knowledge in Ethics," both in [*Science, Morality and Feminist Theory*, ed. M. Hanen and K. Nielsen (University of Calgary Press, 1987)] and Leslie Wilson's "Is a Feminine Ethics Enough?," *Atlantis* (forthcoming).
25. Sherwin, "A Feminist Approach to Ethics."
26. Kathryn Payne Addelson, "Moral Revolution," in Marilyn Pearsall, ed., *Women and Values* (Belmont, CA: Wadsworth 1986), 291-309.
27. Carol Gilligan, *In a Different Voice* (Cambridge, MA: Harvard University Press 1982).
28. Nel Noddings, *Caring* (Berkeley: University of California Press 1984).
29. Annette Baier, "What Do Women Want in a Moral Theory?," *Nous* 19 (March 1985) 53-64, and "Trust and Antitrust," *Ethics* 96 (January 1986) 231-60.
30. Linda Williams presents this position particularly clearly in her invaluable work "But What Will they Mean for Women? Feminist Concerns About the New Reproductive Technologies," No. 6 in the *Feminist Perspective* Series, CRIAW.
31. Marilyn Frye vividly describes the phenomenon of inter-relatedness which supports sexist oppression by appeal to the metaphor of a bird cage composed of thin wires, each relatively harmless in itself, but, collectively, the wires constitute an overwhelming barrier to the inhabitant of the cage. Marilyn Frye, *The Politics of Reality: Essays in Feminist Theory* (Trumansburg, NY: The Crossing Press 1983), 4-7.

19.
"GIVE ME CHILDREN OR I SHALL DIE!": NEW REPRODUCTIVE TECHNOLOGIES AND HARM TO CHILDREN

Cynthia B. Cohen

"Be fruitful and multiply," God urged newly created humans. Those who take this command to heart cherish the opportunity to procreate and nurture children, to pass on their individual traits and family heritage to their offspring. Having children, for many, is a deeply significant experience that offers overall meaning for their lives. Not all who wish to do so, however, can fulfill the biblical injunction to multiply. Those who cannot often experience a terrible sense of loss. Rachel, in Genesis, felt such despair over her failure to conceive that she cried out to Jacob, "Give me children, or I shall die!" Some who echo her cry today turn to the new reproductive technologies.

There are ethical limits, however, to what may be done to obtain long-sought offspring. Having a deep desire and even a need for something does not justify doing anything whatsoever to obtain it. If the means used to bring children into the world were to create substantial harm to others or to these very children, this would provide strong moral reason not to employ them. It would be wrong, for instance, for infertile couples to place women at risk of substantial harm by enticing those who are not in peak physical condition to "donate" eggs with handsome sums of money. By the same token, it would be wrong to use reproductive technologies to create children if this bore a significant chance of producing serious disease and impairments in these very children. Questions are being raised about whether in vitro fertilization (IVF) and other reproductive technologies do, in fact, create serious illness and deficits in a small but significant proportion of children who are born of them. If these technologies were found to do so, it would be wrong to forge ahead with their use.

Yet advocates of procreative liberty reject this seemingly inescapable conclusion. They contend that even if children were born with serious disorders traceable to their origin in the new reproductive technologies, this would not, except in rare cases, provide moral reason to refrain from using them. Those who conclude otherwise, they maintain, do not understand the peculiar sort of substantial harm to which children born of these novel reproductive means are susceptible. Surely, John Robertson and like-minded thinkers claim, it is better to be alive—even with serious disease and deficits—than not. And these children would not be alive, but for the use of the new reproductive techniques. Therefore, they argue, these children cannot be substantially harmed by the use of these means to bring them into the world. Only if they are caused by these technologies to suffer devastating illness that makes life worse than nonexistence can they be said to be substantially harmed by them.

This startling claim raises intriguing questions. What do we mean by substantial harm—particularly when children who might experience it have not yet been conceived? What degree of disease and suffering that a child would experience as a result of the application of these novel means of conception would make it wrong to use them? Would it be wrong if the child's life would be so terrible that nonexistence would be better? Few conditions would be excluded by this standard. Would it be wrong if the child's life would not be awful, but would include major physical impairments, severe mental disability, and/or considerable pain and suffering?

In responding to such questions, we must consider the possibility that different standards of substantial harm may apply to children at the time when we consider conceiving them and after conception and birth. If so, we must develop a standard of substantial harm that applies to children who might be conceived that is distinct from one that applies to those already born—and must explain how children who are not born can be harmed. We must also address the concern that decisions not to conceive children because they would have serious deficits devalue the lives of those already living who were born with such deficits. Finally, we must grapple with the question of what parents and infertility specialists ought to do in the current state of inadequate knowledge about the effects of the new reproductive technologies on the children who result from their use.

THE HARM TO CHILDREN ARGUMENT

To ask what it means to attribute substantial harm to children who result from the new reproductive technologies is not just to pose an interesting abstract question. Studies indicate this may be a very practical, real question, as they raise the possibility that these technologies may create serious deficits in some proportion of the children born of them. To get a sense of the harms at issue, let us consider the claims of critics of the use of these technologies about their effect on the children born of them.

A primary harm that they attribute to the use of the new reproductive technologies is physical damage. Few long-term studies have been undertaken of the kinds and rates of physical diseases and abnormalities incurred by children born of the new reproductive technologies. Moreover, the evidence these investigations provide is conflicting. Australia is the only country that has kept statistics on the condition at birth *and* subsequent progress of children born of IVF since the inception of this technique in the late 1970s. Data from that country indicate that these children are two or three times more likely to suffer such serious diseases as spina bifida and transposition of the great vessels (a heart abnormality). The Australian data also suggest that some drugs used to stimulate women's ovaries to produce multiple oocytes in preparation for IVF increase the risk of serious birth impairments in the resulting children. Other investigations and commentators support this finding.[1] Still other reports, however, suggest that there is no increase in disorders at birth among children resulting from the use of the new reproductive technologies.[2] One small American follow-up study of the health status of children born of IVF and gamete intrafallopian transfer (GIFT) could find no significant differences in the rate of physical or neurological abnormalities in children born of tech-

niques of assisted conception.[3] No controlled study to date, however, has incorporated an adequate sample size or sufficiently long follow-up monitoring period to determine accurately the risk of physical disorders associated with children born of IVF. And little is known about the physiological impact on children who result from such other procedures as embryo freezing, gamete donation, zona drilling, and intracytoplasmic sperm injection.

It is well known that the higher rate of multiple births in IVF due to the implantation of several embryos in the uterus at a time contributes to an increased rate of preterm and low birth-weight babies. This, in turn, is associated with a higher incidence of perinatal, neonatal, and infant mortality in children conceived by IVF than those conceived coitally.[4] In France, for instance, the rates of prematurity and intrauterine growth retardation among IVF births in a two-year period were 16 percent and 14 percent respectively, whereas the expected rates for the general population were 7 percent and 3 percent.[5] An analysis of IVF outcome data from France between 1986 and 1990 indicated that perinatal mortality among IVF births also was higher than that in the general population, even when data were stratified according to gestational number. French neonatologists who had worked to prevent low birth weight, congenital anomalies, and genetic disorders among newborns observed that "[n]ow, we suddenly find our NICU filled with highrisk newborns ... [as a result of the expansion of IVF services]."

Critics also express concern that the new reproductive technologies may jeopardize the psychological and social welfare of the children who result from them, particularly when they involve third parties in donor or surrogacy arrangements and depend on secrecy.[6] These children, they hypothesize, will view themselves as manufactured products, rather than distinctive individuals born of love between a man and a woman.[7] They will be denied the stable sense of identity that comes from knowing their biological heritage and family lineage should their rearing parents differ from their genetic parents.[8] Moreover, the social stigma these children will experience when others learn that they were conceived by these novel means will increase their difficulties, opponents contend. Little research is available on the effect of the use of assisted reproduction on the psychosocial development of the resulting children. In the first controlled study of family relationships and the psychological development of children created by the new reproductive technologies, no group differences in the emotions, behavior, or relationships with parents between children born of assisted reproduction and children conceived naturally or adopted could be found.[9]

One commentator summarizes the issues of harm raised by the use of the new reproductive technologies as follows:

> The technology for both IVF and GIFT as well as adjunct technologies such as zona drilling, embryo freezing, and gamete donation have not been accompanied by careful scrutiny and analysis of the risks involved. Indeed, even when risks are clearly established (as with multiple pregnancy), there has been no discernible attempt to reduce these risks by altering procedures and protocols. There also has been an appalling lack of follow-up studies to determine the long-term health, psychological, and social consequence of these procedures.[10]

In view of the current lack of systematic knowledge about difficulties these methods may create in children born of them, opponents of the new reproductive technologies maintain it is wrong to use them. Those who resort to these techniques, they claim, bear the burden of proof of their safety. They have an obligation to establish whether these ever-increasing methods of assisted reproduction do, in fact, harm a small but significant proportion of children before they are used. For ease of reference, we will call their claims the Harm to Children Argument against the use of the new reproductive technologies.

THE INTEREST IN EXISTING ARGUMENT

The basic response to the Harm To Children Argument by several proponents of the use of the new reproductive technologies,[11] of whom John Robertson is a respected spokesperson, is that even if children born of the new reproductive technologies were to suffer serious impairments as a result of their origin, this would not necessarily render it wrong to use these techniques. We might call this response the Interest in Existing Argument: since it is, in almost all cases, better to be alive than not, and these children would not be alive but for the employment of these techniques, using them to bring these children into the world is justified. Robertson writes:

> [A] higher incidence of birth defects in such offspring would not justify banning the technique in order to protect the offspring, because without these techniques these children would not have been born at all. Unless their lives are so full of suffering as to be worse than no life at all, a very unlikely supposition, the defective children of such a union have not been harmed if they would not have been born healthy.[12]

Only where "from the perspective of the child, viewed solely in light of his interests as he is then situated, any life at all with the conditions of his birth would be so harmful to him that from his perspective he would prefer not to live,"[13] could it be said to be a substantial harm to have been brought into existence by means of the new reproductive technologies.

Robertson here implicitly distinguishes between *devastating harm*—harm that brings such suffering into a person's life that this life is worse than no life at all—from *serious harm*—harm that does not render life worse than death, but that includes such detriments as major physical impairments, severe mental disability, and/or considerable pain and suffering. He labels only the former *substantial harm*. Indeed, at certain points, Robertson maintains that children damaged by their origin in the new reproductive technologies cannot be said to suffer harm at all, since their birth is an overriding benefit.

The Harm to Children Argument is logically flawed, Robertson and like-minded thinkers maintain, because the benefit of life that children born of these techniques receive outweighs almost any detriment they might experience as a result of their origins. Robertson notes:

> Preventing harm would mean preventing the birth of the child whose interests one is trying to protect. Yet a child's interests are hardly protected by preventing the child's existence. If the child has no way to be born or raised free of that harm, a person is not injuring the child by enabling her to be born in the circumstances of concern.[14]

It is not open to children damaged by the use of the new reproductive technologies to live free of impairment, since they could not have existed without the use of these technologies. The alternative for them would have been not to live at all, a state which is not in their interests. Consequently, according to the Interest in Existing Argument, it is, in almost all instances, in the interests of children who might be born of the new reproductive technologies to be brought into the world by these means, even if this would risk serious harm to them.

This argument applies only to children who suffer harm that is a necessary result of the use of these techniques. Thus, if it were claimed that contract surrogacy creates psychological harm for a child because the biological mother and rearing parents would be in a constant state of conflict with each other, the Interest in Existing Argument could not be used in response. This is because the warring trio could behave in a different manner less likely to cause this sort of harm to the child. According to advocates of the Interest in Existing Argument it was not a necessary condition of the child's very existence that the conflict among these various parents occur.

THE HARM OF NOT EXISTING

The Interest in Existing Argument assumes that children with an interest in existing are waiting in a spectral world of nonexistence where their situation is less desirable than it would be were they released into this world. This presupposition is revealed in such observations as "a child's interests are hardly protected by preventing the child's existence" and that it is a disadvantage to such children that they "have no way of being born." In the Interest in Existing Argument children who might be conceived are pictured as pale preexisting entities with an interest in moving into the more full-blooded reality of this world. Their admission into this realm is thwarted by the failure to use available new reproductive technology. This failure negates their interest in existing and thereby harms them.

Before a person exists, however, he or she does not reside in some other domain. Prior to conception, there is *no one who waits to be brought into this world.* Joel Feinberg argues, "Since it is necessary to *be* if one is to *be better off*, it is a logical contradic-

tion to say that someone could be better off though not in existence."[15] To say that it was good for someone already in existence to have been born does imply that his existence in this world is better than his life in some other realm. Nor does it imply that if he had not been caused to exist, this would have been bad for him.[16] Although a wealth of possible children can be conceived, their interests cannot be diminished if they are not. Therefore, it cannot be coherently argued that it is "better" for children to be created by means of the new reproductive technologies, even when this would result in serious disorders to them, since there is no alternative state in which their lot could be worse.

Part of the confusion at the heart of the Interest in Existing Argument stems from an incoherence found in tort actions for "wrongful life," to which this argument has an acknowledged debt. In these suits, children born with impairments claim that their current condition is worse than the state of nonexistence they would have had were it not for negligence on the part of physicians, hospitals or testing laboratories. The wrong done to them, they contend, is not that their impaired condition was negligently caused, but that their very existence was negligently caused. This, they maintain, is a serious injury, since they would have been better off not being born at all. They ask for compensation for the injury of being brought into this world.

In an early wrongful life case, *Gleitman v. Cosgrove*, a child born with impairments whose mother had been told erroneously that her exposure to German measles during pregnancy would not harm the fetus, brought suit for damages for the injury of being born.[17] The traditional method of measuring damages in tort is to compare the condition of the plaintiff before and after an injury and to compensate for the difference. When the putative wrong done to the plaintiff is to have been brought into existence in an impaired state, the court must measure the difference between nonexistence and existence with impairments. In *Gleitman*, the court found it "logically impossible" to "weigh the value of life with impairments against the nonexistence of life itself." We cannot, according to the court, conceptualize a world in which the plaintiff did not exist and ask what benefits and burdens he experienced in that world in order to compare it with his situation in this world.

Even so, the *Gleitman* court concluded that the value of life, no matter how burdened, outweighs the disvalue of not existing, and that damages therefore could not be awarded to the child for "wrongful life." In drawing this conclusion, the court implicitly compared the world of existence with that of nonexistence and declared the former always preferable to the latter. Yet this is precisely the step the court had said it could not take. Similarly, in another leading case, *Berman v. Allan,* the court ruled against recognition of a "wrongful life" claim on grounds that "life—whether experienced with or without a major physical handicap—is more precious than non-life."[18] These courts were concerned that awarding damages for being alive would diminish the high value that the law places on human life. This public policy concern, however, caused them to lapse into incoherence. They claimed that the world of existence cannot be measured against that of nonexistence. However, if existence is better than nonexistence, as they also declared, nonexistence must be conceptually accessible in some sense so that an intelligible comparison can be made between it and existence.

Proponents of the Interest in Existing Argument adopt the two-world view underlying the logically impossible thesis of the early wrongful life cases when they claim that children are harmed if they are not brought out of the world of nonexistence into the world of existence. This leaves them with two problems: (1) explaining how to conceptualize and comprehend nonexistence and (2) justifying the claim that it is better to exist than not. Moreover, their dependence on the wrongful life decisions causes them to overlook an essential feature of their opponents' argument. The Harm to Children Argument is a *before-the-fact* one that applies to the time when a decision must be made about whether to employ the new reproductive technologies. *At this time, unlike the wrongful life cases, no child exists who could be harmed.* The Harm to Children Argument holds that at this preconception time, the morally right decision is not to use such technologies until further research establishes the degree of harm this might do to children who result. The Interest in Existing argument,

however, is an after-the-fact argument meant to apply at a time when children are already born. It must be used as a response to those who object to having already brought children into the world. Since the harm posited by the critics has not yet occurred when the decision is made whether to employ them, it is not an adequate response to say that without these technologies the resulting children would not have been born.[19] That is precisely what is at issue—*whether these children ought to have been conceived and born.*

A further difficulty is that the Interest in Existing Argument justifies allowing the new reproductive technologies to create almost any harm to children conceived as a result of their use—as long as this is not devastating harm in which death is preferable to life with it. As Bonnie Steinbock and Ron McClamrock observe, "Very few lives meet the stringent conditions imposed by the wrongful life analysis.... Even the most dismal sorts of circumstances of opportunity (including, for example ... an extremely high chance of facing an agonizing death from starvation in the early years of life, severe retardation plus quadriplegia) fail to be covered"[20] by the standard of devastating harm. Yet it would strike many as ethically objectionable to proceed with reproductive techniques should such serious, but not devastating harms result from them in a significant proportion of cases.

THE "WRONGFUL LIFE" STANDARD OF SUBSTANTIAL HARM

Those who present the Interest in Existing Argument, adopting the standard applied in wrongful life cases, describe substantial harm as that which, in Robertson's words, puts one in a condition that renders life so "horrible"[21] and so "full of unavoidable suffering" (p. 169) that it is worse than "no life at all."[22] Robertson does not give a more precise definition of substantial harm, nor does he present specific examples of conditions which fall under that rubric in his discussion of harm to children and the new reproductive technologies. Feinberg expands on the "wrongful life" standard of substantial harm:

Surely in most cases of suffering and impairment we think of death as even worse. This is shown by the widespread human tendency to "cling to life at all costs." And even for severe genetic handicaps and inherited maladies, most competent persons who suffer from them will not express regret that they were born in the first place.... In the most extreme cases, however, I think it is rational to prefer not to have come into existence at all, and while I cannot prove this judgment, I am confident that most people will agree that it is at least plausible. I have in mind some of the more severely victimized sufferers from brain malformation, spina bifida, Tay-Sachs disease, polycystic kidney disease, Lesch-Nyhan syndrome, and those who, from whatever cause, are born blind and deaf, permanently incontinent, severely retarded, and in chronic pain or near-total paralysis, with life expectancies of only a few years.[23]

To talk about death, both Feinberg and Robertson assume, is the same as to talk about "not coming into existence at all." They assimilate nonexistence before life and nonexistence after having lived. This is a mistake. *Nonexistence before coming into being* and *nonexistence after having lived* are two distinct concepts.

Lucretius observed that we do not express concern about nonexistence before creation, but we do fear our nonexistence after death. Why is this? The reason we perceive death as bad, Thomas Nagel proposes, is that it causes us to have fewer goods of this life than we would have had if we had continued to live.[24] Frances Kamm further observes that it is not only the absence of future goods in this life that leads us to fear death, but that death "takes away what already was and would have continued to be."[25] Preconception nonexistence, however, does not deprive us of what was ours already. In it there is no particular individual whose life ends and who thereby loses out on life's goods. Consequently, nonexistence before conception and birth does not seem as bad as death. We are indifferent to it.

Several other features of death that are also not characteristic of preconception nonexistence contribute to our assessment of it as bad. Death, for instance, happens to a person, whereas preconception nonexistence does not include an event in which nonexistence happens to a person. Death reveals our vulnerability in that through it a person is destroyed and deprived of life's goods. If a person does not exist, in contrast, this does not reflect negatively on "his" or "her" capacities.[26] Because of significant differences between them, preconception and posthumous nonexistence are qualitatively distinct concepts that are not interchangeable. Death has characteristics that lead us to evaluate it as bad, whereas preconception nonexistence strikes us as neither good nor bad.

Do we, too, fall into the trap of positing a shadowy world of nonexistence by distinguishing between preconception and posthumous nonexistence? We do not claim that either of these forms of nonexistence is a metaphysical locale. Instead, we view both as logical constructs built out of what we know about being alive. For both Nagel and Kamm, the meaning of death is derived from what we know about our existence in this world. The same is true of preconception nonexistence. Although the multitude of children whom it is possible for us to bring into the world do not exist, we can conceptualize certain things about them and what their lives would be like were we to conceive and bear them. We can also comprehend certain things about the negation of their existence were they to be born. That is, we can understand what they would lose if we decided not to conceive them and bring them into the world. Thus we can meaningfully compare preconception nonexistence with life. We can consider children who might be brought into existence and ask whether we ought to conceive them without having to postulate a separate sphere of nonexistence in which they wait as we ponder the question.

While we can make sense of the notion of preconception nonexistence, can we also intelligibly claim that children who have not yet been conceived can have interests? It might be argued that those who do not exist cannot have interests and that therefore possible children can have no interest in not being conceived and brought into the world with serious disorders. Yet possible children can have interests, if these are taken in the sense of what contributes to their good, rather than as psychological states. We can conceive of what would promote their welfare were they to be brought into the world. To deny them such interests is mistakenly to reason by analogy with the dead. It has been supposed that the dead can have no interests because we cannot perform any actions that will affect the condition of their lives.[27] We cannot causally impinge on them for better or worse, it has been argued, for their lives have been completed. But this is not the case with possible children. We can affect them causally for better or worse by our present actions. Thus, we can ascribe to possible children certain interests that can be thwarted or fulfilled by actions that we take.

The interests of children who might be born of the new reproductive technologies are not adequately captured by the "wrongful life" standard. The comparison that parents and physicians must make when they assess whether use of these technologies would negatively affect the good of children who might result is not between *death* and the condition of these children were they to be born with certain deficits. The appropriate comparison is between *preconception nonexistence* and their condition were they to be born with certain deficits. If preconception nonexistence, unlike death, is neither good nor bad, then any life that will be worse than it *will not have to be as bad as the life of devastating deficits set out in the wrongful life standard.* A life with serious, but not devastating deficits, could be bad and therefore worse than preconception nonexistence, which is neither good nor bad. Therefore, we must modify the wrongful life standard of substantial harm to indicate that if new reproductive technologies were shown to cause a significant proportion of children born of them to suffer either devastating *or* serious deficits, they would cause substantial harm to these children and consequently ought not be used.

THE INADEQUATE OPPORTUNITY FOR HEALTH STANDARD OF SUBSTANTIAL HARM

How are we to identify the serious deficits that—along with devastating deficits—would constitute substantial harm to these children? The boundary between moderate, serious, and devastating deficits is sufficiently blurred that reasonable people can disagree about where it lies in particular cases. Many would disagree with Feinberg that children knowingly conceived with such disorders as spina bifida, blindness, deafness, severe retardation, or permanent incontinence should be considered to be suffering from devastating deficits that make their lives worse than death. However, they might well view these dis-

orders as amounting to serious deficits that make their lives worse than preconception nonexistence. What is needed is a conceptual framework that marks off those deficits that have such a negative impact on children that reasonable people would agree that knowingly to conceive children with these disorders would be to impose substantial harm on them in the vast majority of cases.

Laura Purdy suggests that we cause substantial harm to future children and therefore ought not knowingly conceive them "when there is a high risk of transmitting a serious disease or defect [of a sort that would deny them] a normal opportunity for health."[28] At points in Purdy's discussion, as when she states that "every parent should try to ensure normal health for his child," she can be taken to mean that having an abnormal state of health would constitute a disorder sufficiently serious to warrant not conceiving a child who would have it. On this approach, children with a particular biological, chemical, or mental state different from the norm would be said to lack "normal health" and therefore to suffer from a "serious disease or defect" that would justify not conceiving them. Yet it would not strike us as wrong knowingly to conceive children who are not "normal" because they have myopia or albinism. Normality does not appear to provide an adequate standard for deciding that a disorder is a serious deficit that substantially harms a child knowingly conceived with it.

At other points, however, Purdy seems to suggest that the focus for defining a serious deficit that falls under the substantial harm rubric should be on the failure to provide an adequate opportunity for a healthy life, as this is defined within a culture. Here she seems on the right track, for notions of health and disease—for better and for worse—are embedded within a society. What constitutes health and what represents a serious falling away from it varies from culture to culture and changes from time to time. As the notion of health and of an adequate opportunity for health vary according to the cultural context and conditions, so, too, does the meaning of a serious disease or deficit. Moreover, access to health services and the resulting opportunity for health—or lack of it—also affect what is meant by health, serious disorder, and substantial harm.

In our society, children who are color-blind are considered to have only a mild deficit and no diminution of their opportunity for health. However, in certain African cultures in which the capacity to distinguish a great variety of shades of green is needed to function at a minimal level for survival, color blindness is a serious deficit. Children born with this condition in such cultures do not have an adequate opportunity for health because their condition cannot be remedied. Thus, cultural values affect the meanings of health and of serious disorders. Stanley Hauerwas observes that "disease descriptions and remedies are relative to a society's values and needs. Thus 'retardation' might not 'exist' in a society which values cooperation more than competition and ambition."[29] Further, medical practices in different cultures reflect different views of what constitutes health and serious disorders. In Germany children with blood pressure that differs from the norm for their age on both the high and low end are suspected to be at risk of serious disease, whereas in America only high blood pressure is considered an indicator of serious disease.

What makes a disorder serious, however, is not only a matter of cultural needs, expectations, constructions, and practices. Some children are born with remediable conditions that are transformed into serious deficits when they are not ameliorated due to circumstances of injustice and neglect within a culture. The child born with spina bifida to poor parents in the hills of Appalachia has a minimal opportunity for health and a more serious disorder than the child born with this same condition to professional parents in Los Angeles. It might not be unfair to a child knowingly to conceive him or her with paralysis of the lower limbs if that child, once born, would have access to support structures giving him or her adequate mobility.[30] Nor would we have grounds for considering it wrong for parents knowingly to conceive a blind child if that child would receive compensatory education and ameliorative instruments enabling him or her to have an adequate opportunity for health within a society.

This relativity of the notion of health and of an adequate opportunity for health means that no definition of serious disease or disorder amounting to substantial harm that would apply across all cultures, times, and places can be given. Instead, the assessment of serious disease amounting to substantial harm must be made under specific circumstances within particular cultures. It must be defined not only in terms of a given physical or mental condition that damages a child's ability to function within a culture, but also in terms of the failure or inability of a culture to provide a child with access to ameliorative resources.

Sidney Callahan maintains that a principle of proportionality should be applied when making decisions concerning reproduction. This would mean that the lower the risk and gravity of impairment to the child and the more would-be parents, family, and the institutional structures of a society are able and willing to ameliorate the impairment, the less the likelihood that a child would suffer a serious deficit and the more ethically justifiable it would be to conceive him or her. Should the probability and gravity of impairment be great, however, and the would-be-parents, family and social structure unwilling or unable to provide ameliorative measures for the child with such impairment, the higher the likelihood the child would suffer a serious deficit and the less ethically justifiable it would be to conceive that child. We do not end up with a black letter definition of a deficit serious enough to be termed substantial harm on this approach, but one that requires us to consider the nature of the disorder from which the child would suffer, the circumstances into which the child would be brought, and the ameliorative resources available for that child. Under current circumstances in our culture in which children born with disabling disorders have inadequate support, it would be morally questionable, at least, knowingly to conceive a child suffering from some of the deficits listed by Feinberg above.

OBLIGATIONS TO ACTUAL AND POSSIBLE CHILDREN

Although we consider it ethically necessary to provide treatment to keep children alive who have serious illnesses, we do not consider it ethically necessary knowingly to conceive children with those same disorders. Why is this? Why do we assume that our obligations to children who already exist differ from our obligations to children whom we might conceive?

The difference between an actual and possible child and between our evaluations of preconception nonexistence and death help to explain this distinction. Since we view death as an evil in relation to being alive, we tend to maintain that once children are born, only if they suffer devastating harms that make life worse than death would we be justified in not doing what we can to prevent their death. Being alive is better than being dead, except in rare circumstances. However, we do not believe that we have an obligation to do everything we can to conceive and bring into the world possible children who would suffer serious or devastating illness as a result. This is because no one exists who is wronged by not being conceived and also because preconception nonexistence does not strike us as being either bad or good. To fail to actualize a possible child, therefore, does not put that child in a worse situation or wrong that child.

Furthermore, we have no obligation to conceive children if this would detrimentally affect the good of the family or culture into which they would be born. We have no obligation, for instance, to conceive a sixth child if we believe our family can only function adequately with five. And we need not bring children into the world when this would contribute to a problem of overpopulation or of limited resources. It is morally acceptable, indeed, some would say, morally required, that *before* we bring children into the world, we consider not only their well-being were they to be born, but the good of those who would be affected by their birth. *After* birth, however, the interest in existing of the living child comes into play and morally outweighs remnants of a parental or societal interest in not having had that child.

These conclusions may appear to intimate that the lives of children born with serious or even devastating disorders are not valued or valuable. This conclusion does not follow from the preceding argument. Should parents, after receiving convincing evidence that use of the new reproductive technologies would harm the resulting children, decide against employing them, this could say one of two things to living children with serious or devastating disorders. It could suggest that it would have been better for their families if a different child had been born without

these disorders and she was not. Or it could imply that it would have been better for this child to have been born without these disorders.[31] The first implication suggests that it would be better for others if children with these disorders were not born, whereas the second maintains that it would be better for the children themselves if they had not been born with them. The first implies that it is regrettable that these children are alive instead of "normal" children. The second implies that it is regrettable that these children have these disorders. The second implication is the one on which we tend to act. This is exhibited by efforts we make to avoid serious or devastating disorders in children during pregnancy and to treat and care for children with such disorders after they are born. All of this suggests that it is not the children we disvalue, but the disorders that they have sustained. Consequently, it is not necessarily a reproach to disabled children who are already born if decisions are made against knowingly conceiving children who would have the same disabilities.

It is, however, a reproach to us and to our social institutions that once children with serious and devastating disorders are born, we provide woefully insufficient services and resources to them and their families. Does this contradict the claim that we value living children with disabilities and have their interests at heart? Hauerwas provides one perceptive explanation of our ambivalent and complex attitude toward those who live with serious disabilities in the course of discussing those who are developmentally delayed. He observes:

> After all, what we finally seek is not simply to help the retarded better negotiate their disability but to be like us: not retarded. Our inability to accomplish that frustrates and angers us, and sometimes the retarded themselves become the object of our anger. We do not like to be reminded of the limits of our power, and we do not like those who remind us.[32]

We wish to remedy the disabilities with which children may be born, but find it difficult to cope with the recognition of our own vulnerability that they inadvertently call forth. Therefore, we relegate them to a separate domain within the world of existence where we believe unknown others will assist them to meet the special challenges they face. This is uncharitable and unjust. We have a responsibility to overcome our misplaced frustration about being unable to render those who have serious or devastating disorders more like those who do not. We have a responsibility to assist them to make their own way in the world unhampered by our irrational fears.

TAKING HARMS SERIOUSLY

The biblical injunction to multiply does not exhort us to do anything whatsoever to have children. It would be wrong to have children if it were known before conception that the means used to bring this about could inflict serious or devastating deficits on those very children. Yet the logic of the Interest in Existing Argument leads its proponents to brush aside the question whether these technologies might create such serious impairments. The thrust of this argument is that use of the new reproductive technologies provides its own justification—it produces children. This claim disregards the welfare of these children. Moreover, it creates a barrier to more extensive and detailed investigations of the effect of the new reproductive technologies on children born of them.

On the approach presented here, if it were known ahead of time that children conceived with the assistance of the new reproductive technologies would not have an adequate opportunity for health, it would be wrong to use them. Assessment of when and whether this would be the case would be carried out in light of the personal, familial, and social circumstances into which these children would be born. This means that would-be parents who consider resorting to the new reproductive technologies must be informed about the risks these techniques would present to the children born as a result of their use, the means available for ameliorating deficits these children might experience, and what social support would be available should they lack the resources to address such deficits on their own. Only then can they decide whether they ought to proceed with these techniques. To implement this recommendation, evidence for and against the contention that the new reproductive technologies cause serious or devastating physical, psychological, or social harm to the resulting children should be investigated more thoroughly than at present. Because of limited knowledge of the possible effects of these measures on their

children, those who repeat Rachel's cry today face an agonizingly difficult decision when they consider whether to use the new reproductive technologies.

———

Acknowledgments

I am indebted to the faculty and Senior Research Fellows of the Kennedy Institute of Ethics at Georgetown University of their perceptive comments on an earlier draft of this paper and to Michael E. McClure and James L. Mills of the National Institute of Child Health and Human Development for providing extremely helpful references and insights related to medical studies of the status of children born of assisted conception. These individuals are not responsible for the conclusions drawn here.

Notes

1. National Perinatal Statistics Unit, Fertility Society of Australia, *In Vitro Fertilization Pregnancies. Australia and New Zealand 1979-1985,* Sydney, Australia, 1987; Paul L. Lancaster, "Congenital Malformations after In-Vitro Fertilisation," [letter] *Lancet* 2 (1987): 1392-93; see also AIHW National Perinatal Statistics Unit, Fertility Society of Australia, *Assisted Conception in Australia and New Zealand 1990* (Sydney: AIHW National Perinatal Statistics Unit, 1992); Gail Vines, "Shots in the Dark for Infertility," New Scientists 140 (1993) : 13-15; Lene Koch, "Physiological and Psychosocial Risks of the New Reproductive Technologies," in *Tough Choices: In Vitro Fertilization and the Reproductive Technologies,* ed. Patricia Stephenson and Marsden G. Wagner (Philadelphia: Temple University Press. 1993). pp. 122-34.

2. U.B. Wennerholm et al., "Pregnancy Complications and Short-Term Follow Up of Infants Born after In Vitro Fertilization and Embryo Transfer," *Acta Obstetrica et Gynecologicia Scandinavica* 70 (1991): 565-73; B. Rizk et al., "Perinatal Outcome and Congenital Malformations in In-Vitro Fertilization Babies from the Bourn-Hallam Group," *Human Reproduction* 6 (1991): 1259-64; S. Friedler, S. Mashiach, N. Laufer, "Births in Israel Resulting from In-Vitro Fertilization/Embryo Transfer, 1982-1989: National Registry of the Israeli Association for Fertility

Research," *Human Reproduction* 7 (1992): 1159-63; Society for Assisted Reproductive Technology, American Society for Reproductive Medicine, Assisted Reproductive Technology in the United States and Canada, "1993 Results Generated from the American Society for Reproductive Medicine/Society for Assisted Reproductive Technology Registry," *Fertility and Sterility* 64 (1995): 13-21.

3. Norma C. Morin et al., "Congenital Malformations and Psychosocial Development in Children Conceived by In Vitro Fertilization," *Journal of Pediatrics* 115 (1989): 222-27.

4. V. Beral et al., "Outcome of Pregnancies Resulting from Assisted Conception," *British Medical Bulletin* 46, no. 3 (1990): 753-68; I. Craft and T. al-Shawaf, "Outcome and Complications of Assisted Reproduction," *Current Opinion in Obstetrics and Gynecology* 3 (1991): 668-73; Rizk et al., "Perinatal Outcome and Congenital Malformations in In-Vitro Fertilization Babies from the Bourn-Hallam Group"; P. Doyle, V. Beral, and N. Maconochie, "Preterm Delivery, Low Birthweight and Small-for-Gestational-Age in Liveborn Singleton Babies Resulting from In-Vitro Fertilization," *Human Reproduction* 7 (1992): 425-28; Friedler et al., "Births in Israel," pp. 1160-63.

5. Jean-Pierre Relier, Michele Couchard, and Catherine Huon, "The Neo-natologist's Experience of In Vitro Fertilization Risks," *Tough Choices*, pp. 135-143; see also P. Rufat et al., "Task Force Report on the Outcome of Pregnancies and Children Conceived by In Vitro Fertilization (France: 1987 to 1989)," *Fertility and Sterility* 61 (1994): 324-30; FIVNAT (French In Vitro National) "Pregnancies and Births Resulting from In Vitro Fertilization: French National Registry, Analysis of Data 1986 To 1990," *Fertility and Sterility* 64 (1995): 746-56.

6. Cynthia B. Cohen, "Reproductive Technologies: Ethical Issues," in *Encyclopedia of Bioethics,* ed. Warren Thomas Reich (New York: Simon and Schuster Macmillan, 1995), vol. 4, pp. 2233-41; A. Baran and R. Pannor, *Lethal Secrets: The Shocking Consequences and Unsolved Problems of Artificial Insemination* (New York: Warner Books, 1989), D. N. Mushin, J. Spensley, M. Barreda-Hanson, "In Vitro Fertilization Children: Early Psychosocial Development," *Journal of In Vitro Fertilization and Embryo Transfer* 4 (1986): 247-52.

7. Margaret Radin, "Market-Inalienability," *Harvard Law Review* 100 (1987): 1921-36; Sidney Callahan, "The Ethical Challenges of the New Reproductive Technologies," in *Medical Ethics: A Guide for Health Professionals*, ed. J. Monagle and David Thomasma (Rockville, Md.: Aspen, 1988), pp. 26-37.

8. Leon Kass, *Toward a More Natural Science: Biology and Human Affairs* (New York: Free Press, 1985), p. 113; Lisa Sowle Cahill, "The Ethics of Surrogate Motherhood: Biology, Freedom, and Moral Obligation," *Law, Medicine and Health Care* 16, nos. 1-2 (1988): 65-71, at 69; Cynthia B. Cohen, "Parents Anonymous," in *New Ways of Making Babies: The Case of Egg Donation,* ed. Cynthia B. Cohen (Bloomington: Indiana University Press, 1996), forthcoming.

9. Susan Golombok et al., "Parents and Their Children Happy with Assisted Conception," [letter] *British Medical Journal* 307 (1994): 1032.

10. Lene Koch, "Physiological and Psychosocial Risks of the New Reproductive Technologies," p. 128.

11. Ruth F. Chadwick, "Cloning," *Philosophy* 57 (1982): 201-9; John A. Robertson, "Procreative Liberty and the Control of Conception, Pregnancy, and Childbirth," *University of Virginia Law Review* 69 (1983): 405-462, at 434; John A. Robertson, "Embryos, Families, and Procreative Liberty: The Legal Structure of the New Reproduction," *Southern California Law Review* 59 (1986): 942-1041, at 958, 988; John A. Robertson, "Procreative Liberty, Embryos, and Collaborative Reproduction: A Legal Perspective," in *Embryos, Ethics, and Women's Rights: Exploring the New Reproductive Technologies,* ed. E.F. Baruch, A.F. Adamo, Jr., J. Seager (New York: Howarth Press, 1988), pp. 179-194; John A. Robertson, "The Question of Human Cloning," *Hastings Center Report* 24, no. 3 (1994): 6-14; John A. Robertson, *Children of Choice: Freedom and the New Reproductive Technologies* (Princeton, N.J.: Princeton University Press, 1994), pp. 75-76, 110-11, 122-23, 152, 169-70; Ruth Macklin, "Splitting Embryos on the Slippery Slope," *Kennedy Institute of Ethics Journal* 4 (1994): 209-25, at 219-20.

12. Robertson, "Procreative Liberty and the Control of Conception, Pregnancy and Childbirth," p. 434.

13. Robertson, *Children of Choice*, pp. 75-76.

14. Robertson, *Children of Choice*, pp. 75-76.

15. Joel Feinberg, "Wrongful Life and the Counterfactual Element in Harming," *Social Philosophy and Policy* 4 (1988): 145-78, at 158.

16. Derek Parfit, *Reasons and Persons* (Oxford: Oxford University Press, 1985), p. 487.

17. Gleitman v. Cosgrove, 49 N.J. 22, 227 A. 2d 689 (1967).

18. *Berman v. Allan,* 80 N.J. 421, 404 A. 2d 8 (1979).

19. Robertson, *Children of Choice,* pp. 75, 117; "Embryos, Families, and Procreative Liberty," pp. 958, 988.

20. Bonnie Steinbock and Ron McClamrock, "When Is Birth Unfair to the Child?" *Hastings Center Report* 24, no. 6 (1994): 16-22, at 17.

21. Robertson, *Children of Choice*, pp. 82, 85.

22. Robertson, "Procreative Liberty and the Control of Conception, Pregnancy, and Childbirth," p. 434.

23. Feinberg, "Wrongful Life," p. 159.

24. Thomas Nagel, "Death," in *Mortal Questions* (Cambridge: Cambridge University Press: 1979), pp. 1-10.

25. Frances M. Kamm, *Morality, Mortality, Volume I. Death and Whom to Save from It* (New York: Oxford University Press, 1993), p. 40.

26. Kamm, *Morality, Mortality,* p. 40-41.

27. Joan Callahan, "On Harming the Dead," *Ethics* 97 (1987): 341-52; Ernest Partridge, "Posthumous Interests and Posthumous Respect," *Ethics* 91 (1981): 243-64.

28. Laura Purdy, "Genetic Diseases: Can Having Children Be Immoral?" in *Genetics Now: Ethical Issues in Genetic Research,* ed. John Buckly, Jr. (Washington, D. C.: University Press of America, 1978), pp. 25-39, at 25.

29. Stanley Hauerwas, "Suffering the Retarded: Should We Prevent Retardation?" in *Suffering Presence: Theological Reflections on Medicine, the Mentally Handicapped, and the Church,* ed. Stanley Hauerwas (Notre Dame: University of Notre Dame Press, 1986), pp. 159-81.

30. Steinbock and McClamrock, "When Is Birth Unfair to the Child?" and Sidney Callahan, "An Ethical Analysis of Responsible Parenthood," in *Genetic Counseling: Facts, Values, and Norms,* ed. Alexander M. Capron, Marc Lappé, Robert F. Murray (New York: Alan R. Liss, 1979), pp. 217-38.

31. Mary Warnock, "Ethical Challenges in Embryo Manipulation," *British Medical Journal 304* (1992): 1045-49, at 1047.

32. Hauerwas, "Suffering the Retarded," p. 176.

20.
LISTENING TO THE VOICES OF THE INFERTILE

Barbara J. Berg

Ideas are clean. They soar in the serene supernal.
I can take them out and look at them, they fit in
books, they lead me down that narrow way. And in
the morning they are there.
Ideas are straight—
But the world is round, and a messy mortal is my
friend.
Come walk with me in the mud....

— Hugh Prather[1]

There has been much discussion surrounding the
new reproductive technologies. Feminists have
entered this discussion voicing concern over the pervasive influence of pronatalism in our society, the
increasing medicalization of reproduction, the commodification of women and children, the overvalua-
tion of genetic versus social linkages, and the potential exploitation of women. There is much to be
concerned about. But much of the feminist discourse
on this subject has come from the perspective that
these technologies should not be pursued because of
their potentially negative effects on women and children. Although many legitimate concerns have been
raised, complex issues have sometimes been oversimplified and, most disturbing of all, some feminists do not appear to be taking the role of advocating for infertile women so much as speaking for
them. But the infertile have their own voices.

What follows is based upon what I have learned as
a feminist psychologist working with the infertile. I
will attempt to broaden the boundaries of the feminist analysis to include some of these perspectives.
These perspectives can elucidate traditional areas of
focus, such as genetic versus social linkages in parenting, while some newer areas of concern will be
explored, including limitations in access to treatment, lack of funding for preventive health care, sexist medical terminology, and assumptions about psychogenic infertility.

BIOLOGICAL VERSUS ADOPTIVE PARENTHOOD

The pervasive and tenacious pronatalism of our culture has resulted in the view that motherhood is a
woman's *raison d'être*.[2] Although women are
employed outside the home in ever-increasing numbers, being a wife and mother is still viewed as a
woman's primary and central function.[3] Outside
work is acceptable as long as the house is clean and
the husband and children are well tended. Pronatalism has promoted the view that a woman without
husband and children (whether voluntarily or not) is
somehow deficient. Consequently, childless women
continue to be perceived in a pejorative light (i.e., as
selfish). The pronatalist perspective also views having genetically related children as superior to adopting children. The pronatalist motherhood mandate,
then, is that women must bear children for their husbands. Understandably, feminists have rejected this
mandate and affirmed the value of women separate
from spouses and progeny, as well as the value of
social versus genetic ties in parenting.

From an impersonal perspective, it is easy to equate
the value of parenting an adoptive and a biological
child. Both can involve rearing a child from infancy to
adulthood. However, it is undeniable that among the
individuals choosing to rear children, most prefer to
have a biological child. Adoption is usually considered only when a couple[4] is unable to have a biological child. This nearly universal preference (which is
observed among feminists as well as others) reveals
not only a value placed on the genetic linkage but on
other aspects of the experience of parenting a biological child (e.g., the experience of pregnancy and childbirth). Although it may be equally valid and valuable,
the experience of rearing an adopted child is different
from that of rearing a biological child, and it is important to examine these differences.

Our society's emphasis on genetic linkages has
given feminists pause. When genetic connections are

emphasized at the expense of social relationships, the interactions which are truly most meaningful in life have been diminished. Rothman makes a cogent argument for our need to re-examine the importance of our social relationships.[5] She claims that the maternal tie for biological mothers is established by the relationship between the woman and her fetus during gestation. Since the man lacks such a relationship to the growing fetus, the paternal tie is simply reduced to the act of impregnating—a genetic contribution. A societal emphasis upon the genetic tie can deny the importance of the experience of gestation or growing a fetus within one's body, and reduce women to gaining rights to children not as mothers, but essentially as father-equivalents. Thus, the genetic emphasis can be interpreted as the basis for men's control over the children of women. But the desire for biological motherhood is not simply comprised of seeking a genetic tie to a child, it is often comprised of seeking the relational experiences of pregnancy, birth, and nursing as well.[6]

However, interest in the genetic continuity represented by a child need by no means be confined to the child's biological father. When a child is born there is often an intensive search, by biological parents and those around them, for the characteristics in the child which most resemble each parent (e.g., he has his mother's hair or temperament; she's tall or stubborn or bright just like her father). Overall suggests that "in rearing one's genetically related offspring, very real experiences are involved in discerning and appreciating the similarities between oneself and one's children ... there is a sense of continuity and history created by the genetic tie."[7] This need not reflect the eugenic notion that these particular biological characteristics are superior to others; these characteristics may simply symbolize to the parents the child's connection to past generations and the ability to extend that lineage forward into the future. The biological parent is enmeshed in the cycle of life that began in the distant past and now is extending through them into the future. Knowledge of one's ancestors can assist in developing one's identity, whether it is specific to one's ethnic or cultural background/traditions or to the types of individuals from whom one is descended. This is not the only way to form one's identity, but it is an important aspect of

doing so for many individuals. Biological parents may feel that the knowledge of this "genealogical heritage" is an important contribution to give to their children. Additionally, a biological parent may appreciate being an intimate part of the process which creates a new generation in the family.

We can thus interpret the valuing of genetic lineage negatively as an example of eugenics, narcissism, or a way of achieving immortality; or we can make a more neutral or positive interpretation, such as seeing the value of creating a new generation, giving a child a known genealogical heritage, or simply possessing another bond between parent and child which allows parents to weather the invariable strains associated with parenthood. Attachment to lineage, for whatever reason, may not have much intrinsic value, but its value to potential parents may be sufficient to require that we accord it respect.

Adopting parents do not have this automatic connection or linkage to their child. They must be able to love a child who does not represent an extension of their own bodies and genetic lineages, one who has the potential to be quite different from either parent (not that biological children do not continually surprise parents with their differentness). Adopting parents must also cope with more uncertainty about the child's background, such as unfavorable genetic influences (e.g., inherited illnesses), harmful environmental factors during pregnancy (e.g., drug usage), the potential for the biological parent(s) to change their mind(s) about the adoption, and the possibility that the adopted child will later seek out his or her biological parents.

The difficulties associated with adoption have been widely documented. The increasing numbers of young women choosing abortion or electing to continue their pregnancies and keep their children has reduced the availability of children for adoption. Most middle-class white couples seek to adopt white infants (which are the most difficult to obtain) instead of considering non-white infants or children who are older, disabled, and so on. It may be argued that the strong preference for white infants is misplaced, and that these couples should be willing to provide a home for any children who might need one. However, we must understand that the desire of many of these couples may not be the simple reflection of prejudice or bias. The childless couple may feel less able than a couple with parenting experience to face the challenges involved in rearing the child of a different race or an older child (who may have emotional or physical problems). In the case of adopting a child of another race, the parent must struggle with the question of how to retain the child's cultural heritage when the parent does not possess intimate knowledge of the culture or subculture. The childless couples who take on such challenges are to be admired, but the childless couples who know they are not ready for these potential complications should not be criticized. Interestingly, infertile couples can be placed in a double bind. If they do not adopt children of another race they can be characterized as selfish or narrow-minded, but if they do, they may be criticized because they purportedly lack the cultural sensitivity to properly parent a child from a different ethnic heritage.

There is not much support for adoption in our culture. Adopting parents have to make their way through a bewildering array of legal red tape with little guidance. They do not experience the same anticipation and preparation for dealing with an infant that is associated with pregnancy.[8] The pregnant woman becomes a social stimulus for advice concerning childrearing and is "showered" with information and items that can help her adapt to her new role as mother. Adopting parents get much less of this support and preparation for their new role. Because there is so much uncertainty built into the adoption process, it is too often difficult for prospective adopting couples to reach out for support and for others to provide it. As a result, preparation for this transition and the transition itself is often made in seclusion and silence.

Biological parenting is a vastly different experience. First, there is the ability to directly experience pregnancy and childbirth. The process of watching one's own body undergo transformations during pregnancy, establishing emotional connections with the fetus by feeling movements through the abdomen, and giving birth are unique to biological parents. This ability to share in the creation of a child and to experience the early stages of fetal development are highly valued by many individuals. Biological parenting may be especially meaningful to many

because it allows the woman to participate in a remarkable natural process which is unlike any other. With adoption you enter the world of parents, but with childbirth you enter the fertile world.[9] The fertile world encompasses the sisterhood of women who have experienced pregnancy and childbirth, and it establishes a new basis for interaction with others. The sharing of stories related to one's pregnancy and childbirth experiences is an important bonding experience for many women. Childbirth can represent an important milestone in the development of a woman's ability to face fear, pain, and uncertainty.

Feminists understand the value of fertile women striving for a natural childbirth experience which avoids unnecessary medical interventions. But can we understand the value to the infertile woman striving to attain parenthood in a manner that is "as natural as possible"? With adoption, parents receive their child from a stranger in a process which is regulated by lawyers, adoption agencies, and the courts. An individual's ability to parent is scrutinized by various professionals using questionable criteria, and the individual's *social* linkage to the adopted child does not always take precedence in a system that juggles the simultaneous needs of children, biological, and adopting parents.

Although the assisted reproductive technologies (ART) represent a considerable amount of medically related intrusion, they still afford the best approximation to the *natural* processes of conception, gestation, and childbirth available to the infertile. It is important to view adoptive and biological parenting as equally valuable experiences; but it is also important to recognize the many differences between the two and to realize that some individuals may be better suited to one than to the other. An understanding of these two very different parenting experiences makes it inappropriate to simply reduce them to the competing value of genetic versus social linkages.

BIOLOGICAL MOTHERHOOD AND FEMINISM

For all of recorded history, motherhood has often come at a high price—one which has been paid willingly by some, and not so willingly by others. Overall has argued that an infertile woman should not be blamed for her pursuit of infertility treatment because the desire to become a mother is "socially created" in our pronatalist culture.[10] But the social forces that encourage women to bear children cannot entirely explain the desire of some women to become biological mothers and their willingness to pay dearly for this experience. Automatically reducing this desire to an example of effective pronatalist influence is condescending and patronizing toward infertile women as a group and denies the diversity of these women.

In my years of research and clinical experience with the infertile, I have found that most women pursuing medical treatment for infertility are high achievers who have attained remarkable educational and occupational goals. Yet, despite their level of personal accomplishment in these spheres, they also desire to become biological mothers. No matter how much money, prestige, and higher education are touted as signs of personal achievement in our patriarchal society, many women who possess these things still value becoming biological mothers. Even though they have achieved so much in their lives, some still feel that something is missing. To dismiss their desire to experience pregnancy, childbirth, and rearing their own biologically related children is to endorse traditional patriarchal symbols of achievement. Ruth Hubbard seems to suggest that, somehow, a true feminist could not desire motherhood via assisted reproduction: "Some strong, deep feminist consciousness raising might end up being far more therapeutic in the long run than broadening the scope of the technological fix."[11] But using these technologies to achieve biological motherhood does not necessarily reflect that a woman is acting out of mindless socialization. Nor is this incompatible with a feminist consciousness. To claim as much reveals a profound insensitivity to the experience and feelings of infertile women. In fact, the infertile women I have worked with have usually given a great deal of thought to why they want to be biological mothers—often much more thought than fertile women—because they have had to face greater obstacles in order to become biological mothers. As Frost has pointed out, "infertile women sometimes don't hear from the feminist movement that it can be a rational choice to have as well as not to have children."[12]

Let us make sure that when we make a stand against the pronatalist motherhood mandate, we do not oppose mothering. Mothering occurs in many shapes and forms, and we need to embrace this diversity. To dismiss the infertile woman's desire to be a biological mother as simply a pronatalist creation is not even congruent with how we feminists celebrate the wonder of birthing. Feminists have understood childbirth as a way to affirm our uniqueness and power as a gender.[13] Feminists often take inspiration from the tradition of goddess worship, which draws many images of power from the woman giving birth.[14] Since the powerful images of the birth experience can be promoted and affirmed by the feminist community, it hardly seems consistent or reasonable to erect a double standard about the wonders of childbirth when it comes to the infertile.

THE MEDICALIZATION AND COMMODIFICATION OF REPRODUCTION

Other feminist concerns regarding the new reproductive technologies have focused on the extent to which these technologies medicalize reproduction. We have already witnessed the medicalization of pregnancy and childbirth by the introduction of the disease model, fetal monitoring, uterofetal therapy, and cesarean sections. Although, in certain cases, these interventions can be lifesaving, they have represented an increasing tendency for physicians to control childbirth and to view the fetus as a separate patient, often to the detriment of the pregnant woman. In the world of medicalized childbearing fetal rights have become primary; control of the natural process of pregnancy and birth have shifted from pregnant woman to physicians.

Medicalized reproduction carries this tendency one step further. With increasing medical intervention in conception, physicians become viewed as the co-creators of children.[15] The focus of who is responsible for a pregnancy has shifted from the woman to the physicians, who can be congratulated on "getting her pregnant." Since the majority of physicians are still men, this can represent men taking control over the final vestige of power which formerly remained within the female sphere.

When a physician exerts control over the process of hormonal fluctuations, ovulation, transfer of gametes or embryo to the fallopian tube or uterus, placement of sperm and ova in close proximity, and selection of embryos for implantation, this clearly medicalizes conception. For fertile women, these interventions constitute a loss of control over a normal reproductive process, much as a woman undergoing a cesarean section has lost control over her labor. However, for an infertile woman who cannot conceive "naturally," these interventions can represent her only chance at exerting *any* control in reproduction. Further, some of these technologies, such as artificial insemination, expand the reproductive options available to lesbian and single heterosexual women. It is important to realize that many feminists have embraced technology in certain areas of reproduction, such as contraception and abortion, that assist women in avoiding unwanted conception or in terminating an unwanted pregnancy. Although we accept medical interventions in reproduction when they help us resist the pronatalist agenda, some feel less comfortable with medical interventions when they are used to enable procreation. But we must be aware that the acceptance of medical interventions to maximize the choices available to infertile women is not the same as uncritically accepting the medicalization of reproduction.

Related to concerns about the medicalization of reproduction are concerns about the commodification of reproduction and children, which are also raised by feminists.[16] In general, body parts have become increasingly viewed as "products" which can be assigned monetary value and exchanged for financial reimbursement. In human reproductive medicine, sperm has been a purchasable commodity in artificial insemination for decades. Although the amount of money paid for sperm is nominal (e.g., $35), the selling and buying of sperm symbolizes the commodification of life-giving potential. Similarly, reproductive technologies have evolved to the point where one woman can "donate" eggs to another or can have an embryo implanted in her uterus in order to gestate a fetus for herself or someone else. In the latter case, a woman effectively "rents" her womb in serving as a contract mother who is expected to surrender the child at birth. Although oocytes can be given without the expectation of financial compensation (especially if the donor knows the recipient or is already undergoing IVF), in the United States, compensation is typically given for anonymous oocyte donation, with payment ranging between $900 and $1200 per cycle.[17] Contract motherhood arrangements can involve payments in the $10,000 range.[18]

The processes of donating sperm, donating an egg, and using one's womb to gestate a fetus are all quite distinct.[19] For a man to donate sperm, masturbation into a container is all that is required. While this may not be a psychologically comfortable process, it does not involve any physical injury or risk to a man's health. On the other hand, a woman making an egg donation assumes a degree of physical risk. Egg or oocyte donation involves taking injections of powerful hormones for a period of time to promote the simultaneous maturing of several oocytes (egg cells) and then undergoing a surgical procedure where oocytes are aspirated from the ovary through a puncture in the vagina. Finally, a woman who agrees to become a "surrogate" or contract mother may also undergo some hormonal manipulations, will experience an embryo transfer or artificial insemination procedure, may take hormones to maintain the pregnancy, and, of course, is exposed to all the attendant risks of pregnancy and childbirth.[20]

The issue of whether financial reimbursement is ethical and appropriate requires careful consideration. First, there is the question: For what is a prospective "donor" or provider being remunerated? Does the money represent payment for the process of "donation" (e.g., time, effort, pain) or for the gamete/baby? In oocyte donation, donors receive reimbursement for undergoing the process of donation, regardless of whether viable oocytes are obtained.[21] However, in sperm donation, the donors are required to meet specific sperm parameters necessary for the freezing process, and compensation is not provided for this initial screening of the sperm sample.[22] If the donor continues to meet the criteria, then compensation is provided for subsequent sperm samples. Therefore, compensation appears to be provided more for the sperm itself, rather than for the process of providing the sperm. Similarly, compensation in contract motherhood arrangements, which is ostensibly the services of gestation and childbirth, is not provided if the child is not turned over to the infertile couple. Therefore, the payment appears to be for the child and not for the process of gestation. Only oocyte donation appears to circumvent the symbolic purchase of a child or of life-giving potential.

The effects of reimbursement in gamete donation needs further exploration. Financial reimbursement can contribute to the commodification of gametes and of reproduction more generally, as well as potentially lead to exploitation of the economically disadvantaged. Moreover, payment for the "donation" can change the process of giving. The financial payment can alter the meaning of the "donation" for the donor, the recipient, and the child born from such an arrangement. An adult born from artificial insemination by donor (AID) echoes this sentiment when she stated, "No one considers how the child feels when she finds that her natural father was a $25 cup of sperm."[23] At the same time, however, payment makes anonymous donation more viable and circumvents difficulties involved with obtaining known donors. Additionally, if financial incentives are eliminated, those who donate primarily for eugenic reasons may predominate in the remaining pool of donors—a possibility many find repugnant.

If anonymous gamete donors are not used, pressure may be exerted upon infertile individuals to provide friends or family members to assist them in their quest for pregnancy. Friends and family may sympathize with the infertile couple and feel subtle or not-so-subtle pressure to donate. "Known donation" potentially involves all the physical risks detailed previously, but there may be particular long-term psychological risks as well. A harmonious friendship or sibling relationship may be jeopardized at a later point when the donor feels uncomfortable about his or her donation, how the child is being reared, decisions made regarding secrecy versus openness, and so forth. However, when a donor is known to the recipient, greater background information is available (including the medical history, which may be important). Some may argue that family medical history is not always clearly known, even when children are reared with their biological parents. But circumstances may make this information indispensable, and it needs to be available to be gathered whenever possible. Even with anonymous "donors," a great deal of non-identifying information can be obtained and provided to the recipients. For example, the overwhelming majority of sperm donors in a U.S. sample were willing to complete a detailed 12-page questionnaire covering in-depth medical and psychosocial information on themselves which could be made available to the recipient(s) and any resulting children.[24] In Australia, donors can be contacted through a registry when the child reaches 18 years,[25] and 60 percent of a U.S. sample of sperm donors also expressed a willingness to meet the child at age 18.[26] A great deal of information can be obtained from a "donor" while protecting his or her identity. But we do need to remain cognizant that financial incentives might influence the level of a potential "donor's" honesty in responding to queries about his or her background.

Given the paucity of research in this area, it is difficult to ascertain the relative risks and benefits of financial compensation and of using gamete donors known to those seeking pregnancy. We do not understand what it means to be a gamete donor—whether it is similar to donating blood or a kidney, or is more like giving a child up for adoption; and we particularly do not understand whether gender differences exist in the psychology or donation.[27] Further, we know little about the impact that these processes have upon the recipients and the children born as a result of these new technologies. It is inexcusable that we continue experimenting with reproduction with so little attention to the psychological ramifications. Our ignorance is particularly alarming in the case of AID, which has been practiced for over 100 years. The shroud of secrecy veiling the practice of AID needs to be lifted. This is not to say that AID couples should never have the option to maintain privacy regarding their particular method of family-building, but we as a society cannot rely on their silence any longer to avoid what may be an uncomfortable examination of what this process entails for all involved. Furthermore, since other countries, like Australia, appear to have successfully adopted a policy of not allowing payment for sperm donations and since the process of sperm donation does not involve an overwhelming investment of time, physical effort or physical risk, and since, moreover, financial motives might distort testimony on medical history and negatively influence resulting children's perception of themselves, it would be beneficial to explore the feasibility of eliminating payment for sperm donation in this country.

Although there are concerns about the process of gamete donation, they pale in comparison to the psychological, physical, and moral concerns involved with contract motherhood. This practice is the most potentially problematic of all the new technologies. Although such an arrangement may be well-intentioned by all the parties involved, the contract mother is in a perilous legal, physical, and most importantly, moral/psychological position. Contract motherhood will be discussed in greater depth elsewhere in this collection, but it deserves some attention here as well.[28]

Use of terms like *uterine environments* or *incubators* sums up the public status of the contract mother. This derogatory language of dismemberment encourages us to consider the womb instead of the whole woman and to view the woman as somehow loaning the use of her womb for nine months, as if pregnancy only involved the womb. Such language encourages the woman to devalue herself and her social and physical relationship to the fetus. The notion that the contract mother is simply "renting" her womb has been challenged by Rothman, who points out that you can't rent a body part without renting the entire woman, and that "women experience pregnancy with our whole bodies—from the changes in our hair to our swollen ankles—with all of our bodies and perhaps with our souls as well."[29] This process of dissociation is different from what is involved in abortion. In electing abortion, a woman is psychologically refusing to enter into a relationship with a fetus,[30] whereas with contract motherhood a woman is beginning a relationship and severing it at a later point (i.e., birth). As a psychologist, I try to listen non-judgmentally to the voices of the infertile: but the pain expressed by women who have placed children for adoption haunts me. How can we expect women to voluntarily subject themselves to this kind of turmoil? And if a woman does not feel any pain as a contract mother, have we succeeded in having the woman dismember and dissociate herself to the point where she is no longer whole? It is hard enough for most women to place an unwanted child up for adoption; how can we encourage women to voluntarily undergo such a treacherous path? The notion that a woman can predict her level of attachment to her fetus and should be held to a previously signed contract is unacceptable. That a woman should be able to respond with emotional distance to the movements of their fetus, to the changes in her body, and to the birth experience, and, somehow, to deny that this child is hers, is not what we as a society should promote. Further, since many contract mothers already have children, how can we expect these children to cope with the fact that their mother has sold their half-sibling at birth?[31] Surely this can cause anxiety in the children regarding the severing of their relationship to the half-sibling and the stability of their own position in the family. In addition, because contract motherhood arrangements serve to enhance the power of white, fertile, middle- to upper-class men at the expense of lower-class women, there are serious concerns about this practice being classist, sexist, and racist.[32] The potential dangers involved with contract motherhood are so great that it is difficult to see how the potential benefits of this procreative option could outweigh its potential risks and negative implications of the women and children involved.

EXPLOITATION OF WOMEN

> Now men are far beyond the stage at which they expressed their envy of woman's procreative power through couvade, transvestism, subincision. They are beyond merely giving spiritual birth in their baptismal-font wombs, beyond giving physical birth with their electronic fetal monitors, their forceps, their knives. Now they have laboratories.[33]

The potential for women to be exploited with these new technologies is great. Especially since the majority of researchers and clinicians are male, procedures that are unpleasant or risky for women may be approached without sufficient caution. Science for the sake of science tends to take on a life of its own, despite the existence of potential risks or negative side effects. Corea has detailed some of the early experimental efforts in the field of reproductive medicine which illustrate researchers' greater concerns for their own status than for the need to proceed cautiously in order to ensure that the risks to women and future children were minimized.[34] The demands for thorough testing with animal models before procedures were applied to humans were ignored in the scramble to achieve personal scientific status (e.g., to achieve the first IVF birth). It is not difficult to imagine that in the future, the welfare of women may continue to be secondary to the pursuit of medical knowledge about reproduction and furthering the careers of scientific pioneers.

The specter of the new reproductive technologies has also raised much futuristic speculation. The frightening brave new world imagined by Aldous Huxley lurks in the back of our minds.[35] Corea's chilling description of embryo manipulation in the cattle industry leaves one wondering what the future might hold for women submitting to this technology.[36] Concerns have been raised that reproductive technologies can lead to "the objectification of children, impoverishment of meaning in the experience of reproduction, damage to notions of kinship, and the perpetuation of degrading views of women"[37] Indeed, all technological advances have within them the potential for abuse. Just as genetic testing and abortion can result in the selective abortion of female fetuses resulting from the general preference for male children, the new reproductive technologies can be used to harm and exploit women, as in the case of contract motherhood. But for the most part, the new technologies involve minimal "known"[38] risks and can provide important options to individuals and couples experiencing infertility.[39] Feminists have taken a pro-choice stance in the abortion debate. It should be equally important to develop and maintain options for those who are limited in their ability to have biological children. The ability to choose if and when to have children is as important for the infertile woman as it is for the woman with an unwanted pregnancy.

RISK FACTORS FOR INFERTILITY

The forces that contribute to infertility make a pro-choice position even more essential. Epidemiologically, there are three primary risk factors for infertility: being black, being a woman with a lower education level, or being a woman of advanced age.[40] It is thought that the higher rates of sexually transmitted diseases (STDs) in the black population

place blacks at increased risk to experience reduced fecundity. Since the best contraceptive protection against STDs remains the male-controlled condom, women are at a distinct disadvantage in protecting themselves and their fertility. More research needs to be done into what factors—e.g., STDs, IUD use, occupational/environmental hazards, and complications following childbirth or abortion—contribute to the higher incidence of infertility among blacks and women with less education and how infertility, particularly in these populations, can be prevented.

Comparatively, more is known about the risk of infertility in middle-aged women. A woman becomes less fertile with age, and there is a greater possibility of various processes interfering with reproduction (e.g., diseases like endometriosis). Increasingly, however, if a woman is to establish an independent economic position she must pursue educational and occupational goals early in life, even though this coincides with her most fertile biological period. For such a woman, it is at the point when she is established in her career and motherhood will not jeopardize her economic position (e.g., she is able to negotiate maternity leave or afford child care) that she is subject to a much higher probability of infertility.

On the other hand, pregnancy during the most fertile time of a woman's life can have the unfortunate effect of trapping women into lower income levels because there is so little governmental, educational, and occupational support for young mothers. As Rothman argues,[41] if we want to decrease infertility by having women concentrate childbearing in their younger years, we have to make that possible economically. The relationship between pregnancy in young women and the cycle of poverty is well established. As a society, we need to understand how economic forces may serve to create reproductive problems. Unfortunately, as part of the backlash against feminism, conservative forces have attempted to interpret the infertility rates among middle-aged career women as the justifiable punishment for trying to have it all—careers *and* motherhood.[42] But we must be cognizant of the political and economic forces which have contributed to these women's "choice" to delay childbearing.[43]

It has been estimated that as much as 39 percent of infertility is either solely or partially due to iatrogenic factors,[44] which can include pelvic inflammatory disease from IUDs or obstetrical surgery, side effects from drugs like diethylstilbestrol (DES), the aftereffects of cervical conization and cesarean sections, and inadequately treated sexually transmitted diseases.[45] Other factors, such as chemical toxins and nuclear radiation, can also contribute to infertility. As Menning stated over two decades ago, "I think the reproductive organs are the miner's canary of the human species. When our miscarriage rate approaches 40 percent in some areas near illegal chemical waste dumps and nuclear reactors; when our children are born defective, not in the 5 percent range, but in the range of 25 percent where Agent Orange has been sprayed; when our infertility rate approaches 20 percent, as it will be in the 1980s—then I think we as a species are in deep trouble."[46] The infertile have paid a high price for the technologies that we have, and technology may at the very least owe them the children they desire to have. We need to look closer at the ways we can prevent that infertility which is preventable. But for those who are presently infertile, primary prevention is too late: their interests lie in having tertiary treatment options made available to them.

THE SILENCE OF INFERTILE WOMEN

While the issues of pronatalism, medicalization, commodification, and the exploitation of women represent the concerns most often voiced by feminists, there are many others which feminists should begin to consider. Among these, the most important is the relative silence of infertile women, an issue not addressed because the feminist dialogue largely emanates from the perspective of the fertile. Amid the numerous viewpoints raised from various members of ethics committees and feminist conferences on the subject of the new reproductive technologies, the voice least often heard is that of the infertile. Instead of allowing those most affected by these technologies ample time to present their viewpoint, fertile individuals demonstrate an amazing lack of concern for the perspective of those who experience difficulty having children. For example, the Health, Education, and Welfare Ethics Advisory Board on reproductive technology was comprised primarily of clergy, physicians, and lawyers, with no identified

infertile individuals among them.[47] At board hearings, witnesses opposed to IVF were invariably either people who had achieved their families or members of the celibate clergy. B. Menning, an infertile woman, described how "right to lifers" would bear witness at these hearings and preface their comments by telling the number of children they had, as if this were a credential for credibility.[48] But, to the contrary, as she points out, the fact that they had achieved their families makes it unlikely that they understand the pain of childlessness.

Similarly, the feminist literature and proceedings from feminist conferences are replete with academic discourse on potential problems with the new reproductive technologies while scant attention is paid to the perspective of infertile women.[49] Feminist discussion on topics such as the status of African American, Native American, or disabled women would never be conducted in a manner such that the women who have these experiences would be essentially excluded from presenting their viewpoints. Yet, infertile women who seek assisted reproduction are almost always perceived as mindless automatons who have succumbed to the pronatalist agenda and are therefore excluded. Their collective voice, perspective, and varied experiences have somehow been easy to ignore and dismiss.

Reproduction is an area in which nearly everyone feels expert. Infertile individuals are continually assaulted with suggestions to try relaxation, vacationing, alcohol, or adoption to enhance the chances of conception. These suggestions come with great vigor and frequency from fertile individuals who possess no knowledge of the effectiveness of these techniques.[50] The infertile are constantly instructed by others regarding what desires they should have and whether or not they should pursue available reproduction assisting treatments. But the question remains: Who should be making these decisions, fertile individuals or the infertile themselves? Whatever we may learn about the risks and benefits of reproduction-assisting technologies, who is in the better position to make decisions about whether to pursue a particular reproductive technology than infertile women themselves?

The infertile are held to an idealistic standard which is not required of the fertile.[51] Society questions their reasons for having children, their willingness to pursue reproductive technologies, their reluctance to adopt, and their discomfort with adopting "special needs" children. There is a bias against the infertile that is revealed when we picture ourselves questioning the fertile in the same manner. For example, the bias against homosexuals is revealed when we turn typical queries made of them toward heterosexuals (e.g., "When did you first realize you were heterosexual?" or "How did you find each other?"). Similarly, the fertile are not questioned about why they want to have children, or why they don't adopt a child. The desire to have children is rarely challenged unless the individual is having difficulty reproducing. Society doesn't ask fertile parents who are comfortable and confident with parenting to adopt children who need homes. Is it then fair to expect the infertile to live up to an ethical standard which is not applied to the average fertile individual? This double standard based on the vagaries of reproductive ability reveals a form of bias not unlike sexism, racism, ageism, or as I have already suggested, heterosexism (perhaps this should be termed "fertilism"). Interestingly, fertile individuals view adoption as a significantly more acceptable alternative than do infertile individuals.[52] Perhaps attitudes towards adoption are influenced by one's own fertility status and the likelihood of personally pursuing such an alternative.

There have been numerous references to the desperation of the infertile found in everything from scientific journals to the popular media. The depiction of the infertile as desperate can serve the interests of the medical profession, which profits from the provision of infertility treatments.[53] Pfeffer asserts that "the views of the infertile are superfluous; they could in fact prove counterproductive because they may contradict those of their doctor. What is required of the infertile is that they submit in silence to the claim that they are desperate."[54] While desperation among the infertile may help physicians justify their desire to develop reproductive technologies, a denial of such desperation can serve to ease our collective feminist consciousness when we resist the development and use of these technologies. A number of studies have been conducted on the psychological reactions of infertile individuals pursuing infertility

treatment. These data do suggest that the infertile are distressed, but not at psychiatric levels.[55] Problems have been noted in the form of depression and interpersonal alienation, with psychological and marital adjustment particularly declining in the advanced stages of treatment.[56] Interestingly, women felt their femininity was compromised by infertility to a greater degree than men did their masculinity, irrespective of which spouse had the infertility problem.[57] The majority of studies investigating the psychological reaction to infertility are conducted on couples pursuing medical treatment.[58] Therefore, we know little about the distress level of the infertile population that does not actively seek out medical alternatives. Nonetheless, a determination of the average overall distress level in this population may be less important than a recognition that infertility is distressing for some, and that if these individuals find it useful to pursue medical alternatives, these options should be preserved.

THE RIGHT TO REPRODUCE

In addition to the conspicuous silencing of infertile women, there are other issues which merit some consideration, including the question of the right to reproduce, the myth of infertility as a female problem, the diagnosis of psychogenic infertility, the absence of primary prevention, limitations in treatment access, and sexist medical terminology. Let me take this in turn, beginning with the right to reproduce.

Some feminist authors have argued that while women have the right *not* to reproduce, there is no corresponding right *to* reproduce in the sense of a right of access to reproductive technologies.[59] Overall argues that women are entitled to abortion services but that access to reproductive technologies sets the stage for potential exploitation of children and women's bodies. While concern for infertile women who are unable to have children without technological assistance is appropriate, the dangers to the society of women are viewed by Overall as superseding the personal needs of the infertile. But can the good of women as a group really be emphasized over the rights of individual women? The alarming rate of unnecessary cesarean sections and hysterectomies on women has not led us to call for the abolition of cesarean sections and hysterectomies. In fact, the potential harm to the community of women may be much more difficult to prove in the case of reproductive technologies than it is for current known rates of unnecessary gynecological surgery.

The United Nation's Declaration of Human Rights claims that individuals have the right to establish a family; but this does not necessarily mean that services should be promised to the infertile. This right generally refers to fertile persons' ability to exercise their own judgement regarding the number and timing of their children and does not otherwise guarantee procreative options for the infertile. Arguing against the state provision of reproductive technologies, some have claimed that we do not have a right to certain biological capabilities, much as we have no right to certain IQ or blue eyes.[60] Yet, when individuals suffer from a disfiguring condition that does not threaten their health but can be corrected with surgery, we do not deny them access to the medical technology which could alleviate the physical stigma they suffer. The stigma of infertility might be similarly understood. Infertility is not a life-threatening medical condition, but it can potentially be remedied through medical intervention. Treatment which can enable the infertile to bear children is the restoration of a normal aspect of our biology. This is not analogous to the individual who aspires to have an ideally shaped nose or bustline. Infertility treatment is not the augmentation of normal functioning so that an imagined deficiency can conform to some idealistic standard of beauty; it is the restoration of functioning within the normal range. Infertile women do not wish to aspire to some above-average standard of fertility; they simply want to be able to bear a child just as other women do.

ABSENCE OF PRIMARY PREVENTION AND LIMITATIONS IN ACCESS

Infertility is a problem for many in our society. But under the current system, there is little effort made towards primary prevention of infertility from known risk factors. Instead there is a focus on "technological overcompensation," with tertiary treatment only available to those individuals who can afford it.[61] Ineffectual sex education in schools and the lack

of funding for infertility prevention has put present and future generations at risk for reduced fecundity. Sexually transmitted diseases (STDs) account for 20 percent of infertility in the United States and 80 percent of infertility in developing countries.[62] In addition to STDs, other factors associated with infertility include IUDs, illegal abortions, dilation and curettage, frequent douching, occupational/environmental hazards, and smoking.[63] Faludi has noted the irony in the recent U.S. Republican administration's promoting the myth of a serious infertility epidemic while refusing to allocate funds for the prevention of infertility.[64]

Approximately one-third of all couples experiencing infertility seek medical treatment.[65] We know very little about the other two-thirds, since most research concentrates on those seeking treatment.[66] There are many reasons why someone who is infertile might not pursue medical intervention, including lack of desire to have children; limitations on finances, time, and access; and so on. The current rate of infertility has been conservatively estimated at 9 percent of married heterosexual couples in their reproductive years.[67] Actually, although there has been much press given to the "infertility epidemic,"[68] the overall rate of infertility has not changed much since 1965.[69] What has changed is the frequency of certain types of infertility. While the number of couples with primary infertility (i.e., childless) has doubled between 1965 and 1982, this has been offset by the decline in rates of secondary infertility (i.e., couples who have had a child but who are currently unable to have another).[70] This inflation in the rate of primary infertility is thought to be the demographic result of the baby-boom generation reaching their childbearing years. Although the overall rate of infertility has not risen, the demand for infertility services has, which is partially a result of the increase in absolute numbers of couples with primary infertility. The reproductive fundamentalism observed in recent years is centered around the provision of technology in order for white, middle-class heterosexual couples to have babies.[71] However, the mostly white middle- to upper-class couples who pursue infertility treatment are not necessarily the population at greatest risk to develop infertility.[72] As mentioned previously, the infertility rate for African

Americans in one and one-half times that of white couples. Our society is not motivated to address preventable infertility caused by STDs among minorities and the poor in our country, or the infertility caused by the mass sterilization of Third World women and the export of toxic chemicals to Third World countries.

The financial barriers to infertility treatment can prevent many infertile couples from having a child. Since infertility treatments are not typically well covered by insurance policies, couples must be able to personally afford these treatments. Advanced medical techniques like IVF are used by only 10 to 15 percent of all infertile couples.[73] But the cost of just one in vitro fertilization cycle can be several thousand dollars. While some forms of infertility treatment are extremely expensive, many could be handled if we had mandatory insurance policies or a socialized health care system. In essence, infertile couples already pay health insurance premiums for the maternity care and sterilization procedures of fertile individuals, but are expected to cover all their own treatment costs as well.[74] It is ironic that the infertile can receive help in paying for the psychological treatment of depression and anxiety which might result from infertility, but not for the infertility treatment itself.[75] In response to such considerations, some states have already begun to introduce legislation to mandate infertility coverage among insurance carriers.

Some have questioned the ability, wisdom, and morality of society's financially assisting infertile couples in their quest to have biologically related children, especially when resources are already limited for existing children. Interestingly, the cost of pursuing infertility treatment is roughly comparable to the cost of adoption.[76] While there are valid concerns about how our economic resources should be allocated, we must not let social and health programs compete against each other for limited dollars while preventing them from competing with other areas of the budget, such as defense spending. As a society, we need to first prevent what infertility we can and then examine the issues of distributive justice. Genuine procreative choice simply does not exist if economic barriers effectively prohibit treatment options for the infertile of limited means.

THE MYTH OF INFERTILITY AS A FEMALE PROBLEM

Infertility is often assumed to be the result of a woman's faulty biology. However, male factor infertility occurs at a rate comparable to female factor infertility. Infertility is the result of a solitary female factor for 35 percent of couples, a solitary male factor in another 35 percent, combined male and female factors in 20 percent, and a factor or factors whose source is unknown in the remaining 10 percent.[77] The bias towards looking at problems in women partially results from the tradition of contraceptive research, which has usually focused efforts on learning more about the female reproductive system. Since more is known about the female reproductive system, a disproportionately larger number of diagnostic and treatment procedures exist for infertile women than for infertile men.[78] Therefore, men are subjected to fewer of the direct strains of diagnosis and treatment. Even when male factor infertility is diagnosed, many of the treatments still primarily involve women (e.g., artificial insemination, IVF). In the past, the assumption that the problem always existed with the woman led some women being subjected to extensive medical testing even before a simple semen analysis was ordered.[79]

Some of this bias may have resulted from men's reluctance to take responsibility for conception, and it may be compounded by the difficulty men have in dealing with their feelings about their own infertility. Male infertility has been encased in a shroud of secrecy. Even though artificial insemination has been practiced widely for decades, there has been comparatively little public debate about the advisability of using "donor" semen in couples with male factor infertility. The explosion of public attention has only occurred in relation to female infertility in which assisted reproductive technologies such as IVF and contract motherhood have been used. Given sex-role socialization processes, it is not surprising that infertile women are more comfortable than infertile men in sharing their difficulties with others.[80] In fact, some women have reported that they wished they had the infertility problem instead of their husbands;[81] and some fertile women with infertile partners have even assumed the infertile identity for their husbands.[82] Our society as a whole seems more comfortable discussing female infertility than male infertility. Future research needs to be concentrated on developing treatment alternatives for male factor infertility so that women do not continue to remain at the center of most interventions, where they are subjected to all the attendant risks. The debate about the advisability of pursuing reproduction-assisting technologies also needs to include those which involve male factor infertility. In particular, we need to fully understand how the secrecy with envelops male factor infertility impacts on women, men, "donors," and the children created through assisted reproduction technology, particularly AID.

PSYCHOGENIC INFERTILITY

Early attempts to understand the relationship between psychological factors and infertility portrayed psychological factors as the cause of the infertility. This psychogenic infertility model was popularized by Helene Deutsch,[83] who utilized clinical case studies to illustrate how unconscious processes (e.g., unconscious rejection of pregnancy) could lead to infertility. Despite its questionable scientific merit, Deutsch's work helped to establish this approach in the scientific and clinical literature. From there the psychogenic infertility model has found its way into the public psyche, as evidenced in the frequently proffered advice, "Relax and you'll get pregnant."

The psychogenic model has typically been applied when no obvious organic pathology has been identified after an infertility work-up. A few decades ago, this involved approximately 30 to 40 percent of the infertile population.[84] However, advances in diagnostic methods have lowered the estimated percentage of "psychogenic infertility" to 10 percent. The process of diagnosing psychogenic infertility by simply excluding medical factors runs the risk of being limited by the current level of medical knowledge. Case studies used to illustrate psychogenic infertility were typically drawn from an author's psychiatric practice. Since women seek mental health services more frequently than men,[85] women became the focus in the search for unconscious processes that could cause infertility. The precedent for a primary focus on women was thus established. Unfortunately, this conceptual model places the responsibility for infertility squarely upon

the psyche of women and can be interpreted as another form of blaming the victim.[86] This is especially troubling because making a diagnosis of psychogenic infertility is fraught with so much ambiguity; conclusive evidence for the mechanisms of psychogenic infertility has remained elusive. Susan Sontag's analysis of illness as metaphor may be particularly pertinent here.[87] She reminds us that "psychological theories of illness are a powerful means of placing blame on the ill."[88] According to Sontag, "theories that diseases are caused by mental states and can be cured by will power are always an index of how much is not understood about the physical terrain of a disease."[89]

It is interesting that the tendency of professionals to blame the infertile for their infertility has been echoed by the conservative movement and by many infertile women themselves. The recent backlash against women has included the view that infertility is the direct and justifiable result of increased sexual and reproductive choice for women.[90] The tendency of others to blame infertile women has been internalized to some extent as well. Roughly one-third of infertile women have been found to interpret their infertility as punishment for some past mistake.[91]

SEXIST MEDICAL TERMINOLOGY

Some of the medical language used to describe various aspects of reproduction is blatantly sexist and pejorative.[92] The use of this language can exacerbate the distress that many women feel in regard to reproductive events and the medical milieu. Infertile women are especially subject to an array of derogatory diagnostic terms. The woman who has experienced multiple miscarriages may be referred to as a *habitual aborter*, while her miscarriage is labeled a *spontaneous abortion*. This use of the term *abortion* departs from the ordinary colloquial use, which is associated with voluntary termination of an unwanted pregnancy. For the woman who has involuntarily lost a much-desired pregnancy, the use of the term *abortion* can be offensive and demeaning. The term *habitual aborter* makes it sound as if the woman has something comparable to a drug habit over which she can, but does not, exert proper control. Miscarriages might be attributed to an *incompetent cervix* or a *blighted ovum*. Yet, when a man's sperm lacks sufficient motility or adequate morphological shape we do not describe him as possessing incompetent or blighted sperm. The diagnosis of a *blighted ovum* is often made even when the embryonic stage has been reached, suggesting that although both sperm and ovum have united to form the conceptus, the fault is clearly with the woman's ovum. Women having trouble conceiving may be diagnosed with *hostile cervical mucus* or an *inadequate luteal phase*. Meanwhile, the uterus has been identified as a *hostile environment* for the early embryo, while the ovaries are sometimes characterized as *senile*.[93] Descriptive terms like *hostile, inadequate, barren,* and *senile,* are not typically applied to male functioning. Rowland further cautions about the inherent dangers of the language of dismemberment, when women are simply reduced to *uterine environments*. There is simply no question that such language devalues women in general and infertile women in particular. It needs to be rejected as unacceptable and eliminated entirely from the professional vocabulary.

CONCLUSION

A number of feminist authors view reproductive technologies as an aggregated whole. But reproductive technologies are greatly varied, and include practices as different as pergonal treatment, AID, tubal surgery, contract motherhood, and in vitro fertilization. When these are viewed as an aggregate, those approaches which are clearly morally problematic (because, for example, they clearly involve the potential exploitation of women) tend to cast their shadow on the remaining interventions. But each of these interventions needs to be examined separately. Perhaps the reluctance of some analysts to do so reflects an overall discomfort with any treatment that corresponds to the pronatalist agenda. It is important, however, to evaluate the potential value or risk involved in each intervention,[94] much as the different international ethics committees have. In a review of 15 ethics committee statements representing eight different countries, Walters found that the committees uniformly viewed in vitro fertilization to be ethically acceptable, while there was strong opposition to contract motherhood.[95] Even infertile couples, who have more favorable overall attitudes about reproductive interventions than fertile couples do, rate contract motherhood as the least acceptable option.[96] These findings suggest that though atti-

tudes can become much more positive when medical interventions are seen as a "personal necessity," infertile couples still do discriminate among the technological options. Yet, many feminists have been willing to denounce all the reproductive technologies by pointing to problematic practices like contract mother arrangements, even though they have been willing to make distinctions between practices when the technologies are counter to pronatalism. The abuses related to prenatal sex identification and the resulting gynocide of female fetuses in countries such as India and China have not led us to denounce abortion. We are able to distinguish between abortions which allow women to terminate unwanted pregnancies and abortions which are specifically designed to kill an unwanted female fetus. Such distinctions need to be made with the reproduction-assisting technologies as well.

Ultimately, the feminist pro-choice position on reproductive control needs to be extended to the arena of infertility. These new reproductive technologies may require the infertile to make a "Sophie's choice" between two undesirable alternatives (i.e., between remaining infertile or pursuing medical interventions).[97] Similar to the "choice" of amniocentesis, which can make a pregnancy experience more tentative and fraught with anxiety,[98] the technologies change the possibilities and experience of reproduction. Whitbeck notes that "although technologies give us control over certain matters ... they require that we make explicit decisions where formerly we made none. As a result, they change our responsibilities."[99] Yet, it is the infertile (not the physicians, the fertile, the pro-lifers, or even the feminists) who are in the best position to make the choices involved. And this choice represents part of the continuum of options regarding reproduction. As Rothman has argued, "The treatment of infertility needs to be recognized as an issue of self-determination. It is as important an issue for women as access to contraception and abortion, and freedom from forced sterilization."[100]

The specter of the reproductive technologies contains much to be both hopeful and fearful about. It is important for the community of feminists to express their views and be heard in the debate over how these technologies should be applied. But as feminists we should, as we do in so many other areas, make sure that the voices of those most affected, the infertile women, are not kept silent anymore. Theirs is not an easy path to traverse. It is replete with physical, psychological, and moral peril. Let us not condemn their desire to explore this path merely because it would be more comfortable for the rest of us to avoid the dilemmas involved. Let us reach out to our infertile sisters and make our way with care.

Author's Note

I want to thank several individuals for their helpful comments and suggestions on earlier drafts of this chapter: Anne Berg, Terry Caffery, Katherine Schwarz, Paul Weingartner, John Wilson, and most important, Joan Callahan.

Notes

1. H. Prather, *Notes to Myself: My Struggle to Become a Person* (Toronto: Bantam, 1970).

2. N. F. Russo, "The Motherhood Mandate," *Journal of Social Issues* 32 (1976), pp. 143-153.

3. N. Chodorow, *The Reproduction of Mothering: Psychoanalysis and the Sociology of Gender* (Berkeley: University of California Press, 1978); J.H. Williams, *Psychology of Women: Behavior in a Biosocial Context*, 3rd ed., New York: W.W. Norton, 1987).

4. Infertility is usually revealed when a heterosexual couple is unable to conceive or experiences repeated pregnancy loss. Regardless of which member(s) of the couple has the infertility, infertility is essentially a couple's problem. Given the infrequency with which single or homosexual individuals have occasion to discover their infertility, this analysis will deal primarily with the heterosexual couple. Although male reactions to infertility have been generally overlooked and there is a need to learn more about them, this paper will primarily concentrate on the female experience of infertility.

5. B.K. Rothman, *Recreating Motherhood: Ideology and Technology in a Patriarchal Society* (New York: W. W. Norton, 1989).

6. Although mothers with adopted children can attempt to nurse the child, it is much more difficult to establish the nursing relationship, and nursing is rarely done.

7. C. Overall, *Ethics and Human Reproduction: A Feminist Analysis* (Boston: Allen and Unwin, 1987).

8. The time it takes to become an adopting parent can be much longer than for a biological parent, yet adopting parents can reach parenthood with less preparation. When pregnancy occurs, biological parents can be reasonably certain that they will become parents at the end of the gestation period. However, a couple wishing to adopt has little assurance, even if they have passed agency screening and are awaiting the birth of a specific child, that they will get to parent a child. A biological mother who is intending to give her child up for adoption has, and should have, the right to change her mind within a certain period of time after the birth. Nonetheless, this places an enormous burden of uncertainty upon an adopting couple and makes it much more difficult for them to prepare for parenthood. Biological parents do not face this kind of uncertainty and tenuousness in establishing their linkage to the child.

9. Although many medical interventions have the potential to assist infertile women in achieving conception, they may not be able to restore fertility per se. Some interventions can restore fertility permanently, while others can do so temporarily or simply circumvent the problem. (e.g., IVF for blocked fallopian tubes.) Therefore, an infertile woman may still be dependent upon the medical profession if she wants future children. Entering the fertile world refers to the experiential level of knowing pregnancy and childbirth; it does not require that the infertility problem has been permanently corrected.

10. Overall, *Ethics and Human Reproduction*, pp. 137-165.

11. R. Hubbard, "The Case against In Vitro Fertilization," in *The Custom-Made Child? Women-Centered Perspectives,* ed. H.B. Holmes, B.B. Hoskins, and M. Gross (Clifton, NJ: Humana, 1981), pp. 259-262.

12. C. Frost, "Feminism and Infertility," *Resolve, Inc. Newsletter* (December, 1980) p. 5.

13. E.F. Kittay, "Womb Envy: An Explanatory Concept," in *Mothering: Essays in Feminist Theory*, ed. J. Treblicott (Rowman and Allanheld, 1984).

14. J. Campbell, *The Power of Myth*, ed. B.S. Flowers and B. Moyers (NY: Doubleday, 1988).

15. E.H. Baruch, "A Womb of His Own," in *Embryos, Ethics, and Women's Rights: Exploring the New*

Reproductive Technologies, ed. E.H. Baruch, A.F. D'Adamo Jr., and J. Seager (New York: Haworth, 1988), pp. 135-139.

16. Rothman, *Recreating Motherhood,* pp. 65-84.

17. L.R. Schover et al., "Psychological Follow-up of Women Evaluated as Oocyte Donors," *Human Reproduction 6* (1991), pp. 1487-1491.

18. Rothman, *Recreating Motherhood,* p. 236.

19. In the United States, donors are typically paid for their gametes, whether the latter are sperm or oocytes. Therefore, the connotations of the word "donation" may not be entirely appropriate to this type of financially based transaction. It is important, however, to note that while "donors" are being paid for their gametes, this may not be the principal reason they donated their gametes. More research needs to be done on the motivations of gamete donors and how financial reimbursement influences the practice.

20. Although the term "surrogate mother" enjoys more common usage, this term implies that this woman is not the *real* mother. Since the woman can be either the gestational and/or genetic mother, the term "contract mother" is a more parsimonious term and will be used throughout the text.

21. Lewis, personal communication (March, 1992).

22. Centola, personal communication (March, 1992).

23. R. Rowland, "Decoding Reprospeak,*" Ms. Magazine I* (1991), pp. 38-41.

24. P.P. Mahlstedt and K.A. Probasco, "Sperm Donors: Their Attitudes toward Providing Medical and Psychosocial Information for Recipient Couples and Donor Offspring," *Fertility and Sterility 56* (1991), pp. 747-753.

25. P.P. Mahlstedt and D.A. Greenfeld, "Assisted Reproductive Technology with Donor Gametes: The Need for Patient Preparation," *Fertility and Sterility 52* (1989), pp. 908-914.

26. Mahlstedt and Probasco, pp. 747-753.

27. Little is known about how the act of "donating" gametes affects the "donor." I am currently conducting a study of male and female gamete providers to investigate their differing motivations and feelings of connectedness to their gametes.

28. See also Overall, *Ethics and Human Reproduction,* pp. 111-136; Rothman, *Recreating Motherhood,* pp. 229-245.

29. Rothman, *Recreating Motherhood,* p. 20.

30. Rothman, *Recreating Motherhood* pp. 106-124.

31. See the discussion in J.C. Callahan, "The Contract Motherhood Debate," *Journal of Clinical Ethics* 4:1 (1993), pp. 82-91.

32. Callahan, p. 86.

33. G. Corea, *The Mother Machine: Reproductive Technologies from Artificial Insemination to Artificial Wombs* (New York: Harper and Row, 1985).

34. Corea, *The Mother Machine,* pp. 99-186.

35. A. Huxley, *Brave New World* (New York: Harper and Row, 1932).

36. Corea, *The Mother Machine,* pp 59-98.

37. M.A. Ryan, "The Argument for Unlimited Procreative Liberty: A Feminist Critique," *Hastings Center Report* (July/August, 1990), pp. 6-12.

38. Since the technologies have been developed so recently it is hard to assess what long-term impact they may have.

39. S.A. Salladay, "Ethics and Reproductive Technology," in Holmes, Hoskins, and Gross, eds., *The Custom-Made Child?* pp. 241-248.

40. Office of Technology Assessment, *Infertility: Medical and Social Choices* (OTA-BA-358) (Washington, D.C.: U.S. Government Printing Office, 1988). The term "advanced age" refers to a woman's reproductive years. Although chronologically a woman who is 40 years old is middle-aged, reproductively speaking she is close to menopause and is nearing the end of her reproductive years

41. Rothman, *Recreating Motherhood,* p. 147.

42. S. Faludi, *Backlash: the Undeclared War against American Women* (New York: Crown, 1991); J.C. Shattuck and K.K. Schwartz "Walking the Line between Feminism and Infertility: Implications for Nursing, Medicine and Patient Care," *Health Care for Women International* 12 (1991), pp. 331-339.

43. Rothman, *Recreating Motherhood,* p. 147.

44. Corea, *The Mother Machine,* p. 147.

45. Corea, *The Mother Machine,* p. 147.

46. B. Menning, "In Defense of In Vitro Fertilization," in Holmes, Hoskins, and Gross, eds., *The Custom-Made Child?* pp. 263-267.

47. B.B. Hoskins, "Manipulative Reproductive Technologies Discussion: Part II," in Holmes, Hoskins, and Gross, eds., *The Custom-Made Child?* pp. 275-280.

48. Menning, "In Defense of," pp. 263-267.

49. It is difficult to discern whether particular authors have experienced infertility problems. But the frequency with which authors fail to identify themselves as infertile suggests that they have not experienced these problems and may be counted among the fertile.

50. B.E. Menning, *Infertility: A Guide for the Childless Couple,* 2nd ed. (New York: Prentice-Hall, 1988).

51. I recognize that not all infertile individuals wish to have children. The infertile I am talking about here are those who *are* unhappy because of their infertility.

52. L.J. Halman, A. Abbey, and R.M. Andrews, "Attitudes about Infertility Interventions among Fertile and Infertile Couples," *American Journal of Public Health 82* (1992), pp. 191-194.

53. Corea, *The Mother Machine*, pp. 172-173; N. Pfeffer, "Artificial Insemination, In-Vitro Fertilization, and the Stigma of Infertility," in *Reproductive Technologies: Gender, Motherhood, and Medicine,* ed. F.M. Stanworth (Minneapolis: University of Minnesota Press, 1987), pp. 81-97.

54. Pfeffer, "Artificial Insemination," p. 91.

55. B.J. Berg and J.F. Wilson, "Psychiatric Morbidity in the Infertile Population: A Reconceptualization," *Fertility and Sterility 53* (1990), pp. 654-661.

56. B.J. Berg and J.F. Wilson, "Psychological Functioning across Stages of Treatment for Infertility," *Journal of Behavioral Medicine* 14 (1991), pp. 11-26.

57. B.J. Berg, J.F. Wilson, and P.J. Weingartner, "Psychological Sequelae of Infertility Treatment: The Role of Gender and Sex-Role Identification," *Social Science and Medicine 33* (1991), pp. 1071-1080.

58. B.J. Berg, "Psychological Sequelae to Infertility: A Critical Review of the Literature," unpublished manuscript (1993).

59. Overall, *Ethics and Human Reproduction*, pp. 166-196.

60. Hubbard, "The Case," pp. 259-262.

61. Overall, *Ethics and Human Reproduction*, pp. 137-165.

62. Office of Technology Assessment, *Infertility*, pp. 85-96.

63. Office of Technology Assessment, *Infertility*, pp. 85-96.

64. Faludi, *Backlash*, pp. 27-35.

65. Office of Technology Assessment, *Infertility*, pp. 49-60.

66. Berg, "Psychological Sequelae."

67. Office of Technology Assessment, *Infertility*, pp. 49-60.

68. Faludi, *Backlash*, pp. 27-35.

69. Office of Technology Assessment, *Infertility*, pp. 49-60.

70. Office of Technology Assessment, *Infertility,* pp. 49-60.

71. J.G. Raymond, "International Traffic in Reproduction," *Ms. Magazine I* (1991), pp. 29-33.

72. Office of Technology Assessment, *Infertility*, pp. 49-60.

73. Office of Technology Assessment, *Infertility*, p.7

74. J.S. Fox, "Infertility Insurance Update" (Serono Symposia USA pamphlet, 1991).

75. Overall, *Ethics and Human Reproduction,* p.147.

76. Office of Technology Assessment, *Infertility*, pp. 49-60.

77. Menning, *Infertility*, p. 5.

78. Office of Technology Assessment, *Infertility*, pp. 49-60.

79. Frost, p. 5.

80. Berg, Wilson, and Weingartner, "Psychological Sequelae," pp. 1071-1080.

81. C. Crowe, "'Women Want it': In-Vitro Fertilization and Women's Motivations for Participation," *Women's Studies International Forum 8* (1985), PP. 547-552.

82. J.D. Czyba and M. Chevret, "Psychological Reactions of Couples to Artificial Insemination with Donor Sperm," *International Journal of Fertility 24* (1979) pp. 240-245.

83. H. Deutsch, *Psychology of Women: Volume II, Motherhood* (New York: Grune and Stratton, 1945), pp. 106-125

84. M.D. Mazor, "Barren Couples," *Psychology Today 12* (1979), pp. 101-112.

85. Williams, *Psychology of Women*, pp. 445-463.

86. Frost, p. 5.

87. S. Sontag, *Illness as Metaphor and AIDS and Its Metaphors* (New York: Doubleday, Anchor Books, 1990), pp. 55-57.

88. Sontag, *Illness as Metaphor,* p. 57.

89. Sontag, p. 55.

90. Faludi, *Backlash* pp. 27-35; M. Sandelowski, "Sophie's Choice: A Metaphor for Infertility," *Health Care for Women International 7* (1986), pp. 439-453.

91. Berg, Wilson, and Weingartner, "Psychological Sequelae," pp. 1071-1080.

92. B.J. Berg, "Sexism and Medical Terminology," Letters to the Editor, *Women's Health Issues 2* (in press); Menning, "In Defense of," pp. 263-267.

93. Rowland, pp. 38-41.

94. Ryan, pp. 6-12; Rothman, *Recreating Motherhood*, pp. 140-151.

95. L. Walters, "Ethics and New Reproductive Technologies: An International Review of Committee Statements," *The Hastings Center Report* (1987), pp. 3-22.

96. Halman, Abbey, and Andrews, "Attitudes," pp. 193-194.

97. Sandelowski, "Sophie's Choice," pp. 439-453.

98. B.K. Rothman, *The Tentative Pregnancy: Prenatal Diagnosis and the Future of Motherhood* (New York: Viking, 1986).

99. C. Whitbeck, "Ethical Issues Raised by the New Medical Technologies," in *Women and New Reproductive Technologies: Medical, Psychosocial, Legal, and Ethical Dilemmas,* ed. J. Rodin and A. Collins (Hillsdale, NJ: Lawrence Erlbaum, 1991), pp. 49-64.

100. Rothman, *Recreating Motherhood,* p. 140.

21.
A CASE FOR PERMITTING ALTRUISTIC SURROGACY

Brenda M. Baker

Canada's Royal Commission on New Reproductive Technologies[1] (1993) comes down hard on all forms of pre-conception or surrogacy arrangements[2]—commercial practices involving the cooperation or management of third parties for profit, contractual agreements whether commercial or noncommercial, and noncommercial arrangements, including informal surrogacy arrangements undertaken by close relatives or friends. Commercial arrangements are rejected for several major reasons. Most seriously, they are held to commodify children and treat them as products that can be bought and sold, as means to serve the ends of others. Commercial surrogacy is held to harm surrogates directly or indirectly, and other women generally by exploiting women who are economically and socially less advantaged, reducing the autonomy of gestational mothers with regard to their own pregnancies, and subordinating them to the wishes of infertile couples and to objectionable practices of overmedicalization. It is also said to deny them the opportunity to be responsive to their psychological and emotional experiences during their pregnancies. It is thought to place heavy stress on family relations and to be potentially disruptive for resulting children and their "social" parents. The commission also regards surrogacy as harming society in that it diminishes the dignity of women's reproductive capacities and the inherent value of children by commodifying them, reinforces social attitudes that define women's status and social role in terms of motherhood, and encourages a "market production" model of procreation and of children. Contractual surrogacy arrangements are rejected because they are potentially coercive and exploitative, and wrongly require the gestational mother to give up certain legitimate moral claims in relation to her pregnancy and prospective child, in addition to some of the reasons given above.

One might have thought that the commission would look differently at noncommercial pre-conception arrangements, which involve no third parties in the business of arranging and overseeing agreements and no payments to them. But although the commission expresses sympathy for those who wish to have a family but cannot do so by either the standard means or adoption, it does not speak in favor of permitting any noncommercial arrangements but instead holds that these "should not be undertaken, sanctioned or encouraged." The commissioners' view is that despite the sincere motivation in altruistic surrogacy undertakings, the arrangement "still results in the commodification of a child and of the reproductive process"; the report continues "no one should have the right to make a 'gift' of another human being" (Minister of Government Services Canada 1993, chap. 23, 689). The commissioners also worry about the potential for family members to coerce women into serving as surrogates. They object to the idea that the health risks of pregnancy are borne by one woman for the benefit of another, and express concern about damage to family relations and about confusion on the part of the child.

In this essay, I maintain that the commission's arguments against noncommercial forms of surrogacy are either not well-taken or else not as strong as it believes. Where these have some weight, they can nonetheless be counterbalanced by other considerations so as to make a case for the permissibility or acceptability of altruistic surrogacy, as a practice that is compatible with major values that women share and wish to see recognized in society. Although I am concerned to provide reasons to permit a noncommercial practice of surrogacy, a larger purpose in writing this essay is to stimulate further discussion of such a practice on its own merits. This is a question worth closer exploration, even if a decision is made to prohibit commercial surrogacy agreements and enforceable pre-conception contracts.[3] I shall use the term "altruistic surrogacy" to refer to surrogacy arrangements in which the surrogate is not paid for her services and is motivated mainly by a desire to help an infertile couple to have a child of their own; I will assume that in such arrangements, medical and other expenses incurred by the gestation and birth of the child would be covered by some other source than the surrogate or her family.

My argument is developed in three stages. I first critically assess the objections of the commission to unpaid surrogacy. Here I show that several of the commission's objections, if accepted, would constitute objections to certain practices of gifting that we think worthy and wish to retain, such as organ donation and blood donation as well as adoption. I then outline some positive reasons for permitting altruistic surrogacy. Finally, I consider two important worries that certain feminists have to a practice of altruistic surrogacy. I argue that neither is sufficient to disallow a practice of unpaid surrogacy, though both may warrant monitoring any practice.

The practice of surrogacy can be imagined to take many possible social forms, exhibiting varying degrees of commercialization, public or private regulation, legal modeling, formality, and informality. One can reject certain forms of surrogate practice while endorsing other forms. For instance, one can reject commercial surrogacy while thinking that surrogacy is a legitimate subject for contractual agreements, and one can reject both these frameworks while still thinking that noncommercial practices of surrogate parenting should be permitted or even encouraged. And within each of these categories, there is a large variety of distinct normative configurations that the practice could take; some of these normative practices may be much more defensible than others. For example, a practice of surrogacy contracts could provide that such contracts be voidable if the gestational mother experiences a change of heart, or that a waiting period after birth be required before the birth mother's decision to give up her parental rights to the child becomes final, or that any decision about aborting a fetus is one that should rest with the surrogate alone. It is possible that certain serious worries that one might have about the use of contract

law to govern surrogate agreements could be laid to rest by ensuring that one or more of these conditions is obtained. If the commission had looked more closely at how some of the worries they canvass and the values they want to protect might have been addressed by regulating certain practices of surrogacy appropriately, I expect they would not have reached the fairly sweeping negative conclusions that they did reach about all forms of surrogacy.

Let me begin by taking up the commission's suggestion that even noncommercial surrogacy results in commodification of children and the reproductive process. It is uncertain just what the charge of commodification comes to here, since the matter of payment is excluded, by definition, in these cases. There are no commodities here in the sense of objects of commercial exchanges, such as buying and selling. If the objection is that any transfer of newborn children from a parent to another prospective parent whether biologically related or not, or that any conception or pregnancy where it is intended that the ensuing infant be cared for by someone other than the gestational mother, amounts to commodification, then it is too quick. The objection would imply that the practice of adoption entails some objectionable commodification of children, despite the fact that adoption law forbids any payment for children precisely in order to avoid treating them as commodities. There are many circumstances in which things or rights to things are transferred from one person to another, as in gift-giving, donations in response to need, appointments to positions, and so on, and these transfers are not regarded as commodity transfers. It is true, of course, that there are some transfers of rights or authority over persons that we do object to as wrongly commodifying persons. This would be the case, for example, of a cultural practice of paternal giving of young women as property to their husbands-to-be. Our objection to this practice as commodifying persons, however, turns on the failure of the practice to respect the moral rights (and capabilities) of these women as persons to self-determination. In the case of altruistic surrogacy (and adoption), as long as care is taken to secure the informed and voluntary consent of the parties, there is no objectionable disregard of the surrogate or treatment of her merely as a means or as property, nor do we have reason to regard the child as having its interests or choices disregarded. Surrogacy can be thought of as the consensual provision of a valuable service for another, and the transfer of the child is governed by the idea that its interests will be well met by transferring parental responsibility for it.

Nonetheless, it might be thought that there is a deeper concern which these remarks do not sufficiently address. There is a (not well articulated) line of argument in the commission's report which focuses on the children who are the "subjects" of pre-conception arrangements, and contends that these are treated as objects whose disposition is for the benefit of the contracting couple and the gestational mother. The objection would be that surrogacy arrangements, whether commercial or noncommercial, involve the creation and the transfer of children not for their own benefit, but for the benefit of the adult caretakers involved. This amounts to an objectification of children, a treating of them as objects or things, and is a stage in the direction of their commodification.[4] This concern is not removed by the removal of commercial interests or by ensuring that the women participants are respected as autonomous and protected from exploitation. Even where the child is given to another out of generosity or love, one might worry that the child is being treated as an object. This may explain the commission's remark that "no one should have the right to make a 'gift' of another human being," a claim which is certainly true of adult human beings and of children of most ages.

We might try to develop this line of objection in a way that differentiates pre-conception arrangements from blood or organ donation and from adoption. Doing so might reveal disanalogies between cases that I treated above as similar. In the case of organ or blood donation, what is given is something that is recognizably an object although it is also a necessary means to life for the recipient, whereas in surrogacy what is given is actually a living individual, a human being with a life of its own. The transfer of the child from the gestational mother to the social parents is an essential feature of surrogacy, and this may be thought to constitute an unacceptable objectification of the child. In the case of adoption or foster-parenting, there is already in existence a child or potential child whose needs and interests should predominate

in finding for it a caretaker that it now lacks, whereas in the case of surrogacy the situation seems reversed, in that a child who would not otherwise have existed is created in order to satisfy the needs and interests of already existing adults.

How should we respond to these concerns? I think their objective is to claim that surrogate arrangements treat the child involved as an object in some morally undue or morally objectionable way. I do not think that this conclusion follows from most of the observations just presented, although the issues are complex and cannot be entirely resolved here. Some responses seem in order. First, no surrogacy practice need regard children as objects or property with which one can do whatever one wishes. The social parents, and often the birth mother, are bound by obligations of parenthood. Nor does the fact that a practice permits a child to be transferred at birth under certain strict conditions imply that children in general are in any way objects that may be regularly and appropriately transferred between adults. It does not imply that we can make gifts of human beings, generally speaking. Second, in altruistic surrogacy the social parents have hopes and aspirations for their child and want a good life for it; and the surrogate mother is willing to gestate the child only because she appreciates the joys of parenting and believes that the child will have a good life in a loving family setting with parents who want it very much. So although a new life is created in surrogacy, in contrast with the cases of adoption, foster-parenting, or other custodial transfers, a governing idea remains that of securing the interests of a child in enjoying a fulfilling and satisfying life. Third, if there is something morally objectionable about creating a child because doing so will fulfill certain interests or wishes that existing adults have in doing so,[5] then we must say that natural biological reproduction in traditional families is morally suspect. For it is simply not true that biological parents have children purely for the sake of the children themselves; they have them for a wide variety of personal reasons, such as continuing the family line, expressing their love for one another through creating and raising a family, wishing to experience new personal relationships with their children, providing siblings for their other children, and so on. While it is not part of this essay to defend the traditional biological family, it is reasonable to point out that a criterion for an acceptable practice of reproduction which casts suspicion on reproduction in the normal biological family is probably too demanding. Finally, there are reasons to think that both the desire and the capacity to foster the best interests of resulting children would be greater within a practice of altruistic surrogacy than it would be in natural families, where some children are unexpected and unwanted and adults are not screened for parenting suitability.

Is there some other interpretation of surrogate parenting relationships which could lend credence to worries about undue objectification of either the children or the women involved?

Perhaps one reading could pose problems: suppose surrogacy, altruistic or not, inclines a woman to regard herself as a "reproductive vessel" and to separate herself from her developing fetus by regarding it not as "her own prospective child" but as a child who belongs to and is transferable to another at birth. The commission seems to have such a view in mind when it speaks of surrogacy as "placing women in the situation of alienating aspects of themselves that should be inherently inalienable."

This claim of the commission should be regarded with skepticism. The argument is similar to a more general argument posed by the Quebec Council for the Status of Women to the effect that reproductive technologies threaten to fragment the reproductive process and to alienate women from their own reproductive capacity. But the increasing ability provided by technology to control and separate different phases of female reproduction does not always make for the fragmentation of "mothering," as contraception and abortion witness. These have given women much more control over their roles as mothers, and have allowed women to regard mothering as one, but only one, important role in which their aspirations for themselves may be fulfilled. Being able to distinguish and separate themselves from their reproductive capacities has been for most women a liberating experience contributing to an enlarged sense of personal autonomy, rather than an alienating experience. So if the commission thinks that the whole sequence of reproduction should be an "inherently inalienable" aspect of a woman's self-understanding, then I must disagree.

But perhaps surrogacy specifically "fragments maternity" in an unacceptable way, by distancing women from the children they are carrying for others? Any general worry of this sort underestimates the diversity of attitudes that women can assume toward their individual pregnancies and ignores the evidence we have about women's motivations for becoming surrogates. Studies of existing surrogacy programs have found that surrogates are usually women with families of their own who wish to re-experience the joy and ease of being pregnant but who do not want to raise another child themselves. They are strongly motivated by empathy with the infertile couple (woman), having found the experience of having children to be very important in their own lives, and they desire to help another couple share this special experience.[6] They find the experience of surrogate motherhood a source of pride, confidence, and control; they receive satisfaction and an enhanced sense of self-worth from having accomplished something they think to be of tremendous value, the gestation of a child, with the result that a high percentage of them wish to repeat the surrogate experience. If we can accept these as facts,[7] then I think we should acknowledge that for some women, the separation between being pregnant and raising the child of that pregnancy as one's own that surrogacy incorporates presents an opportunity to be welcomed and enjoyed. It would be moralistic to deny the legitimacy of this perspective as being uncaring or insufficiently maternal;[8] while it may be the perspective of a small minority of women, these same women are deeply supportive of families and children. It is better to embrace this diversity within women's experience and to model our ideas about women's reproductive identity accordingly.[9]

My point here is that we have no reason to think that a practice of noncommercial surrogacy harms the women who participate in it by "commodifying" their reproduction or alienating them from self-affirming experiences. It is a separate argument that any practice of noncommercial surrogacy may be harmful to other women than the direct participants, or inimical to the aspirations of women generally—but I will look briefly at that position later.

The other objections raised by the commission to altruistic surrogacy include the potential for coercion by the woman's family, potential for damage to family relations, and the fact that health risks are borne by one person/woman for the benefit of another. All of these are equally well objections to many forms of organ donation, to participation in nontherapeutic experimental research for the welfare of others, and to adoption and foster-parenting. But we have thus far looked on these practices as permissible despite these risks. Our way of dealing with the associated risks and potential for abuse has been to regulate or monitor these in certain ways, but not to prohibit them outright. Barring further argument, the objections mentioned supply reasons for carefully monitoring or regulating a practice of unpaid surrogacy, but they are not enough to show that unpaid surrogacy should not be allowed.

I now want to move away from the commission's objections to identify some features that give us reasons to permit and even to welcome noncommercial surrogacy. Some of these also highlight certain advantages it has over a practice of commercial surrogacy. After making a positive case for altruistic surrogacy, I look at several objections to permitting it as a practice, and assess their strength.

Why should altruistic surrogacy be a permissible form of action for women in a society? Well, most obviously because it is a contribution that women are uniquely equipped to make, one that is evidently fulfilling for a certain subset of women, and one that brings large benefits in that it can satisfy very strong desires had by some infertile couples and infertile women that at present cannot be met by other social means. Permitting altruistic surrogacy should result in greater recognition of the variety of life choices that different women can and do make, by increasing the range of highly desirable choices for a minority of women. But beyond this, surrogate parenting is undeniably an altruistic and beneficent form of behavior, and a society ought to permit and welcome altruistic interactions among its citizens. There are many economic and structural features of our contemporary materialist culture which tend to discourage altruistic and benevolent relationships among individuals, of any gender, and there is too little, rather than too much, sustained action animated by care for the good of others. This is a strong prima facie reason for permitting altruistic surrogacy,

though of course it is not the only value that will need to be weighed.

In addition, because altruistic surrogacy excludes commercial elements, it enables us to appreciate differently what is of value in surrogacy. An interesting analogy here is that of blood and organ donation, where it has been argued that the introduction of the market diminishes the value of what is given by associating it with a "price" that is always "less than" the priceless life-saving gift that blood or a human organ is.[10] A system of voluntary blood donation can be thought of, Peter Singer suggests, as a form of "institutionalized generosity" which affirms certain bonds and common interdependencies between strangers in a community. In a similar way, a practice of noncommercial surrogacy highlights the indispensability of a person's gestational role to anyone's enjoyment of parenting and children, and it allows us to see surrogacy as expressing a relationship of mutual understanding and generosity between the surrogate and the infertile couple. Of course, there are many differences between the blood donor system and surrogacy. The former is anonymous, whereas in existing "open" surrogacy programs, the interpersonal relationship between surrogate and prospective parents is personal and quite intimate. One likely explanation for this difference is that a close relationship grounded in mutual liking and sympathy is important as a framework and support for the lengthy and psychologically complicated process of pregnancy, in contrast with the relatively undemanding giving of blood. Although the relationships established by surrogacy are more personal than those between blood and organ donors and recipients, a practice of surrogacy is able to extend well beyond familial relationships and to bring together persons who were formerly strangers. Moreover, it has the potential to extend its reach beyond conventional family forms to single-sex couples, lesbians, and others.

Much could be said here about the advantages as well as the possible drawbacks of such a practice, but I confine myself to underlining three strengths of altruistic surrogacy's emphasis on relationship and on the importance of what is being given. One strength is that the idea of a personal relationship is a much better model than either that of a contract or that of a commercial transaction for understanding and addressing the complexities and uncertainties of the process involved in gestation and the participants' attitudes to that. Because pregnancy is a culturally value-laden and comprehensive physiological condition which may have significant and sometimes unpredictable emotional and attitudinal effects on the women experiencing it, it is important that prospective parents and surrogates have a framework in which these experiences can be properly acknowledged and conflicts appropriately resolved. Contracts could be made unenforceable against sincere changes of mind that surrogates undergo or subject to post-birth ratification by surrogates; but although these policies would alleviate some feminist objections to the contract model, I am not convinced that the contract model is as well-suited for thinking about surrogacy as is the model of a personal and mutually beneficial helping relationship. The latter incorporates moral, psychological, and expressive dimensions that the former lacks. Second, altruistic surrogacy supports the view that gestation is an indispensable process which can be donated to and shared with others but is not something to be bought, or simply to be compensated for. Third, permitting altruistic surrogacy may help remove it from the control of medicalized reproductive technologies and place it more firmly in the hands of women, with medicine playing an ancillary role. This would reduce the undue "medicalization" of these women's experiences.

Having outlined some reasons for permitting a social practice of noncommercial surrogacy, I turn to look at some objections that can be raised to such a practice. The most important objection to consider is, I think, one posed by feminists who hold that permitting or encouraging altruistic surrogacy will disadvantage women by reinforcing/perpetuating the cultural and patriarchal stereotype of them as nurturant, caring, and self-sacrificial which has historically been responsible for women's inequality. Janice Raymond has developed this criticism in her thought-provoking "Reproductive Gifts and Gift Giving: The Altruistic Woman" (1990). I outline and discuss here only the major lines of her criticism. She begins by questioning the idea that altruistic surrogacy is morally acceptable simply because it avoids the commodification and exploitation

involved in commercial surrogacy. What we should really be considering is the acceptability of surrogacy itself. In order to assess the value of an altruistic practice, Raymond says, we need to consider it in relation to the larger cultural, social, and economic values and structures in which it functions. Altruistic surrogacy must be viewed in the light of the cultural norm that regards women as giving, self-sacrificing, and accessible to meet the needs of others before their own (Raymond 1990, 8-9). This norm of women's altruism is in fact the expression of a male-generated ideology which holds that women are expected to or have a duty to act selflessly and to meet the needs of others; it serves men and disadvantages women. Raymond cites with approval Catharine MacKinnon's remark that "women value care because men have valued us according to the care we give them" (MacKinnon 1987, 29, quoted in Raymond), and she rejects both Gilligan's feminine ethics of care and altruistic surrogacy because these perpetuate traditional male-imposed norms that have oppressed women under the guise of a "moral celebration" of their altruism.

I agree that it is important to consider the surrounding sociocultural ideology and patterns of wealth and power in a society when thinking about the acceptability of a form of altruistic practice. As Susan Sherwin perceptively notes, we have to be alive to the political dimension of gender experiences, practices, and traits when these exist in a sexist culture; concern and caring for the needs of others can be seen as "the survival skills of an oppressed group that lives in close contact with its oppressors" (Sherwin 1992, 50). And it is true, given our history of gender inequality, that altruistic surrogacy looks problematic in a way that blood and organ donation do not, since the latter would apply to members of all genders and economic classes, whereas altruistic surrogacy would apply only to a group in society which has historically assumed almost all of the responsibility for caring of others and whose work has been undervalued. Nonetheless, although these facts of history and ideology warrant caution, I do not think they warrant prohibiting altruistic surrogacy, for the following reasons.

Raymond's reason for disallowing altruistic surrogacy, namely, that allowing it will perpetuate male-imposed stereotypes of women as giving and self-sacrificing, is too inclusive. The same pattern of argument would result in the restriction or prohibition of all sorts of behavior for the reason that allowing them might well have the indirect effect of perpetuating some objectionable gender stereotype or inequality in our society. Should women be discouraged or prevented from entering the caring professions, from raising children, from entering service roles, from volunteer work, because these may have the effect of reinforcing in some quarters objectionable stereotypes of women? No doubt women should be made fully aware of the cultural history of gender-specific roles and gender stereotyping and its effects, but we do not think their subsequent choices should be limited or proscribed. Some tighter connection between the behavior and detrimental effects on women is needed to justify its prohibition.

Another reason is that women rightly value their caring experiences and relationships and think that they embody genuinely worthwhile activities as well as socially important ones.[11] They do not want to deny the value of these, but to bring society to a public recognition of their value and to encourage others to incorporate more such activities in their lives. If women are to bring what is valuable in their own experience into the broader public domain, it is reasonable for them to support opportunities for engaging in other-regarding behavior and beneficent relationships as long as these are properly respectful of the persons involved and of equitable relations between the sexes.

Raymond's criticism of altruistic surrogacy sometimes confuses the view that it should be permissible or acceptable with the view that altruistic behavior is a normative expectation that women should meet. Raymond rightly rejects the view that women have a duty to act selflessly, and that "women's lives should exemplify moral purity and self-sacrifice, whereas men may live by the more minimal rational standards of moral obligation" (Harrison 1983, 29-30, quoted in Raymond 1990, 8). The position under examination, however, is simply that of keeping open certain possibilities of action for women by permitting altruistic surrogacy; there is no reason to take this as imposing any expectation on women, or any norm or duty. Of course, feminists are well aware of the ways in which theoretical possibilities of action can sometimes be socially transformed into normatively charged expectations. But in the case of altruistic surrogacy this seems unlikely, because it will probably be attractive to only a few women and because it entails the kind of commitment that is already recognized as going generously beyond duty.

The view that altruistic surrogacy should be socially permissible is compatible with our maintaining, as feminists, that our and society's first priority should be to establish greater gender equality, and to secure greater opportunities for women to achieve excellence and final satisfaction through work as part of that objective. Given that as a first priority, the opportunity to become a surrogate could be regarded as like the opportunity to become a mother or a homemaker, that is, as possibilities we would want to hold open for women given the diversity of their interests and aspirations. Providing these opportunities would be subordinate to our primary social aim, to improve the perception of and the position of women in society. In this connection, it is likely that permitting only noncommercial surrogacy might slow its spread as a practice, giving us more time to decide on how far reproductive relationships should be restructured so as to improve women's prospects.

Another objection to altruistic surrogacy focuses on risks inherent in its being practiced informally, without professional guidance and direction. Given the importance of protecting the well-being of the child at the center of such relationships, and the duration, emotional significance, and uncertainties of the process of gestation, it would seem irresponsible simply to leave the maintenance of the surrogacy relation to the parties themselves. In response to this concern, I think we must agree that any practice of surrogacy, including an altruistic one, will need to be regulated in a variety of ways. Regulation is importantly different from commercialization, however. Regulations will be needed to determine such matters as eligibility to participate in a surrogacy arrangement (e.g., evidence of infertility in couples, fertility in potential surrogates, suitability to assume parental responsibilities, stability in the surrogate's spousal and family situation, etc.), to specify needed medical procedures governing conception and pregnancy, and to determine how costs will be allocated. There will also need to be legal provisions that protect certain rights for the surrogate and the prospective parents, and ensure the interests of the child in having a secure parentage. These regulations could be administered by existing institutions such as the public health care system or family law. There will also need to be some coordinating body, perhaps attached to a public health care system, which serves to bring together interested parties, facilitates the making of individual agreements, oversees the process, provides resources for resolving difficulties, and so on. This sounds like a lot of regulation. But it is reasonable to require that the practice protect vulnerable individuals and meet standards of social equity by making the practice widely accessible and establishing uniform standards that apply universally. A regulated practice of noncommercial surrogacy should be able to avoid the serious inequities in access that are a feature of commercial programs, where costs to couples begin at about $45,000, only about $10,000 of which goes to the surrogates themselves.

More interesting but troubling is whether a practice of surrogacy needs the assistance of some psychological and ideological "orchestration" in order to run smoothly. Helena Ragoné says that existing commercial surrogacy programs encourage both surrogates and couples to act toward each other in certain stylized or ideal ways. Surrogates are encouraged to develop a "heightened degree of caring, empathy, and consideration for their couples" and "a sense of responsibility and mission as well" while couples are advised about the importance of creating the image of being a loving and devoted couple who would be ideal parents (Ragoné 1994, 40, 42). Ragoné's explanation is that these serve to "normalize or standardize surrogacy by reinforcing certain culturally embedded ideas that participants share" in "culturally palatable ways" (41), namely, that surrogacy, despite being paid work, is a selfless loving act expressing ideals of motherhood. These actions look like a kind of ideological manipulation of the principals by third parties who (whatever their enthusiasm about surrogacy) stand to profit from them. It is hard to know how much this "structural and social matrix" may be needed to offset the commercial nature of these programs themselves, or how much it may be the promotional product of those who have a

commercial interest in seeing their programs flourish. But if such tendencies turn out to be inherent in any regulated practice of surrogacy, even noncommercial practices, this might be a fatal objection to them. Until we have some experience with a noncommercial but regulated practice, we will not know whether such tendencies are endemic and, if so, rectifiable, or not.

Many other questions can be raised about an altruistic surrogacy practice, such as whether it would be too small in numbers to meet the desires of infertile couples for genetically related children and how much moral weight should be given to this should it turn out to be a fact. My purpose here has been the more limited one of showing that the fears outlined by the Royal Commission and by some feminist thinkers are not sufficient to justify prohibiting a noncommercial practice of surrogacy and that there are a number of positive moral reasons for permitting such a practice both as an expression of (some) women's experience and of generosity toward others.

Notes
I would like to thank Mary Wyart Sindlinger and Nicole Wyatt for valuable research assistance in preparing this essay, and Laura Shanner and the editor and a referee of *Hypatia* for helpful comments on an earlier draft.

1. Minister of Government Services Canada (1993). Pre-conception arrangements are discussed in vol. 2, chap 23.
2. Throughout this essay I use the terms "surrogacy," "surrogate mother," and so on. These terms have been criticized by some feminists as misnomers because they suggest that true biological/gestational mothers of children are in fact "substitutes" or "surrogates" for the social mother and that contracting mothers have the role of "mere receptacles" when really they have important emotional and biological ties to the child. A criticism of this sort is made in Gouvernement du Quebec (May 1989, chap 4.1.1), which proposes to use instead the terminology of "preconception contract" and "contracting mother." For purposes of the argument of my essay, however, the language of contract is not more helpful or appropriate, so I have chosen to stay with the terminol-

ogy of "surrogacy" while eschewing any attempt to diminish the vital biological, gestational, social, and emotional roles played by surrogate mothers.

3. This essay does not, however, take a stand on the acceptability or unacceptability of commercial or contractual forms of surrogacy arrangement. A case can be made for thinking that an appropriately structured practice of contractual surrogacy may benefit surrogates in the long run by giving them additional power, protections, and standing. See Andrews (1988) and Gostin (1990). And there is an extensive literature devoted to debating the merits of a commercial surrogacy practice for the advancement of women. Recent discussions include Anderson (1990), Ameston (1992), Satz (1992). Although this essay does not address these issues, it is hoped that a careful look at altruistic surrogacy will provide a useful vantage point for considering the other possible social forms that the practice of surrogacy can take.

4. I am indebted to Laura Shanner, who commented on a version of this paper at the Canadian Society for Women in Philosophy 1994 Conference, for articulating this important line of argument. The argument is clearly in keeping with the commission's concern to ensure that the reproductive policies we adopt serve to protect the most vulnerable members of society.

5. This appears to be the argument of Krimmel (1983). He regards surrogate parenting as immoral because it involves desiring the child "as a means for attaining some other end," including an altruistic end, rather than viewing it as a unique individual personality to be desired in its own right (36). Krimmel's position is criticized by Tong (1990).

6. An intelligent and perceptive analysis of the motivational factors leading to women's participation in paid surrogate programs in the United States is developed by Ragoné (1994, chap. 2). Ragoné's study confirms, while proposing a far more sophisticated interpretation of, motivational patterns found in earlier studies such as Franks (1981) and Parker (1983).

7. The argument of this essay does depend on its being the case that some women's interests and motivations for surrogacy are of this positive kind. Should further studies show that many or most women who participate in such arrangements come later to regret intensely having done so, that would undermine the case for an unpaid surrogacy practice.

8. Nonetheless, it is important to take seriously the idea that parents owe certain responsibilities of care to those whom they create. Nelson and Nelson (1989) argue that such obligations arise from the causal fact of creating a vulnerable individual who needs care, and these are misrepresented by a surrogacy practice that tries to discharge such obligations by finding suitable "social parents" for these children. The argument merits closer consideration, but appears to tie parental obligations too tightly to biology and to make them so stringent that they are virtually indefeasible. I owe these critical observations to Nicole Wyatt.

9. It is ironic that the argument against surrogacy as fragmenting women's reproduction and alienating women from their reproductive experience appears to reinforce a view of women as committed to the bearing and raising of children. This is the very kind of picture of women that many feminists have tried to dispel.

10. "If blood is a commodity with a price, to give blood means merely to save someone money. Blood has a cash value of a certain number of dollars, and the importance of the gift will vary with the wealth of the recipient. If blood cannot be bought, however,... blood becomes a very special kind of gift, and giving it means providing for strangers, without hope of reward, something they cannot buy and without which they may die. This gift relates strangers in a manner that is not possible when blood is a commodity" (Singer 1978, 211; cf. Titmuss 1970).

11. One of the distinctive contributions of feminist theorizing has been to draw attention to the importance of cooperative personal relationships and of caring in our self-understandings and our conceptions of a good human life. See especially Gilligan (1980), Noddings (1984), Kittay and Meyers (1987), Calhoun (1988), and Sherwin (1992).

References

Anderson, Elizabeth. 1990. "Is Women's Labor a Commodity?" *Philosophy and Public Affairs* 19, 1: 71-92.

Andrews, Lori B. 1988. "Surrogate Motherhood: The Challenge to Feminists," *Law, Medicine and Health Care* 16, 1-2: 72-80. Reprinted in *Surrogate Motherhood*. See Gostin 1990.

Arneson, Richard J. 1992. "Commodification and Commercial Surrogacy," *Philosophy and Public Affairs* 21, 2: 132-64.

Calhoun, Cheshire. 1988. "Justice, Care, and Gender Bias," *Journal of Philosophy* 85, 9: 451-63.

Franks, Darrell D. 1981. "Psychiatric Evaluation of Women in Surrogate Mother Programs," *American Journal of Psychiatry* 138, 10: 1978-9.

General Opinion of the *Conseil du Status de la Femme* in regard to new reproductive technologies. 1989. Gouvernement du Quebec.

Gilligan, Carol. 1980. *In a Different Voice*. Cambridge: Harvard University Press.

Gostin, Larry. 1990. *Surrogate Motherhood*. Bloomington: Indiana University Press.

Harrison, Beverly Wildung. 1983. *Our Right to Choose: Toward a New Ethic of Abortion*. Boston: Beacon Press.

Kittay, E. Feder and Diana T. Meyers, eds. 1987. *Women and Moral Theory*. Totowa, N.J.: Rowman and Littlefield.

Krimmel, Herbert T. 1983. "The Case Against Surrogate Parenting," *The Hastings Center Report* 13, 5: 35-39.

MacKinnon, Catharine. 1987. *Feminism Unmodified*. Cambridge: Harvard University Press.

Nelson, Hilde Lindemann, and James Lindemann Nelson. 1989. "Cutting Motherhood in Two: Some Suspicions Concerning Surrogacy," *Hypatia* 4, 3: 85-94.

Noddings, Nel. 1984. *Caring: A Feminist Approach to Ethics and Moral Education*. Berkeley: University of California Press.

Parker, Philip J. 1983. "Motivation of Surrogate Mothers: Initial Findings," *Clinical and Research Reports, American Journal of Psychiatry* 140, 1: 117-18.

Minister of Government Services Canada. 1993. *Proceed with Care: Final Report of the Royal Commission on New Reproductive Technologies*. 2 vols.

Ragoné, Helena. 1994. *Surrogate Motherhood: Conceptions in the Heart*. Boulder: Westview Press.

Raymond, Janice. 1990. "Reproductive Gifts and Gift-giving: The Altruistic Woman," *The Hastings Center Report* Nov/Dec: 7-11 .

Satz, Debra. 1992. "Markets in Women's Reproductive Labor," *Philosophy and Public Affairs* 21, 2: 107-31.

Sherwin, Susan. 1992. *No Longer Patient*. Philadelphia: Temple University Press.

Singer, Peter. 1978. "Rights and the Market," in John Arthur and William Shaw, eds, *Justice and Economic Distribution*. Englewood Cliffs, N.J.: Prentice Hall.

Titmuss, Richard M. 1970. *The Gift Relationship*. London: Allen and Unwin.

Tong, Rosemarie.1990. "The Overdue Death of a Feminist Chameleon: Taking a Stand on Surrogacy Arrangements," *Journal of Social Philosophy* 21, 2-3: 40-56.

CHAPTER FIVE

FETAL RIGHTS?

22.
WHY ABORTION IS IMMORAL

Don Marquis

The view that abortion is, with rare exceptions, seriously immoral has received little support in the recent philosophical literature. No doubt most philosophers affiliated with secular institutions of higher education believe that the anti-abortion position is either a symptom of irrational religious dogma or a conclusion generated by seriously confused philosophical argument. The purpose of this essay is to undermine this general belief. The essay sets out an argument that purports to show, as well as any argument in ethics can show, that abortion is, except possibly in rare cases, seriously immoral, that it is in the same moral category as killing an innocent adult human being.

The argument is based on a major assumption. Many of the most insightful and careful writers on the ethics of abortion—such as Joel Feinberg, Michael Tooley, Mary Anne Warren, H. Tristram Engelhardt, Jr., L.W. Sumner, John T. Noonan, Jr., and Philip Devine[1]—believe that whether or not abortion is morally permissible stands or falls on whether or not a fetus is the sort of being whose life it is seriously wrong to end. The argument of this essay will assume, but not argue, that they are correct.

Also, this essay will neglect issues of great importance to a complete ethics of abortion. Some anti-abortionists will allow that certain abortions, such as abortion before implantation or abortion when the life of a woman is threatened by a pregnancy or abortion after rape, may be morally permissible. This essay will not explore the casuistry of these hard cases. The purpose of this essay is to develop a general argument for the claim that the overwhelming majority of deliberate abortions are seriously immoral.

I

A sketch of standard anti-abortion and pro-choice arguments exhibits how those arguments possess certain symmetries that explain why partisans of those positions are so convinced of the correctness of their own positions, why they are not successful in convincing their opponents, and why, to others, this issue seems to be unresolvable. An analysis of the nature of this standoff suggests a strategy for surmounting it.

Consider the way a typical anti-abortionist argues. She will argue or assert that life is present from the moment of conception or that fetuses look like babies or that fetuses possess a characteristic such as a genetic code that is both necessary and sufficient for being human. Anti-abortionists seem to believe that (1) the truth of all of these claims is quite obvious, and (2) establishing any of these claims is sufficient to show that abortion is morally akin to murder.

A standard pro-choice strategy exhibits similarities. The pro-choicer will argue or assert that fetuses are not persons or that fetuses are not rational agents or that fetuses are not social beings. Pro-choicers seem to believe that (1) the truth of any of these claims is quite obvious, and (2) establishing any of these claims is sufficient to show that an abortion is not a wrongful killing.

In fact, both the pro-choice and the anti-abortion claims do seem to be true, although the "it looks like a baby" claim is more difficult to establish the earlier the pregnancy. We seem to have a standoff. How can it be resolved?

As everyone who has taken a bit of logic knows, if any of these arguments concerning abortion is a good argument, it requires not only some claim characterizing fetuses, but also some general moral principle that ties a characteristic of fetuses to having or not having the right to life or to some other moral characteristic that will generate the obligation or the lack of obligation not to end the life or a fetus. Accordingly, the arguments of the anti-abortionist and the pro-choicer need a bit of filling in to be regarded as adequate.

Note what each partisan will say. The anti-abortionist will claim that her position is supported by such generally accepted moral principles as "It is always prima facie seriously wrong to end the life of a baby." Since these are generally accepted moral principles her position is certainly not obviously wrong. The pro-choicer will claim that her position is supported by such plausible moral principles as "Being a person is what gives an individual intrinsic moral worth" or "It is only seriously prima facie wrong to take the life of a member of the human community." Since these are generally accepted moral principles, the pro-choice position is certainly not obviously wrong. Unfortunately, we have again arrived at a standoff.

Now, how might one deal with this standoff? The standard approach is to try to show how the moral principles of one's opponent lose their plausibility under analysis. It is easy to see how this is possible. On the one hand, the anti-abortionist will defend a moral principle concerning the wrongness of killing which tends to be broad in scope in order that even fetuses at an early stage of pregnancy will fall under it. The problem with broad principles is that they often embrace too much. In this particular instance, the principle "It is always prima facie wrong to take a human life" sees to entail that it is wrong to end the existence of a living human cancer-cell culture, on the grounds that the culture is both living and human. Therefore, it seems that the anti-abortionist's favored principle is too broad.

On the other hand, the pro-choicer wants to find a moral principle concerning the wrongness of killing which tends to be narrow in scope in order that fetuses will *not* fall under it. The problem with narrow principles is that they often do not embrace enough. Hence, the needed principles such as "It is prima facie seriously wrong to kill only persons" or "It is prima facie wrong to kill only rational agents" do not explain why it is wrong to kill infants or young children or the severely retarded or even perhaps the severely mentally ill. Therefore, we seem again to have a standoff. The anti-abortionist charges, not unreasonably, that pro-choice principles concerning killing are too narrow to be acceptable; the pro-choicer charges, not unreasonably, that anti-abortionist principles concerning killing are too broad to be acceptable.

Attempts by both sides to patch up the difficulties in their positions run into further difficulties. The anti-abortionist will try to remove that problem in her position by reformulating her principle concerning killing in terms of human beings. Now we end up with: "It is always prima facie seriously wrong to end the life of a human being." This principle has the advantage of avoiding the problem of the human cancer-cell culture counterexample. But this advantage is purchased at a high price. For although it is clear that a fetus is both human and alive, it is not at all clear that a fetus is a human *being*. There is at least something to be said for the view that something becomes a human being only after a process of development, and that therefore first trimester fetuses and perhaps all fetuses are not yet human beings. Hence, the anti-abortionist, by this move has merely exchanged one problem of another.[2]

The pro-choicer fares no better. She may attempt to find reasons why killing infants, young children, and the severely retarded is wrong which are independent of her major principle that is supposed to explain the wrongness of taking human life, but which will not also make abortion immoral. This is no easy task. Appeals to social utility will seem satisfactory only to those who resolve not to think of the enormous difficulties with a utilitarian account of the wrongness of killing and the significant social costs of preserving the lives of the unproductive.[3] A pro-choice strategy that extends the definition of "person" to infants or even to young children seems just as arbitrary as an anti-abortion strategy that extends the definition of "human being" to fetuses. Again, we find symmetries in the two positions and we arrive at a standoff.

There are even further problems that reflect symmetries in the two positions. In addition to counterexample problems, or the arbitrary application problems that can be exchanged for them, the standard anti-abortionist principle "It is prima facie seriously wrong to kill a human being," or one of its variants, can be objected to on the grounds of ambiguity. If "human being" is taken to be a *biological* category, the anti-abortionist is left with the problem of explaining why a merely biological category should make a moral difference. Why, it is asked, is it any more reasonable to base a moral conclusion on the number of chromosomes in one's cells than on the color of one's skin?[4] If "human being," on the other hand, is taken to be a *moral* category, then the claim that a fetus is a human being cannot be taken to be a premise in the anti-abortion argument, for it is precisely what needs to be established. Hence, either the anti-abortionist's main category is a morally irrelevant, merely biological category, or it is of no use to the anti-abortionist in establishing (noncircularly, of course) that abortion is wrong.

Although this problem with the anti-abortionist position is often noticed, it is less often noticed that the pro-choice position suffers from an analogous problem. The principle "Only persons have the right to life" also suffers from an ambiguity. The term "person" is typically defined in terms of psychological characteristics, although there will certainly be disagreement concerning which characteristics are most important. Supposing that this matter can be settled, the pro-choicer is left with the problem of explaining why *psychological* characteristics should make a *moral* difference. If the pro-choicer should attempt to deal with this problem by claiming that an explanation is not necessary, that in fact we do treat such a cluster of psychological properties as having moral significance, the sharp-witted anti-abortionist should have a ready response. We do treat being both living and human as having moral significance. If it is legitimate for the pro-choicer to demand that the anti-abortionist provide an explanation of the connection between the biological character of being a human being and the wrongness of being killed (even though people accept this connection), then it is legitimate for the anti-abortionist to demand that the pro-choicer provide an explanation of the connection between psychological criteria for being a person and the wrongness of being killed (even though that connection is accepted).[5]

Feinberg has attempted to meet this objection (he calls psychological personhood "commonsense personhood"):

The characteristics that confer commonsense personhood are not arbitrary bases for rights and duties, such as race, sex or species membership; rather they are traits that make sense out of rights and duties and without which those moral attributes would have no point or function. It is because people are conscious; have a sense out of their personal identities; have plans, goals, and projects; experience emotions; are liable to pains, anxieties, and frustrations; can reason and bargain, and so on—it is because of these attributes that people have values and interests, desires and expectations of their own, including a stake in their own futures. And a personal well-being of a sort we cannot ascribe to unconscious or nonrational beings. Because of their developed capacities they can assume duties and responsibilities and can have and make claims on one another. Only because of their sense of self, their life plans, their value hierarchies, and their stakes in their own futures can they be ascribed fundamental rights. There is nothing arbitrary about these linkages.[6]

The plausible aspects of this attempt should not be taken to obscure its implausible features. There is a great deal to be said for the view that being a psychological person under some description is a necessary condition for having duties. One cannot have a duty unless one is capable of behaving morally, and a being's capability of behaving morally will require having a certain psychology. It is far from obvious, however, that having rights entails consciousness or rationality as Feinberg suggests. We speak of the rights of the severely retarded or the severely mentally ill, yet some of these persons are not rational. We speak of the rights of the temporarily unconscious. The New Jersey Supreme Court based their decision in the Quinlan case on Karen Ann Quinlan's right to privacy, and she was known to be permanently unconscious at that time. Hence, Feinberg's claim that having rights entails being conscious is, on its face, obviously false.

Of course, it might not make sense to attribute rights to a being that would never in its natural history have certain psychological traits. This modest connection between psychological personhood and moral personhood will create a place for Karen Ann Quinlan and the temporarily unconscious. But then it makes a place for fetuses also. Hence, it does not serve Feinberg's pro-choice purposes. Accordingly, it seems that the pro-choicer will have as much difficulty bridging the gap between psychological personhood and personhood in the moral sense as the anti-abortionist has bridging the gap between being a biological human being and being a human being in the moral sense.

Furthermore, the pro-choicer cannot any more escape her problem by making person a purely moral category that the anti-abortionist could escape by the analogous move. For if person is a moral category, the pro-choicer is left without the resources for establishing (noncircularly, of course) the claim that a fetus is not a person, which is an essential premise in her argument. Again, we have both a symmetry and a standoff between pro-choice and anti-abortion views.

Passions in the abortion debate run high. There are both plausibilities and difficulties with the standard positions. Accordingly, it is hardly surprising that partisans of either side embrace with fervor the moral generalizations that support the conclusions they preanalytically favor, and reject with disdain the moral generalizations of their opponents as being subject to inescapable difficulties. It is easy to believe that the counterexamples to one's own moral principles are merely temporary difficulties that will dissolve in the wake of further philosophical research, and that the counterexamples to the principles of one's opponents are as straightforward as the contradiction between A and O propositions in traditional logic. This might suggest to an impartial observer (if there are any) that the abortion issue is unresolvable.

There is a way out of this apparent dialectible quandary. The moral generalizations of both sides are not quite correct. The generalizations hold for the most part, for the usual cases. This suggests that they are all *accidental* generalizations, that the moral claims made by those on both sides of the dispute do not touch on the *essence* of the matter.

This use of the distinction between essence and accident is not meant to invoke obscure metaphysical categories. Rather, it is intended to reflect the rather atheoretical nature of the abortion discussion. If the generalization a partisan in the abortion dispute adopts were derived from the reason why ending the life of a human being is wrong, then there could not be exceptions to that generalization unless

some special case obtains in which there are even more powerful countervailing reasons. Such generalizations would not be merely accidental generalizations; they would point to, or be based upon, the essence of the wrongness of killing, what it is that makes killing wrong. All this suggests that a necessary condition of resolving the abortion controversy is a more theoretical account of the wrongness of killing. After all, if we merely believe, but do not understand, why killing adult human beings such as ourselves is wrong how could we conceivably show that abortion is either immoral or permissible?

II

In order to develop such an account, we can start from the following unproblematic assumption concerning our own case: it is wrong to kill *us*. Why is it wrong? Some answers can be easily eliminated. It might be said that what makes killing us wrong is that a killing brutalizes the one who kills. But the brutalization consists of being inured to the performance of an act that is hideously immoral; hence, the brutalization does not explain the immorality. It might be said that what makes killing us wrong is the great loss others would experience due to our absence. Although such hubris is understandable, such an explanation does not account for the wrongness of killing hermits, or those whose lives are relatively independent and whose friends find it easy to make new friends.

A more obvious answer is better. What primarily makes killing wrong is neither its effect on the murderer nor its effect on the victim's friends and relative, but its effect on the victim. The loss of one's life is one of the greatest losses one can suffer. The loss of one's life deprives one of all the experiences, activities, projects, and enjoyments that would otherwise have constituted one's future. Therefore, killing someone is wrong, primarily because the killing inflicts (one of) the greatest possible losses on the victim. To describe this as the loss of life can be misleading, however. The change in my biological state does not by itself make killing me wrong. The effect of the loss of my biological life is the loss to me of all those activities, projects, experiences, and enjoyments which would otherwise have constituted my future personal life. These activities, projects, experiences, and enjoyments are either valuable for their own sakes or are means to something else that is valuable for its own sake. Some parts of my future are not valued by me now, but will come to be valued by me as I grow older and as my values and capacities change. When I am killed, I am deprived both of what I now value which would have been part of my future personal life, but also what I would come to value. Therefore, when I die, I am deprived of all of the value of my future. Inflicting this loss on me is ultimately what makes killing me wrong. This being the case, it would seem that what makes killing *any* adult human being prima facie seriously wrong is the loss of his or her future.[7]

How should this rudimentary theory of the wrongness of killing be evaluated? It cannot be faulted for deriving an "ought" from an "is" for it does not. The analysis assumes that killing me (or you, reader) is prima facie seriously wrong. The point of the analysis is to establish which natural property ultimately explains the wrongness of the killing, given that it is wrong. The point of the analysis is to establish which natural property ultimately explains the wrongness of the killing, given that it is wrong. A natural property will ultimately explain the wrongness of killing, only if (1) the explanation fits with our intuitions about the matter and (2) there is not other natural property that provides the basis for a better explanation of the wrongness of killing. This analysis rests on the intuition that what makes killing a particular human or animal wrong is what it does to that particular human or animal. What makes killing wrong is some natural effect or other of the killing. Some would deny this. For instance, a divine-command theorist in ethics would deny it. Surely this denial is, however, one of those features of divine-command theory which renders it so implausible.

The claim that what makes killing wrong is the loss of the victim's future is directly supported by two considerations. In the first place this theory explains why we regard killing as one of the worst of crimes. Killing is especially wrong, because it deprives the victim of more than perhaps any other crime. In the second place, people with AIDS or cancer who know they are dying believe, of course, that dying is a very bad thing for them. They believe that the loss of a future to them that they would otherwise have experienced is what makes their premature death a very bad thing for them. A better theory of the wrongness of killing would require a different natural property associated with killing which better fits with the attitudes of the dying. What could it be?

The view that what makes killing wrong is the loss to the victim of the value of the victim's future gains additional support when some of its implications are examined. In the first place, it is incompatible with the view that it is wrong to kill only beings who are biologically human. It is possible that there exists a different species from another planet whose members have a future like ours. Since having a future like that is what makes killing someone wrong, this theory entails that it would be wrong to kill members of such a species. Hence, this theory is opposed to the claim that only life that is biologically human has great moral worth, a claim which many anti-abortionists have seemed to adopt. This opposition, which this theory has in common with personhood theories, seems to be a merit of the theory.

In the second place, the claim that the loss of one's future is the wrong-making feature of one's being killed entails the possibility that the futures of some actual nonhuman mammals on our own planet are sufficiently like ours that it is seriously wrong to kill them also. Whether some animals do have the same right to life as human beings depends on adding to the account of the wrongness of killing some additional account of just what it is about my future or the futures of other adult human beings which makes it wrong to kill us. No such additional account will be offered in this essay. Undoubtedly, the provision of such an account would be a very difficult matter. Undoubtedly, any such account would be quite controversial. Hence, it surely should not reflect badly on this sketch of an elementary theory of the wrongness of killing that it is indeterminate with respect to some very difficult issues regarding animal rights.

In the third place, the claim that the loss of one's future is the wrong-making feature of one's being killed does not entail, as sanctity of human life theories do, that active euthanasia is wrong. Persons who are severely and incurably ill, who face a future of pain and despair, and who wish to die will not have suffered a loss if they are killed. It is, strictly speaking, the value of a human's future which makes killing wrong in this theory. This being so, killing does not necessarily wrong some persons who are sick and dying. Of course there may be other reasons for a prohibition of active euthanasia, but this is another matter. Sanctity-of-human-life theories seem to hold that active euthanasia is seriously wrong even in an individual case where there seems to be good reason for it independently of public policy considerations. This consequence is most implausible, and it is a plus for the claim that the loss of a future of value is what makes killing wrong that it does not share this consequence.

In the fourth place, the account of the wrongness of killing defended in this essay does straightforwardly entail that it is prima facie seriously wrong to kill children and infants, for we do presume that they have futures of value. Since we do believe that it is wrong to kill defenseless little babies, it is important that a theory of the wrongness of killing easily account for this. Personhood theories of the wrongness of killing, on the other hand, cannot straightforwardly account for the wrongness of killing infants and young children.[8] Hence, such theories must add special ad hoc accounts of the wrongness of killing the young. The plausibility of such ad hoc theories seems to be a function of how desperately one wants such theories to work. The claim that the primary wrong-making feature of a killing is the loss to the victim of the value of its future accounts for the wrongness of killing young children and infants directly; it makes the wrongness of such acts as obvious as we actually think it is. This is a further merit of this theory. Accordingly, it seems that this value of a future-like-ours theory of the wrongness of killing shares strengths of both sanctity-of-life and personhood accounts while avoiding weaknesses of both. In addition, it meshes with a central intuition concerning what makes killing wrong.

The claim that the primary wrong-making feature of a killing is the loss to the victim of the value of its future has obvious consequences for the ethics of abortion. The future of a standard fetus includes a set of experiences, projects, activities, and such which are identical with the futures of adult human beings and are identical with the futures of young children. Since the reason that is sufficient to explain why it is wrong to kill human beings after the time of birth is a reason that also applies to fetuses, it follows that abortion is prima facie seriously morally wrong.

This argument does not rely on the invalid inference that, since it is wrong to kill persons, it is wrong to kill potential persons also. The category that is morally central to this analysis is the category of having a valuable future like ours; it is not the category of personhood. The argument to the conclusion that abortion is prima facie seriously morally wrong proceeded independently of the notion of person or potential person or any equivalent. Someone may wish to start with this analysis in terms of the value of a human future, conclude that abortion is, except perhaps in rare circumstances, seriously morally wrong, infer that fetuses have the right to life, and then call fetuses "persons" as a result of their having the right to life. Clearly, in this case, the category of person is being used to state the *conclusion* of the analysis rather than to generate the *argument* of the analysis.

The structure of this anti-abortion argument can be both illuminated and defended by comparing it to what appears to be the best argument for the wrongness of the wanton infliction of pain on animals. This latter argument is based on the assumption that it is prima facie wrong to inflict pain on me (or you, reader). What is the natural property associated with the infliction of pain which makes such infliction wrong? The obvious answer seems to be that the infliction of pain causes suffering and that suffering is a misfortune. The suffering caused by the infliction of pain is what makes the wanton infliction of pain on other adult humans causes suffering. The wanton infliction of pain on animals causes suffering. Since causing suffering is what makes the wanton infliction of pain wrong and since the wanton infliction of pain on animals causes suffering, it follows that the wanton infliction of pain on animals is wrong.

This argument for the wrongness of the wanton infliction of pain on animals shares a number of structural features with the argument for the serious prima facie wrongness of abortion. Both arguments start with an obvious assumption concerning what it is wrong to do to me (or you, reader). Both then look for the characteristic or the consequence of the wrong action which makes the action wrong. Both recognize that the wrong-making feature of these immoral actions is a property of actions sometimes directed at individuals other than postnatal human beings. If the structure of the argument for the wrongness of the wanton infliction of pain on animals is sound, then the structure of the argument for the prima facie serious wrongness of abortion is also sound, for the structure of the two arguments is the same. The structure common to both is the key to the explanation of how the wrongness of abortion can be demonstrated without recourse to the category of person. In neither argument is that category crucial.

This defense of an argument for the wrongness of abortion in terms of a structurally similar argument for the wrongness of the wanton infliction of pain on animals succeeds only if the account regarding animals is the correct account. Is it? In the first place, it seems plausible. In the second place, its major competition is Kant's account. Kant believed that we do not have direct duties to animals at all, because they are not persons. Hence, Kant had to explain and justify the wrongness of inflicting pain on animals on the grounds that "he who is hard in his dealings with animals becomes hard also in his dealing with men."[9] The problem with Kant's account is that there seems to be no reason for accepting this latter claim unless Kant's account is rejected. If the alternative to Kant's account is accepted, then it is easy to understand why someone who is indifferent to inflicting pain on animals is also indifferent to inflicting pain on humans, for one is indifferent to what makes inflicting pain wrong in both cases. But, if Kant's account is accepted, there is not intelligible reason why one who is hard in his dealings with animals (or crabgrass of stones) should also be hard in his dealings with men. After all, men are persons: animals are no more persons than crabgrass or stones. Persons are Kant's crucial moral category. Why, in short, should a Kantian accept the basic claim in Kant's argument?

Hence, Kant's argument for the wrongness of inflicting pain on animals rests on a claim that, in a world of Kantian moral agents, is demonstrably false. Therefore, the alternative analysis, being more plausible anyway, should be accepted. Since this alternative analysis has the same structure as the anti-abortion argument being defended here, we have further support for the argument for the immorality of abortion being defended in this essay.

Of course, this value of a future-like-ours argument, if sound, shows only that abortion is prima facie wrong, not that it is wrong in any and all circumstances. Since the loss of the future to a standard fetus, if killed, is, however, at least as great a loss as the loss of the future to a standard adult human being who is killed, abortion, like ordinary killing, could be justified only by the most compelling reasons. The loss of one's life is almost the greatest misfortune that can happen to one. Presumably abortion could be justified in some circumstances, only if the loss consequent on failing to abort would be at least as great. Accordingly, morally permissible abortions will be rare indeed unless, perhaps, they occur so early in pregnancy that a fetus is not yet definitely an individual. Hence, this argument should be taken as showing that abortion is presumptively very seriously wrong, where the presumption is very strong—as strong as the presumption that killing another adult human being is wrong.

III

How complete an account of the wrongness of killing does the value of a future-like-ours account have to be in order that the wrongness of abortion is a consequence? This account does not have to be an account of the necessary conditions for the wrongness of killing. Some persons in nursing homes may lack valuable human futures, yet it may be wrong to kill them for other reasons. Furthermore, this account does not obviously have to be the sole reason killing is wrong where the victim did have a valuable future. This analysis claims only that, for any killing where the victim did have a valuable future like ours, having that future by itself is sufficient to create the strong presumption that the killing is seriously wrong.

One way to overturn the value of a future-like-ours argument would be to find some account of the wrongness of killing which is at least as intelligible and which has different implications for the ethics of abortion. Two rival accounts possess at least some degree of plausibility. One account is based on the obvious fact that people value the experience of living and wish for the valuable experience to continue.

Therefore, it might be said, what makes killing wrong is the discontinuation of that experience for the victim. Let us call this the *discontinuation account*.[10] Another rival account is based upon the obvious fact that people strongly desire to continue to live. This suggests that what makes killing us so wrong is that it interferes with the fulfillment of a strong and fundamental desire, the fulfillment of which is necessary for the fulfillment of any other desires we might have. Let us call this the *desire account*.[11]

Consider first the desire account as a rival account of the ethics of killing which would provide the basis for rejecting the anti-abortion position. Such an account will have to be stronger than the value of a future-like-ours account of the wrongness of abortion if it is to do the job expected of it. To entail the wrongness of abortion, the value of a future-like-ours account has only to provide a sufficient, but not a necessary condition for the wrongness of killing. The desire account, on the other hand, must provide us also with a necessary condition for the wrongness of killing in order to generate a pro-choice conclusion on abortion. The reason for this is that presumably the argument from the desire account moves from the claim that what makes killing wrong is interference with a very strong desire to the claim that abortion is not wrong because the fetus lacks a strong desire to live. Obviously, this inference fails if someone's having the desire to live is not a necessary condition of its being wrong to kill that individual.

One problem with the desire account is that we do regard it as seriously wrong to kill persons who have little desire to live or who have no desire to live or, indeed, have a desire not to live. We believe it is seriously wrong to kill the unconscious, the sleeping, those who are tired of life, and those who are suicidal. The value-of-a-human-future account renders standard morality intelligible in these cases; these cases appear to be incompatible with the desire account.

The desire account is subject to a deeper difficulty. We desire life, because we value the goods of this life. The goodness of life is not secondary to our desire for it. If this were not so, the pain of one's own premature death could be done away with merely by an appropriate alteration in the configuration of one's desires. This is absurd. Hence, it would seem that it is the loss of the goods of one's future, not the interference with the fulfillment of a strong desire to life, which accounts ultimately for the wrongness of killing.

It is worth noting that, if the desire account is modified so that it does not provide a necessary, but only a sufficient, condition for the wrongness of killing, the desire account is compatible with the value of a future-like-ours account. The combined accounts will yield an anti-abortion ethic. This suggests that one can retain what is intuitively plausible about the desire account without a challenge to the basic argument of this essay.

It is also worth noting that, if future desires have moral force in a modified desire account of the wrongness of killing, one can find support for an anti-abortion ethic even in the absence of a value of a future-like-ours account. If one decides that a morally relevant property, the possession of which is sufficient to make it wrong to kill some individual, is the desire at some future time to live—one might decide to justify one's refusal to kill suicidal teenagers on these grounds, for example—then, since typical fetuses will have the desire in the future to live, it is wrong to kill typical fetuses. Accordingly, it does not seem that a desire account of the wrongness of killing can provide a justification of a pro-choice ethic of abortion which is nearly as adequate as the value of a human-future justification of an anti-abortion ethic.

The discontinuation account looks more promising as an account of the wrongness of killing. It seems just as intelligible as the value of a future-like-ours account, but it does not justify an anti-abortion position. Obviously, if it is the continuation of one's activities, experiences, and projects, the loss of which makes killing wrong, then it is not wrong to kill fetuses for that reason, for fetuses do not have experiences, activities, and projects to be continued or discontinued. Accordingly, the discontinuation account does not have the anti-abortion consequences that the value of a future-like-ours account has. Yet it seems as intelligible as the value of a future-like-ours account, for when we think of what would be wrong with our being killed, it does seem as if it is the discontinuation of what makes our lives worthwhile which makes killing us wrong.

Is the discontinuation account just as good an account as the value of a future-like-ours account? The discontinuation account will not be adequate at all, if it does not refer to the *value* of the experience that may be discontinued. One does not want the discontinuation account to make it wrong to kill a patient who begs for death and who is in severe pain that cannot be relieved short of killing. (I leave open the question of whether it is wrong for other reasons.) Accordingly, the discontinuation account must be more than a bare discontinuation account. It must make some reference to the positive value of the patient's experiences. But, by the same token, the value of a future-like-ours account cannot be a bare future account either. Just having a future surely does not itself rule out killing the above patient. This account must make some reference to the value of the patient's future experiences and projects also. Hence, both accounts involve the value of experiences, projects, and activities. So far we still have symmetry between the accounts.

The symmetry fades, however, when we focus on the time period of the value of experiences, etc., which has moral consequences. Although both accounts leave open the possibility that the patient in our example may be killed, this possibility is left open only in virtue of the utterly bleak future for the patient. It makes no difference whether the patient's immediate past contains intolerable pain, or consists in being in a coma (which we can imagine is a situation of indifference), or consists in a life of value. If the patient's future is a future of value, we want our account to make it wrong to kill the patient. If the patient's future is intolerable, whatever his or her immediate past, we want our account to allow killing the patient. Obviously, then, it is the value of the patient's future which is doing the work in rendering the morality of killing the patient intelligible.

This being the case, it seems clear that whether one has immediate past experiences or not does no work in the explanation of what makes killing wrong. The addition the discontinuation account makes to the value of a human future account is otiose. Its addition to the value-of-a-future account plays no role at all in rendering intelligible the wrongness of killing. Therefore, it can be discarded with the discontinuation account of which it is a part.

IV

The analysis of the previous section suggests that alternative general accounts of the wrongness of killing are either inadequate or unsuccessful in getting around the anti-abortion consequences of the value of a future-like-ours argument. A different strategy for avoiding the anti-abortion consequences involve limiting the scope of the value of a future argument. More precisely, the strategy involves arguing that fetuses lack a property that is essential for the value-of-a-future argument (or for any anti-abortion argument) to apply to them.

One move of this sort is based upon the claim that a necessary condition of one's future being valuable is that one values it. Value implies a valuer. Given this one might argue that, since fetuses cannot value their futures, their futures are not valuable to them. Hence, it does not seriously wrong them deliberately to end their lives.

This move fails, however, because of some ambiguities. Let us assume that something cannot be of value unless it is valued by someone. This does not entail that my life is of no value unless it is valued by me. I may think, in a period of despair, that my future is of no worth whatsoever, but I may be wrong because others rightly see value—even great value— in it. Furthermore, my future can be valuable to me even if I do not value it. This is the case when a young person attempts suicide, but is rescued and goes on to significant human achievements. Such young people's futures are ultimately valuable to them, even though such futures do not seem to be valuable to them at the moment of attempted suicide. A fetus' future can be valuable to it in the same way. Accordingly, this attempt to limit the anti-abortion argument fails.

Another similar attempt to reject the anti-abortion position is based on Tooley's claim that an entity cannot possess the right to life unless it has the capacity to desire its continued existence. It follows that, since fetuses lack the conceptual capacity to desire to continue to live, they lack the right to life. Accordingly, Tooley concludes that abortion cannot be seriously prima facie wrong.[12]

What could be the evidence for Tooley's claim? Tooley once argued that individuals have a prima facie right to what they desire and that the lack of the capacity to desire something undercuts the basis of one's right to it.[13] This argument plainly will not succeed in the context of the analysis of this essay, however, since the point here is to establish the fetus' right to life on other grounds. Tooley's argument assumes that the right to life cannot be established in general on some basis other than the desire for life. This position was considered and rejected in the preceding section.

One might attempt to defend Tooley's basic claim on the grounds that, because a fetus cannot apprehend continued life as a benefit, its continued life cannot be a benefit or cannot be something it has a right to or cannot be something that is in its interest. This might be defended in terms of the general proposition that, if an individual is literally incapable of caring about or taking an interest in some X, then one does not have a right to X or X is not a benefit or X is not something that is in one's interest.[14]

Each member of this family of claims seems to be open to objections. As John C. Stevens has pointed out, one may have a right to be treated with a certain medical procedure (because of a health insurance policy one has purchased), even though one cannot conceive of the nature of the procedure.[15] And, as Tooley himself has pointed out, persons who have been indoctrinated, or drugged, or rendered temporarily unconscious may be literally incapable of caring about or taking an interest in something that is in their interest or is something to which they have a right, or is something that benefits them. Hence, the Tooley claim that would restrict the scope of the value of a future-like-ours argument is undermined by counterexamples.[16]

Finally, Paul Bassen[17] has argued that, even though the prospects of an embryo might seem to be a basis for the wrongness of abortion, an embryo cannot be a victim and therefore cannot be wronged. An embryo cannot be a victim, he says, because it lacks sentience. His central argument for this seems to be that, even though plants and the permanently unconscious are alive, they clearly cannot be victims. What is the explanation of this? Bassen claims that the explanation is that their lives consists of mere metabolism and mere metabolism is not enough to ground victimizability. Mentation is required.

The problem with this attempt to establish the absence of victimizability is that both plants and the permanently unconscious clearly lack what Bassen calls "prospects" or what I have called "a future life like ours." Hence, it is surely open to one to argue that the real reason we believe plants and the permanently unconscious cannot be victims is that killing them cannot deprive them of a future life like ours; the real reason is not their absence of present mentation.

Bassen recognizes that his view is subject to this difficulty, and he recognizes that the case of children seems to support this difficulty, for "much of what we do for children is based on prospects." He argues, however, that, in the case of children and in other such cases, "potentiality comes into play only where victimizability has been secured on other grounds."[18]

Bassen's defense of this view is patently question-begging, since what is adequate to secure victimizability is exactly what is at issue. His examples do not support his own view against the thesis of this essay. Of course, embryos can be victims: when their lives are deliberately terminated, they are deprived of their futures of value, their prospects. This makes them victims, for it directly wrongs them.

The seeming plausibility of Bassen's view stems from the fact that paradigmatic cases of imagining someone as a victim involve empathy, and empathy requires mentation of the victim. The victims of flood, famine, rape, or child abuse are all persons with whom we can empathize. That empathy seems to be part of seeing them as victims.[19]

In spite of the strength of these examples, the attractive intuition that a situation in which there is victimization requires the possibility of empathy is subject to counterexamples. Consider a case that Bassen himself offers: "Posthumous obliteration of an author's work constitutes a misfortune for him only if he had wished his work to endure."[20] The conditions Bassen wishes to impose upon the possibility of being victimized here seem far too strong. Perhaps this author, due to his unrealistic standards of excellence and his low self-esteem, regarded his work as unworthy of survival, even though it possessed genuine literary merit. Destruction of such work would surely victimize its author. In such a case, empathy with the victim concerning the loss is clearly impossible.

Of course, Bassen does not make the possibility of empathy a necessary condition of victimizability; he requires only mentation. Hence, on Bassen's actual view, this author, as I have described him, can be a victim. The problem is that the basic intuition that renders Bassen's view plausible is missing in the author's case. In order to attempt to avoid counterexamples, Bassen has made his thesis too weak to be supported by the intuitions that suggested it.

Even so, the mentation requirement on victimizability is still subject to counterexamples. Suppose a severe accident renders me totally unconscious for a month, after which I recover. Surely killing me while I am unconscious victimizes me, even though I am incapable of mentation during that time. It follows that Bassen's thesis fails. Apparently, attempts to restrict the value of a future-like-ours argument so that fetuses do not fall within its scope do not succeed.

V

In this essay, it has been argued that the correct ethic of the wrongness of killing can be extended to fetal life and used to show that there is a strong presumption that any abortion is morally impermissible. If the ethic of killing adopted here entails, however, that contraception is also seriously immoral, then there would appear to be a difficulty with the analysis of this essay.

But this analysis does not entail that contraception is wrong. Of course, contraception prevents the actualization of a possible future of value. Hence, it follows from the claim that futures of value should be maximized that contraception is prima facie immoral. This obligation to maximize does not exist, however; furthermore, nothing in the ethics of killing in this paper entails that it does. The ethics of killing in this essay would entail that contraception is wrong only if something were denied a human future of value by contraception. Nothing at all is denied such a future by contraception, however.

Candidates for a subject of harm by contraception fall into four categories: (1) some sperm or other, (2) some ovum or other, (3) a sperm and an ovum separately, and (4) a sperm and an ovum together. Assigning the harm to some sperm is utterly arbitrary, for no reason can be given for making a sperm the subject of harm rather than an ovum. Assigning the harm to

some ovum is utterly arbitrary, for no reason can be given for making an ovum the subject of harm rather than a sperm. One might attempt to avoid these problems by insisting that contraception deprives both the sperm and the ovum separately of a valuable future like ours. On this alternative, too many futures are lost. Contraception was supposed to be wrong, because it deprived us of one future of value, not two. One might attempt to avoid this problem by holding that contraception deprives the combination of sperm and ovum of a valuable future like ours. But here the definite article misleads. At the time of contraception, there are hundreds of millions of sperm, one (released) ovum and millions of possible combinations of all of these. There is not actual combination at all. Is the subject of the loss to be a merely possible combination? Which one? This alternative does not yield an actual subject of harm either. Accordingly, the immorality of contraception is not entailed by the loss of a future-like-ours argument simply because there is no nonarbitrarily identifiable subject of the loss in the case of contraception.

VI

The purpose of this essay has been to set out an argument for the serious presumptive wrongness of abortion subject to the assumption that the moral permissibility of abortion stands or falls on the moral status of the fetus. Since a fetus possesses a property, the possession of which in adult human beings is sufficient to make killing an adult human being wrong, abortion is wrong. This way of dealing with the problem of abortion seems superior to other approaches to the ethics of abortion, because it rests on an ethics of killing which is close to self-evident, because the crucial morally relevant property clearly applies to fetuses, and because the argument avoids the usual equivocations on "human life," "human being," or "person." The argument rests neither on religious claims nor on Papal dogma. It is not subject to the objection of "speciesism." Its soundness is compatible with the moral permissibility of euthanasia and contraception. It deals with our intuitions concerning young children.

Finally, this analysis can be viewed as resolving a standard problem—indeed, *the* standard problem—concerning the ethics of abortion. Clearly, it is wrong to kill adult human beings. Clearly, it is not wrong to end the life of some arbitrarily chosen single human cell. Fetuses seem to be like arbitrarily chosen human cells in some respects and like adult humans in other respects. The problem of the ethics of abortion is the problem of determining the fetal property that settles this moral controversy. The thesis of this essay is that the problem of the ethics of abortion, so understood, is solvable.

Notes

1. Joel Feinberg, "Abortion," in *Matters of Life and Death: New Introductory Essays in Moral Philosophy,* ed. Tom Regan (New York: Random House, 1986), pp. 256-93; Michael Tooley, "Abortion and Infanticide," *Philosophy and Public Affairs,* II, no. 1 (1972), pp. 37-65; idem, *Abortion and Infanticide* (New York: Oxford, 1984); Mary Anne Warren, "On the Moral and Legal Status of Abortion," *The Monist* 57, no. 1 (1973), pp. 43-61; Tristram Engelhardt Jr., "The Ontology of Abortion," *Ethics* 84, no. 3 (1974), pp. 217-34; L.W. Sumner, *Abortion and Moral Theory* (Princeton: University Press, 1981); John T. Noonan Jr., "Almost Absolute Value in History," in *The Morality of Abortion: Legal and Historical Perspective,* ed. Noonan (Cambridge: Harvard, 1970); and Philip Devine, *The Ethics of Homicide* (Ithaca: Cornell University Press, 1978).

2. For interesting discussions of this issue, see Warren Quinn, "Abortion: Identity and Loss," *Philosophy and Public Affairs* 13, no. 1 (1984), pp. 24-54; and Lawrence C. Becker, "Human Being: the Boundaries of the Concept," *Philosophy and Public Affairs* 4, no. 4 (1975), pp. 334-59.

3. See, e.g., Don Marquis, "Ethics and The Elderly: Some Problems," in *Aging and the Elderly: Humanistic Perspectives in Gerontology,* ed. Stuart Spicker, Kathleen Woodwark, and David Van Tassel (Atlantic Highlands, NJ: Humanities Press, 1978) pp. 341-55.

4. See Warren, "Moral and Legal Status"; and Tooley, "Abortion and Infanticide."

5. This seems to be the fatal flaw in Warren's treatment of this issue.

6. Feinberg, "Abortion," p. 270.

7. I have been most influenced on this matter by Jonathan Glover, *Causing Death and Saving Lives* (New York: Penguin, 1977), chap. 3; and Robert Young, "What is So Wrong with Killing People?" *Philosophy* 54, no. 210 (1979), pp. 515-28.

8. Feinberg, Tooley, Warren, and Engelhardt have all dealt with this problem.

9. Immanuel Kant, "Duties to Animals and Spirits," in *Lectures on Ethics,* trans. Louis Infeld (New York: Harper, 1963), p. 239.

10. I am indebted to Jack Bricke for raising this objection.

11. Presumably a preference utilitarian would press such an objection. Tooley once suggested that his account has such a theoretical underpinning; "Abortion and Infanticide," pp. 46-47.

12. Tooley, "Abortion and Infanticide," pp. 46-47.

13. Ibid., pp. 44-45.

14. Donald VanDeVeer seems to think this is self-evident; see his "Whither Baby Doe?" in Regan, *Matters of Life and Death,* p. 233.

15. John C. Stevens, "Must the Bearer of a Right Have the Concept of That to Which He Has A Right?" *Ethics* 95, no. 1 (1984), pp. 68-74.

16. See Tooley, "Abortion and Infanticide," pp. 47-49.

17. Paul Bassen, "Present Sakes and Future Prospects: The Status of Early Abortion," Philosophy and Public Affairs 11, no. 4 (1982), pp. 322-26.

18. Ibid., p. 333.

19. Note carefully the reasons he gives on the bottom of ibid., p. 316.

20. Ibid., p. 318.

23.
A THIRD WAY

Wayne Sumner

The established views have failed on both the intuitive and theoretical levels. Their conceptions of the moral status of the fetus, if they are not shallow and arbitrary, violate widely shared moral convictions concerning contraception and infanticide. The conservative's defense of a restrictive policy violates equally widely shared convictions concerning the individual's right of self-defense against threats to life, liberty, or personal integrity. Moreover, both views are underdetermined by their own moral theories. Liberals have been unable to ground their view of the fetus in a theory of rights, whereas conservatives have been served even less well by a natural-law morality that not only fails to support their view of the fetus but would lead from that view to a moderate abortion policy.

The demise of the established views deprives us of our familiar reference points in the abortion landscape. It is the simplicity of these views that has rendered them easy to grasp and thus easy to market in the public forum. Unfortunately, it is also that simplicity—especially their uniform views of the fetus—which has proved to be their fatal weakness. When confronted with a problem as complex as that of abortion, we have some initial reason to suspect simple solutions. Our critique of the established views has amply justified this suspicion. We need a view of abortion responsive to all of the elements whose conjunction renders the problem of abortion so perplexing and so divisive. Such a view cannot be a simple one.

If an alternative to the established views is to be developed, three tasks must be successfully completed. The first is to construct this third way and to show how it is essentially different from both of the positions it supersedes. The indispensable ingredient at this stage is a criterion of moral standing that will generate a view of the fetus and thus a view of abortion (including an abortion policy). The second task is to defend this view on the intuitive level by showing that it coheres better than either of its predecessors with our considered moral judgments both on abortion itself and on cognate issues. Then, finally, the view must be given a deep structure by grounding it in a moral theory. This chapter will undertake the first two tasks by outlining a position on the abortion problem and justifying it by appeal to moral intuitions. The more daunting theoretical challenge will be confronted in the two succeeding chapters.

SPECIFICATIONS

Although our critique has produced negative results, it will also point the way to a more constructive outcome. The established views have failed in certain specific respects. Collating their points of weakness will provide us with guidelines for building a more satisfactory alternative. It will be convenient to divide these guidelines into two categories corresponding to the two ingredients that complicate the problem of abortion: the nature of the fetus and the implications of the mother/fetus relationship.

The conservative view, and also the more naive versions of the liberal view, select a precise point (conception, birth, etc.) as the threshold of moral standing, implying that the transition from no standing to full standing occurs abruptly. In doing so they rest more weight on these sudden events than they are capable of bearing. A view that avoids this defect will allow full moral standing to be acquired gradually. It will therefore attempt to locate not a threshold point, but a threshold period or stage.

Both of the established views attribute a uniform moral status to all fetuses, regardless of their dissimilarities. Each, for example, counts a newly conceived zygote for precisely as much (or as little) as a full-term fetus, despite the enormous differences between them. A view that avoids this defect will assign moral status differentially, so that the threshold stage occurs sometime during pregnancy.

A consequence of the uniform approach adopted by both of the established views is that neither can attach any significance to the development of the fetus during gestation.[1] Yet this development is the most obvious feature of gestation. A view that avoids this defect will base the (differential) moral standing of the fetus at least in part on its level of development. It will thus assign undeveloped fetuses a moral status akin to that of ova and spermatozoa, whereas it will assign developed fetuses a moral status akin to that of infants.

So far, then, an adequate view of the fetus must be gradual, differential and developmental. It must also be derived from a satisfactory criterion of moral standing. The conditions of adequacy for such a criterion were set out in Section 5: it must be general (applicable to beings other than fetuses), it must connect moral standing with the empirical properties of such beings, and it must be morally relevant. Its moral relevance is partly testable by appeal to intuition, for arbitrary or shallow criteria will be vulnerable to counterexamples. But the final test of moral relevance is grounding in a moral theory. An adequate view of the fetus promises a morally significant division between early abortions (before the threshold stage) and late abortions (after the threshold stage). It also promises borderline cases (during the threshold stage). Wherever that stage is located, abortions that precede it will be private matters, since the fetus will at that stage lack moral standing. Thus the provisions of the liberal view will apply to early abortions: they will be morally innocent (as long as the usual conditions or maternal consent, etc., are satisfied) and ought to be legally unregulated (except for rules equally applicable to all other medical procedures). Early abortion will have the same moral status as contraception.

Abortions that follow the threshold stage will be interpersonal matters, since the fetus will at that stage possess moral standing. The provisions of Thomson's argument will apply to late abortions: they must be assessed on a case-by-case basis and they ought to be legally permitted only on appropriate grounds. Late abortions will have the same moral status as infanticide, except for the difference made by the physical connection between fetus and mother.

A third way with abortion is thus a moderate and differential view, combining elements of the liberal view for early abortions with elements of (a weakened version of) the conservative view for late abortions. The policy that a moderate view will support is a moderate policy, permissive in the early stages of pregnancy and more restrictive (though not as restrictive as conservatives think appropriate) in the later stages. So far as the personal question of the moral evaluation of particular abortions is concerned, there is no pressing need to resolve the borderline cases around the threshold stage. But a workable abortion policy cannot tolerate this vagueness and will need to establish a definite time limit beyond which the stipulated grounds will come into play. Although the precise location of the time limit will unavoidably be somewhat arbitrary, it will be defensible as long as it falls somewhere within the threshold stage. Abortion on request up to the time limit and only for cause thereafter: these are the elements of a satisfactory abortion policy.

A number of moderate views may be possible, each of them satisfying all of the foregoing constraints. A particular view will be defined by selecting (a) a criterion of moral standing, (b) the natural characteristics whose gradual acquisition during normal fetal development carries with it the acquisition of moral standing, and (c) a threshold stage. Of these three steps, the first is the crucial one, since it determines both of the others.

A CRITERION OF MORAL STANDING

We have thus far assumed that for a creature to have moral standing is for it to have a right to life. Any such right imposes duties on moral agents; these duties may be either negative (not to deprive the creature of life) or positive (to support the creature's life). Possession of a right to life implies at least some immunity against attack by others, and possibly also some entitlement to the aid of others. As the duties may vary in strength, so may the corresponding rights. To have some moral standing is to have some right to life, whether or not it may be overridden by the rights of others. To have full moral standing is to have the strongest right to life possessed by anyone, the right to life of the paradigm person. Depending on one's moral theory, this right may or may not be inviolable and indefeasible and thus may or may not impose absolute duties on others.

Although this analysis of moral standing will later be broadened, it will still suffice for our present purposes. To which creatures should we distribute (some degree of) moral standing? On which criterion should we base this distribution? It may be easier to answer these questions if we begin with the clear case and work outward to the unclear ones. If we can determine why we ascribe full standing to the paradigm case, we may learn what to look for in other creatures when deciding whether or not to include them in the moral sphere.

The paradigm bearer of moral standing is an adult human being with normal capacities of intellect, emotion, perception, sensation, decision, action, and the like. If we think of such a person as a complex bundle of natural properties, then in principle we could employ as a criterion any of the properties common to all normal and mature members of our species. Selecting a particular property or set of properties will define a class of creatures with moral standing, namely, all (and only) those who share that property. The extension of that class will depend on how widely the property in question is distributed. Some putative criteria will be obviously frivolous and will immediately fail the tests of generality or moral relevance. But even after excluding the silly candidates, we are left with a number of serious ones. There are four that appear to be the most serious: we might attribute full moral standing to the paradigm person on the ground that he/she is (a) intrinsically valuable, (b) alive, (c) sentient, or (d) rational. An intuitive test of the adequacy of any of these candidates will involve first enumerating the class of beings to whom it will distribute moral standing and then determining whether that class either excludes creatures that upon careful reflection we believe ought to be included or includes creatures that we believe ought to be excluded. In the former case the criterion draws the boundary of the moral sphere too narrowly and fails as a necessary condition of moral standing. In the later case the criterion draws the boundary too broadly and fails as a sufficient condition. (A given criterion may, of course, be defective in both respects.)

Beings may depart from the paradigm along several different dimensions, each of which presents us with unclear cases that a criterion must resolve. These cases may be divided into seven categories: (1) inanimate objects (natural and artificial); (2) non-human terrestrial species of living things (animals and plants); (3) nonhuman extraterrestrial species of living things (should there be any); (4) artificial "life forms" (androids, robots, computers); (5) grossly defective human beings (the severely and permanently retarded or deranged); (6) human beings at the end of life (especially the severely and permanently senile or comatose); (7) human beings at the beginning of life (fetuses, infants, children). Since the last context is the one in which we wish to apply a criterion, it will here be set aside. This will enable us to settle on a criterion without tailoring it specially for the problem of abortion. Once a criterion has established its credentials in other domains, we will be able to trace out its implications for the case of the fetus.

The first candidate for criterion takes a direction rather different from that of the remaining three. It is a commonplace in moral philosophy to attribute to (normal adult) human beings a special worth or value or dignity in virtue of which they possess (among other rights) a full right to life. This position implies that (some degree of) moral standing extends just as far as (some degree of) this intrinsic value, a higher degree of the latter entailing a higher degree of the former.[2] We cannot know which things have moral standing without being told which things have intrinsic worth (and why)—without, that is, being offered a theory of intrinsic value. What is unique about this criterion, however, is that it is quite capable in principle of extending moral standing beyond the class of living beings, thus embracing such inanimate objects as rocks and lakes, entire landscapes (or indeed worlds), and artifacts. Of course, nonliving things cannot literally have a right to *life*, but it would be simple enough to generalize to a right to (continued) *existence*, where this might include both a right not to be destroyed and a right to such support as is necessary for that existence. A criterion that invokes intrinsic value is thus able to define a much more capacious moral sphere than is any of the other candidates.

Such a criterion is undeniably attractive in certain respects: how else are we to explain why it is wrong to destroy priceless icons or litter the moon even when doing so will never affect any living, sentient, or rational being?[3] But it is clear that it cannot serve our present purpose. A criterion must connect moral standing with some property of things whose presence or absence can be confirmed by a settled, objective, and public method of investigation. The property of being intrinsically valuable is not subject to such verification. A criterion based on intrinsic value cannot be applied without a theory of intrinsic value. Such a theory will supply a criterion of intrinsic value by specifying the natural properties of things in virtue of which they possess such value. But if things have moral standing in virtue of having intrinsic value, and if they have intrinsic value in virtue of having some natural property, then it is that natural property which is serving as the real criterion of moral standing, and the middle term of intrinsic value is eliminable without loss. A theory of intrinsic value may thus entail a criterion of moral standing, but intrinsic value cannot itself serve as that criterion.

There is a further problem confronting any attempt to ground moral rights in the intrinsic worth of creatures. One must first be certain that this is not merely a verbal exercise in which attributing intrinsic value to things is just another way of attributing intrinsic moral standing to them. Assuming that the relation between value and rights is synthetic, there are then two possibilities: the value in question is moral or it is nonmoral. If it is moral, the criterion plainly fails to break out of the circle of moral properties to connect them with the nonmoral properties of things. But if it is nonmoral, it is unclear what it has to do with moral rights. If there are realms of value, some case must be made for deriving moral duties toward things from the non-moral value of these things.

The remaining three candidates for a criterion of moral standing (life, sentience, rationality) all satisfy the verification requirement since they all rest standing on empirical properties of things. They may be ordered in terms of the breadth of the moral spheres they define. Since rational beings are a proper subset of sentient beings, which are a proper subset of living beings, the first candidate is the weakest and will define the broadest sphere, whereas the third is the strongest and will define the narrowest sphere.[4] In an interesting recent discussion, Kenneth

Goodpaster (1978) has urged that moral standing be accorded to all living beings, simply in virtue of the fact that they are alive.[5] Although much of his argument is negative, being directed against more restrictive criteria, he does provide a positive case for including all forms of life within the moral sphere.[6]

Let us assume that the usual signs of life—nutrition, metabolism, spontaneous growth, reproduction—enable us to draw a tolerably sharp distinction between animate and inanimate beings, so that all plant and animal species, however primitive, are collected together in the former category. All such creatures share the property of being *teleological systems*: they have functions, ends, directions, natural tendencies, and so forth. In virtue of their teleology such creatures have needs, in a nonmetaphorical sense—conditions that must be satisfied if they are to thrive or flourish. Creatures with needs can be benefited or harmed; they are benefited when their essential needs are satisfied and harmed when they are not. It also makes sense to say that such creatures have a good: the conditions that promote their life and health are good for them, whereas those that impair their normal functioning are bad for them. But it is common to construe morality as having essentially to do with benefits and harms or with the good of creatures. So doing will lead us to extend moral standing to all creatures capable of being benefited and harmed, that is, all creatures with a good. But this condition will include all organisms (and systems of organisms), and so life is the only reasonable criterion of moral standing.

This extension of moral standing to plants and to the simpler animals is of course highly counterintuitive, since most of us accord the lives of such creatures no weight whatever in our practical deliberations. How could we conduct our affairs if we were to grant protection of life to every plant and animal species? Some of the more extreme implications of this view are, however, forestalled by Goodpaster's distinction between a criterion of inclusion and a criterion of comparison.[7] The former determines which creatures have (some) moral standing and thus locates the boundary of the moral sphere; it is Goodpaster's contention that life is the proper inclusion criterion. The latter is operative entirely within the moral sphere and enables us to assign different grades of moral standing to different creatures in virtue of some natural property that they may possess in different degrees. Since all living beings are (it seems) equally alive, life cannot serve as comparison criterion. Goodpaster does not provide such a criterion, though he recognizes its necessity. Thus his view enables him to affirm that all living creatures have (some) moral standing but to deny that all such creatures have equal standing. Though the lives of all animate beings deserve consideration, some deserve more than others. Thus, for instance, higher animals might count for more than lower ones, and all animals might count for more than plants.

In the absence of a criterion of comparison, it is difficult to ascertain just what reforms Goodpaster's view would require in our moral practice. How much weight must human beings accord to the lives of lichen or grass or bacteria or insects? When are such lives more important than some benefit for a higher form of life? How should we modify our eating habits, for example? There is a problem here that extends beyond the incompleteness and indeterminacy of Goodpaster's position. Suppose that we have settled on a comparison criterion; let it be sentience (assuming that sentience admits of degrees in some relevant respect). Then a creature's ranking in the hierarchy of moral standing will be determined by the extent of its sentience: nonsentient (living) beings will have minimal standing, whereas the most sentient beings (human beings, perhaps) will have maximal standing. But then we are faced with the obvious question: if sentience is to serve as the comparison criterion, why should it not also serve as the inclusion criterion? Conversely, if life is the inclusion criterion, does it not follow that nothing else can serve as the comparison criterion, in which case all living beings have equal standing? It is difficult to imagine an argument in favor of sentience as a comparison criterion that would not also be an argument in favor of it as an inclusion criterion.[8] Since the same will hold for any other comparison criterion, Goodpaster's view can avoid its extreme implications only at the price of inconsistency.

Goodpaster's view also faces consistency problems in its claim that life is necessary for moral standing. Beings need not be organisms in order to be teleological systems, and therefore to have needs, a good, and the capacity to be benefited and harmed. If these conditions are satisfied by a tree (as they surely are), then they are equally satisfied by a car. In order to function properly most machines need periodic maintenance; such maintenance is good for them, they are benefited by it, and they are harmed by its neglect. Why then is being alive a necessary condition of moral standing? Life is but an (imperfect) indicator of teleology and the capacity to be benefited and harmed. But Goodpaster's argument then commits him to treating these deeper characteristics as the criterion of moral standing, and thus to according standing to many (perhaps most) inanimate objects.[9] This inclusion of (at least some) non-living things should incline us to re-examine Goodpaster's argument—if the inclusion of all living things has not already done so. The connection between morality and the capacity to be benefited and harmed appears plausible, so what has gone wrong? We may form a conjecture if we again consider our paradigm bearer of moral standing. In the case of a fully normal adult human being, it does appear that moral questions are pertinent whenever the actions of another agent promise to benefit or threaten to harm such a being. Both duties and rights are intimately connected with benefits and harms. The kinds of acts that we have a (strict) duty not to do are those that typically cause harm, whereas positive duties are duties to confer benefits. Liberty-rights protect autonomy, which is usually thought of as one of the chief goods for human beings, and the connection between welfare-rights and benefits is obvious. But if we ask what counts as a benefit or a harm for a human being, the usual answers take one or both of the following directions:

(1) *The desire model.* Human beings are benefited to the extent that their desires (or perhaps their considered and informed desires) are satisfied; they are harmed to the extent that these desires are frustrated.

(2) *The experience model.* Human beings benefited to the extent that they are thought to have experiences that they like or find agreeable; they are harmed to the extent that they are brought to have experiences that they dislike or find disagreeable.

We need not worry at this stage whether one of these models is more satisfactory than the other. On both models benefits and harms for particular persons are interpreted in terms of the psychological states of those persons, in terms, that is, of their interests or welfare. Such states are possible only for beings who are conscious or sentient. Thus, if morality has to do with the promotion and protection of interests or welfare, morality can concern itself only with beings who are conscious or sentient.[10] No other beings can be beneficiaries or victims *in the morally relevant way.* Goodpaster is not mistaken in suggesting that nonsentient beings can be benefited and harmed. But he is mistaken in suggesting that morality has to do with benefits and harms as such, rather than with a particular category of them. And that can be seen the more clearly when we realize that the broadest capacity to be benefited and harmed extends not only out to, but beyond the frontier of life. Leaving my lawn mower out in the rain is bad for the mower, pulling weeds is bad for the weeds, and swatting mosquitoes is bad for the mosquitoes; but there are no moral dimensions to any of these acts unless the interests or welfare of some sentient creature is at stake. Morality requires the existence of sentience in order to obtain a purchase on our actions.

The failure of Goodpaster's view has thus given us some reason to look to sentience as a criterion of moral standing. Before considering this possibility directly, it will be helpful to turn to the much narrower criterion of rationality.[11] The rational/nonrational boundary is more difficult to locate with certainty than the animate/inanimate boundary, since rationality (or intelligence) embraces a number of distinct but related capacities for thought, memory, foresight, language, self-consciousness, objectivity, planning, reasoning, judgment, deliberation, and the like.[12] It is perhaps possible for a being to possess some of these capacities and entirely lack others, but for simplicity we will assume that the higher-order cognitive processes are typically owned as a bundle.[13] The bundle is possessed to one extent or another by normal adult human beings, by adolescents and older children, by persons suffering from the milder cognitive disorders, and by some other animal species (some primates and cetaceans for example). It is not possessed to any appreciable extent by fetuses and infants, by the severely retarded or disordered, by the irreversibly comatose, and by most other animal species. To base moral standing on rationality is thus to deny it alike to most nonhuman beings and to many human beings. Since the implications for fetuses and infants have already been examined, they will be ignored in the present discussion. Instead we will focus on why one might settle on rationality as a criterion in the first place.

That rationality is sufficient for moral standing is not controversial (though there are some interesting questions to be explored here about forms of artificial intelligence). As a necessary condition, however, rationality will exclude a good many sentient beings—just how many, and which ones, to be determined by the kind and the stringency of the standards employed. Many will find objectionable this constriction of the sphere of moral concern. Because moral standing has been defined in terms of the right to life, to lack moral standing is not necessarily to lack all rights. Thus one could hold that, although we have no duty to (nonrational) animals to respect their lives, we do have a duty to them not to cause them suffering. For the right not to suffer, one might choose a different (and broader) criterion—sentience, for example. (However, if this is the criterion appropriate for that right, why is it not also the criterion appropriate for the right to life?) But even if we focus strictly on the (painless) killing of animals, the implications of the criterion are harsh. Certainly we regularly kill nonhuman animals to satisfy our own needs or desires. But the justification usually offered for these practices is either that the satisfaction of those needs and desires outweighs the costs to the animals (livestock farming, hunting, fishing, trapping, experimentation) or that no decent life would have been available for them anyway (the killing of stray dogs and cats). Although some of these arguments doubtless are rationalizations, their common theme is that the lives of animals do have some weight (however slight) in the moral scales, which is why the practice of killing animals is one that requires moral justification (raises moral issues). If rationality is the criterion of moral standing, and if (most) nonhuman animals are nonrational, killing such creatures could be morally questionable only when it impinges on the interests of rational beings (as where animals are items of property). In no case could killing an animal be a wrong against it. However callous and chauvinistic the common run of our treatment of animals may be, still the view that killing a dog or a horse is morally no more serious (ceteris paribus) than weeding a garden can be the considered judgment of only a small minority.

The standard that we apply to other species we must in consistency apply to our own. The greater the number of animals who are excluded by that standard, the greater the number of human beings who will also be excluded. In the absence of a determinate criterion it is unclear just where the moral line will be drawn on the normal/abnormal spectrum: will a right to life be withheld from mongoloids, psychotics, the autistic, the senile, the profoundly retarded? If so, killing such persons will again be no wrong *to them*. Needless to say, most such persons (in company with many animals) are sentient and capable to some extent of enjoyable and satisfying lives. To kill them is to deprive them of lives that are of value to them. If such creatures are denied standing, this loss will be entirely discounted in our moral reasoning. Their lack of rationality may ensure that their lives are less full and rich than ours, that they consist of simpler pleasures and more basic enjoyments. But what could be the justification for treating their deaths as though they cost them nothing at all?

There is a tradition, extending back at least to Kant, that attempts just such a justification. One of its modern spokesmen is A.I. Melden (1977), who treats the capacity for moral agency as the criterion of moral standing. This capacity is manifested by participation in a moral community—a set of beings sharing allegiance to moral rules and recognition of one another's integrity. Rights can be attributed only to beings with whom we can have such moral intercourse, thus only to beings who have interests similar to ours, who show concern for the well-being of others, who are capable of uniting in cooperative endeavors, who regulate their activities by a sense of right and wrong, and who display the characteristically moral emotions of indignation, remorse, and guilt.[14] Rationality is a necessary condition (though not a sufficient one) for possessing this bundle of capacities. Melden believes that of all living creatures known to us only human beings are capable of moral agency.[15] Natural rights, including the right to life, are thus human rights.

We may pass over the obvious difficulty of extending moral standing to all human beings on this basis (including the immature and abnormal) and focus on the question of why the capacity for moral agency should be thought necessary for possession of a right to life. The notion of a moral community to which Melden appeals contains a crucial ambiguity.[16] On the one hand it can be thought of as a community of moral agents—the bearers of moral duties. Clearly to be a member of such a community one must be capable of moral agency. On the other hand a moral community can be thought of as embracing all beings to whom moral agents owe duties—the bearers of moral rights. It cannot simply be assumed that the class of moral agents (duty-bearers) is coextensive with the class of moral patients (right-bearers). It is quite conceivable that some beings, (infants, nonhuman animals) might have rights though they lack duties (because incapable of moral agency). The capacity for moral agency is (trivially) a condition of having moral duties. It is not obviously also a condition of having moral rights. The claim that the criterion for rights is the same as the criterion for duties is substantive and controversial. The necessity of defending this claim is merely concealed by equivocating on the notion of a moral community.

Beings who acknowledge one another as moral agents can also acknowledge that (some) creatures who are not themselves capable of moral agency nonetheless merit (some) protection of life. The more we reflect on the function of rights, the stronger becomes the inclination to extend them to such creatures. Rights are securities for beings who are sufficiently autonomous to conduct their own lives but who are also vulnerable to the aggression of others and dependent upon these others for some of the necessaries of life. Rights protect the goods of their owners and shield them from evils. We ascribe rights to one another because we all alike satisfy these minimal conditions of autonomy, vulnerability, and dependence. In order to satisfy these conditions a creature need not itself be capable of morality: it need only possess interests that can be protected by rights. A higher standard thus seems appropriate for possession of moral duties than for possession of moral rights. Rationality appears to be the right sort of criterion for the former, but something less demanding (such as sentience) is better suited to the latter.

A criterion of life (or teleology) is too weak, admitting classes of beings (animate and inanimate) who are not suitable loci for moral rights; being alive is necessary for having standing, but it is not sufficient. A criterion of rationality (or moral agency) is too strong, excluding classes of beings (human and nonhuman) who are suitable loci for rights; being rational is sufficient for having standing, but it is not necessary. A criterion of sentience (or consciousness) is a promising middle path between these extremes.[17] Sentience is the capacity for feeling or affect. In its most primitive form it is the ability to experience sensations of pleasure and pain, and thus the ability to enjoy and suffer. Its more developed forms include wants, aims, and desires (and thus the ability to be satisfied and frustrated); attitudes, tastes, and values; and moods, emotions, sentiments, and passions. Consciousness is a necessary condition of sentience, for feelings are states of mind of which their owner is aware. But it is not sufficient; it is at least possible in principle for beings to be conscious (percipient, for instance, or even rational) while utterly lacking feelings. If rationality embraces a set of cognitive capacities, then sentience is rooted in a being's affective and conative life. It is in virtue of being sentient that creatures have interests, which are compounded either out of their desires or out of the experiences they find agreeable (or both). If morality has to do with the protection and promotion of interests, it is a plausible conjecture that we owe moral duties to all those beings capable of having interests. But this will include all sentient creatures.

Most animal species, like all plant species, are (so far as we can tell) utterly nonsentient. Like consciousness, sentience emerged during the evolutionary process as a means of permitting more flexible behavior patterns and thus of aiding survival. Biologically it is marked by the emergence in the first vertebrates of the forebrain (the primitive ancestor of the human cerebral hemispheres).[18] As far can be determined, even the simple capacity for pleasure and pain is not possessed by invertebrate animals.[19] If this is the case, then the phylogenetic threshold of moral standing is the boundary between invertebrates and vertebrates.

Like rationality, and unlike life, it makes sense to think of sentience as admitting of degrees. Within any given mode, such as the perception of pain, one creature may be more or less sensitive than another. But there is a further sense in which more developed (more rational) creatures possess a higher degree of sentience. The expansion of consciousness and of intelligence opens up new ways of experiencing the world, and therefore new ways of being affected by the world. More rational beings are capable of finding either fulfilment or frustration in activities and states of affairs to which less developed creatures are, both cognitively and affectively, blind. It is in this sense of a broader and deeper sensibility that a higher being is capable of a richer, fuller, and more varied existence. The fact that sentience admits of degrees (whether of sensitivity or sensibility) enables us to employ it both as an inclusion criterion and as a comparison criterion of moral standing. The animal kingdom presents us with a hierarchy of sentience. Nonsentient beings have no moral standing; among sentient beings the more developed have greater standing than the less developed, the upper limit being occupied by the paradigm of a normal adult human being. Although sentience is the criterion of moral standing, it is also possible to explain the relevance of rationality. The evolutionary order is one of ascending intelligence. Since rationality expands a creature's interests, it is a reliable indicator of the degree of moral standing which that creature possesses. Creatures less rational than human beings do not altogether lack standing, but they do lack full standing.

An analysis of degrees of standing would require a graded right to life, in which the strength of the right varied inversely with the range of considerations capable of overriding it. The details of any such analysis will be complex and need not be worked out here. However, it seems that we are committed to extending (some) moral standing to all vertebrate animals, and also to counting higher animals for more than lower. Thus we should expect the higher vertebrates (mammals) to merit greater protection of life than the lower (fish, reptiles, amphibia, birds) and we should also expect the higher mammals (primates, cetaceans) to merit greater protection of life than the lower (canines, felines, etc.). Crude as this division may be, it seems to accord reasonably well with most people's intuitions that in our moral reasoning paramecia and horseflies count for nothing, dogs and cats count for something, chimpanzees and dolphins count for more, and human beings count for most of all.

A criterion of sentience can thus allow for the gradual emergence of moral standings in the order of nature. It can explain why no moral issues arise (directly) in our dealings with inanimate objects, plants, and the simpler forms of animal life. It can also function as a moral guideline in our encounters with novel life forms on other planets. If the creatures we meet have interests and are capable of enjoyment and suffering, we must grant them some moral standing. We thereby constrain ourselves not to exploit them ruthlessly for our own advantage. The kind of standing that they deserve may be determined by the range and depth of their sensibility, and in ordinary circumstances this will vary with their intelligence. We should therefore recognize as equals beings who are as rational and sensitive as ourselves. The criterion also implies that if we encounter creatures who are rational but nonsentient—who utterly lack affect and desire—nothing we can do will adversely affect such creatures (in morally relevant ways). We would be entitled, for instance, to treat them as a species of organic computer. The same obviously holds for forms of artificial intelligence; in deciding whether to extend moral standing to sophisticated machines, the question (as Bentham put it) is not whether they can reason but whether they can suffer.

A criterion of sentience also requires gentle usage of the severely abnormal. Cognitive disabilities and disorders may impair a person's range of sensibility, but they do not generally reduce that person to the level of a nonsentient being. Even the grossly retarded or deranged will still be capable of some forms of enjoyment and suffering and thus will still possess (some) moral standing in their own right. This standing diminishes to the vanishing point only when sentience is entirely lost (irreversible coma) or never gained in the first place (anencephaly).[20] If all affect and responsivity are absent, and if they cannot be engendered, then (but only then) are we no longer dealing with a sentient creature. This verdict accords well with the contemporary trend toward defining death in terms of the permanent loss of cerebral functioning.[21] Although such patients are in one obvious sense still alive (their blood circulates and is oxygenated), in the morally relevant sense they are now beyond our reach, for we can cause them neither good nor ill. A criterion of life would require us to continue treating them as beings with (full?) moral standing, whereas a criterion of rationality would withdraw that standing when reason was lost even though sensibility should remain. Again a criterion of sentience enables us to find a middle way.

Fastening upon sentience as the criterion for possession of a right to life thus opens up the possibility of a reasonable and moderate treatment of moral problems other than abortion, problems pertaining to the treatment of nonhuman animals, extraterrestrial life, artificial intelligence, "defective" human beings, and persons at the end of life. We need now to trace out its implications for the fetus.

THE MORALITY OF ABORTION
The adoption of sentience as a criterion determines the location of a threshold of moral standing. Since sentience admits of degrees, we can in principle construct a continuum ranging from fully sentient creatures at one extreme to completely nonsentient creatures at the other. The threshold of moral standing is that area of the continuum through which sentience fades into non-sentience. In phylogenesis the continuum extends from homo sapiens to the simple animals and plants, and the threshold area is the boundary between vertebrates and invertebrates. In pathology the continuum extends from the fully normal to the totally incapacitated, and the threshold area is the transition from consciousness to unconsciousness. Human ontogenesis also presents us with a continuum from adult to zygote. The threshold area will be the stage at which sentience first emerges, but where is that to be located?

A mental life is built upon a physical base. The capacity for sentience is present only when the necessary physiological structures are present. Physiology, and in particular neurophysiology, is our principal guide in locating a threshold in the phylogenetic continuum. Like a stereo system, the brain of our paradigm sentient being is a set of connected components.[22] These components may be roughly sorted into three groups: forebrain (cerebral hemispheres, thalamus, hypothalamus, amygdala), midbrain (cerebellum), and brainstem (upper part of the spinal cord, pineal and pituitary glands). The brainstem and midbrain play no direct role in the individual's conscious life; their various parts regulate homeostasis (temperature, respiration, heartbeat, etc.), secrete hormones, make reflex connections, route nerves, coordinate motor activities, and so on. All of these functions can be carried on in the total absence of consciousness. Cognitive, perceptual, and voluntary motor functions are all localized in the forebrain, more particularly in the cerebral cortex. Sensation (pleasure/pain), emotion, and basic drives (hunger, thirst, sex, etc.) are controlled by subcortical areas in the forebrain. Although the nerves that transmit pleasure/pain impulses are routed through the cortex, their ultimate destination is the limbic system (amygdala, hypothalamus). The most primitive forms of sentience are thus possible in the absence of cortical activity.

Possession of particular neural structures cannot serve as a criterion of moral standing, for we cannot rule out encounters with sentient beings whose structures are quite different from ours. But in all of the species with which we are familiar, the components of the forebrain (or some analogues) are the minimal conditions of sentience. Thus the evolution of the forebrain serves as an indicator of the kind and degree of sentience possessed by a particular animal species. When we turn to human ontogenesis we may rely on the same indicator.

The normal gestation period for our species is 280 days from the onset of the last menstrual period to birth.[23] This duration is usually divided into three equal trimesters of approximately thirteen weeks each. A zygote has no central nervous system of any sort. The spinal cord makes its first appearance early in the embryonic period (third week), and the major divisions between forebrain, midbrain, and brainstem are evident by the end of the eighth week. At

the conclusion of the first trimester virtually all of the major neural components can be clearly differentiated and EEG activity is detectable. The months to follow are marked chiefly by the growth and elaboration of the cerebral hemispheres, especially the cortex. The brain of a seven-month fetus is indistinguishable, at least in its gross anatomy, from that of a newborn infant. Furthermore, by the seventh month most of the neurons that the individual's brain will contain during its entire lifetime are already in existence. In the newborn the brain is closer than any other organ to its mature level of development.

There is no doubt that a newborn infant is sentient—that it feels hunger, thirst, physical pain, the pleasure of sucking, and other agreeable and disagreeable sensations. There is also no doubt that a zygote, and also an embryo, are presentient. It is difficult to locate with accuracy the stage during which feeling first emerges in fetal development.[24] The structure of the fetal brain, including the cortex, is well laid down by the end of the second trimester. But there is reason to expect the more primitive and ancient parts of that brain to function before the rest. The needs of the fetus dictate the order of appearance of neural functions. Thus the brainstem is established and functioning first, since it is required for the regulation of heartbeat and other metabolic processes. Since the mammalian fetus develops in an enclosed and protected environment, cognition and perception are not essential for survival and their advent is delayed. It is therefore not surprising that the cortex, the most complex part of the brain and the least important to the fetus, is the last to develop to an operational level.

Simple pleasure/pain sensations would seem to occupy a medial position in this priority ranking. They are localized in a part of the brain that is more primitive than the cortex, but they could have little practical role for a being that is by and large unable either to seek pleasurable stimuli or to avoid painful ones. Behavioral evidence is by its very nature ambiguous. Before the end of the first trimester, the fetus will react to unpleasant stimuli by flinching and withdrawing. However, this reaction is probably a reflex that is entirely automatic. How are we to tell when mere reflex has crossed over into consciousness? The information we now possess does not enable us to date with accuracy the emergence of fetal sentience. Of some judgments, however, we can be reasonably confident. First-trimester fetuses are clearly not yet sentient. Third-trimester fetuses probably possess some degree of sentience, however minimal. The threshold of sentience thus appears to fall in the second trimester.[25] More ancient and primitive than cognition, the ability to discriminate simple sensations of pleasure and pain is probably the first form of consciousness to appear in the ontogenetic order. Further, when sentience emerges it does not do so suddenly. The best we can hope for is to locate a threshold stage or period in the second trimester. It is at present unclear just how far into that trimester this stage occurs.

The phylogenetic and pathological continua yield us clear cases at the extremes and unclear cases in the middle. The ontogenetic continuum does the same. Because there is no quantum leap into consciousness during fetal development, there is no clean and sharp boundary between sentient and nonsentient fetuses. There is therefore no precise point at which a fetus acquires moral standing. More and better information may enable us to locate the threshold stage ever more accurately, but it will never collapse that stage into a point. We are therefore inevitably confronted with a class of fetuses around the threshold stage whose sentience, and therefore whose moral status, is indeterminate.

A criterion based on sentience enables us to explain the status of other putative thresholds. Neither conception nor birth marks the transition from a presentient to a sentient being. A zygote has not one whit more consciousness than the gametes out of which it is formed. Likewise, although a neonate has more opportunity to employ its powers, it also has no greater capacity for sensation than a full-term fetus. Of thresholds located during gestation, quickening is the perception of fetal movement that is probably reflex and therefore preconscious. Only viability has some relevance, though at one remove. For reasons given earlier, it cannot serve as a criterion. But a fetus is viable when it is equipped to survive in the outside world. A being that is aware of, and can respond to, its own inner states is able to communicate its needs to others. This ability is of no use in utero but may aid survival in an extrauterine environment. A fetus is therefore probably sentient by the conventional stage of viability (around the end of the second trimester). Viability can therefore serve as a (rough) indicator of moral standing.

Our common moral consciousness locates contraception and infanticide in quite different moral categories. This fact suggests implicit recognition of a basic asymmetry between choosing not to create a new life in the first place and choosing to destroy a new life once it has been created.[26] The boundary between the two kinds of acts is the threshold at which that life gains moral protection. Since gametes lack moral standing, contraception (however it is carried out) merely prevents the creation of a new person. Since an infant has moral standing, infanticide (however it is carried out) destroys a new person. A second-trimester threshold of moral standing introduces this asymmetry into the moral assessment of abortion. We may define an early abortion as one performed sometime during the first trimester or early in the second, and a late abortion as one performed sometime late in the second trimester or during the third. An early abortion belongs in the same moral category as contraception: it prevents the emergence of a new being with moral standing. A late abortion belongs in the same moral category as infanticide: it terminates the life of a new being with moral standing. The threshold of sentience thus extends the morality of contraception forward to cover early abortion and extends the morality of infanticide backward to cover late abortion. One of the sentiments voiced by many people who contemplate the problem of abortion is that early abortions are importantly different from late ones. The abortion techniques of the first trimester (the IUD, menstrual extraction, vacuum aspiration) are not to be treated as cases of homicide. Those employed later in pregnancy (saline induction, hysterotomy) may, however, have a moral quality approaching that of infanticide. For most people, qualms about abortion are qualms about late abortion. It is a virtue of the sentience criterion that it explains and supports this differential approach.

The moral issues raised by early abortion are precisely those raised by contraception. It is for early abortions that the liberal view is appropriate. Since the fetus at this stage has no right to life, early abortion (like contraception) cannot violate its rights. But if it violates no one's rights, early abortion (like contraception) is a private act. There are of course significant differences between contraception and early abortion, since the former is generally less hazardous, less arduous, and less expensive. A woman has, therefore, good prudential reasons for relying on contraception as her primary means of birth control. But if she elects an early abortion, then, whatever the circumstances and whatever her reasons, she does nothing immoral.[27]

The moral issues raised by late abortion are similar to those raised by infanticide. It is for late abortions that (a weakened form of) the conservative view is appropriate. Since the fetus at this stage has a right to life, late abortion (like infanticide) may violate its rights. But if it may violate the fetus' rights, then late abortion (like infanticide) is a public act. There is, however, a morally significant difference between late abortion and infanticide. A fetus is parasitic upon a unique individual in a manner in which a newborn infant is not. That parasitic relation will justify late abortion more liberally than infanticide, for they do not occur under the same circumstances.

Since we have already explored the morality of abortion for those cases in which the fetus has moral standing, the general approach to late abortions is clear enough. Unlike the simple and uniform treatment of early abortion, only a case-by-case analysis will here suffice. We should expect a serious threat to the woman's life or health (physical or mental) to justify abortion, especially if that threat becomes apparent only late in pregnancy. We should also expect a risk of serious fetal deformity to justify abortion, again especially if that risk becomes apparent (as it usually does) only late in pregnancy. On the other hand, it should not be necessary to justify abortion on the ground that pregnancy was not consented to, since a woman will have ample opportunity to seek an abortion before the threshold stage. If a woman freely elects to continue a pregnancy past that stage, she will thereafter need a serious reason to end it.

A differential view of abortion is therefore liberal concerning early abortion and conservative (in an extended sense) concerning late abortion. The status of the borderline cases in the middle weeks of the second trimester is simply indeterminate. We cannot say of them with certainty either that the fetus has a

right to life or that it does not. Therefore we also cannot say either that a liberal approach to these abortions is suitable or that a conservative treatment of them is required. What we can say is that, from the moral point of view, the earlier an abortion is performed the better. There are thus good moral reasons, as well as good prudential ones, for women not to delay their abortions.

A liberal view of early abortion in effect extends a woman's deadline for deciding whether to have a child. If all abortion is immoral, her sovereignty over that decision ends at conception. Given the vicissitudes of contraception, a deadline drawn that early is an enormous practical burden. A deadline in the second trimester allows a woman enough time to discover that she is pregnant and to decide whether to continue the pregnancy. If she chooses not to continue it, her decision violates neither her duties nor any other being's rights. From the point of view of the fetus, the upshot of this treatment of early abortion is that its life is for a period merely probationary; only when it has passed the threshold will that life be accorded protection. If an abortion is elected before the threshold, it is as though from the moral point of view that individual had never existed.

Settling on sentience as a criterion of moral standing thus leads us to a view of the moral status of the fetus, and of the morality of abortion, which satisfies the constraints set out in Section 15. It is gradual, since it locates a threshold stage rather than a point and allows moral standing to be acquired incrementally. It is differential, since it locates the threshold stage during gestation and thus distinguishes the moral status of newly conceived and full-term fetuses. It is developmental, since it grounds the acquisition of moral standing in one aspect of the normal development of the fetus. And it is moderate, since it distinguishes the moral status of early and late abortions and applies each of the established views to that range of cases for which it is appropriate.

AN ABORTION POLICY

A differential view of the morality of abortion leads to a differential abortion policy—one that draws a legal distinction between early and late abortions. If we work within the framework of a liberal social theory, then it is understood that the state has no right to interfere in the private activities of individuals. An early abortion is a private act—or, rather, a private transaction between a woman and her physician. No regulation of this transaction will be legitimate unless it is also legitimate for other contractual arrangements between patients and physicians. It might be quite in place for the state to require that abortions be performed by qualified (perhaps licensed) personnel in properly equipped (perhaps licensed) facilities: whether or not this is so will depend on whether the state is in general competent to regulate trade in medical skills. Both the decision to abort and the decision to use contraceptives are private ones on which a woman ought to seek medical advice and medical assistance. There is no justification in either case for restricting access to that advice or that assistance.

An abortion policy must therefore be permissive for early abortions. There is at this stage no question of inquiring into a woman's reason for seeking an abortion. Her autonomy here is absolute; the simple desire not to have a child (or not to have one now) is sufficient. Grounds for abortion become pertinent only when we turn to late abortions. Since virtually all such abortions will result in the death of a being that has a right to life (though not all will violate that right), the state has a legitimate role to play in governing trade in abortion at this stage. Legal grounds for late abortion are a special case of conditions for justifiable homicide. As much as possible (allowing for the unique relation between mother and fetus) these grounds should authorize abortion when killing would also be justified in relevantly similar cases not involving fetuses. Two general conditions for justifiable homicide will be applicable to abortions: self-defense and euthanasia.

The usual legal grounds for abortion provided by moderate policies may be divided into four categories:[28] (a) therapeutic (threat to maternal life or health); (b) eugenic (risk of fetal abnormality); (c) humanitarian (pregnancy due to the commission of a crime, such as rape or incest); (d) socioeconomic (poverty, family size, etc.). If a moderate treatment of late abortion is coupled (as it should be) with a permissive treatment of early ones, only the first two categories are necessary. Therapeutic grounds for abortion follow from a woman's right of self-defense. The threat, however, must be serious in two different respects: the injury in prospect must be more than trivial and the probability of its occurrence must be more than trivial and the probability of its occurrence must be greater than normal. The risks generally associated with pregnancy will not here suffice. Further, there must be good medical reason not to delay until the fetus has a better chance of survival, and every effort must be made to save the fetus' life if this is possible.[29] Thus late abortion for therapeutic reasons ought to be reserved for genuine medical emergencies in which no other course of action would qualify as proper care of the mother. In many putatively moderate policies therapeutic grounds for abortion (especially mental health clauses) are interpreted so liberally as to cover large numbers of cases that are not by any stretch of the imagination medical emergencies. This is the standard device whereby a policy moderate in principle becomes permissive in practice. Since the policy here advanced is permissive in principle (for early abortions), a strict interpretation of the therapeutic grounds for late abortions will be mandatory.

The same strictures will apply to eugenic grounds. Where there is a substantial risk of some severe anomaly (rubella, spina bifida, Tay-Sachs disease, etc.), abortion may be the best course of action for the fetus. This is not obviously the case for less severe defects (Down's syndrome, dwarfism, etc.). Again there will be no justification for an interpretation of eugenic grounds so elastic that it permits abortion whenever the child is unwanted (because, say, it is the "wrong" sex). A rough rule of thumb is that late abortion for reasons of fetal abnormality is permissible only in those cases in which euthanasia for defective newborns would also be permissible. Probability will play a different role in the two kinds of case, since prenatal diagnosis of these conditions is often less certain than postnatal. But against this reason for delay we must balance the anguish of a woman carrying a fetus who may turn out at birth to be grossly deformed. Since diagnostic techniques such as ultrasound and amniocentesis cannot be employed until the second trimester, a permissive treatment of early abortions will not eliminate the need for late abortions on eugenic grounds.

Both therapeutic and eugenic grounds can be alleged for a wide range of abortions. Some of these cases will be clearly justified, others will be just as clearly unjustified, and the remainder will just be hard cases. There is no formula that can be applied mechanically to decide the hard cases. We should look to a statute for only the most perfunctory statement of justifying grounds for abortion. Particular decisions (the analogue of case law) are best undertaken by persons with the relevant medical expertise. This might be a hospital or clinic committee established especially to monitor late abortions or an "ethics committee" with broader responsibilities. In either case, establishing the right sort of screening mechanism is the best means of ensuring that the justifying grounds are given a reasonable application.

There is no need for any special notice of humanitarian grounds. It is doubtful indeed whether incest ought to be a crime, except in those cases in which someone is being exploited. In any case, any woman who has become pregnant due to incestuous intercourse will have ready access to an early abortion. If she declines this opportunity and if there is no evidence of genetic abnormality, she may not simply change her mind later. The same obviously applies to pregnancy due to rape, including statutory rape. The practical problems should be approached by providing suitable counseling.

A permissive policy for early abortions will also render socioeconomic grounds redundant. Since social constraints do not normally create an emergency for which abortion is the only solution, and since women will be able to terminate pregnancies at will in the early stages, there is no need for separate recognition of social or economic justifications for abortion.

An adequate abortion policy is thus a conjunction of a permissive policy for early abortions and a moderate policy for late abortions. The obvious remaining question is where to draw the boundary between the two classes of cases. When we are dealing with the morality of abortion, borderline fuzziness is both inevitable and tolerable. Many moral problems turn on factors that are matters of degree. Where such factors are present, we cannot avoid borderline cases whose status is unclear or indeterminate. It is a defect in a moral theory to draw sharp lines where there are none, or to treat hard cases as though they

were easy. But what makes for good morals may also make for bad law. An abortion policy must be enforceable and so must divide cases as clearly as possible. A threshold stage separating early from late abortions must here give way to a cutoff point.

Since there is no threshold point in fetal development, any precise upper limit on the application of a permissive policy will be to some extent arbitrary. Clearly it must be located within the threshold period, thus sometime in the second trimester. Beyond this constrain the choice of a time limit may be made on pragmatic grounds. If a permissive policy for early abortions is to promote their autonomy, women must have time to discover that they are pregnant and to decide on a course of action. This factor will tend to push the cutoff point toward the end of the second trimester. On the other hand, earlier abortions are substantially safer and more economical of scarce medical resources than later ones. This factor will tend to pull the cutoff point toward the beginning of the second trimester. Balancing these considerations would incline one toward a time limit located sometime around the midpoint of pregnancy. But it should not be pretended that there is a unique solution to this policy problem. Differential policies may legitimately vary (within constraints) in their choice of a boundary between permissiveness and moderation.

Since abortion is a controversial matter, a society's abortion policy ought to include a "conscience clause" that allows medical personnel with conscientious objections to avoid involvement in abortions.[30] It is in general preferable not to require doctors and nurses to perform tasks that deeply offend their moral principles, at least as long as others are willing to meet patients' needs. But it should be stated plainly that dissenting scruples are here being honored, not because they are correct (for they are not), but because a pluralistic society thrives when it promotes as much mutual respect of values as is compatible with the common good. The position of hospitals may be quite different. Any institution that is publicly funded is obliged to provide a suitably wide range of public services. Individual persons may opt out of performing abortions without thereby rendering abortions unavailable, but if entire hospitals do so, substantial numbers of women may have no meaningful access to this service. Whether abortions ought to be subsidized by government medical insurance plans is a question of social justice that cannot be answered without investigating the moral basis of compulsory social welfare programs in general. However, once a society has installed such a plan, there is no justification for omitting abortions from the list of services covered by it.[31]

The abortion policy here proposed is not novel: a differential policy with a time limit in the second trimester is already in operation in a number of countries.[32] But these policies seem usually to have been settled on as compromises between the opposed demands of liberals and conservatives rather than as matters of principle. Such compromises are attractive to politicians, who do not seek any deeper justification for the policies they devise. But there is a deeper justification for this policy. Although it does define a middle ground between the established views, it has not been defended here as the outcome of a bargaining procedure. Instead it has been advanced as the only policy congruent with an adequate criterion of moral standing and proper recognition of both a woman's right to autonomy and a fetus' right to life. A differential policy does not mediate between alternatives both of which are rationally defensible; instead it supersedes alternatives both of which have been discredited.

Notes

1. Both Tooley (1973) and Warren (1978) allow moral standing to be acquired gradually in the normal course of human development. But since both believe that such standing is only acquired after birth, neither attributes any importance to prenatal development— except as the groundwork of postnatal development.

2. Tom Regan appears to defend this position in his (unpublished) essay "Sumner on the Wrongness of Killing" (however, see note 9, below). Basing moral standing on intrinsic value also seems to be implied by the ideal utilitarianism of Moore and Rashdall.

3. On the other hand, why should we assume that all wrongs are moral wrongs?

4. Or so we shall assume, though it is certainly possible that some (natural or artificial) entity might display signs of intelligence but no signs of either sentience or

life. We might, for instance, create forms of artificial intelligence before creating forms of artificial life.

5. Goodpaster employs the locution "moral considerability" where we are speaking of moral standing. The notions are identical, except for the fact that Goodpaster explicitly refrains from restricting moral considerability to possession of rights, let alone to the right to life. Nothing in the assessment of Goodpaster's view will hang on the issue of rights, and the notion of moral standing will later be generalized so as to drop essential reference to rights.

6. In the paragraph to follow I have stated that case in my own words.

7. These are my terms; Goodpaster distinguishes between a criterion of moral considerability and a criterion of moral significance (p. 311). It is odd that when Goodpaster addresses the practical problems created by treating life as an inclusion criterion (p. 324) he does not appeal to the inclusion/comparison distinction. Instead he invokes the quite different distinction between its being reasonable to attribute standing to a creature and its being (psychologically and causally) possible to act on that attribution. One would have thought the question is not what we *can* bring ourselves to do but what we *ought* to bring ourselves to do, and that the inclusion/comparison distinction is precisely designed to help us answer this question.

8. Goodpaster does not defend separating the two criteria but merely says "we should not expect that the criterion for having 'moral standing' at all will be the same as the criterion for adjudicating competing claims to priority among beings that merit that standing" (p. 311). Certainly inclusion and comparison criteria can be different, as in Mill's celebrated evaluation of pleasures. For Mill every pleasure has some value simply in virtue of being a pleasure (inclusion), but its relative value is partly determined by its quality or kind (comparison). All of this is quite consistent (despite claims to the contrary by some critics) because every pleasure has some quality or other. Goodpaster's comparison criterion threatens to be narrower than his inclusion criterion; it certainly will be if degrees of standing are based on sentience, since many living things have no sentience at all. It is inconsistent to base degrees of standing on (variations) in a property and also to extend (some) standing to beings who lack that property entirely.

9. Tom Regan (1976), who argues that moral standing should be distributed on the basis of possession of a good (or the capacity to be benefited and harmed), explicitly accepts the implication that inanimate things may have standing. Regan sometimes fails to distinguish between "*x* has a good (can be benefited and harmed)" and "the existence of *x* is good (has intrinsic value)." Thus his apparent endorsement of both an intrinsic value and a benefit/harm criterion.

10. Goodpaster (1978) does not shrink, from attributing interests to nonsentient organisms, and Regan (1976) does not shrink, from attributing interests to both nonsentient organisms and artifacts. Both authors assume that if a being has needs, a good, and a capacity to be benefited and harmed, then that being has interests. There is much support for this assumption in the dictionary definitions of both "interest" and "welfare," though talk of protecting the interests or welfare of plants or machines seems contrived and strained. But philosophers and economists have evolved technical definitions of "interest" and "welfare" that clearly tie these notions to the psychological states of sentient beings. It is the existence of beings with interests or welfare *in this sense* that is a necessary condition of the existence of moral issues.

11. Rationality is the basis of Kant's well-known distinction between persons (ends in themselves) and mere things (means). It is also advanced as a criterion by Tooley (1973), Donagan (1977), and Warren (1978).

12. Possession of a capacity at a given time does not entail that the capacity is being manifested or displayed at that time. A person does not lose the capacity to use language, for instance, in virtue of remaining silent or being asleep. The capacity remains as long as the appropriate performance could be elicited by the appropriate stimuli. It is lost only when this performance can no longer be evoked (as when the person has become catatonic or comatose). Basing moral standing on the possession of some capacity or set of capacities does not therefore entail silly results, such as that persons lose their rights when they fall asleep. This applies of course, not only to rationality but also to other capacities, such as sentience.

13. The practical impact of basing moral standing on rationality will, however, depend on which particular capacities are treated as central. Practical rationality (the ability to adjust means to ends, and vice versa) is,

for instance, much more widely distributed through the animal kingdom than is the use of language.

14. Melden (1977), p. 204. Melden rejects rationality as a criterion of standing (p. 187), but only on the ground that a being's rationality does not ensure its possessing a sense of morality. Clearly rationality is a necessary condition of moral agency. Thus a criterion of moral agency will not extend standing beyond the class of rational beings.

15. Whether or not this is so will depend on how strong the conditions of moral agency are. Certainly many nonhuman species display altruism, if we mean by this a concern for the well-being of conspecifics and a willingness to accept personal sacrifices for their good. On p. 199 Melden enumerates a number of features of our lives that are to serve as the basis of our possession of rights; virtually all mammals display all of these features.

16. The same ambiguity infects the argument in Fox (1978), who wishes to deny rights to nonhuman animals.

17. In their several ways, Feinberg (1974), Regan (1975), and Singer (1975) have all defended the possession of interests (and thus sentience) as the criterion of moral standing.

18. See, for example, Rose (1976), chap. 6 Psychologists and physiologists tend to use the term "consciousness" to cover perception and such higher-order cognitive processes as thought and language use, rather than sensation. In this sense conscious activities in human beings are localized in the cerebral cortex, an area of the brain that we share with most mammals. Sensation (pleasure/pain) and emotion are rooted in the limbic system, an evolutionarily more ancient part of the brain present in most vertebrates.

19. See Snyder (1977). For an outline of the physiology of pain sensation, see Melzack (1973), chap. 4. The transmission of pain requires mechanisms present only in animals with a central nervous system.

20. The definition of irreversible coma in Harvard Medical School (1968) includes complete unreceptivity and unresponsivity. Anencephaly is the total absence of the cerebral hemispheres; anencephalic fetuses or neonates never survive.

21. See Veatch (1976), especially chaps. 1 and 2.

22. For an accessible account of brain structures and functions, see Rose (1976).

23. Standard accounts of fetal development may be found in Patten and Carlson (1974), and Torrey and Feduccia (1979). For the prenatal development of the brain, see also Rose (1976), chap. 7.

24. This is a question to which embryologists seem not to address themselves.

25. The view in Pluhar (1977) agrees with that defended here in basing the moral standing of the fetus on what Pluhar calls "simple consciousness" (as opposed to reflexive consciousness or self-consciousness). However, he argues that the potential for simple consciousness also qualifies its owner for moral standing; it would appear, then, that he attributes (some degree of) such standing to all fetuses. Pluhar is effectively criticized on this point by Daniels (1979). See also Carrier (1975).

26. The asymmetry is easily accounted for by a rights theory, since only the latter act can violate anyone's right to life.

27. Unless there are circumstances (such as extreme underpopulation) in which contraception would also be immoral.

28. I here adapt the categories used in World Health Organization (1971), p. 6.

29. For convenience I here count as abortions procedures undertaken at or beyond the conventional point of viability (which in some jurisdictions is set as early as twenty weeks). In cases of genuine medical emergency, the desire to save the life of the fetus can be manifested by preferring hysterotomy to saline induction.

30. There is a good account of the debate on a conscience clause for the 1967 British Abortion Act in St. John-Stevas (1967-1968).

31. If abortion should be omitted on the ground that most pregnancies can be easily avoided, then treatment for lung cancer must also be omitted since most cases of lung cancer can be even more easily avoided. There is no justification for restricting a woman's access to abortion by requiring the consent of the father. Until men learn to become pregnant, if a man wishes to father a child he must find a woman willing to carry and bear it. Parental consent is a slightly more complicated issue, since it raises questions about the competence of minors. In most cases a girl who is mature enough to be sexually active is also mature enough to decide on an abortion; in any case no parental consent regulation is justified for abortion that is not also justified for all comparable forms of minor surgery.

32. Notably the United States, Great Britain, France, Italy, Sweden, the Soviet Union, China, India, Japan, and most of the countries of Eastern Europe. The cut-off points in these jurisdictions vary from the beginning to the end of the second trimester.

24.
THE MORAL SIGNIFICANCE OF BIRTH

Mary Anne Warren

English common law treats the moment of live birth as the point at which a legal person comes into existence. Although abortion has often been prohibited, it has almost never been classified as homicide. In contrast, infanticide generally is classified as a form of homicide, even where (as in England) there are statutes designed to mitigate the severity of the crime in certain cases. But many people—including some feminists—now favor the extension of equal legal rights to some or all fetuses (S. Callahan 1984, 1986). The extension of legal personhood to fetuses would not only threaten women's right to choose abortion, but also undermine other fundamental rights. I will argue that because of these dangers, birth remains the most appropriate place to mark the existence of a new legal person.

SPEAKING OF RIGHTS

In making this case, I find it useful to speak of moral as well as legal rights. Although not all legal rights can be grounded in moral rights, the right to life can plausibly be so construed. This approach is controversial. Some feminist philosophers have been critical of moral analyses based upon rights. Carol Gilligan (1982), Nel Noddings (1984), and others have argued that women tend to take a different approach to morality, one that emphasizes care and responsibility in interpersonal relationships rather than abstract rules, principles, or conflicts of rights. I would argue, however, that moral rights are complementary to a feminist ethics of care and responsibility, not inconsistent or competitive with it. Whereas caring relationships can provide a moral ideal, respect for rights provides a moral floor—a minimum protection for individuals which remains morally binding even where appropriate caring relationships are absent or have broken down (Manning 1988). Furthermore, as I shall argue, social relationships are part of the foundation of moral rights.

Some feminist philosophers have suggested that the very concept of a moral right may be inconsistent with the social nature of persons. Elizabeth Wolgast (1987, 41-42) argues convincingly that this concept has developed within an atomistic model of the social world, in which persons are depicted as self-sufficient and exclusively self-interested individuals whose relationships with one another are essentially competitive. As Wolgast notes, such an atomistic model is particularly inappropriate in the context of pregnancy, birth, and parental responsibility. Moreover, recent feminist research has greatly expanded our awareness of the historical, religious, sociological, and political forces that shape contemporary struggles over reproductive rights, further underscoring the need for approaches to moral theory that can take account of such social realities (Harrison 1983; Luker 1984; Petchesky 1984).

But is the concept of a moral right necessarily incompatible with the social nature of human beings? Rights are indeed individualistic, in that they can be ascribed to individuals, as well as to groups. But respect for moral rights need not be based upon an excessively individualistic view of human nature. A more socially perceptive account of moral rights is possible, provided that we reject two common assumptions about the theoretical foundations of moral rights. These assumptions are widely accepted by mainstream philosophers, but rarely stated and still more rarely defended.

The first is what I shall call the intrinsic-properties assumption. This is the view that the only facts that can justify the ascription of basic moral rights[1] or moral standing[2] to individuals are facts about *the intrinsic properties of those individuals*. Philosophers who accept this view disagree about which of the intrinsic properties of individuals are relevant to the ascription of rights. They agree, however, that relational properties—such as being loved, or being part of a social community or biological ecosystem—cannot be relevant.

The second is what I shall call the single-criterion assumption. This is the view that there is some single property, the presence or absence of which divides the world into those things which have moral rights or moral standing, and those things which do not. Christopher Stone (1987) locates this assumption within a more general theoretical approach, which he calls "moral monism." Moral monists believe that the goal of moral philosophy is the production of a coherent set of principles, sufficient to provide definitive answers to all possible moral dilemmas. Among these principles, the monist typically assumes, will be one that identifies some key property which is such that, "Those beings that possess the key property count morally ... [while those] things that lack it are all utterly irrelevant, except as resources for the benefit of those things that do count" (1987, 13).

Together, the intrinsic-properties and single-criterion assumptions preclude any adequate account of the social foundations of moral rights. The intrinsic-properties assumption requires us to regard all personal or other relationships among individuals or groups as wholly irrelevant to basic moral rights. The single-criterion assumption requires us to deny that there can be a variety of sound reasons for ascribing moral rights, and a variety of things and beings to which some rights may appropriately be ascribed. Both assumptions are inimical to a feminist approach to moral theory, as well as to approaches that are less anthropocentric and more environmentally adequate. The prevalence of these assumptions helps to explain why few mainstream philosophers believe that birth can in any way alter the infant's moral rights.

THE DENIAL OF THE MORAL SIGNIFICANCE OF BIRTH

The view that birth is irrelevant to moral rights is shared by philosophers on all points of the spectrum of moral views about abortion. For the most conservative, birth adds nothing to the infant's moral rights, since all of those rights have been present since conception. Moderates hold that the fetus acquires an equal right to life at some point after conception but before birth. The most popular candidates for this

point of moral demarcation are (1) the stage at which the fetus becomes viable (i.e., capable of surviving outside the womb, with or without medical assistance), and (2) the stage at which it becomes sentient (i.e., capable of having experiences, including that of pain). For those who hold a view of this sort, both infanticide and abortion at any time past the critical stage are forms of homicide, and there is little reason to distinguish between them either morally or legally.

Finally, liberals hold that even relatively late abortion is sometimes morally acceptable, and that at no time is abortion the moral equivalent of homicide. However, few liberals wish to hold that infanticide is not—at least sometimes—morally comparable to homicide. Consequently, the presumption that being born makes no difference to one's moral rights creates problems for the liberal view of abortion. Unless the liberal can establish some grounds for a general moral distinction between late abortion and early infanticide, she must either retreat to a moderate position on abortion, or else conclude that infanticide is not so bad after all.

To those who accept the intrinsic-properties assumption, birth can make little difference to the moral standing of the fetus/infant. For birth does not seem to alter any intrinsic property that could reasonably be linked to the possession of a strong right to life. Newborn infants have very nearly the same intrinsic properties as do fetuses shortly before birth. They have, as L.W. Sumner (1983, 53) says, "the same size, shape, internal constitution, species membership, capacities, level of consciousness, and so forth."[3] Consequently, Sumner says, infanticide cannot be morally very different from late abortion. In his words, "Birth is a shallow and arbitrary criterion of moral standing, and there appears to be no way of connecting it to a deeper account" (52).

Sumner holds that the only valid criterion of moral standing is the capacity for sentience (136). Prenatal neurophysiology and behavior suggest that human fetuses begin to have rudimentary sensory experiences at some time during the second trimester of pregnancy. Thus, Sumner concludes that abortion should be permitted during the first trimester but not thereafter, except in special circumstances (152).[4]

Michael Tooley (1983) agrees that birth can make no difference to moral standing. However, rather than rejecting the liberal view of abortion, Tooley boldly claims that neither late abortion nor early infanticide is seriously wrong. He argues that an entity cannot have a strong right to life unless it is capable of desiring its own continued existence. To be capable of such a desire, he argues, a being must have a concept of itself as a continuing subject of conscious experience. Having such a concept is a central part of what it is to be a person, and thus the kind of being that has strong moral rights (41). Fetuses certainly lack such a concept, as do infants during the first few months of their lives. Thus, Tooley concludes, neither fetuses nor newborn infants have a strong right to life, and neither abortion nor infanticide is an intrinsic moral wrong.

These two theories are worth examining, not only because they illustrate the difficulties generated by the intrinsic-properties and single-criterion assumptions, but also because each includes valid insights that need to be integrated into a more comprehensive account. Both Sumner and Tooley are partially right. Unlike "genetic humanity"—a property possessed by fertilized human ova—sentience and self-awareness are properties that have some general relevance to what we may owe another being in the way of respect and protection. However, neither the sentience criterion nor the self-awareness criterion can explain the moral significance of birth.

THE SENTIENCE CRITERION

Both newborn infants and late-term fetuses show clear signs of sentience. For instance, they are apparently capable of having visual experiences. Infants will often turn away from bright lights, and those who have done intrauterine photography have sometimes observed a similar reaction in the late-term fetus when bright lights are introduced in its vicinity. Both may respond to loud noises, voices, or other sounds, so both can probably have auditory experiences. They are evidently also responsive to touch, taste, motion, and other kinds of sensory stimulation.

The sentience of infants and late-term fetuses makes a difference to how they should be treated, by contrast with fertilized ova or first-trimester fetuses. Sentient beings are usually capable of experiencing painful as well as pleasurable or affectively neutral sensations.[5] While the capacity to experience pain is

valuable to an organism, pain is by definition an intrinsically unpleasant experience. Thus, sentient beings may plausibly be said to have a moral right not to be deliberately subjected to pain in the absence of any compelling reason. For those who prefer not to speak of rights, it is still plausible that a capacity for sentience gives an entity some moral standing. It may, for instance, require that its interests be given some consideration in utilitarian calculations, or that it be treated as an end and never merely as a means.

But it is not clear that sentience is a sufficient condition for moral equality, since there are many clearly-sentient creatures (e.g., mice) to which most of us would not be prepared to ascribe equal moral standing. Sumner examines the implications of the sentience criterion primarily in the context of abortion. Given his belief that some compromise is essential between the conservative and liberal viewpoints on abortion, the sentience criterion recommends itself as a means of drawing a moral distinction between early abortion and late abortion. It is, in some ways, a more defensible criterion than fetal viability.

The 1973 *Roe v. Wade* decision treats the presumed viability of third-trimester fetuses as a basis for permitting states to restrict abortion rights in order to protect fetal life in the third trimester, but not earlier. Yet viability is relative, among other things, to the medical care available to the pregnant woman and her infant. Increasingly sophisticated neonatal intensive care has made it possible to save many more premature infants than before, thus altering the average age of viability. Someday it may be possible to keep even first-trimester fetuses alive and developing normally outside the womb. The viability criterion seems to imply that the advent of total ectogenesis (artificial gestation from conception to birth) would automatically eliminate women's right to abortion, even in the earliest stages of pregnancy. At the very least, it must imply that as many aborted fetuses as possible should be kept alive through artificial gestation. But the mere technological possibility of providing artificial wombs for huge numbers of human fetuses could not establish such a moral obligation. A massive commitment to ectogenesis would probably be ruinously expensive, and might prove contrary to the interests of parents and children. The viability criterion forces us to make a hazardous leap from the technologically possible to the morally mandatory.

The sentience criterion at first appears more promising as a means of defending a moderate view of abortion. It provides an intuitively plausible distinction between early and late abortion. Unlike the viability criterion, it is unlikely to be undermined by new biomedical technologies. Further investigation of fetal neurophysiology and behavior might refute the presumption that fetuses begin to be capable of sentience *at some point in the second trimester*. Perhaps this development occurs slightly earlier or slightly later than present evidence suggests. (It is unlikely to be much earlier or much later.) However, that is a consequence that those who hold a moderate position on abortion could live with; so long as the line could still be drawn with some degree of confidence, they need not insist that it be drawn exactly where Sumner suggests.

But closer inspection reveals that the sentience criterion will not yield the result that Sumner wants. His position vacillates between two versions of the sentience criterion, neither of which can adequately support his moderate view of abortion. The strong version of the sentience criterion treats sentience as a sufficient condition for having full and equal moral standing. The weak version treats sentience as sufficient for having some moral standing, but not necessarily full and equal moral standing.

Sumner's claim that sentient fetuses have the same moral standing as older human beings clearly requires the strong version of the sentience criterion. On this theory, any being which has even minimal capacities for sensory experience is the moral equal of any person. If we accept this theory, then we must conclude that not only is late abortion the moral equivalent of homicide, but so is the killing of such sentient nonhuman beings as mice. Sumner evidently does not wish to accept this further conclusion, for he also says that "sentience admits of degrees ... [a fact that] enables us to employ it both as an inclusion criterion and as a comparison criterion of moral standing" (144). In other words, all sentient beings have some moral standing, but beings that are more highly sentient have greater moral standing than do less highly sentient beings. This weaker version of

the sentience criterion leaves room for a distinction between the moral standing of mice and that of sentient humans—provided, that is, that mice can be shown to be less highly sentient. However, it will not support the moral equality of late-term fetuses, since the relatively undeveloped condition of fetal brains almost certainly means that fetuses are less highly sentient than older human beings.

A similar dilemma haunts those who use the sentience criterion to argue for the moral equality of nonhuman animals. Some animal liberationists hold that all sentient beings are morally equal, regardless of species. For instance, Peter Singer (1981, 111) maintains that all sentient beings are entitled to equal consideration for their comparably important interests. Animal liberationists are primarily concerned to argue for the moral equality of vertebrate animals, such as mammals, birds, reptiles and fish. In this project, the sentience criterion serves them less well than they may suppose. On the one hand, if they use the weak version of the sentience criterion then they cannot sustain the claim that all nonhuman vertebrates are our moral equals—unless they can demonstrate that they are all sentient *to the same degree* that we are. It is unclear how such a demonstration would proceed, or what would count as success. On the other hand, if they use the strong version of the sentience criterion, then they are committed to the conclusion that if flies and mosquitos are even minimally sentient then they too are our moral equals. Not even the most radical animal liberationists have endorsed the moral equality of such invertebrate animals,[6] yet it is quite likely that these creatures enjoy some form of sentience.

We do not really know whether complex invertebrate animals such as spiders and insects have sensory experiences, but the evidence suggests that they may. They have both sense organs and central nervous systems, and they often act as if they could see, hear, and feel very well. Sumner says that all invertebrates are probably nonsentient, because they lack certain brain structures—notably forebrains—that appear to be essential to the processing of pain in vertebrate animals (143). But might not some invertebrate animals have neurological devices for the processing of pain that are different from those of vertebrates, just as some have very different organs for the detection of light, sound, or odor? The capacity to feel pain is important to highly mobile organisms which guide their behavior through perceptual data, since it often enables them to avoid damage or destruction. Without that capacity, such organisms would be less likely to survive long enough to reproduce. Thus, if insects, spiders, crayfish, or octopi can see, hear, or smell, then it is quite likely that they can also feel pain. If sentience is the sole criterion for moral equality, then such probably sentient entities deserve the benefit of the doubt.

But it is difficult to believe that killing invertebrate animals is as morally objectionable as homicide. That an entity is probably sentient provides a reason for avoiding actions that may cause it pain. It may also provide a reason for respecting its life, a life which it may enjoy. But it is not a sufficient reason for regarding it as a moral equal. Perhaps an ideally moral person would try to avoid killing any sentient being, even a fly. Yet it is impossible in practice to treat the killing of persons and the killing of sentient invertebrates with the same severity.

Even the simplest activities essential to human survival (such as agriculture, or gathering wild foods) generally entail some loss of invertebrate lives. If the strong version of the sentience criterion is correct, then all such activities are morally problematic. And if it is not, then the probable sentience of late-term fetuses and newborn infants is not enough to demonstrate that either late abortion or infanticide is the moral equivalent of homicide. Some additional argument is needed to show that either late abortion or early infanticide is seriously immoral.

THE SELF-AWARENESS CRITERION

Although newborn infants are regarded as persons in both law and common moral conviction, they lack certain mental capacities that are typical of persons. They have sensory experiences, but, as Tooley points out, they probably do not yet think, or have a sense of who they are, or a desire to continue to exist. It is not unreasonable to suppose that these facts make some difference to their moral standing. Other things being equal, it is surely worse to kill a self-aware being that wants to go on living than one that has never been self-aware and that has no such prefer-

ence. If this is true, then it is hard to avoid the conclusion that neither abortion nor infanticide is quite as bad as the killing of older human beings. And indeed many human societies seem to have accepted that conclusion.

Tooley notes that the abhorrence of infanticide which is characteristic of cultures influenced by Christianity has not been shared by most cultures outside that influence (315-322). Prior to the present century, most societies—from the gatherer-hunter societies of Australia, Africa, North and South America, and elsewhere, to the high civilizations of China, India, Greece, Rome, and Egypt—have not only tolerated occasional instances of infanticide but have regarded it as sometimes the wisest course of action. Even in Christian Europe there was often a defacto toleration of infanticide—so long as the mother was married and the killing discreet. Throughout much of the second millennium in Europe, single women whose infants failed to survive were often executed in sadistic ways, yet married women whose infants died under equally suspicious circumstances generally escaped legal penalty (Piers 1978, 45-46). Evidently, the sanctions against infanticide had more to do with the desire to punish female sexual transgressions than with a consistently held belief that infanticide is morally comparable to homicide.

If infanticide has been less universally regarded as wrong than most people today believe, then the self-awareness criterion is more consistent with common moral convictions than it at first appears. Nevertheless, it conflicts with some convictions that are almost universal, even in cultures that tolerate infanticide. Tooley argues that infants probably begin to think and to become self-aware at about three months of age, and that this is therefore the stage at which they begin to have a strong right to life (405-406). Perhaps this is true. However the customs of most cultures seem to have required that a decision about the life of an infant be made within, at most, a few days of birth. Often, there was some special gesture or ceremony—such as washing the infant, feeding it, or giving it a name—to mark the fact that it would thenceforth be regarded as a member of the community. From that point on, infanticide would not be considered, except perhaps under unusual circumstances. For instance, Margaret Mead gives this account of birth and infanticide among the Arapesh people of Papua New Guinea:

> While the child is being delivered, the father waits within ear-shot until its sex is determined. when the midwives call out to him. To this information he answers laconically, "Wash it," or "Do not wash it." If the command is "Wash it," the child is to be brought up. In a few cases when the child is a girl and there are already several girl-children in the family, the child will not be saved, but left, unwashed, with the cord uncut, in the bark basin on which the delivery takes place. (Mead [1935] 1963, 32-33)

Mead's account shows that among the Arapesh infanticide is at least to some degree a function of patriarchal power. In this, they are not unusual. In almost every society in which infanticide has been tolerated, female infants have been the most frequent victims. In patriarchal, patrilineal and patrilocal societies, daughters are usually valued less than sons, e.g., because they will leave the family at marriage, and will probably be unable to contribute as much as sons to the parents' economic support later. Female infanticide probably reinforces male domination by reducing the relative number of women and dramatically reinforcing the social devaluation of females.[7] Often it is the father who decides which infants will be reared. Dianne Romaine has pointed out to me that this practice may be due to a reluctance to force women, the primary caregivers, to decide when care should not be given. However, it also suggests that infanticide often served the interests of individual men more than those of women, the family, or the community as a whole.

Nevertheless, infanticide must sometimes have been the most humane resolution of a tragic dilemma. In the absence of effective contraception or abortion, abandoning a newborn can sometimes be the only alternative to the infant's later death from starvation. Women of nomadic gatherer-hunter societies, for instance, are sometimes unable to raise an infant born too soon after the last one, because they can neither nurse nor carry two small children.

But if infanticide is to be considered, it is better that it be done immediately after birth, before the bonds of love and care between the infant and the mother (and other persons) have grown any stronger than they may already be. Postponing the question of the infant's acceptance for weeks or months would be cruel to all concerned. Although an infant may be little more sentient or self-aware at two weeks of age than at birth, its death is apt to be a greater tragedy—not for it, but for those who have come to love it. I suspect that this is why, where infanticide is tolerated, the decision to kill or abandon an infant must usually be made rather quickly. If this consideration is morally relevant—and I think it is—then the self-awareness criterion fails to illuminate some of the morally salient aspects of infanticide.

PROTECTING NONPERSONS

If we are to justify a general moral distinction between abortion and infanticide, we must answer two questions. First, why should infanticide be discouraged, rather than treated as a matter for individual decision? And second, why should sentient fetuses not be given the same protections that law and common sense morality accord to infants? But before turning to these two questions, it is necessary to make a more general point.

Persons have sound reasons for treating one another as moral equals. These reasons derive from both self-interest and altruistic concern for others—which, because of our social nature, are often very difficult to distinguish. Human persons—and perhaps all persons—normally come into existence only in and through social relationships. Sentience may begin to emerge without much direct social interaction, but it is doubtful that a child reared in total isolation from human or other sentient (or apparently sentient) beings could develop the capacities for self-awareness and social interaction that are essential to personhood. The recognition of the fundamentally social nature of persons can only strengthen the case for moral equality, since social relationships are undermined and distorted by inequalities that are perceived as unjust. There may be many nonhuman animals who have enough capacity for self awareness and social interaction to be regarded as persons, with equal basic moral rights. But, whether or not this is true, it is certainly true that if any things have full and equal basic moral rights then persons do.

However we cannot conclude that, because all persons have equal basic moral rights, it is always wrong to extend strong moral protections to beings that are not persons. Those who accept the single-criterion assumption may find that a plausible inference. By now, however, most thoughtful people recognize the need to protect vulnerable elements of the natural world—such as endangered plant and animal species, rainforests, and rivers—from further destruction at human hands. Some argue that it is appropriate, as a way of protecting these things, to ascribe to them legal if not moral rights (Stone 1974). These things should be protected not because they are sentient or self-aware, but for other good reasons. They are irreplaceable parts of the terrestrial biosphere, and as such they have incalculable value to human beings. Their long-term instrumental value is often a fully sufficient reason for protecting them. However, they may also be held to have inherent value, i.e., value that is independent of the uses we might wish to make of them (Taylor 1986). Although destroying them is not murder, it is an act of vandalism which later generations will mourn.

It is probably not crucial whether or not we say that endangered species and natural habitats have a moral right to our protection. What is crucial is that we recognize and act upon the need to protect them. Yet certain contemporary realities argue for an increased willingness to ascribe rights to impersonal elements of the natural world. Americans, at least, are likely to be more sensitive to appeals and demands couched in terms of rights than those that appeal to less familiar concepts, such as inherent value. So central are rights to our common moral idiom, that to deny that trees have rights is risk being thought to condone the reckless destruction of rainforests and redwood groves. If we want to communicate effectively about the need to protect the natural world—and to protect it for its own sake as well as our own—then we may be wise to develop theories that permit us to ascribe at least some moral rights to some things that are clearly not persons.

Parallel issues arise with respect to the moral status of the newborn infant. As Wolgast (1987, 38) argues, it is much more important to understand our responsibilities to protect and care for infants than to insist that they have exactly the same moral rights as older human beings. Yet to deny that infants have equal basic moral rights is to risk being thought to condone infanticide and the neglect and abuse of infants. Here too, effective communication about human moral responsibilities seems to demand the ascription of rights to beings that lack certain properties that are typical of persons. But, of course, that does not explain why we have these responsibilities towards infants in the first place.

WHY PROTECT INFANTS?

I have already mentioned some of the reasons for protecting human infants more carefully than we protect most comparably-sentient nonhuman beings. Most people care deeply about infants, particularly—but not exclusively—their own. Normal human adults (and children) are probably "programmed" by their biological nature to respond to human infants with care and concern. For the mother, in particular, that response is apt to begin well before the infant is born. But even for her it is likely to become more intense after the infant's birth. The infant at birth enters the human social world, where, if it lives, it becomes involved in social relationships with others, of kinds that can only be dimly foreshadowed before birth. It begins to be known and cared for, not just as a potential member of the family or community, but as a socially present and responsive individual. In the words of Loren Lomasky (1984, 172), "birth constitutes a quantum leap forward in the process of establishing ... social bonds." The newborn is not yet self-aware, but it is already (rapidly becoming) a social being.

Thus, although the human newborn may have no intrinsic properties that can ground a moral right to life stronger than that of a fetus just before birth, its emergence into the social world makes it appropriate to treat it as if it had such a stronger right. This, in effect, is what the law has done, through the doctrine that a person begins to exist at birth. Those who accept the intrinsic-properties as assumption can only regard this doctrine as a legal fiction. However, it is a fiction that we would have difficulty doing without. If the line were not drawn at birth, then I think we would have to draw it at some point rather soon thereafter, as many other societies have done.

Another reason for condemning infanticide is that, at least in relatively privileged nations like our own, infants whose parents cannot raise them can usually be placed with people who will love them and take good care of them. This means that infanticide is rarely in the infant's own best interests, and would often deprive some potential adoptive individual or family of a great benefit. It also means that the prohibition of infanticide need not impose intolerable burdens upon parents (especially women). A rare parent might think it best to kill a healthy[8] infant rather than permitting it to be reared by others, but a persuasive defense of that claim would require special circumstances. For instance, when abortion is unavailable and women face savage abuses for supposed sexual transgressions, those who resort to infanticide to conceal an "illegitimate" birth may be doing only what they must. But where enforcement of the sexual double standard is less brutal, abortion and adoption can provide alternatives that most women would prefer to infanticide.

Some might wonder whether adoption is really preferable to infanticide, at least from the parent's point of view. Judith Thomson (1971, 66) notes that "a woman may be utterly devastated by the thought of a child, a bit of herself, put out for adoption and never seen or heard of again." From the standpoint of narrow self-interest, it might not be irrational to prefer the death of the child to such a future. Yet few would wish to resolve this problem by legalizing infanticide. The evolution of more open adoption procedures which permit more contact between the adopted child and the biological parent(s) might lessen the psychological pain often associated with adoption. But that would be at best a partial solution. More basic is the provision of better social support for child-rearers, so that parents are not forced by economic necessity to surrender their children for adoption.

These are just some of the arguments for treating infants as legal persons, with an equal right to life. A more complete account might deal with the effects of the toleration of infanticide upon other moral norms. But the existence of such effects is unclear. Despite a tradition of occasional infanticide, the Arapesh appear in Mead's descriptions as gentle people who treat their children with great kindness and affection. The case against infanticide need not rest upon the questionable claim that the toleration of infanticide inevitably leads to the erosion of other moral norms. It is enough that most people today strongly desire that the lives of infants be protected, and that this can now be done without imposing intolerable burdens upon individuals or communities.

But have I not left the door open to the claim that infanticide may still be justified in some places, e.g., where there is severe poverty and a lack of accessible adoption agencies or where women face exceptionally harsh penalties for "illegitimate" births? I have, and deliberately. The moral case against the toleration of infanticide is contingent upon the existence of morally preferable options. Where economic hardship, the lack of contraception and abortion, and other forms of sexual and political oppression have eliminated all such options, there will be instances in which infanticide is the least tragic of a tragic set of choices. In such circumstances, the enforcement of extreme sanctions against infanticide can constitute an additional injustice.

WHY BIRTH MATTERS

I have defended what most regard as needing no defense, i.e., the ascription of an equal right to life to human infants. Under reasonably favorable conditions that policy can protect the rights and interests of all concerned, including infants, biological parents, and potential adoptive parents.

But if protecting infants is such a good idea, then why is it not a good idea to extend the same strong protections to sentient fetuses? The question is not whether sentient fetuses ought to be protected: of course they should. Most women readily accept the responsibility for doing whatever they can to ensure that their (voluntarily continued) pregnancies are successful, and that no avoidable harm comes to the fetus. Negligent or malevolent actions by third parties which result in death or injury to pregnant women or their potential children should be subject to moral censure and legal prosecution. A just and caring society would do much more than ours does to protect the health of all its members, including pregnant women. The question is whether the law should accord to late-term fetuses *exactly the same* protections as are accorded to infants and older human beings.

The case for doing so might seem quite strong. We normally regard not only infants, but all other post-natal human beings as entitled to strong legal protections *so long as they are either sentient or capable of an eventual return to sentience*. We do not also require that they demonstrate a capacity for thought, self-awareness, or social relationships before we conclude that they have an equal right to life. Such restrictive criteria would leave too much room for invidious discrimination. The eternal propensity of powerful groups to rationalize sexual, racial, and class oppression by claiming that members of the oppressed group are mentally or otherwise "inferior" leaves little hope that such restrictive criteria could be applied without bias. Thus, for human beings past the prenatal stage, the capacity for sentience—or for a return to sentience—may be the only pragmatically defensible criterion for the ascription of full and equal basic rights. If so, then both theoretical simplicity and moral consistency may seem to require that we extend the same protections to sentient human beings that have not yet been born as to those that have.

But there is one crucial consideration which this argument leaves out. It is impossible to treat fetuses *in utero* as if they were persons without treating women as if they were something less than persons. The extension of equal rights to sentient fetuses would inevitably license severe violations of women's basic rights to personal autonomy and physical security. In the first place, it would rule out most second-trimester abortions performed to protect the woman's life or health. Such abortions might sometimes be construed as a form of self-defense. But the right to self-defense is not usually taken to mean that one may kill innocent persons just because their continued existence poses some threat to one's own life or health. If abortion must be justified as self-defense, then it will rarely be performed until the woman is already in extreme danger, and perhaps not even then. Such a policy would cost some women their lives, while others would be subjected to needless suffering and permanent physical harm.

Other alarming consequences of the drive to extend more equal rights to fetuses are already apparent in the United States. In the past decade it has become increasingly common for hospitals or physicians to obtain court orders requiring women in labor to undergo cesarean sections, against their will, for what is thought to be the good of the fetus. Such an extreme infringement of the woman's right to security against physical assault would be almost unthinkable once the infant has been born. No parent or relative can legally be forced to undergo any surgical procedure, even possibly to save the life of a child, once it is born. But pregnant women can sometimes be forced to undergo major surgery, for the supposed benefit of the fetus. As George Annas (1982, 16) points out, forced cesareans threaten to reduce women to the status of inanimate objects—containers which may be opened at the will of others in order to get at their contents.

Perhaps the most troubling illustration of this trend is the case of Angela Carder, who died at George Washington University Medical Center in June 1987, two days after a court-ordered cesarean section. Ms. Carder had suffered a recurrence of an earlier cancer, and was not expected to live much longer. Her physicians agreed that the fetus was too undeveloped to be viable, and that Carder herself was probably too weak to survive the surgery. Although she, her family, and the physicians were all opposed to a cesarean delivery, the hospital administration—evidently believing it had a legal obligation to try to save the fetus—sought and obtained a court order to have it done. As predicted, both Carder and her infant died soon after the operation.[9] This woman's rights to autonomy, physical integrity, and life itself were forfeit—not just because of her illness, but because of her pregnancy.

Such precedents are doubly alarming in the light of the development of new techniques of fetal therapy. As fetuses come to be regarded as patients, with rights that may be in direct conflict with those of their mothers, and as the *in utero* treatment of fetuses becomes more feasible, more and more pregnant women may be subjected against their will to dangerous and invasive medical interventions. If so, then we may be sure that there will be other Angela Carders.

Another danger in extending equal legal protections to sentient fetuses is that women will increasingly be blamed, and sometimes legally prosecuted, when they miscarry or give birth to premature, sick, or abnormal infants. It is reasonable to hold the care-takers of infants legally responsible if their charges are harmed because of their avoidable negligence. But when a woman miscarries or gives birth to an abnormal infant, the cause of the harm might be traced to any of an enormous number of actions or circumstances which would not normally constitute any legal offense. She might have gotten too much exercise or too little, eaten the wrong foods or the wrong quantity of the right ones, or taken or failed to take certain drugs. She might have smoked, con-sumed alcohol, or gotten too little sleep. She might have "permitted" her health to be damaged by hard work, by unsafe employment conditions, by the lack of affordable medical care, by living near a source of industrial pollution, by a physically or mentally abu-sive partner, or in any number of other ways.

Are such supposed failures on the part of pregnant women potentially to be construed as child abuse or negligent homicide? If sentient fetuses are entitled to the same legal protections as infants, then it would seem so. The danger is not a merely theoretical one. Two years ago in San Diego, a woman whose son was born with brain damage and died several weeks later was charged with felony child neglect. It was said that she had been advised by her physician to avoid sex and illicit drugs, and to go to the hospital immediately if she noticed any bleeding. Instead, she had allegedly had sex with her husband, taken some inappropriate drug, and delayed getting to the hospi-tal for what might have been several hours after the onset of bleeding.

In this case, the charges were eventually dismissed on the grounds that the child protection law invoked had not been intended to apply to cases of this kind. But the multiplication of such cases is inevitable if the strong legal protections accorded to infants are extended to sentient fetuses. A bill recently intro-duced in the Australian state of New South Wales would make women liable to criminal prosecution if they are found to have smoked during pregnancy, eaten unhealthful foods, or taken any other action which can be shown to have adversely affected the development of the fetus (*The Australian*, July 5, 1988, 5). Such an approach to the protection of fetus-es authorizes the legal regulation of virtually every aspect of women's public and private lives, and thus

is incompatible with even the most minimal right to autonomy. Moreover, such laws are apt to prove counterproductive, since the fear of prosecution may deter poor or otherwise vulnerable women from seek-ing needed medical care during pregnancy. I am not suggesting that women whose apparent negligence causes prenatal harm to their infants should always be immune from criticism. However, if we want to improve the health of infants we would do better to provide the services women need to protect their health, rather than seeking to use the law to punish those whose prenatal care has been less than ideal.

There is yet another problem, which may prove temporary but which remains significant at this time. The extension of legal personhood to sentient fetus-es would rule out most abortions performed because of severe fetal abnormalities, such as Down syn-drome or spina bifida. Abortions performed follow-ing amniocentesis are usually done in the latter part of the second trimester, since it is usually not possi-ble to obtain test results earlier. Methods of detecting fetal abnormalities at earlier stages, such as chorion biopsy, may eventually make late abortion for rea-sons of fetal abnormality unnecessary; but these methods are not yet widely available.

The elimination of most such abortions might be a consequence that could be accepted, were the soci-ety willing to provide adequate support for the hand-icapped children and adults who would come into being as a result of this policy. However, our society is not prepared to do this. In the absence of adequate communally-funded care for the handicapped, the prohibition of such abortions is exploitative of women. Of course, the male relatives of severely handicapped persons may also bear heavy burdens. Yet the heaviest portion of the daily responsibility generally falls upon mothers and other female rela-tives. If fetuses are not yet persons (and women are), then a respect for the equality of persons should lead to support for the availability of abortion in cases of severe fetal abnormality.[10]

Such arguments will not persuade those who deeply believe that fetuses are already persons, with equal moral rights. How, they will ask, is denying legal equality to sentient fetuses different from deny-ing it to any other powerless group of human beings? If some human beings are more equal than others, then how can any of us feel safe? The answer is twofold.

First, pregnancy is a relationship different from any other, including that between parents and already-born children. It is not just one of innumerable situations in which the rights of one individual may come into conflict with those of another; it is probably the *only* case in which the legal personhood of one human being is necessarily incompatible with that of another. Only in pregnancy is the organic functioning of one human individual biologically inseparable from that of another. This organic unity makes it impossible for others to provide the fetus with medical care or any other presumed benefit, except by doing something to or for the woman. To try to "protect" the fetus other than through her cooperation and consent is effectively to nullify her right to autonomy, and potentially to expose her to violent physical assaults such as would not be legally condoned in any other type of case. The uniqueness of pregnancy helps to explain why the toleration of abortion does not lead to the disenfranchisement of other groups of human beings, as opponents of abortion often claim. For biological as well as psychological reasons, "It is all but impossible to extrapolate from attitudes towards fetal life attitudes toward [other] existing human life" (D. Callahan 1970, 474).

But, granting the uniqueness of pregnancy, why is it *women's* rights that should be privileged? If women and fetuses cannot both be legal persons then why not favor fetuses, e.g., on the grounds that they are more helpless, or more innocent, or have a longer life expectancy? It is difficult to justify this apparent bias towards women without appealing to the empirical fact that women are already persons in the usual, non-legal sense—already thinking, self-aware, fully social beings—and fetuses are not. Regardless of whether we stress the intrinsic properties of persons, or the social and relational dimensions of personhood, this distinction remains. Even sentient fetuses do not yet have either the cognitive capacities or the richly interactive social involvements typical of persons.

This "not yet" is morally decisive. It is wrong to treat persons as if they do not have equal basic rights. Other things being equal, it is worse to deprive persons of their most basic moral and legal rights than

to refrain from extending such rights to beings that are not persons. This is one important element of truth in the self-awareness criterion. If fetuses were already thinking, self-aware, socially responsive members of communities, then nothing could justify refusing them the equal protection of the law. In that case, we would sometimes be forced to balance the rights of the fetus against those of the woman, and sometimes the scales might be almost equally weighted. However, if women are persons and fetuses are not, then the balance must swing towards women's rights.

CONCLUSION

Birth is morally significant because it marks the end of one relationship and the beginning of others. It marks the end of pregnancy, a relationship so intimate that it is impossible to extend the equal protection of the law to fetuses without severely infringing women's most basic rights. Birth also marks the beginning of the infant's existence as a socially responsive member of a human community. Although the infant is not instantly transformed into a person at the moment of birth, it does become a biologically separate human being. As such, it can be known and cared for as a particular individual. It can also be vigorously protected without negating the basic rights of women. There are circumstances in which infanticide may be the best of a bad set of options. But our own society has both the ability and the desire to protect infants, and there is no reason why we should not do so.

We should not, however, seek to extend the same degree of protection to fetuses. Both late-term fetuses and newborn infants are probably capable of sentience. Both are precious to those who want children; and both need to be protected from a variety of possible harms. All of these factors contribute to the moral standing of the late-term fetus, which is substantial. However, to extend equal legal rights to fetuses is necessarily to deprive pregnant women of the rights to personal autonomy, physical integrity, and sometimes life itself. *There is room for only one person with full and equal rights inside a single human skin.* That is why it is birth, rather than sentience, viability, or some other prenatal milestone that must mark the beginning of legal personhood.

Notes

My thanks to Helen Heise, Dianne Romaine, Peter Singer, and Michael Scriven for their helpful comments on earlier versions of this paper.

1. Basic moral rights are those that are possessed equally by all persons, and that are essential to the moral equality of persons. The intended contrast is to those rights which arise from certain special circumstances—for instance, the right of a person to whom a promise has been made that that promise be kept. (Whether there are beings that are not persons but that have similar basic moral rights is one of the questions to be addressed here.)

2. "Moral standing," like "moral status" is a term that can be used to refer to the moral considerability of individuals, without being committed to the existence of moral rights. For instance, Sumner (1983) and Singer (1981) prefer these terms because, as utilitarians, they are unconvinced of the need for moral rights.

3. It is not obvious that a newborn infant's "level of consciousness" is similar to that of a fetus shortly before birth. Perhaps birth is analogous to an awakening, in that the infant has many experiences that were previously precluded by its prenatal brain chemistry or by its relative insulation within the womb. This speculation is plausible in evolutionary terms, since a rich subjective mental life might have little survival value for the fetus, but might be highly valuable for the newborn, e.g., in enabling it to recognize its mother and signal its hunger, discomfort, etc. However, for the sake of the argument I will assume that the newborn's capacity for sentience is generally not very different from that of the fetus shortly before birth.

4. It is interesting that Sumner regards fetal abnormality and the protection of the woman's health as sufficient justifications for late abortion. In this, he evidently departs from his own theory by effectively differentiating between the moral status of sentient fetuses and that of older humans—who presumably may not be killed just because they are abnormal or because their existence (through no fault of their own) poses a threat to someone else's health.

5. There are evidently some people who, though otherwise sentient, cannot experience physical pain. However, the survival value of the capacity to experience pain makes it probable that such individuals are the exception rather than the rule among mature members of sentient species.

6. There is at least one religion, that of the Jains, in which the killing of any living thing—even an insect—is regarded as morally wrong. But even the Jains do not regard the killing of insects as morally equivalent to the killing of persons. Laypersons (unlike mendicants) are permitted some unintentional killing of insects—though not of vertebrate animals or persons—when this is unavoidable to the pursuit of their profession (See Jaini 1979, 171-3).

7. Marcia Guttentag and Paul Secord (1983) argue that a shortage of women benefits at least some women, by increasing their "value" in the marriage market. However, they also argue that this increased value does not lead to greater freedom for women; on the contrary, it tends to coincide with an exceptionally severe sexual double standard, the exclusion of women from public life, and their confinement to domestic roles.

8. The extension of equal basic rights to infants need not imply the absolute rejection of euthanasia for infant patients. There are instances in which artificially extending the life of a severely compromised infant is contrary to the infant's own best interests. Competent adults or older children who are terminally ill sometimes rightly judge that further prolongation of their lives would not be a benefit to them. While infants cannot make that judgment for themselves, it is sometimes the right judgment for others to make on their behalf.

9. See *Civil Liberties* 363 (Winter 1988), 12, and Lawrence Lader, "Regulating Birth: Is the State Going Too Far?" *Conscience* IX: 5 (September/October, 1988), 5-6.

10. It is sometimes argued that using abortion to prevent the birth of severely handicapped infants will inevitably lead to a loss of concern for handicapped persons. I doubt that this is true. There is no need to confuse the question of whether it is good that persons be born handicapped with the very different question of whether handicapped persons are entitled to respect, support, and care.

References

Annas, George. 1982. "Forced Cesareans: The Most Unkindest Cut of All," *Hastings Center Report* 12, 3: 16-17, 45.

The Australian, Tuesday, July 5, 1988, 5.

Callahan, Daniel. 1970. *Abortion: Law, Choice and Morality*. New York: Macmillan.

Callahan, Sydney. 1984. "Value choices in abortion," in Sydney Callahan and Daniel Callahan, eds., *Abortion: Understanding Differences*. New York and London: Plenum Press.

Callahan, Sydney. 1986. "Abortion and the Sexual Agenda," *Commonweal*, April 25: 232-38.

Gilligan, Carol. 1981. *In a Different Voice: Psychological Theory and Women's Development*. Cambridge, Mass.: Harvard University Press.

Guttentag, Marcia, and Paul Secord. 1983. *Too Many Women: The Sex Ratio Question*. Beverly Hills: Sage Publications.

Harrison, Beverly Wildung. 1983. *Our Right to Choose: Toward a New Ethic of Abortion*. Boston Beacon Press.

Jaini, Padmanab S. 1979. *The Jaina Path of Purification*. Berkeley, Los Angeles, London: University of California Press.

Lomasky, Loren. 1984. "Being a Person—Does It Matter?" in Joel Feinberg, ed., *The Problem of Abortion*. Belmont, California.

Luker, Kristen. 1984. *Abortion and the Politics of Motherhood*. Berkeley, Los Angeles and London: University of California Press.

Manning, Rita. 1988. *Caring For and Caring About*. Paper presented at conference entitled *Explorations in Feminist Ethics*, Duluth, Minnesota. October 8.

Mead, Margaret. [1935] 1963. *Sex and Temperament in Three Primitive Societies*. New York: Morrow Quill Paperbacks.

Noddings, Nel. 1984. *Caring: A Feminine Approach to Ethics and Moral Education*. Berkeley, Los Angeles and London: University of California Press.

Petchesky, Rosalind Pollack. 1984. *Abortion and Women's Choice*. New York, London: Longman.

Piers, Maria W. 1978. *Infanticide*. New York: W.W. Norton and Company.

Singer, Peter. 1981. *The Expanding Circle: Ethics and Sociobiology*. New York: Farrar, Straus and Giroux.

Stone, Christopher. 1974. *Should Trees Have Standing: Towards Legal Rights for Natural Objects*. Los Altos: William Kaufman.

Stone, Christopher. 1987. *Earth and Other Ethics*. New York: Harper & Row.

Sumner, L.W. 1983. *Abortion and Moral Theory*. Princeton, N.J.: Princeton University Press.

Taylor, Paul W. 1986. *Respect for Nature: A Theory of Environmental Ethics*. Princeton, N.J.: Princeton University Press.

Thomson, Judith Jarvis. 1971. "A Defense of Abortion," *Philosophy and Public Affairs* 1, 1: 47-66.

Tooley, Michael. 1983. *Abortion and Infanticide*. Oxford: Oxford University Press.

Wolgast, Elizabeth. 1987. *The Grammar of Justice*. Ithaca and London: Cornell University Press.

25.
ABORTION THROUGH A FEMINIST ETHICS LENS

Susan Sherwin

Abortion has long been a central issue in the arena of applied ethics, but, the distinctive analysis of feminist ethics is generally overlooked in most philosophic discussions. Authors and readers commonly presume a familiarity with the feminist position and equate it with liberal defences of women's right to choose abortion, but, in fact, feminist ethics yields a different analysis of the moral questions surrounding abortion than that usually offered by the more familiar liberal defenders of abortion rights. Most feminists can agree with some of the conclusions that arise from certain non-feminist arguments on abortion, but they often disagree about the way the issues are formulated and the sorts of reasons that are invoked in the mainstream literature.

Among the many differences found between feminist and non-feminist arguments about abortion, is the fact that most non-feminist discussions of abortion consider the questions of the moral or legal permissibility of abortion in isolation from other questions, ignoring (and thereby obscuring) relevant connections to other social practices that oppress women. They are generally grounded in masculinist conceptions of freedom (e.g., privacy, individual choice, individuals' property rights in their own bodies) that do not meet the needs, interests, and intuitions of many of the women concerned. In contrast, feminists seek to couch their arguments in moral concepts that support their general campaign of overcoming injustice in all its dimensions, including those inherent in moral theory itself.[1] There is even disagreement about how best to understand the moral question at issue: non-feminist arguments focus exclusively on the morality and/or legality of performing abortions, whereas feminists insist that other questions, including ones about accessibility and delivery of abortion services must also be addressed.

Although feminists welcome the support of non-feminists in pursuing policies that will grant women control over abortion decisions, they generally envision very different sorts of policies for this purpose than those considered by non-feminist sympathizers. For example, Kathleen McDonnell (1984) urges feminists to develop an explicitly "'feminist morality' of abortion .... At its root it would be characterized by the deep appreciations of the complexities of life, the refusal to polarize and adopt simplistic formulas" (p. 52). Here, I propose one conception of the shape such an analysis should take.

WOMEN AND ABORTION

The most obvious difference between feminist and non-feminist approaches to abortion can be seen in the relative attention each gives to the interests and experiences of women in its analysis. Feminists consider it self-evident that the pregnant woman is a subject of principal concern in abortion decisions. In most non-feminist accounts, however, not only is she not perceived as central, she is rendered virtually invisible. Non-feminist theorists, whether they support or oppose women's right to choose abortion, focus almost all their attention on the moral status of the developing embryo or the fetus.

In pursuing a distinctively feminist ethics, it is appropriate to begin with a look at the role of abortion in women's lives. Clearly, the need for abortion can be very intense; women have pursued abortions under appalling and dangerous conditions, across widely diverse cultures and historical periods. No one denies that if abortion is not made legal, safe, and accessible, women will seek out illegal and life-threatening abortions to terminate pregnancies they cannot accept. Anti-abortion activists seem willing to accept this price, but feminists judge the inevitable loss of women's lives associated with restrictive abortion policies to be a matter of fundamental concern.

Although anti-abortion campaigners imagine that women often make frivolous and irresponsible decisions about abortion, feminists recognize that women have abortions for a wide variety of reasons. Some women, for instance, find themselves seriously ill and incapacitated throughout pregnancy; they cannot continue in their jobs and may face enormous difficulties in fulfilling their responsibilities at home. Many employers and schools will not tolerate pregnancy in their employees or students, and not every woman is able to put her job, career, or studies on hold. Women of limited means may be unable to take adequate care of children they have already borne and they may know that another mouth to feed will reduce their ability to provide for their existing children. Women who suffer from chronic disease, or who feel too young, or too old, or who are unable to maintain lasting relationships may recognize that they will not be able to care properly for a child at this time. Some who are homeless, or addicted to drugs, or who are diagnosed as carrying the AIDS virus may be unwilling to allow a child to enter the world under such circumstances. If the pregnancy is a result of rape or incest, the psychological pain of carrying it to term may be unbearable, and the woman may recognize that her attitude to the child after birth will always be tinged with bitterness. Some women have learned that the fetuses they carry have serious chromosomal anomalies and consider it best to prevent them from being born with a condition bound to cause suffering. Others, knowing the fathers to be brutal and violent, may be unwilling to subject a child to the beatings or incestuous attacks they anticipate; some may have no other realistic way to remove the child (or themselves) from the relationship.

Or a woman may simply believe that bearing a child is incompatible with her life plans at this time, since continuing a pregnancy is likely to have profound repercussions throughout a woman's entire life. If the woman is young, a pregnancy will very likely reduce her chances of education and hence limit her career and life opportunities: "The earlier a woman has a baby, it seems, the more likely she is to drop out of school; the less education she gets, the more likely she is to remain poorly paid, peripheral to the labour market, or unemployed, and the more children she will have—between one and three more than her working childless counterpart" (Petchesky

1984, p. 150). In many circumstances, having a child will exacerbate the social and economic forces already stacked against her by virtue of her sex (and her race, class, age, sexual orientation, or the effects of some disability, etc.). Access to abortion is a necessary option for many women if they are to escape the oppressive conditions of poverty.

Whatever the reason, most feminists believe that a pregnant woman is in the best position to judge whether abortion is the appropriate response to her circumstances. Since she is usually the only one able to weigh all the relevant factors, most feminists reject attempts to offer any general abstract rules for determining when abortion is morally justified. Women's personal deliberations about abortion include contextually defined considerations reflecting her commitment to the needs and interests of everyone concerned—including herself, the fetus she carries, other members of her household, etc. Because there is no single formula available for balancing these complex factors through all possible cases, it is vital that feminists insist on protecting each woman's right to come to her own conclusions. Abortion decisions are, by their very nature, dependent on specific features of each woman's experience; theoretically dispassionate philosophers and other moralists should not expect to set the agenda for these considerations in any universal way. Women must be acknowledged as full moral agents with the responsibility for making moral decisions about their own pregnancies.[2] Although I think that it is possible for a woman to make a mistake in her moral judgment on this matter (i.e., it is possible that a woman may come to believe that she was wrong about her decision to continue or terminate a pregnancy), the intimate nature of this sort of decision makes it unlikely that anyone else is in a position to arrive at a more reliable conclusion; it is, therefore, improper to grant others the authority to interfere in women's decisions to seek abortions.

Feminist analysis regards the effects of unwanted pregnancies on the lives of women individually and collectively as a central element in the moral evaluation of abortion. Even without patriarchy, bearing a child would be a very important event in a woman's life. It involves significant physical, emotional, social, and (usually) economic changes for her. The ability to exert control over the incidence, timing, and frequency of child-bearing is often tied to her ability to control most other things she values. Since we live in a patriarchal society, it is especially important to ensure that women have the authority to control their own reproduction.[3] Despite the diversity of opinion among feminists on most other matters, virtually all feminists seem to agree that women must gain full control over their own reproductive lives if they are to free themselves from male dominance.[4] Many perceive the commitment of the political right wing to opposing abortion as part of a general strategy to reassert patriarchal control over women in the face of significant feminist influence (Petchesky 1980, p. 112).

Women's freedom to choose abortion is also linked with their ability to control their own sexuality. Women's subordinate status often prevents them from refusing men sexual access to their bodies. If women cannot end the unwanted pregnancies that result from male sexual dominance, their sexual vulnerability to particular men can increase, because caring for an(other) infant involves greater financial needs and reduced economic opportunities for women.[5] As a result, pregnancy often forces women to become dependent on men. Since a woman's dependence on a man is assumed to entail that she will remain sexually loyal to him, restriction of abortion serves to channel women's sexuality and further perpetuates the cycle of oppression.

In contrast to most non-feminist accounts, feminist analyses of abortion direct attention to the question of how women get pregnant. Those who reject abortion seem to believe that women can avoid unwanted pregnancies by avoiding sexual intercourse. Such views show little appreciation for the power of sexual politics in a culture that oppresses women. Existing patterns of sexual dominance mean that women often have little control over their sexual lives. They may be subject to rape by strangers, or by their husbands, boyfriends, colleagues, employers, customers, fathers, brothers, uncles, and dates. Often, the sexual coercion is not even recognized as such by the participants, but is the price of continued "good will"—popularity, economic survival, peace, or simple acceptance. Few women have not found themselves in circumstances where they do not feel free to refuse

a man's demands for intercourse, either because he is holding a gun to her head or because he threatens to be emotionally hurt if she refuses (or both). Women are socialized to be compliant and accommodating, sensitive to the feelings of others, and frightened of physical power; men are socialized to take advantage of every opportunity to engage in sexual intercourse and to use sex to express dominance and power. Under such circumstances, it is difficult to argue that women could simply "choose" to avoid heterosexual activity if they wish to avoid pregnancy. Catherine MacKinnon neatly sums it up: "the logic by which women are supposed to consent to sex [is]: preclude the alternatives, then call the remaining option 'her choice'" (MacKinnon 1989, p. 192).

Nor can women rely on birth control alone to avoid pregnancy. There simply is no form of reversible contraception available that is fully safe and reliable. The pill and the IUD are the most effective means offered, but both involve significant health hazards to women and are quite dangerous for some. No woman should spend the 30 to 40 years of her reproductive life on either form of birth control. Further, both have been associated with subsequent problems of involuntary infertility, so they are far from optimum for women who seek to control the timing of their pregnancies.

The safest form of birth control involves the use of barrier methods (condoms or diaphragms) in combination with spermicidal foams or jelly. But these methods also pose difficulties for women. They may be socially awkward to use: young women are discouraged from preparing for sexual activity that might never happen and are offered instead romantic models of spontaneous passion. (Few films or novels interrupt scenes of seduction for the fetching of contraceptives.) Many women find their male partners unwilling to use barrier methods of contraception and they do not have the power to insist. Further, cost is a limiting factor for many women. Condoms and spermicides are expensive and are not covered under most health care plans. There is only one contraceptive option which offers women safe and fully effective birth control: barrier methods with the back-up option of abortion.[6]

From a feminist perspective, a central moral feature of pregnancy is that it takes place in *women's bodies* and has profound effects on *women's* lives. Gender-neutral accounts of pregnancy are not available; pregnancy is explicitly a condition associated with the female body.[7] Because the need for abortion is experienced only by women, policies about abortion affect women uniquely. Thus, it is important to consider how proposed policies on abortion fit into general patterns of oppression for women. Unlike non-feminist accounts, feminist ethics demands that the effects on the oppression of women be a principal consideration when evaluating abortion policies.

THE FETUS

In contrast, most non-feminist analysts believe that the moral acceptability of abortion turns on the question of the moral status of the fetus. Even those who support women's right to choose abortion tend to accept the central premise of the anti-abortion proponents that abortion can only be tolerated if it can be proved that the fetus is lacking some criterion of full personhood.[8] Opponents of abortion have structured the debate so that it is necessary to define the status of the fetus as either valued the same as other humans (and hence entitled not to be killed) or as lacking in all value. Rather than challenging the logic of this formulation, many defenders of abortion have concentrated on showing that the fetus is indeed without significant value (Tooley 1972, Warren 1973); others, such as Wayne Sumner (1981), offer a more subtle account that reflects the gradual development of fetuses whereby there is some specific criterion that determines the degree of protection to be afforded them which is lacking in the early stages of pregnancy but present in the later stages. Thus, the debate often rages between abortion opponents who describe the fetus as an "innocent," vulnerable, morally important, separate being whose life is threatened and who must be protected at all costs, and abortion supporters who try to establish some sort of deficiency inherent to fetuses which removes them from the scope of the moral community.

The woman on whom the fetus depends for survival is considered as secondary (if she is considered at all) in these debates. The actual experiences and responsibilities of real women are not perceived as morally relevant (unless they, too, can be proved innocent by establishing that their pregnancies are a result of rape or incest). It is a common assumption of both defenders and opponents of women's right to choose abortion that many women will be irresponsible in their choices. The important question, though, is whether fetuses have the sort of status that justifies interfering in women's choices at all. In some contexts, women's role in gestation is literally reduced to that of "fetal containers"; the individual women disappear or are perceived simply as mechanical life-support systems.[9]

The current rhetoric against abortion stresses the fact that the genetic make-up of the fetus is determined at conception and the genetic code is incontestably human. Lest there be any doubt about the humanity of the fetus, we are assailed with photographs of fetuses at various stages of development demonstrating the early appearance of recognizably human characteristics, e.g., eyes, fingers, and toes. The fact that the fetus in its early stages is microscopic, virtually indistinguishable from other primate fetuses to the untrained eye, and lacking in the capacities that make human life meaningful and valuable is not deemed relevant by the self-appointed defenders of fetuses. The anti-abortion campaign is directed at evoking sympathetic attitudes towards this tiny, helpless being whose life is threatened by its own mother; it urges us to see the fetus as entangled in an adversarial relationship with the (presumably irresponsible) woman who carries it. We are encouraged to identify with the "unborn child" and not with the (selfish) woman whose life is also at issue.

Within the non-feminist literature, both defenders and opponents of women's right to choose abortion agree that the difference between a late-term fetus and a newborn infant is "merely geographical" and cannot be considered morally significant. But a fetus inhabits a woman's body and is wholly dependent on her unique contribution to its maintenance while a newborn is physically separate though still in need of a lot of care. One can only view the distinction between being in or out of a woman's womb as morally irrelevant if one discounts the perspective of the pregnant woman; feminists seem to be alone in recognizing her perspective as morally important.[10]

Within anti-abortion arguments, fetuses are identified as individuals; in our culture which views the (abstract) individual as sacred, fetuses *qua* individuals should be honoured and preserved. Extraordinary claims are made to try to establish the individuality and moral agency of fetuses. At the same time, the women who carry these fetal individuals are viewed as passive hosts whose only significant role is to refrain from aborting or harming their fetuses. Since it is widely believed that the woman does not actually have to *do* anything to protect the life of the fetus, pregnancy is often considered (abstractly) to be a tolerable burden to protect the life of an individual so like us.[11]

Medicine has played its part in supporting these sorts of attitudes. Fetal medicine is a rapidly expanding specialty, and it is commonplace in professional medical journals to find references to pregnant women as "fetal environments." Fetal surgeons now have at their disposal a repertory of sophisticated technology that can save the lives of dangerously ill fetuses; in light of such heroic successes, it is perhaps understandable that women have disappeared from their view. These specialists see fetuses as their patients, not the women who nurture them. Doctors perceive themselves as the *active* agents in saving fetal lives and, hence, believe that they are the ones in direct relationship with the fetuses they treat.

Perhaps even more distressing than the tendency to ignore the woman's agency altogether and view her as a purely passive participant in the medically controlled events of pregnancy and childbirth is the growing practice of viewing women as genuine threats to the well-being of the fetus. Increasingly, women are viewed as irresponsible or hostile towards their fetuses, and the relationship between them is characterized as adversarial (Overall 1987, p. 60). Concern for the well-being of the fetus is taken as licence for doctors to intervene to ensure that women comply with medical "advice." Courts are called upon to enforce the doctors' orders when moral pressure alone proves inadequate, and women are being coerced into undergoing unwanted Caesarean deliveries and technologically monitored hospital births. Some states have begun to imprison women for endangering their fetuses through drug abuse and other socially unacceptable behaviours. An Australian state recently introduced a bill that makes women liable to criminal prosecution "if they

are found to have smoked during pregnancy, eaten unhealthful foods, or taken any other action which can be shown to have adversely affected the development of the fetus" (Warren 1989, p. 60).

In other words, physicians have joined with anti-abortionist activists in fostering a cultural acceptance of the view that fetuses are distinct individuals, who are physically, ontologically, and socially separate from the women whose bodies they inhabit, and who have their own distinct interests. In this picture, pregnant women are either ignored altogether or are viewed as deficient in some crucial respect and hence subject to coercion for the sake of their fetuses. In the former case, the interests of the women concerned are assumed to be identical with those of the fetus; in the latter, the women's interests are irrelevant because they are perceived as immoral, unimportant, or unnatural. Focus on the fetus as an independent entity has led to presumptions which deny pregnant women their roles as active, independent, moral agents with a primary interest in what becomes of the fetuses they carry. Emphasis on the fetus's status has led to an assumed licence to interfere with women's reproductive freedom.

A FEMINIST VIEW OF THE FETUS

Because the public debate has been set up as a competition between the rights of women and those of fetuses, feminists have often felt pushed to reject claims of fetal value in order to protect women's claims. Yet, as Addelson (1987) has argued, viewing abortion in this way "tears [it] out of the context of women's lives" (p. 107). There are other accounts of fetal value that are more plausible and less oppressive to women.

On a feminist account, fetal development is examined in the context in which it occurs, within women's bodies rather than in the imagined isolation implicit in many theoretical accounts. Fetuses develop in specific pregnancies which occur in the lives of particular women. They are not individuals housed in generic female wombs, nor are they full persons at risk only because they are small and subject to the whims of women. Their very existence is relational, developing as they do within particular women's bodies, and their principal relationship is to the women who carry them.

On this view, fetuses are morally significant, but their status is relational rather than absolute. Unlike other human beings, fetuses do not have any independent existence; their existence is uniquely tied to the support of a specific other. Most non-feminist commentators have ignored the relational dimension of fetal development and have presumed that the moral status of fetuses could be resolved solely in terms of abstract metaphysical criteria of personhood. They imagine that there is some set of properties (such as genetic heritage, moral agency, self-consciousness, language use, or self-determination) which will entitle all who possess them to be granted the moral status of persons (Warren 1973, Tooley 1972). They seek some particular feature by which we can neatly divide the world into the dichotomy of moral persons (who are to be valued and protected) and others (who are not entitled to the same group privileges); it follows that it is a merely empirical question whether or not fetuses possess the relevant properties.

But this vision misinterprets what is involved in personhood and what it is that is especially valued about persons. Personhood is a social category, not an isolated state. Persons are members of a community; they develop as concrete, discrete, and specific individuals. To be a morally significant category, personhood must involve personality as well as biological integrity.[12] It is not sufficient to consider persons simply as Kantian atoms of rationality; persons are all embodied, conscious beings with particular social histories. Annette Baier (1985) has developed a concept of persons as "second persons" which helps explain the sort of social dimension that seems fundamental to any moral notion of personhood:

A person, perhaps, is best seen as one who was long enough dependent upon other persons to acquire the essential arts of personhood. Persons essentially are *second* persons, who grow up with other persons.... The fact that a person has a life *history*, and that a people collectively have a history depends upon the humbler fact that each person has a childhood in which a cultural heritage is transmitted, ready for adolescent rejection and adult discriminating selection and contribution. Persons come after and before other persons. (p. 84-85; her emphasis.)

Persons, in other words, are members of a social community which shapes and values them, and personhood is a relational concept that must be defined in terms of interactions and relationships with others.

A fetus is a unique sort of being in that it cannot form relationships freely with others, nor can others readily form relationships with it. A fetus has a primary and particularly intimate relationship with the woman in whose womb it develops; any other relationship it may have is indirect, and must be mediated through the pregnant woman. The relationship that exists between a woman and her fetus is clearly asymmetrical, since she is the only party to the relationship who is capable of making a decision about whether the interaction should continue and since the fetus is wholly dependent on the woman who sustains it while she is quite capable of surviving without it.

However much some might prefer it to be otherwise, no one else can do anything to support or harm a fetus without doing something to the woman who nurtures it. Because of this inexorable biological reality, she bears a unique responsibility and privilege in determining her fetus's place in the social scheme of things. Clearly, many pregnancies occur to women who place very high value on the lives of the particular fetuses they carry, and choose to see their pregnancies through to term despite the possible risks and costs involved; hence, it would be wrong of anyone to force such a woman to terminate her pregnancy under these circumstances. Other women, or some of these same women at other times, value other things more highly (e.g., their freedom, their health, or previous responsibilities which conflict with those generated by the pregnancies), and choose not to continue their pregnancies. The value that women ascribe to individual fetuses varies dramatically from case to case, and may well change over the course of any particular pregnancy. There is no absolute value that attaches to fetuses apart from their relational status determined in the context of their particular development.

Since human beings are fundamentally relational beings, it is important to remember that fetuses are characteristically limited in the relationships in which they can participate; within those relationships, they can make only the most restricted "contributions."[13] After birth, human beings are capable of a much wider range of roles in relationships with an infinite variety of partners; it is that very diversity of possibility and experience that leads us to focus on the abstraction of the individual as a constant through all her/his relationships. But until birth, no such variety is possible, and the fetus is defined as an entity within a woman who will almost certainly be principally responsible for it for many years to come.

No human, and especially no fetus, can exist apart from relationships; feminist views of what is valuable about persons must reflect the social nature of their existence. Fetal lives can neither be sustained nor destroyed without affecting the women who support them. Because of a fetus's unique physical status—*within* and dependent on a particular woman—the responsibility and privilege of determining its specific social status and value must rest with the woman carrying it. Fetuses are not persons because they have not developed sufficiently in social relationships to be persons in any morally significant sense (i.e., they are not yet second persons). Newborns, although just beginning their development into persons, are immediately subject to social relationships, for they are capable of communication and response in interaction with a variety of other persons. Thus, feminist accounts of abortion stress the importance of protecting women's right to continue as well as to terminate pregnancies as each sees fit.

FEMINIST POLITICS AND ABORTION

Feminist ethics directs us to look at abortion in the context of other issues of power and not to limit discussion to the standard questions about its moral and legal acceptability. Because coerced pregnancy has repercussions for women's oppressed status generally, it is important to ensure that abortion not only be made legal but that adequate services be made accessible to all women who seek them. This means that within Canada, where medically approved abortion is technically recognized as legal (at least for the moment), we must protest the fact that it is not made available to many of the women who have the greatest need for abortions: vast geographical areas offer no abortion services at all, but unless the women of those regions can afford to travel to urban clinics, they have no meaningful right to abortion. Because women

depend on access to abortion in their pursuit of social equality, it is a matter of moral as well as political responsibility that provincial health plans should cover the cost of transport and service in the abortion facilities women choose. Ethical study of abortion involves understanding and critiquing the economic, age, and social barriers that currently restrict access to medically acceptable abortion services.[14]

Moreover, it is also important that abortion services be provided in an atmosphere that fosters women's health and well-being; hence, the care offered should be in a context that is supportive of the choices women make. Abortions should be seen as part of women's overall reproductive health and could be included within centres that deal with all matters of reproductive health in an open, patient-centred manner where effective counselling is offered for a wide range of reproductive decisions.[15] Providers need to recognize that abortion is a legitimate option so that services will be delivered with respect and concern for the physical, psychological, and emotional effects on a patient. All too frequently, hospital-based abortions are provided by practitioners who are uneasy about their role and treat the women involved with hostility and resentment. Increasingly, many anti-abortion activists have personalized their attacks and focussed their attention on harassing the women who enter and leave abortion clinics. Surely requiring a woman to pass a gauntlet of hostile protesters on her way to and from an abortion is not conducive to effective health care. Ethical exploration of abortion raises questions about how women are treated when they seek abortions;[16] achieving legal permission for women to dispose of their fetuses if they are determined enough to manage the struggle should not be accepted as the sole moral consideration.

Nonetheless, feminists must formulate their distinctive response to legislative initiatives on abortion. The tendency of Canadian politicians confronted by vocal activists on both sides of the abortion issue has been to seek "compromises" that seem to give something to each (and, thereby, also deprives each of important features sought in policy formation). Thus, the House of Commons recently passed a law (Bill C-43) that allows a woman to have an abortion only if a doctor certifies that her physical, mental, or emotional health will be otherwise threatened. Many non-feminist supporters of women's right to choose consider this a victory and urge feminists to be satisfied with it, but feminists have good reason to object. Besides their obvious objection to having abortion returned to the Criminal Code, feminists also object that this policy considers doctors and not women the best judges of a woman's need for abortion; feminists have little reason to trust doctors to appreciate the political dimension of abortion or to respond adequately to women's needs. Abortion must be a woman's decision, and not one controlled by her doctor. Further, experience shows that doctors are already reluctant to provide abortions to women; the opportunity this law presents for criminal persecution of doctors by anti-abortion campaigners is a sufficient worry to inhibit their participation.[17] Feminists want women's decision-making to be recognized as legitimate, and cannot be satisfied with a law that makes abortion a medical choice.

Feminists support abortion on demand because they know that women must have control over their reproduction. For the same reason, they actively oppose forced abortion and coerced sterilization, practices that are sometimes inflicted on the most powerless women, especially those in the Third World. Feminist ethics demands that access to voluntary, safe, effective birth control be part of any abortion discussion, so that women have access to other means of avoiding pregnancy.[18]

Feminist analysis addresses the context as well as the practice of abortion decisions. Thus, feminists also object to the conditions which lead women to abort wanted fetuses because there are not adequate financial and social supports available to care for a child. Because feminist accounts value fetuses that are wanted by the women who carry them, they oppose practices which force women to abort because of poverty or intimidation. Yet, the sorts of social changes necessary if we are to free women from having abortions out of economic necessity are vast; they include changes not only in legal and health-care policy, but also in housing, child care, employment, etc. (Petchesky 1980, p. 112). Nonetheless, feminist ethics defines reproductive freedom as the condition under which women are able to make truly voluntary choices about their reproductive lives, and these many dimensions are implicit in the ideal.

Clearly, feminists are not "pro-abortion," for they are concerned to ensure the safety of each pregnancy to the greatest degree possible; wanted fetuses should not be harmed or lost. Therefore, adequate pre- and post-natal care and nutrition are also important elements of any feminist position on reproductive freedom. Where anti-abortionists direct their energies to trying to prevent women from obtaining abortions, feminists seek to protect the health of wanted fetuses. They recognize that far more could be done to protect and care for fetuses if the state directed its resources at supporting women who continue their pregnancies, rather than draining away resources in order to police women who find that they must interrupt their pregnancies. Caring for the women who carry fetuses is not only a more legitimate policy than is regulating them; it is probably also more effective at ensuring the health and well-being of more fetuses.

Feminist ethics also explores how abortion policies fit within the politics of sexual domination. Most feminists are sensitive to the fact that many men support women's right to abortion out of the belief that women will be more willing sexual partners if they believe that they can readily terminate an unwanted pregnancy. Some men coerce their partners into obtaining abortions the women may not want.[19] Feminists understand that many women oppose abortion for this very reason, being unwilling to support a practice that increases women's sexual vulnerability (Luker 1984, p. 209-15). Thus, it is important that feminists develop a coherent analysis of reproductive freedom that includes sexual freedom (as women choose to define it). That requires an analysis of sexual freedom that includes women's right to refuse sex; such a right can only be assured if women have equal power to men and are not subject to domination by virtue of their sex.[20]

In sum, then, feminist ethics demands that moral discussions of abortion be more broadly defined than they have been in most philosophic discussions. Only by reflecting on the meaning of ethical pronouncements on actual women's lives and the connections between judgments on abortion and the conditions of domination and subordination can we come to an adequate understanding of the moral status of abortion in our society. As Rosalind Petchesky

(1980) argues, feminist discussion of abortion "must be moved beyond the framework of a 'woman's right to choose' and connected to a much broader revolutionary movement that addresses all of the conditions of women's liberation" (p. 113).

———

Notes

*Earlier versions of this paper were read to the Department of Philosophy, Dalhousie University and to the Canadian Society for Women in Philosophy in Kingston. I am very grateful for the comments received from colleagues in both forums; particular thanks go to Lorraine Code, David Braybrooke, Richmond Campbell, Sandra Taylor, Terry Tomkow and Kadri Vihvelin for their patience and advice.

1. For some idea of the ways in which traditional moral theory oppresses women, see Morgan (1987) and Hoagland (1988).
2. Critics continue to want to structure the debate around the *possibility* of women making frivolous abortion decisions and hence want feminists to agree to setting boundaries on acceptable grounds for choosing abortion. Feminists ought to resist this injunction, though. There is no practical way of drawing a line fairly in the abstract; cases that may appear "frivolous" at a distance, often turn out to be substantive when the details are revealed, i.e., frivolity is in the eyes of the beholder. There is no evidence to suggest that women actually make the sorts of choices worried critics hypothesize about: e.g., a woman eight months pregnant who chooses to abort because she wants to take a trip or gets in "a tiff" with her partner. These sorts of fantasies, on which demands to distinguish between legitimate and illegitimate personal reasons for choosing abortion chiefly rest, reflect an offensive conception of women as irresponsible; they ought not to be perpetuated. Women, seeking moral guidance in their own deliberations about choosing abortion, do not find such hypothetical discussions of much use.
3. In her monumental historical analysis of the early roots of Western patriarchy, Gerda Lerner (1986) determined that patriarchy began in the period from 3100 to 600 B.C. when men appropriated women's sexual and reproductive capacity; the earliest states entrenched patriarchy by institutionalizing the sexual and procreative subordination of women to men.
4. There are some women who claim to be feminists against choice in abortion. See, for instance, Callahan (1987), though few spell out their full feminist program. For reasons I develop in this paper, I do not think this is a consistent position.
5. There is a lot the state could do to ameliorate this condition. If it provided women with adequate financial support, removed the inequities in the labour market, and provided affordable and reliable childcare, pregnancy need not so often lead to a woman's dependence on a particular man. The fact that it does not do so is evidence of the state's complicity in maintaining women's subordinate position with respect to men.
6. See Petchesky (1984), especially Chapter 5, "Considering the Alternatives: The Problems of Contraception," where she documents the risks and discomforts associated with pill use and IUD's and the increasing rate at which women are choosing the option of diaphragm or condom with the option of early legal abortions as backup.
7. See Zillah Eisenstein (1988) for a comprehensive theory of the role of the pregnant body as the central element in the cultural subordination of women.
8. Thomson (1971) is a notable exception to this trend.
9. This seems reminiscent of Aristotle's view of women as "flower pots" where men implant the seed with all the important genetic information and the movement necessary for development and women's job is that of passive gestation, like the flower pot. For exploration of the flower pot picture of pregnancy, see Whitbeck (1973) and Lange (1983).
10. Contrast Warren (1989) with Tooley (1972).
11. The definition of pregnancy as a purely passive activity reaches its ghoulish conclusion in the increasing acceptability of sustaining brain-dead women on life support systems to continue their functions as incubators until the fetus can be safely delivered. For a discussion of this new trend, see Murphy (1989).
12. This apt phrasing is taken from Petchesky (1986), p. 342.
13. Fetuses are almost wholly individuated by the women who bear them. The fetal "contributions" to the relationship are defined by the projections and

interpretations of the pregnant woman in the latter stages of pregnancy if she chooses to perceive fetal movements in purposeful ways (e.g., "it likes classical music, wine, exercise").

14. Some feminists suggest we seek recognition of the legitimacy of non-medical abortion services. This would reduce costs and increase access dramatically, with no apparent increase in risk, provided that services were offered by trained, responsible practitioners concerned with the well-being of their clients. It would also allow the possibility of increasing women's control over abortion. See, for example McDonnell (1984), chap. 8.

15. For a useful model of such a centre, see Wagner and Lee (1989).

16. See CARAL/Halifax (1990) for women's stories about their experiences with hospitals and free-standing abortion clinics.

17. The Canadian Medical Association has confirmed those fears. In testimony before the House of Commons committee reviewing the bill, the CMA reported that over half the doctors surveyed who now perform abortions expect to stop offering them if the legislation goes through. Since the Commons passed the bill, the threats of withdrawal of service have increased. Many doctors plan to abandon their abortion service once the law is introduced, because they are unwilling to accept the harassment they anticipate from anti-abortion zealots. Even those who believe that they will eventually win any court case that arises, fear the expense and anxiety involved as the case plays itself out.

18. Therefore, the Soviet model, where women have access to multiple abortions but where there is no other birth control available, must also be opposed.

19. See CARAL/Halifax (1990), p. 20-21, for examples of this sort of abuse.

20. It also requires that discussions of reproductive and sexual freedom not be confined to "the language of control and sexuality characteristic of a technology of sex" (Diamond and Quinby 1988, p. 197), for such language is alienating and constrains women's experiences of their own sexuality.

References

Addelson, Kathryn Pyne. 1987. "Moral Passages," in Eva Feder Kittay and Diana T. Meyers, eds., *Women and Moral Theory*. Totowa, N.J.: Rowman & Littlefield.

Baier, Annette. 1985. *Postures of the Mind: Essays on Mind and Morals*. Minneapolis: University of Minnesota Press.

Callahan, Sidney. 1987. "A Pro-life Feminist Makes Her Case," *Utne Reader* (March/April): 104-14.

CARAL/Halifax. 1990 *Telling Our Stories: Abortion Stories from Nova Scotia*. Halifax: CARAL/Halifax (Canadian Abortion Rights Action League).

Daly, Mary. 1973. *Beyond God the Father: Toward a Philosophy of Women's Liberation*. Boston: Beacon Press.

Diamond, Irene, and Lee Quinby. 1988. "American Feminism and the Language of Control," in Irene Diamond and Lee Quinby, eds., *Feminism and Foucault: Reflections on Resistance*. Boston: Northeastern University Press.

Eisenstein, Zillah R. 1988. *The Female Body and the Law*. Berkeley: University of California Press.

Hoagland, Sara Lucia. 1988. *Lesbian Ethics: Toward New Value*. Palo Alto, Calif.: Institute of Lesbian Studies.

Lange, Lynda. 1983. "Woman is Not a Rational Animal: On Aristotle's Biology of Reproduction," in Sandra Harding and Merill B. Hintickka, eds., *Discovering Reality: Feminist Perspectives on Epistemology, Metaphysics, Methodology, and Philosophy of Science*. Dordrecht, Holland: D. Reidel.

Lerner, Gerda. 1986. *The Creation of Patriarchy*. New York: Oxford.

Luker, Kristin. 1984. *Abortion and the Politics of Motherhood*. Berkeley: University of California Press.

MacKinnon, Catherine. 1989. *Toward a Feminist Theory of the State*. Cambridge, Mass.: Harvard University Press.

McDonnell, Kathleen. 1984. *Not an Easy Choice: A Feminist Re-examines Abortion*. Toronto: The Women's Press.

McLaren, Angus, and Arlene Tigar McLaren. 1986. *The Bedroom and the State: The Changing Practices and Politics of Contraception and Abortion in Canada, 1880-1980)*. Toronto: McClelland and Stewart.

Morgan, Kathryn Pauly. 1987. "Women and Moral Madness," in Marsha Hanen and Kai Nielsen, eds., *Science, Morality and Feminist Theory. Canadian Journal of Philosophy*, Supplementary Volume 13: 201-26.

Murphy, Julien S. 1989 "Should Pregnancies Be Sustained in Brain-dead Women?: A Philosophical Discussion of Postmortem Pregnancy," in Kathryn Srother Ratcliff et al., eds., *Healing Technology: Feminist Perspectives*. Ann Arbor: The University of Michigan Press.

Overall, Christine. 1987. *Ethics and Human Reproduction: A Feminist Analysis* Winchester, Mass.: Allen & Unwin.

Petchesky, Rosalind Pollack. 1980. "Reproductive Freedom: Beyond 'A Woman's Right to Choose,'" in Catharine R. Stimpson and Ethel Spector Person, eds., *Women: Sex and Sexuality*. Chicago: University of Chicago Press.

—. 1984. *Abortion and Woman's Choice: The State, Sexuality, and Reproductive Freedom*. Boston: Northeastern University Press.

Sumner, L.W. 1981. *Abortion and Moral Theory*. Princeton: Princeton University Press.

Thomson, Judith Jarvis. 1971. "A Defense of Abortion," *Philosophy and Public Affairs*, 1: 47-66.

Tooley, Michael. 1972. "Abortion and Infanticide," *Philosophy and Public Affairs*, 2, 1 (Fall): 37-65.

Van Wagner, Vicki, and Bob Lee. 1989. "Principles into Practice: An Activist Vision of Feminist Reproductive Health Care," in Christine Overall, ed., *The Future of Human Reproduction*. Toronto: The Women's Press.

Warren, Mary Anne. 1973. "On the Moral and Legal Status of Abortion," *The Monist*, 57: 43-61.

—. 1989. "The Moral Significance of Birth," *Hypatia*, 4, 2 (Summer): 46-65.

Whitbeck, Carolyn. 1973. "Theories of Sex Difference," *The Philosophic Forum*, 5, 1-2 (Fall/Winter 1973-74): 54-80.

26.
MORAL OBLIGATIONS TO THE NOT-YET BORN: THE FETUS AS PATIENT

Thomas H. Murray

The health of the not-yet-born child—the fetus intended to be brought to live birth—periodically emerges as a subject of concern. From dramatic interventions such as fetal surgery through drugs and special diets on to efforts to get pregnant women to abstain from alcohol and tobacco or to bar them from workplaces possibly toxic to developing fetuses, there has been a recent surge of ideas on how to prevent, ameliorate, or remedy damage to the not-yet-born.

Many things might be done *with, by* or *to* a pregnant woman to benefit her not-yet-born child. They range from the most physically intrusive to the least, from the most technologically sophisticated to mundane efforts at education and persuasion, from those with clearly established benefit to the fetus to those of highly uncertain benefit. The ethical issues raised by interventions of all kinds designed to aid a fetus share essential features. Once some form of fetal surgery becomes established, the case of a woman who refuses it will raise many of the same moral questions as that of a woman whose alcoholism threatens her fetus's health to a point where incarceration or institutionalization are being considered. Although different in several respects, both of the cases require asking how far the state—and physicians as agents of the state—ought to go in coercively intervening in the life of a woman in order to benefit her fetus. And both presume at least a tentative answer to a difficult ethical question: What is the moral status of a fetus?

To answer such a question sensibly and with a modicum of wisdom is our ultimate goal. A burgeoning literature on fetal therapies, fetal surgery, fetal rights, and maternal-fetal conflicts has enlivened the argument. While technologically sophisticated interventions like fetal surgery are receiving the most attention, they will probably be relevant to only a minute proportion of all pregnancies. Yet most of the ethical questions raised by fetal surgery are equally pertinent to a host of other, less glamorous means to the same end. Some sample questions include the following:

- How far should we go in getting diabetic women to manage their disease during pregnancy?: Should we inform them of the consequences to their fetus? Should we try to persuade them gently? Browbeat them? If they refuse to cooperate should we initiate civil or criminal proceedings to try and coerce them? Should we try to institutionalize them as has been done in some cases of drug addicted mothers, and then perhaps strip them of their children once they are born?
- What about a mother suspected of using drugs—legal or illegal—that might deleteriously affect the fetus? What of the mother who smokes or drinks? How hard do we try to discourage her smoking or drinking during pregnancy? If she continues to do either or both heavily, at what point if any do we move beyond persuasion to coercion?
- If we think that low levels of a potentially embryotoxic or fetotoxic substance are present in a workplace, should all pregnant women be kept out? What about "potentially pregnant," that is, nonsterile women? Many United States companies have "Fetal Protection Policies" that do just that.[1]

KEY ISSUES

Given the present, chaotic state of the debate over fundamental issues of ethics, law, and public policy regarding the fetus, offering simple answers to questions such as the ones just asked would require ignoring even more important questions. It is more valuable in the long run to clarify some of the fundamental issues now. Five are discussed in this article.

1. Whether there are any moral duties to a fetus.
2. Whether viability affects those duties.
3. How the concept of duties to a fetus is frequently misused.
4. What pitfalls must be avoided in moving from moral judgments to public policy.
5. The importance of the social and historical context of the current debate.

DO WE HAVE MORAL DUTIES TO A FETUS?

The moral status of those fetuses who will never be born alive is problematic. Right-to-life advocates claim that even the fertilized ovum is a person, entitled to all the protections and respect due every person. Many other people, including many of those with qualms about abortion, believe that the fetus, especially in its early stages of development, has a lesser moral stature than adults, infants, or even late-term fetuses. No consensus exists on such fetuses. Fortunately, we can discuss the fetus as patient without becoming bogged down in the mire of the abortion debate. All we need is a simple distinction between those fetuses destined bo be brought to live birth, and those who will not know extrauterine life.

The Not-Yet-Born Child

The situation is quite different for fetuses who will be born alive. A few theorists argue that the fetus, or even the infant and young child, has no moral status, or else an inferior one.[2] Some writers, while not directly addressing the question, argue that whatever moral claims the fetus might have are always secondary to those of the woman in whose body the fetus lies.[3] Nonetheless, there is good reason to believe that we have moral obligations to the fetus destined to be born, who we will call the not-yet-born child to distinguish it from both the already-born child and from the fetus who will not be born alive. Further, this view has considerable popular support, as evidenced by the efforts aimed at preserving fetal health through antenatal medical care, public health education of pregnant women, and the like.

The Timing of a Harm is Irrelevant

Imagine two different cases. In the first, a man assaults a woman with the intention of inflicting grave harm on her fetus. He succeeds, causing permanent, irreparable—but not fatal—damage to the fetus's spinal cord, resulting in paralysis. In the second case, all the circumstances are identical, except that the man attacks an infant rather than a fetus, with the same result—permanent, irreparable paralysis. Was the first act any less wrong than the second? In both cases, lifelong harm was done to humans who, whatever your beliefs about when personhood begins, would eventually cross that line and attain full moral status.

My thesis, in short, is that the timing of a harm, in itself, is not morally relevant. An act resulting in harm to a not-yet-born person (who will eventually be a full-fledged person according to everyone's moral theory) is as great a harm as if it were done later. The morally relevant factors are the usual ones: the actor's intentions; excuses; mitigating circumstances, and so on. In practice, a fetus is rarely harmed intentionally; typically, harm to a fetus occurs as a result of intentional or unintentional harm to its mother. The lack of intention to harm then is what affects our judgment about the wrongness of the act, and not the fact that it was a not-yet-born person who was harmed. We would judge unintended harm to a child or adult in a similar manner. The debate over the ethics of abortion aside, then, we can talk sensibly and without inherent contradiction about moral duties to the fetus destined to become a person—to the not-yet-born person. There will be duties to avoid harm, and there may be duties to render aid.

We can discuss moral duties to not-yet-born persons without becoming hopelessly trapped in the abortion debate. Before moving on to discuss the scope of our duties to the fetus, we need to consider whether viability affects these duties.

THE MORAL RELEVANCE OF VIABILITY

Viability is, at best, a slippery concept. For one thing it is a moving front. As our ability to save younger and smaller newborns improves, the so-called age of viability is reached earlier. Physicians frequently use viability as a statistical concept: the age at which some unspecified percentage of newborns will survive. Sometimes the concept is used with reference to specific infants. We could describe survival possibilities as a probabilistic function of weight or gestational age. For example, the BW or GA 10 would be the birthweight or gestational age at which 10 per cent of infants survive. The GA 50 would be the level at which 50 per cent live, and so on. These numbers would change as our ability to save these infants change.

Viability and Abortion

The central question is whether our moral obligations to the fetus change as a function of viability. Viability as a determinant of our duties to a fetus was given great importance by its inclusion in the well-known Supreme Court abortion decision, *Roe v. Wade*.[4] The complex ruling says in its summary: "For the stage subsequent to viability, the State in promoting its interest in the potentiality of human life may, if it chooses, regulate, and even proscribe, abortion except where it is necessary, in appropriate medical judgment, for the preservation of the life or health of the mother."[5]

Viability serves as a threshold in *Roe v. Wade*. Even though the Court uses the ambiguous phrase "potentiality of human life," behind their decision must lie some notion of the fetus growing in legal and presumably moral stature as it approaches term. Otherwise, there would be no justification for linking the State's interest in protecting that potential life with viability which, at the time of that decision (1973), roughly coincided with the end of the second trimester for most fetuses.

Attempting to uncover the moral reasoning underlying a legal decision can be perilous because one may simply be wrong and because it may encourage the unfortunate tendency to see moral disapproval as a sufficient reason for taking legal action, something we will take up later. Bearing that caution in mind, we nonetheless must try to determine what moral ideas underlie the legal reasoning in *Roe v. Wade*. The court appears to believe that, prior to viability, whatever claim the fetus may have not to be killed is outweighed by a woman's right to choose whether or not to bear and give birth to a child, with all that those activities bring in their wake. After viability, the fetus's increasing nearness to actual rather than

merely potential life strengthens its moral claim against being killed to the point where it overrides the mother's right to choose not to bear a child, though not so far as to force her to risk her own life in doing so.

Viability Is Irrelevant for Nonfatal Harms

In other words, for the problem of deciding whether a woman can abort her fetus, it may be important to know what the fetus's moral status is *at that particular moment*: whether or not it is a person or how close it is to becoming a full-fledged person may be important in this context. In stark contrast, the fetus's moral standing at that moment in its development is not relevant to judging our duties to avoid or avert nonfatal harms, since, as far as we know, the fetus will some day be a full person, and the timing of such nonlethal harms is not pertinent to determining their wrongfulness. Interestingly, the law itself seems to agree.

Until 1946, a child injured prenatally then born alive but impaired rarely found a court willing to sustain a suit for damages. But in that year began what Prosser, who wrote the standard reference work on tort law, called "the most spectacular abrupt reversal of a well settled rule in the whole history of the law of torts. The child, provided that he is born alive, is permitted to maintain an action for the consequences of prenatal injuries, and if he dies of such injuries after birth an action will lie for his wrongful death."[6] Prosser believed that the earlier denials of claims on behalf of children injured while they were still fetuses were based on invalid reasoning, and he approved of the reversal.

With the concept of prenatal injuries established as a valid one, does it matter whether the fetus was viable at the time of injury? Some courts have required that the fetus have been viable, or at least "quickened" at the time of injury.[7] But many courts have rejected viability as a relevant factor in determining whether the born child may recover from prenatal injury.[8] One critic of the concept of fetal rights says pointedly: "[V]iability is a meaningless distinction in the fetal rights context because the state's interest in the health of its future citizens is equally strong throughout pregnancy."[9] Prosser himself says, "[c]ertainly the [previable] infant may be no less injured; and all logic is in favor of ignoring the stage at which it occurs." Acknowledging that proving injury early in pregnancy might be difficult, he concludes, "[t]his, however, goes to proof rather than principle; and if, as is undoubtedly the case there are injuries as to which reliable medical proof is possible, it makes no sense to deny recovery on any such arbitrary basis."[10] The moral principle, that is, does not depend on the arbitrary criterion of viability.

While most cases have focused on recovering damages for harms already done, a number of recent cases attempt to prevent harm by affecting the pregnant woman's behavior, even to the point of outright coercion. The forced caesarean cases discussed elsewhere in this volume are one sort of example.[11] In another case (reported by a newspaper) a physician accused a woman, seven months pregnant, of endangering her fetus's development by abusing drugs. The woman was ordered to enter a drug rehabilitation program and undergo regular urinalyses until the child was born.[12] Whether this is a reasonable response to the problem is the subject of the next section.

MISUSING THE IDEA OF DUTIES TO A FETUS

A recurrent theme in this essay is the danger of making moral judgments or public policy without sufficient regard for context. Just this sort of misuse of the concept of duties to a fetus occurs with unsettling frequency.

The Dangers of Oversimplifying Moral Decisions

The moral world we inhabit is one marked by a multiplicity of interests and duties. We are certainly entitled to give good moral weight to our own interests. Then there are duties to those with whom we have special relationships, relationships that prescribe even strenuous moral duties in certain domains. Finally, we have duties to "strangers"—those with whom no special moral relationship exists. Most significant moral decisions have implications for many of these interests and relationships simultaneously. For example, a woman who must decide whether to place her fetus at risk of harm by working in a factory with low levels of a suspected fetotoxin must weigh her own interests in having a job with the psychological and material benefits that may bring against the risks imposed on

herself as well as her fetus. She must also consider possible benefits to her fetus that the job makes possible, such as improved nutrition for herself and prenatal care facilitated by health insurance. Then there may be others dependent on her working: a spouse, other children, perhaps elderly parents. When we portray the ethical dimensions of her decision as beginning and ending with the question of whether or not she has duties to avoid exposing her fetus to risks, we rip such a complex decision out of its moral, as well as its social and political, context. Yet, this is commonly done. Or, not much better, the woman's "right" to do whatever she desires is counterposed to the fetus's right to protection from harm. Once the problem is framed this way, giving a nuanced answer becomes impossible. A more complex view of the moral life, one that encompasses a multiplicity of legitimate moral concerns, of interests and duties, of roles and relationships, allows us to frame the question in a way that can be answered, if not more easily, at least more satisfactorily.

Warning of Fearful Consequences

In a clash of rights, complex issues can become stripped of their nuances and turned into simplistic all-or-none contests. On either extreme, we can imagine bleak consequences. If, on the one hand, we give pre-eminence to the fetus's right to avoid being harmed, then must pregnant women structure every detail of their lives in order to avoid all suspected risks to their not-yet-born child? Such an attitude appears to have influenced some companies to adopt so-called "Fetal Protection Policies," or FPPs, that deny employment opportunities to women.[13] Fears of what would happen should fetal rights gain the upper hand generate a litany of nightmarish possibilities:

A woman could be held civilly or criminally liable for fetal injuries caused by accidents resulting from maternal negligence, such as automobile or household accidents. She could also be held liable for any behavior during her pregnancy having potentially adverse effects on her fetus, including failure to eat properly, using prescription, non-prescription and illegal drugs, smoking, drinking alcohol, exposing herself to infectious disease or to any workplace hazards, engaging in immoderate exercise or sexual intercourse, residing at high altitudes for prolonged periods, or using a general anesthetic or drugs to induce rapid labor during delivery. If the current trend in fetal rights continues, pregnant women would live in constant fear that any accident or "error" in judgment could be deemed "unacceptable" and become the basis for a criminal prosecution by the state or a civil suit....[14]

On the other hand, if we give full sway to the woman's right to control her body, can we even level moral criticism against a case such as the one of a woman who at 40 weeks gestation, in labor with abruptio placenta with fetal distress, refused a caesarean section? After the infant was delivered stillborn, she explained to a nurse that "the death of the fetus solved complicated personal problems."[15] The language of rights in conflict may not permit us to give full and weighty consideration to a host of factors that we believe are important in making moral judgments. Examining relationships, legitimate interests, and duties may give us a more adequate picture of the moral choices people face.

Obligations to the Not-Yet-Born Are Not All Or None

Take, for example, the case of the woman who must decide whether to accept a job that might pose some risk to her fetus. Let us suppose that she intends to bring the child to birth, so we do not have to worry about the ethics of abortion. As far as we know, this is a not-yet-born child; therefore the woman has some obligation to avoid harming it while it is still a fetus. What is the scope and intensity of this obligation? Must she refuse the job?

Because of the link between most discussions of the fetus's moral status and abortion, there is an unfortunate tendency to think of our obligations to the fetus as all-or-none. But there are other creatures dependent on us, to whom we have obligations, but where those duties do not unequivocally overwhelm all other considerations—our children for example. We certainly have a duty to do what is reasonable to protect our young children from harm. That requires keeping them from known and probable dangers. But we are not required to sacrifice everything else to this task. We should teach them not to play in busy streets, and offer them a protected play-area. But

must we build crash-proof barriers around their playground, strong enough to stop a cement truck run wild? Obviously not. That would be beyond "reasonable" responsibility. Anytime we take them in a car, there is a risk of injury or death. Responsible parents should provide a secure carseat for their infant or toddler. But we are not forbidden from going for a drive, even though no matter how carefully we drive there is always the distinct possibility of an accident.

What is it that makes certain risks reasonable, and others the kind that responsible parents would not take? The probability of harm and its severity should it occur are certainly relevant. Also significant is the importance of the purpose for which the risk is run and the avoidability of the risk. If we want the children to see their grand-parents, a long car ride may be unavoidable. And exposing our child to the considerable risks of cytotoxic drugs is clearly justifiable if and only if our purpose is to treat them for cancer.

My purpose here is to put us on more familiar ground than the exotic situations in which questions of fetal status typically arise. Two points come out of the discussion. First, whatever moral duties we might have to a fetus—a not-yet-born child—they may equal but not exceed our duties to already-born children. The circumstances of a fetus's physical enclosure within and link to its mother's body confuses many discussions. This linkage may mean that a broader range of actions might affect the fetus, and the facts of the case will be accordingly affected. But the same moral considerations apply equally to both the not-yet-born and the already-born—considerations such as intentions, probability and severity of risk, and duties to others. Second, duties to the not-yet-born, like duties to the already-born, are usually just one of many factors to be considered in judging the moral acceptability of an act.

Another advantage of discussing our obligations to the not-yet-born and already-born together is that it enables us to talk about fathers and not just mothers. To the extent that cultural blinders distort our view of a mother's responsibility to her fetus, then looking at a case with comparable morally relevant features, but one that asks about a father's responsibility to his child, may restore some moral clarity.

A Father-Child Analogy

Take the plausible case of a man who lost his job in the oil fields of west Texas. He has two children counting on him for support; his wife is also out of work. An offer comes of a job in a petrochemical plant near Houston. Taking that job will mean moving his family to a part of Texas crawling with petrochemical complexes where toxic releases into the air, ground, and water are not unknown, and where the risk of cancer is somewhat, though not drastically, higher than in their current community. There are a number of good reasons to take the job. He will be able to afford better food, clothing, and housing for his family and himself. Being unemployed threatens his sense of self-worth, which depresses him and incidentally also makes him a less thoughtful parent and spouse. Like most unemployed Americans, when he lost his job he also lost his health insurance; the new job will assure better access to health care for himself and his family. Perhaps the schools are better in the new community. Suppose he accepts the job even though he knows and regrets the increased risk that will mean for his children. Decisions such as this are all-things-considered choices: by their nature they involve weighing and balancing many things. Would we say that this man's choice was immoral? That he should not have exposed his children to the slightly increased risk of cancer whatever else was involved? It would make better sense to say that he made a responsible, morally defensible decision, even if we share his regret about the increased risk to which his children as well as his wife and himself will be exposed.

How was this man's decision any different from that of a woman who chooses to accept a job, knowing that her fetus will be exposed to some low but nonetheless increased risk of harm because of exposures there? Perhaps she too is without health insurance. Perhaps having a job is important to her sense of self-worth. Perhaps there are other children and a spouse at home who are dependent on her. The fact that she carries a fetus within her, a not-yet-born child, that she has moral duties to protect that fetus from harm, and that the workplace increases slightly the probability of harm does not make her decision immoral. Exactly the same considerations were relevant to the man's decision. To the extent that the morally relevant factors are comparable—and in this case they might well be identical—the decisions are equally justified. And if the circumstances vary, at least we know the kinds of morally significant considerations that will influence our judgments.[16] Whether it is a man or a woman is not relevant. Nor, I have argued, does it matter whether it is a not-yet-born or already-born child.

FROM ETHICAL JUDGMENTS TO PUBLIC POLICY

We do not ban all conduct we regard as morally suspect, nor do we compel people to carry out every moral duty. Many things are left to personal conscience, to moral suasion, or to social pressure. For good reasons, including moral ones, we are reluctant to allow the state to force its view of correct conduct on individuals unless the harm to be avoided is grave, especially when doing so requires coercion, bodily invasion, or incarceration. These means are among the most repugnant and are reserved for extreme circumstances. If we conclude then that a woman morally ought to quit smoking during pregnancy, moderate or eliminate her consumption of alcohol, and do likewise with caffeine, this does not automatically justify heavy-handed state intervention to assure that she does these things. Some wrongs are minimally so. The state should not exercise its often great power on such things. Sometimes the effort to correct a wrong itself creates new moral problems. The moral and other costs of enforcement may outweigh the good that might be done.

The fetus becomes a "patient" when its welfare becomes the physician's concern. The obstetrician caring for a mother and not-yet-born child has two patients. In much the way that a pediatrician advises parents about their newborn's diet, monitors the infant's health, and prescribes needed medication or other therapeutic interventions, an obstetrician routinely does the same for the mother and the fetus-patient. How extensive is the obstetrician's duty to assure that the fetus-patient's welfare is being protected?

The "Child-As-Maximum" Principle

One useful guideline might be called the "child-as-maximum" principle. The principle says that our obligations to ensure the fetus's welfare can equal but not exceed our obligations to a born child. If a pediatrician would not be obliged to do more than try to persuade parents to do a certain thing—say observe a special diet—then under conditions of comparable burdens and benefits, obstetricians cannot be obliged to do more to protect a fetus, although they may be required to do less.

One inescapable difference between the obstetrician's and the pediatrician's case is of course that the former's second patient, the fetus, is encased in the body of the first patient, the mother. All interventions directed at the fetus literally must go through its mother. The burdens created, therefore, generally will be much greater, as will be the potential for morally wronging one person in the effort to aid another. This is why the child-as-maximum principle emphasizes that our duties to a born child constitute an upperbound for our duties to a not-yet-born child rather than a strict equivalence. A drug that might benefit a fetus but that will be harmful to the mother can be refused. That same drug for that same being, now born, should probably be administered. The pediatrician in the latter instance is justified in pushing harder for consent from the parents than was the obstetrician.

A Variety of Needs, a Range of Interventions

One study shows that women who smoke a pack of cigarettes or more a day have babies on average about 180 gm smaller at birth than women who do not smoke. The same study found that women who drank twenty or more beers per month sacrificed roughly 100 gm of birthweight, while those who consumed 300 or more grams of caffeine daily (three or four cups of coffee or seven cola beverages) had babies 40 to 50 gm smaller on average.[17] What should physicians do? When the risks are small, we usually employ education and persuasion. That is the typical and appropriate response to maternal smoking, diet, nutritional supplements, and the like. These anchor one end of a continuum of possible "interventions." We can move to stronger measures, such as New York City has done, by requiring that signs be posted in public places serving alcohol warning pregnant women that alcohol may endanger their fetus's health. This is a public policy that relies as much on shame as on the educative effect of the signs.

Beyond this is a broad range of more traditionally "medical" interventions: managing maternal dia-

betes in pregnancy[18]; placing women with PKU on low-phenylalanine diets when they wish to become pregnant[19]; treating fetal methylmelonic acidemia by giving vitamin B-12 to the mother[20]; treating congenital hypothyroidism by injections into the amniotic fluid[21]; drug therapy for fetal ventricular tachycardia,[22] and other possibilities.

There are surgical routes as well. In addition to the familiar exchange transfusions for erythroblastosis fetalis, a variety of still-experimental fetal surgeries are under triculomegaly,[23] diaphragmatic hernia,[24] and hematopoietic stem cell transplantation for severe immunologic deficiencies.[25] (The law and ethics of fetal surgery have been amply discussed elsewhere.)[26]

Our ethical analysis of any proposed interventions to benefit a fetus intended to be brought to birth should include at least the following considerations:

1. How certain is the benefit to the fetus? (Is the intervention experimental? Is it well-established? Does it carry substantial risks to the fetus?)
2. How great are the benefits? (Will a successful intervention make a large or small difference in the fetus's prognosis?)
3. How intrusive, coercive, or harmful will it be to the mother?
4. Will anything be lost or gained by waiting until after the child is born?

Even if we are convinced that the mother has a moral responsibility to agree to the intervention, the question of how far we should go in attempting to persuade or coerce her raises an entirely new set of issues at the intersection of ethics and public policy. Once we move to the level of policy, political and historical considerations become very important. At this point, a brief look at another era's concern for the health of the not-yet-born is appropriate.

ALCOHOL AND "RACE-DECAY" IN EDWARDIAN ENGLAND

This is not the first time that parental behavior has been held responsible for harm to the not-yet-born or the already-born. The oldest prenatal health advice of which I am aware is in the Old Testament. In

Judges 13:7 the mother of Samson is told "Behold, thou shalt conceive and bear a son: and drink no wine or strong drink."

Many women today are fearful and suspicious of the movement towards ascribing moral status to the fetus. For women who aspire to compete in the economic marketplace on an equal footing with men, those fears and suspicions have substantial historical validity. Past social movements to protect helpless infants and not-yet-born children have had something less than pure and altruistic motives. One illuminating example comes from England at the turn of the century—the Edwardian era.

In the first decade of this century, England found itself losing its empire abroad and awash with immigrants at home: immigrants, moreover, whose children were more likely to survive infancy than their British neighbors. A number of laypeople and physicians believed they understood the problem—alcohol. A campaign to arouse public ire against parents who drank flourished in the first decade of the 1900s. While it was directed largely against women who drank, men came in for their share of the blame as well. Indeed, one highly influential Swiss study reported that 78 per cent of women unable to breastfeed had fathers who drank, heavily. But for the most part women were faulted.

In 1906, a British physician wrote:

Undoubtedly much of the high infant mortality is due to alcoholism, and conditions directly ... or indirectly arising from this morbid condition. The widespread prevalence of alcoholism among women, especially during the reproductive period of life, is one of the most important factors making for racial-decay.[27]

"Race-decay" is but one of many dubious reasons given for worrying about women and drink. George Sims, a prominent journalist of the time, had a related concern: "What can be the future of our Empire, if on a falling birth rate 120,000 infants continue to die annually in the first year of their lives ...!"[28] And he knew the cause: "Bad motherhood is the first great cause of our appalling infant morality."[29] No less an exemplar of success than Andrew Carnegie, the American industrialist, pointed to the drunken worker as a central threat to British productivity.[30]

For the most part, this was a campaign waged by the upper classes, including a number of male physicians, against working class women. They were not doing their national duty by outreproducing the immigrants—Jews, Italians, Scots, and Irish. Theophilus Hyslop, a physician active in the anti-drink movement, referred to immigrants derogatorily and declared that if the British worker would give up alcohol, he could "drive the foreigner from our midst."[31]

Perhaps Dr. Robert Jones best expressed the sentiment feared by contemporary women: "Women are now the companions of men in ... industrial pursuits, and the freedom to work on equal terms with men has caused ... the same depressing physical and mental influences ..., for which stimulants offer a temporary relief."[32] Women, that is, as vessels of reproduction, as the assurers of racial integrity, as the saviors of the empire, as the protectors of the innocent must be made to look after their offspring, and not be contaminated in the labor marketplace.

Many women understand any contemporary movement emphasizing their biologic role as bearers of children to be a threat to their economic liberty and equality—"fetal rights" being no exception. The need to control reproduction so that they could compete in the job market emerged as a major theme among pro-choice activists in Kristin Luker's study of anti- and pro-abortion activists. Conversely, having and raising children were crucial sources of self-value for many who worked against abortion.[33] Because it focuses attention on women's reproductive capacities, it is not surprising that the trend toward regarding the fetus as a patient has evoked concern and controversy. And with the long history of efforts to keep women in roles defined by and in the interests of men, it is no less surprising that women regard the current trend with suspicion. Legitimate concerns for fetal rights can also be carried along by other, questionable, motives and may carry with them other destructive social consequences.

CONCLUSIONS

Five points emerge from this analysis. First, we can discuss moral duties to the fetus destined to be born—to the not-yet-born child—without logical contradiction and without becoming hopelessly mired in debate over abortion.

Second, whether the fetus is viable may be regarded as morally significant in the context of abortion decisions, but it is not directly relevant to our duties to not-yet-born children. This is so because of the irrelevance of the timing of a harm.

Third, that we do have moral duties to fetuses, viable and previable alike, may not have the horrendous consequences for women that is typically thought. Our common error has been to focus exclusively on a pregnant woman's duty to avoid harming her fetus, without regard for the multitude of other moral considerations she ought to include in her decision. A more complex and adequate view of the moral life understands that in such decisions a host of factors may be relevant such as promises made, the woman's own interests, her obligations to other family members, and the welfare of her not-yet-born child. Seeing the mother's moral relationship to the fetus as morally analogous to a fathers's relationship to his child will help avoid oversimplification.

Fourth, establishing that women have moral duties to their not-yet-born children does not justify automatically coercive public policies to force them to fulfill those obligations. Again, the analogy to fathers and children may be helpful. The state must be very cautious in using its power to enforce particular notions of maternal duties. Effective enforcement might necessitate forcible invasion of a woman's body or prolonged incarceration. These are usually "last resorts" used only under very restricted circumstances. We must be careful to assure that they are not used more casually against pregnant women.

Fifth, women have ample reason to be suspicious of the growing tendency to focus on the welfare of the fetus-as-patient and, by implication, on the woman's role as bearer of children. Historically, movements allegedly directed toward aiding fetuses and children have often been motivated as much by other, less praiseworthy concerns, including racism, and especially by men's fear of women's political, social, and economic equality.

Rather than arguing of "fetal rights," let us use the less heated language of moral obligations to not-yet-born children. We must not oversimplify complex moral decisions, especially our tendency to focus on a pregnant woman's obligations to her not-yet-born child as the only morally important factor in her decisions. We would not tolerate such oversimplification when discussing parents' duties toward their children, and we must not tolerate it in the difficult decisions we now face regarding the welfare of the not-yet-born. History provides forceful reminders of the dangers of thinking of women as mere "vessels of reproduction." Finally, we must continue the work of clarifying our obligations toward both the fetus destined to be born and the mother who retains her full moral individuality and interests, and in whose body that developing person exists for a time.

Notes

1. US Congress, Office of Technology Assessment: Reproductive Health Hazards in the Workplace. US Government Printing Office: Washington, DC, 1985.
2. Tooley M.: Abortion and Infanticide. New York, Oxford University Press, 1983.
3. Engelhardt H.T.: The Foundation of Bioethics. New York, Oxford, 1986.
4. Roe v Wade, 410 U. S. 113, 1973.
5. Ibid.
6. Prosser W.L.: Handbook of the Law of Torts. Edition 3. St Paul, MN, West Publishing Co, 1964.
7. Ibid.
8. Keeton W.P., Dobbs D., Keeton R., et al: Prosser and Keeton on the Law of Torts. Edition 5. Mineola, NY, West Publishing Co, 1984.
9. Johnsen D.E.: The creation of fetal rights: Conflicts with women's constitutional rights to liberty, privacy, and equal protection. Yale Law J 95:599-625, 1986.
10. See note 6.
11. Strong C.: Ethical conflicts between mother and fetus in obstetrics. Clin Perinatol 14(2).
12. Shaw M.W.: Conditional prospective rights of the fetus. J Leg Med 5:63-116, 1984.
13. US Congress, Office of Technology Assessment: Reproductive Health Hazards in the Workplace. US Government Printing Office: Washington, DC, 1985.
14. Johnsen D.E.: The creation of fetal right: Conflicts with women's constitutional rights to liberty, privacy, and equal protection. Yale Law J 95:599-625, 1986.
15. Leiberman J.R., Mazor M., Chaim W., et al: The fetal right to live. Obstet Gynecol 53:515-517, 1979.

16. Murray T.H.: Who do fetal protection policies really protect? Tech Rev 88(7):12-13, 20, 1985.

17. Kuzma J.W., Sokol R.J.: Maternal drinking behavior and decreased intrauterine growth. Alcohol Clin Exp Res 6:396-402, 1982.

18. Gabbe S.G.: Management of diabetes mellitus in pregnancy. AM J Obstet Gynecol 153:824-827, 1985.

19. Robertson J.A., Schulman J.D.: PKU women and pregnancy: The limits of reproductive autonomy. Unpublished manuscript.

20. Schulman J.D.: Prenatal treatment of biochemical disorders. Sem Perinatol 9:75-78, 1985.

21. Weiner S., Scharf J.F., Bolognese P.J., et al: Antenatal diagnosis and treatment of fetal goiter. J Reprod Med 24:39-42, 1980.

22. Kleinman C.S., Copel J.A., Weinstein E.M., et al: In utero diagnosis and treatment of fetal supra-ventricular tachycardia. Sem Perinatol 9:113-129, 1985.

23. Clewell W.H., Meier P.R., Manchester D.K., et al: Ventriculomegaly: Evaluation and management. Sem Perinatol 9:98-102, 1985.

24. Harrison M.R., Adzick N.S., Nakayama D.K., et al: Fetal diaphragmatic hernia: Fatal but fixable. Sem Parinatol 9:103-112, 1985.

25. Simpson T.J., Golbus M.S.: In utero fetal hematopoietic stem cell transplantation. Sem Perinatol 9:68-74, 1985.

26. Fletcher, J.C.: Ethical considerations in and beyond experimental fetal therapy. Sem Perinatol 9:130-135, 1985; Murray TH: Ethical issues in fetal surgery. Bull Am Col Surg 70(6):6-10, 1985; Robertson JA: Legal issues in fetal therapy. Sem Perinatol 9:136-142, 1985.

27. Gutzke D.W.: "The cry of the children": The Edwardian medical campaign against maternal drinking. Br J Addiction 79:71-84, 1984.

28. Ibid.

29. Ibid.

30. Ibid.

31. Ibid.

32. Ibid.

33. Luker K.: Abortion and the Politics of Motherhood. University of California, Berkeley, 1984.

CHAPTER SIX

SCREENING AND TREATMENT
OF "DISABLED" NEWBORNS

27.
PRENATAL DIAGNOSIS: REPRODUCTIVE CHOICE? REPRODUCTIVE CONTROL?

Abby Lippman

Reproductive technology probably dates back to the seventeenth century and the first use of forceps during labour.[1] Since then, various other technical tools and procedures have been applied to the whole process of reproduction from conception (or its prevention) through delivery, with recent developments such as in vitro fertilization, embryo transfer and surrogate motherhood attracting growing attention in professional and lay literature. Unfortunately, the focus on these dramatic and overtly controversial procedures appears to have distracted attention from other technical interventions in pregnancy that, because of their widespread use, may have even more impact on our attitudes and social policies with respect to pregnancy and to pregnant women. These are the techniques used for prenatal diagnosis.

In speaking of prenatal diagnosis, I am referring generically to all the methods and techniques that can be used to obtain information about a fetus during pregnancy. Included are already widely-used procedures such as amniocentesis and ultrasonography, methods currently under assessment such as chorionic villi sampling, and methods under development such as fetal cell sorting.

Recent biomedical discoveries and technological developments have rapidly expanded both our genetic knowledge and our ability to obtain information about the fetus in utero, vastly increasing the possibilities for prenatal diagnosis. This expansion in the availability and application of prenatal diagnosis and the widespread adoption of these specific reproductive technologies by professionals have not been accompanied—much less preceded—by thoughtful deliberation about their social policy implications. However, because some form of prenatal diagnosis is here to stay, and because all women planning a pregnancy are already potential candidates for prenatal

diagnosis, it is still important to identify some of the implications that appear especially problematic.

Prenatal diagnosis had its beginning in the development of tests for couples at known, quantifiable risk for having children with certain specific genetic disorders that would interfere with their health or intelligence. Most of these disorders were considered "serious." Although "serious" was never rigorously defined, it was rapidly accepted as a physician-imposed criterion for testing.[2]

This orientation primarily to genetic conditions whose severity and consequences were generally agreed upon, and for which there was no effective treatment, now seems less and less the case given the enormous broadening, over the years, of the scope of conditions considered appropriate for prenatal diagnosis. With many of the tests that can now be carried out, we can identify fetuses with conditions that have little effect on, or uncertain implications for, postnatal health and functioning. Often we can tell if the fetus has the relevant genes that increase its susceptibility to some illness, but not whether it will be exposed to the environmental circumstances that will interact with these genes to actually create a problem. As well, we can sometimes give a fetus a general diagnostic label—neural tube defect, for example—but we cannot tell how serious its disability will actually be. We can diagnose conditions for which effective treatment is available and can also detect a number of conditions that are not even genetic.

To date, this expansion has resulted largely from the choices physicians and scientists have made about the tests they would develop and make available. These choices have resulted in some selected conditions being labelled not only as "serious," but as "undesirable": undesirable enough to warrant testing and the possible abortion of affected fetuses.

Before further expansion occurs, it is timely to consider carefully both the conditions we want to have diagnosed and the process by which we want decisions about access to testing to be made.

To begin these difficult and complicated tasks of establishing objectives for prenatal diagnosis programs[3] and defining a decision-making process, we might first try to learn why we seek knowledge about the fetus. Unlike mountains, climbed just because "they are there," information about the fetus ought not necessarily be sought or provided just because we can do so. Thus, what is it we want to predict—and why? Are there any basic objectives of testing we can agree on that will prevent its banalization?[4] This question is becoming increasingly pertinent as information about fetal status can be obtained earlier and earlier, and at less and less risk to the pregnancy, perhaps even at no risk at all, if fetal cells in the mother's blood can be found and analyzed. Are there principles regarding prenatal testing that we should honour, irrespective of the nature of the test or when it is carried out? For example, what if we can do prenatal diagnosis even before there is a pregnancy by examining an egg fertilized in vitro? What ground rules would we want to see in place?

Answering these questions will require us to determine the kind of information we want to obtain and the responses to this information we will tolerate as individuals and as a society. Can we harness the technologies and apply only those that conform to our common values, limiting the diagnoses we will make? Or will we continue as we have been doing, letting our ability to make diagnoses early in pregnancy lead automatically to extensions in what is called "undesirable," changing our values as we redefine what we consider to be a "disability" whenever our technical skills expand the list of diagnosable conditions? Past experience does not lead to optimism. But we must at least begin to consider the objectives of testing and insure that choices about its extension or restriction reflect the social and moral values not only of the health professionals who will provide the testing, but also of the women who will seek it.

Adding urgency to this need for open, broad-based consideration of the objectives of prenatal diagnosis are not only the recent developments allowing earlier testing for a longer list of conditions but, perhaps more importantly, the changing emphases in health care and especially the growing popularity of what is called "predictive medicine." Predictive medicine involves the search for genetic or other markers that identify individuals who will develop some disorder in the future. It may also involve the search for markers that identify those who are only predisposed to develop some disability; those who will develop the condition only if the circumstances (for example, some environmental or occupational exposure) are "right." Both kinds of markers—for diseases *and* for predisposition—can now be diagnosed in the fetus. This means we must be concerned not only about objectives of prenatal diagnosis that reflect obviously malign eugenic policies, but also about those that may originate in more insidious, but no less dangerous, programs to identify, while still in utero, children who are "susceptible," so that they may postnatally experience "preventive" measures aimed at minimizing the harmful effects of their genetic characteristics.

For example, depending on the condition, testing is now or will probably soon be available to identify those who, after birth, may be at greater than average risk for the development of a disorder of adult onset, a disorder such as diabetes, heart disease, cancer or mental illness; a disorder likely triggered by some gene-environment combination. Once again, the early identification of those thought to be genetically susceptible is not just to gather this knowledge for its own sake. Rather, it can be a basis for suggesting to these individuals behaviours and lifestyles that are believed to decrease their probability of future disability. As such, it sounds fairly benign and, properly used, employing interventions of known effectiveness, it may be. But the predictive information could also be used as a basis for *prescribing* a path for each individual to follow (what jobs to avoid or favour and what habits to avoid) to prevent future disability, with, for example, penalties for non-observance of the guidelines, discrimination in hiring or refusals of insurance for those with known susceptibilities.

Knowledge of an individual's susceptibilities prenatally could result either in establishing the "best" program to decrease future risks after birth, or in deciding to abort the "susceptibles" because of the added burden this special programming could entail. Unfortunately, we and our children are *all* susceptible to something. Consequently, all fetuses are potential candidates for screening for predictive purposes, and we must not be seduced by this seemingly rational approach to dealing with health problems before closely questioning its assumptions. As currently practised, predictive medicine emphasizes primarily how the individual must act to reduce her probability of later disability. Do we accept this approach, or shall we favour the alternative and look at how the environment can be changed to accommodate the most susceptible among us? The latter appears politically disfavoured today, but it *is* a choice.

Another worrisome aspect of uncritically expanding prenatal diagnosis in the guise of predictive medicine is that the mass screening programs being established to test pregnant women will call into question many more pregnancies than will actually later be diagnosed as affected.[5] These are the initial "false positives"—fetuses who are at first thought to be affected but are later shown by confirmatory diagnostic tests to be unaffected. We have no solid data on the effects of early knowledge of fetal status on the individual subsequently born or on her family, but it is not unreasonable to be concerned about them.[6] What does it mean to a woman to have her fetus' health called into question, however temporarily, early in pregnancy? Can the anxiety this may create have an effect either physiologically, on the pregnancy itself, or socially, on parent-infant relations? What does it mean to the child born subsequently to have had her health questioned? To know she might not have been born had she not met certain standards?[7] Are we at risk of creating an entire generation of "vulnerable children" among those who were "false positives" on an initial battery of screening tests?[8] Or among those who are selected to be born? Even if a false positive diagnosis per se only rarely causes a problem, the number of false positives in most screening programs is likely to be sufficiently large to make this an important concern. Certainly, any policies implemented in the context of predictive medicine using the new genetic technologies must take this factor into consideration. A separate question is how often women will take action,

usually by choosing abortion, following the provisional results of screening tests without waiting for diagnostic confirmation.

To date, reproductive technologies used for prenatal diagnosis have been developed as a "professional resource." Professionals alone have set the context for their use by assuming the power to decide when and by whom they will be used.[9] As well, professionals have defined those situations in which they will permit "consumer" input and, in particular, have specified those procedures which members of the public can request or reject.

The breadth of these definitions has then determined how much opportunity there is for individual autonomy.[10] For example, amniocentesis for fetal diagnosis, supposedly a means for enhancing women's reproductive choices, is not available to all women, though this would appear to be a logical albeit debatable consequence of an autonomy argument.[11] It is allowed to women over thirty-five years of age, who can choose whether to be tested in most jurisdictions, but it is not allowed to women under thirty-five who may also want testing. Similarly, amniocentesis is allowed to be chosen by women wishing to diagnose trisomy 21 (Down's syndrome), but it is not made available in Canada (or the United States) to those wanting to learn fetal sex in the absence of a specific medical need for this information. By contrast, ultrasound screening, most often overlooked as an approach to prenatal diagnosis, is frequently carried out with *no* input from women, some of whom might reject this testing if they had a choice.

So far, professionals alone have established the criteria for access to all these techniques and it is appropriate to question not merely the criteria but the entire process of decision-making. Who should establish objectives and criteria for prenatal diagnosis, through what processes, and how do we want policies made in this domain? Again, none of this has ever truly been the subject of public discussion that it should be.[12] Even if the techniques used for prenatal diagnosis are "professional resources"[13] insofar as licence to use them is concerned and even though, to date, professionals alone have decided on their use, these decisions about their actual application are rarely, if ever, strictly medical. For example, the almost universal choice of thirty-five years as *the* minimum age requirement for entry to prenatal diagnosis has no clear biological or other medical justification; it is, in fact, a strictly arbitrary threshold probably chosen for economic reasons.[14]

Recent non-medical developments which physicians have labelled as threats to their professional control[15] highlight other social-policy factors that influence the application of prenatal diagnostic techniques. Unfortunately, these developments—cost containment requirements, profit motive, government regulation, fear of medical malpractice suits[16]—are unsuitable bases on which to establish criteria for testing. Paradoxically, they may further exclude women from the process of decision-making on both individual and policy levels, and tighten rather than relax medical constraints on them. The opportunities for decision-making by pregnant women may be threatened even more than those of their physicians—as has already occurred with respect to decision-making in other areas of genetic medicine.

Thus, in the field of genetic screening, the progression from viewing a test as voluntary to viewing it as mandatory has tended to be fairly rapid. This transition is most evident with respect to newborn screening: professionals viewed its benefits as so far outweighing its costs as to require that all infants be tested for selected disorders, even when the efficacy of some interventions was unproven. In this situation, overt professional paternalism replaced individual autonomy with few exceptions.[17]

More subtle transitions have occurred as a procedure gains wide use. In these situations—and amniocentesis for women thirty-five years and over is again an example—the use of the procedure itself establishes a standard of care to which other professionals believe they must adhere to avoid litigation. In turn, this very availability is interpreted by the lay public as meaning that the test is routine and sanctioned and "must" be done.

This leads to further restraint on the contribution of pregnant women to decision-making about prenatal diagnostic techniques, a restraint reinforced by the trend towards "defensive medicine"—the tendency of physicians to make clinical decisions based as much on the possibility of a future lawsuit should

something go wrong as on the chance that the test results will lead to some effective intervention.[18] Here, two factors are especially relevant in the context of prenatal diagnosis. First, since most parents in our society wish—and may even be led to expect—that their babies will always be healthy, the birth of an infant with a disability leads to a search for and explanation and, perhaps, for someone—self or other—to blame for what has apparently "gone wrong." Physicians are aware of this and, in their desire to insure that they are blameless, may routinely suggest prenatal testing to all patients. A. R. Feinstein suggests that this strategy of choosing the option "whose wrong result will cause the least chagrin" is commonly applied in clinical decision-making, and it would certainly appear to apply here.[19] Second, the very availability of a prenatal test may pressure physicians to offer it to insure that their practice conforms with local standards of care for legal purposes.

Given this context, the use of prenatal diagnosis may come less and less to reflect either physicians' efforts to reduce the birth prevalence of some disorders or women's control over the quality of the children they bear, both previous (though arguable) justifications of prenatal diagnosis.[20] Instead, the techniques may be integrated into obstetric practice by physicians who merely want to comply with perceived medical-legal standards of care. One effect of this will be to trivialize the implications of these new techniques and this is, I suggest, the situation now with the extensive—and still growing—use of ultrasound. The latter is *not* recommended for routine use since its efficacy has not been demonstrated,[21] but it is nonetheless so used, probably as a component of a defensive, if not "aggressive," medical approach. This attitude may also explain how ultrasound has become the first method of prenatal diagnosis for which informed consent is not obtained. Physicians alone determine when and by whom it will be used.

So it would not be surprising if public discussion and open processes of policy evaluation for other prenatal technologies continued to be precluded by the quick and universal application of newly-developing diagnostic approaches by physicians wishing either to "keep up" with colleagues or to avoid any possibility of a law suit, should a patient who was not tested subsequently give birth to a child with some disability that a test might have identified. In fact, professional association advisories and state regulations requiring physicians to inform all pregnant women of maternal serum alpha-fetoprotein screening tests seem to have been enacted in the United States just to protect physicians, rather than out of concern for the pregnant woman.[22] A similar trend in Canada is not unlikely. And, given the growing frequency in both countries of court-ordered obstetric interventions often requested to protect health professionals, one must ask if mandatory prenatal diagnosis and other attempts to regulate women's behaviour during pregnancy are really unlikely.

Furthermore, while professionals may still insist that prenatal diagnosis is voluntary, and though *they* may be able to distinguish between "routinely" making prenatal diagnosis available for patients to accept or reject and "routinely" testing everyone,[23] this distinction may be too subtle for most of us to recognize.[24] How often do patients really feel they can themselves decide about having a test the physician recommends? How many women can reject tests "recommended" by their physicians, especially if the advice is couched in terms suggesting the tests are "for the baby's good."[25] There may be alternatives, but is there truly a choice for the woman whose physician "recommends"—or even mentions—prenatal diagnosis? For many women, the answer is clear. Already, when asked why they decided to have amniocentesis, they respond: "I didn't have a choice." Unfortunately, they often don't.

Given that prenatal diagnostic techniques will continue to be developed—and not just for serious disabling conditions—and that at least some women will continue to request them, we need to change the process of decision-making about the individual and collective use of this technology if fetal testing is to "work" to serve the needs of women and to provide them with real choices, not hypothetical alternatives. To start, prenatal diagnosis needs to be seen *not* apart from, but as a component of, a social policy that guarantees comprehensive care for all pregnant women and all children. This should include a guarantee of adequate care for those born with a disability and for their families. This means limiting, if not severing, the connection between prenatal diagnosis and genet-

ic medicine, and viewing these interventions as part of an array of potential health services for women.

In this context, the basis for, and effects of, prenatal diagnosis could be compared with those of other "preventive" programs to assess their relative impacts on the health and wellbeing of children and parents. Such an exercise would help de-mystify prenatal diagnosis. And, by making us directly confront its role versus, for example, the role of nutritional supplementation, parent education or anti-smoking interventions in the improvement of reproductive health, it would require us to explicitly consider its objectives. Perhaps if prenatal diagnosis were seen in this broader, more appropriate context as a possible addition to, rather than as a substitute for, caring, relevant and effective preventive and health promotion services, its objectives and its social and policy implications could be clarified and ways found for it to truly begin to simultaneously expand women's choices and women's control.

Notes

1. A. Oakley, *Becoming a Mother* (New York, Schocken Books, 1979), p. 16.

2. Among the several possible explanations of this, two seem most relevant. 1) Prenatal diagnosis carries some risk to the fetus. Thus, physicians may have been unwilling to jeopardize a clinically normal pregnancy in the absence of what was, to them, a compelling reason to do so, such as a serious fetal abnormality. 2) Abortion has historically (if myopically) been isolated as *the* ethical or sociopolitical question of paramount importance with regard to prenatal diagnosis, perhaps because the prenatal diagnosis technology available has meant that any resultant pregnancy terminations would have to be carried out in the second trimester. Health professionals, the gatekeepers for prenatal diagnosis, may have considered only "serious" disabilities to be compelling justifications for the procedure this late in pregnancy. In addition, the fact that only "serious" fetal abnormalities are legally accepted grounds for abortion in many countries, though not in Canada, may also explain why seriousness or severity become grounds for access to testing.

3. There has never really been a broad-based attempt to define the objectives of prenatal diagnosis. This has not impeded the establishment and proliferation of guidelines or criteria for access to testing, however.

4. B.K. Rothman, *The Tentative Pregnancy: Prenatal Diagnosis and the Future of Motherhood* (New York, Viking Press, 1986).

5. This is because these screening tests, for technical reasons, can almost never be a hundred percent accurate in detecting either the affected or the unaffected pregnancies; there is usually some overlap in the test results for these two groups.

6. A preliminary study of parents of infants screened in the newborn period failed to reveal increased anxiety or depression in those awaiting confirmatory tests after an initial abnormal test (J.R. Sorenson, H.L. Levy, T.W. Mangione and S.J. Sepe, "Parental Response to Repeat Testing of Infant with 'False Positive' Results in a Newborn Screening Program," *Pediatrics*, vol. 73 (1984), pp. 183-187), but the generalizability of these results to the prenatal period is unknown.

7. J. Fletcher, "The Brink: The Parent-Child Bond in the Genetic Revolution," *Theological Studies*, vol. 33 (1972), pp. 457-485.

8. J.C. Levy, "Vulnerable Children: Parents' Perspectives and the Use of Medical Care," *Pediatrics*, vol 65. (1980), pp. 956-963.

9. A. Oakley, "The History of Ultrasonography in Obstetrics," *Birth*, vol. 13 (1986), pp. 8-13.

10. D. Dickson, "Public Interest Criteria for Technology," *Gene Watch*, vol. 4, no. 3 (May/June 1987), pp. 1-2; 14-15.

11. A. Lippman, "Access to Prenatal Screening Services: Who Decides?" *Canadian Journal of Women and the Law*, vol 1 (1986), pp. 434-445.

12. President's Commission for the Study of Ethical Problems in Medicine, *Screening and Counselling for Genetic Conditions* (Washington, US Government Printing Office, 1983).

13. Oakley, op. cit.

14. Lippman, op. cit.

15. S. Elias and G.J. Annas, "Routine Prenatal Genetic Screening," *New England Journal of Medicine,* vol. 317 (1987), pp. 1407-1409

16. Ibid.

17. It is possible, though arguable, that screening programs carried out in high schools in Quebec or through health maintenance organizations in the United States reflect a similar paternalism via professional control.

18. This is "defensive" medicine on the individual level. It is probably not stretching the term too far to suggest that defensive medicine on the societal level is reflected in the growing reliance on cost-benefit arguments to support medical interventions. Here, early screening "defends" the public purse against future medical costs of care of the disabled.

19. A.R. Feinstein, "The Chagrin Factor and Qualitative Decision Analysis," *Archives of Internal Medicine,* vol. 145. (1985), pp. 1257-1259.

20. Lippman, op. cit.

21. Consensus Conference, "The Use of Diagnostic Ultrasound Imaging During Pregnancy," *Journal of the American Medical Association*, vol 252 (1984), pp. 669-672.

22. S. Elias and G. J. Annas, "Maternal serum AFP: Educating physicians and the public,"*American Journal of Public Health*, vol. 75 (1985), pp. 1374-1375.

23. Elias and Annas, op.cit.

24. M.H. Shearer, "Does This Work? We Don't Know, But It Pays," *Birth*, vol. 14 (June 1987), pp. 73-74.

25. Ibid.

28.
LOVING FUTURE PEOPLE

Laura M. Purdy

Moral philosophers often wonder what a better world would look like.[1] It seems clear that eradicating war and poverty and building ecologically sustainable economies, among other things, would improve life immensely for many people. Only achieving such goals will enable us to provide the clean water, nutritious food, safe shelter, education, and medical care essential for human welfare; by themselves, these goods would go far toward helping people fashion satisfying lives. We will not have a morally bearable world until everybody enjoys them.

In the United States and elsewhere, individuals in increasing numbers lack these basic prerequisites for a decent life, and our first priority should be to create a floor of well-being with respect to them below which no one would be allowed to fall.

Prominent among requisite policies would be promoting justice for women. Most, if not all societies, define women in such a way that it seems right to subordinate us to men; the resultant inequality of burdens and benefits is still being documented. A just society would get rid of this inequality. To recommend such a state of affairs is not to embrace a libertarian moral theory, but rather to assert the importance of women's equal autonomy within a more caring and egalitarian society.

Although many details of this just society remain to be worked out, feminists are sketching out its main lines. They include truly equal education that equips us to take up whatever work suits our talents and interests, sufficient compensation for all occupations to enable us to live independently of men if we wish, and the right to determine whether and when we will have children. They assume social support for those decisions, including the resources necessary for bearing and rearing healthy children. The gap between the conditions in which most women now live and this feminist utopia is huge. At present, many women lack the equal educational and work opportunities that would help guarantee decent living conditions—including a safe environment and appropriate medical care—for themselves and their children. Justice requires getting closer to this ideal.

Having reached this conclusion, the main work of the moral philosopher qua philosopher is done: moral or political exhortation is not part of the job description.[2] However, there remain a few problems to mop up. Among them is the question of possible moral limits on women's reproductive rights.[3]

THE RIGHT TO REPRODUCE

Although there is no explicit constitutional right to procreate, it is generally assumed that such a right is implied by other fundamental constitutional rights. It is also assumed that it is, in any case, morally justifiable to assert such a right, and that this right should be protected by law. Certainly, the assumption that individuals have a right to control their own bodies is deeply embedded in the Anglo-American intellectual tradition, and that right, because of reproductive biology, might reasonably be taken to imply for women, if not for men, a moral right to reproduce that should be protected by law. At present there are significant legal limits on women's reproductive rights, and, given the contemporary political climate, more are likely to be forthcoming. I believe that such legal limitations are unjustifiable.[4] It does not follow, though, that there are no *moral* limits on reproduction.

The right to reproduce is one of those moral rights that has been more assumed than argued for; it could, no doubt, be traced back to earlier days when human existence was more threatened by underpopulation than overpopulation.[5] The whole network of expectations and assumptions about reproduction is usually taken for granted and viewed as obvious, natural, and legitimate. However, cultural changes and technological developments have begun to inspire more serious scrutiny of these issues, even if a good deal of it still seems to me to be tied to fairly parochial "popular wisdom."[6]

The most plausible case for recognizing a moral right to reproduce comes, it seems to me, from a utilitarian moral theory coupled with the desire for children.[7] As I have suggested elsewhere, it is good, other things being equal, for desires to be satisfied.[8] Unfortunately, the potential for harm via reproduction means that very often things are not equal. Seeking to satisfy the urge to reproduce may increase the suffering created by overpopulation, contribute to the failure to meet the needs of existing children, channel women into rigid and narrow social roles, promote technologies that harm women, and bring to existence children who are more likely than average to lead miserable lives.[9]

If we are consistent in our concern about human happiness, it seems clear that we must attend to the welfare of future people. For the most part, it is possible to envision social policies that will further the good of both existing persons and the interests of future ones[10]; but here, sharp conflicts may emerge between the desires of the former and the interests of the latter. Most people want children, and they want their own children—that is, children who carry their own genetic material.

Some 15 years ago, I began wondering whether it is ever wrong to have children and wrote a paper arguing that if you are at risk for a serious illness like Huntington's disease, a good case can be made against your procreating; that paper still provokes animated—and highly emotional—discussion. And, despite the proliferation of fascinating new questions in biomedical ethics, this core issue still haunts us, returning again and again in different guises; its most recent incarnations involve "fetal abuse," neonatal AIDS, and genetic therapy.[11]

I originally claimed that although there is good reason to reject legal interference in individual decisions about reproduction, we need much more open discussion of the ethical dimensions of such decisions, for exercising your legal rights can sometimes be morally wrong. Since we ought to try to provide every child with at least a normal opportunity for a good life, and since we do not harm possible people if we prevent them from existing, we ought to try to prevent the birth of those with a significant risk of living worse than normal lives. I then went on to argue that Huntington's disease presents such a risk.[12]

My argument has been attacked on various grounds connected with the particularities of Huntington's disease.[13] A second objection could be based on women's privacy rights: women have only just been achieving some measure of control over our bodies, and this control is by no means either secure or universal; we should therefore encourage society to keep its nose out of these matters, even to the point of withholding moral evaluation of the reproductive decisions women make. While this concern is extremely important, we should nonetheless be wary of asserting the necessity for such an extreme suspension of judgment where there is potential for serious harm to others.[14]

Two other objections have emerged against the position that procreation is sometimes irresponsible. One comes from philosophers who hold that it is morally permissible to create children unless there is reason to think that they would prefer death to the life they live. The other comes from disability rights activists who hold that it is, among other things, bias against disabled people, not well-grounded moral argument, which motivates such recommendations. I shall be concentrating here on the second case, except where the two intersect.[15]

ARGUMENTS FROM DISABILITY

Marsha Saxton and Adrienne Asch argue against abortion for disability.[16] Both also distinguish between abortion for disability and the attempt to avoid conception on those grounds. Asch writes:

> Although I have serious moral qualms about selective abortion for sex or disability, I do not have moral objections—albeit social and psychological ones—to deciding not to conceive if one knows that one's offspring will be of one sex or will have a certain disability. I consider women who refrain from childbearing and rearing for these reasons to be misguided, possibly depriving themselves of the joys of parenthood by their unthinking acceptance of the values of a society still deeply sexist and ambivalent about people with disabilities (p. 321).

Neither Asch nor Saxton reject abortion in general, but they clearly think that aborting an existing fetus is morally worse than failing to conceive one.[17] Yet is seems to me that their arguments, if sound, are as telling against failing to conceive as against aborting. For this reason, and because more general questions about abortion would quickly obscure the specific question I want to consider here, my argument will focus simply on the question of what we want for future people.[18]

One of the clearest and most powerful messages to come from both Asch and Saxton is that much suffering of disabled persons arises not from their disabilities but from the social response to their disabilities. The United States is, in many ways, an uncaring society, which, despite its relative wealth, tolerates a great deal of preventable misery on the part of those who must depend more than normal on community resources. Support is often both miserly and, because of the influence of special interests and erroneous preconceptions about the needs of individuals with disabilities, not offered in the form that would be most useful to them.[19]

Asch and Saxton are certainly right here: it is clear that the plight of disabled persons would be much improved if each had all the help possible. And, such help should be available: we waste billions on the military and other boondoggles, whereas a fraction of that amount would enable us to create a society that would meet people's needs far better.

Quite apart from our evaluation of disabilities themselves, however, this nasty state of affairs raises the question of the extent to which we ought to take into account socially imposed obstacles to satisfying lives when we try to judge whether it is morally right to bring a particular child into the world. As a dyed-in-the-wool consequentialist, I cannot ignore the probable difficulties that await children with special problems. It seems to me that only the truly rich can secure the well-being of those with the most serious problems. Given the costs and other difficulties of guaranteeing good care, even very well-to-do individuals might well wonder whether their offspring will get the care they need after their own deaths. This question is still more acute for those who aren't so well off—the vast majority of the U. S. population. Furthermore, it would be unwise to forget that many women are at risk for divorce and its financial aftermath.[20] Although the solution is obvious—more

social responsibility for individual needs—it's beginning to look as though none of us will see that come about in our lifetimes. It seems to me that this consideration should be, in the case of some decisions about future children, decisive.

Other facets of the inadequacy of the social response to disabled people involve common habits, attitudes, and values. Ignorance leads even basically nice people to behave in hurtful ways; less good-hearted ones may be thoughtless or cruelly unsympathetic. In addition, apparently innocent values we hold make life difficult. "[W]e, especially in the United States, live in a culture obsessed with health and well-being. We value rugged self-reliance, athletic prowess, and rigid standards of beauty. We incessantly pursue eternal youth," writes Saxton (p. 303). Certainly, excessive admiration for independence, along with athleticism and narrow conceptions of beauty, make life more painful than it need be for many; they are especially problematic for some disabled people. They constrict the range of prized achievement and characteristics in unjustifiable and harmful ways, and could often be traced, I suspect, to unexamined gender-, race-, or class-based prejudice. It would therefore be desirable to see much of the energy now directed toward promoting these values channeled instead toward others, such as intellectual or artistic achievement, creating warm and supportive emotional networks, and opening our eyes to the beauty of a wide variety of body types. Unfortunately, our culture doesn't seem to be moving in that direction. It's all very well to believe that such social values shouldn't count, but that doesn't do much to lessen their impact on our children.[21]

Furthermore, there are serious objections to lumping health and well-being together with these other suspect values. Good health and the feeling of well-being it helps engender are significant factors in a happy life. They enable people to engage in a wide variety of satisfying activities, and to feel good while they are doing them. When they are absent, our suffering is caused not by our consciousness of having failed to live up to some artificial social value but by the intrinsic pain or limitation caused by that absence.

Denigrating these values is doubly mistaken. First, denying the worth of goals that can be achieved only partially (if at all) by some people would seem to require us to exclude from the arena of desirable traits many otherwise plausible candidates.[22] Perhaps more importantly, it also denies the value of less-than-maximal achievement of such values, and hence undermines the primary argument in favor of allocating social resources to help people cope with special problems. If health and well-being aren't valuable, what moral case is there for eradicating the social obstacles Asch and Saxton complain of so bitterly? Surely it is just their importance that obligates us to provide the opportunity to help people reach the highest levels of which they are capable. If health and well-being are of no special value, what is wrong with letting people languish in pain, or sit in the street with a tin cup when a prosthetic leg or seeing-eye dog could make them independent?

Secondly, it is important to resist the temptation to identify with our every characteristic. Members of oppressed groups quite rightly want to change society's perception of the features that oppressors latch onto as the mark of their alleged inferiority.[23] Such is the source of such slogans as "Black is beautiful!", of the emphasis on gay pride, and of the valorizing of women's nurturing capacity. However fitting this approach may be in some cases, its appropriateness for every characteristic does not follow. Moral failings are one obvious example.

More generally, we need to think through more carefully any leap from qualities to persons. First, qualities must be evaluated on independent grounds, not on the basis of their connection with us. Then, it is important to keep in mind that to value some characteristic isn't necessarily to look with contempt upon those who lack it. Such an equation would suggest, among other things, that teachers always (ought to) have contempt for their pupils. And, on the one hand, we may admire diametrically opposed characteristics that could not, by their very nature, be found in a single individual. Consider your widely read couch potato friend: do you really have contempt for her because she isn't Mikhail Baryshnikov? Or the converse? On the other, our assessment of and liking for individuals is not determined in any obvious way by whether they exemplify our favorite traits. Don't we all know people who, given their characteristics, ought to be our dearest friends—yet we just don't

click? And don't we all have friends who don't meet our "standards" at all?

None of this is to deny that it might be appropriate in some contexts for disability rights activists to downplay the effects of certain impairments. It might be helpful, for example, to forcefully remind able-bodied individuals that people with physical problems are people first and foremost. That would help reinforce the point that, like other citizens with special difficulties, their needs should be secured as unobtrusively and respectfully as possible, and that they ought not to be viewed as mere objects of pity.

THE DEMANDS OF LOVE

Perhaps the worry here is that since some disabled people cannot become healthy or fully able no matter what we do, society will—in a fit of pique—declare that it is not worth doing anything at all. But that would be true only if the help were motivated by a quasi-aesthetic perfectionism.

Doubts and questions about the motivation of those who argue for preventing certain births lurk continuously in the wings here. There are indeed those who seek "perfection" in others. Their desire for it, their narrow and rigid standards, and their utter lack of human empathy with those who fail to "measure up" justifies wariness: it would be inexcusable to ignore the lessons of history or to allow ourselves to be taken in by those who seek to camouflage their bigotry with lofty rationalizations. However, it would be equally inexcusable to dismiss the possibility that a caring and coherent position can lead, by an altogether different route, to the same conclusion that it is wrong to knowingly bring some children into the world.[24]

When I look into my heart to see what it says about this matter I see, I admit, emotions I would rather not feel—reluctance to face the burdens society must bear, unease in the presence of some disabled persons. But most of all, what I see there are the demands of love: to love someone is to care desperately about their welfare and to want for them only good things. The thought that I might bring to life a child with serious physical or mental problems when I could, by doing something different, bring forth one without them, is utterly incomprehensible to me. Isn't that what love means?

Appeals to love in ethics generally are unhelpful. The exhortation to love or care for another doesn't usually tell you what to do: for example, it may be that the best way to help an alcoholic mate is to leave the relationship, even if that causes a lot of suffering. Nor does an appeal to love tell us how to resolve conflicts of interest: it suggests that even legitimate interests of our own must always be subordinated to those of others. Until everybody takes that approach, this leads to rather lopsided relationships.

Where the appeal to love and care does have enormous power, however, is in the quite common conflict between our own desires and the welfare of others, where those desires either fail to constitute a legitimate interest, or where the disparity between the two is clear. Thus, if your life could be saved by someone's pulling a hair from my head, love would dictate allowing the pulling, despite my legitimate interest in protecting my body from attack.

So to say that love is relevant here is to say that there is sometimes a disparity between a future person's interest in a healthy body and the interest in procreation. Defending that viewpoint requires showing that the moral right to reproduce is relatively weak and that the moral right to a healthy body is relatively strong.[25] Given the potential for harm to another that reproduction involves, it seems to me that the presumed right to reproduce one's genetically related offspring is indeed the weakest element in the right to control your body. Although this claim clearly needs more argument, I will concentrate here on the argument for healthy bodies—the claim that people are better off without disease or special limitation, and that this interest is sufficiently compelling in some cases to justify the judgment that reproducing would be wrong.

Disagreement about my claim could be about ends or means. That is, it could be about the value of health pure and simple, or it could be about its value in comparison to the means necessary to procure it. Surely, it is hard to disagree about the former: if you could ensure good health for everyone at no cost, say by pushing an easily accessible button, then failing to push it would be indefensible. But that doesn't, of course, determine the lengths to which we should be prepared to go if ensuring or trying to ensure good health takes more than that. It seems that Asch and

Saxton are in the odd position of holding that it is generally questionable to try to avoid health problems by altering reproductive behavior, but that we should go to great lengths to repair or compensate for health problems once children with them are born.[26]

This position appropriately emphasizes how much suffering from disability and disease is unnecessary, arising as it does from our failure as individuals and as a society to take away their sting. Clearly, greater social responsibility would cause some health problems simply to dissolve, just as early surgery can repair a heart valve leaving no trace of disease, or wheelchair ramps can open up new worlds; others, like diabetes, once life-threatening, could become relatively minor irritations. Frustration at the blindness, inertia, and selfishness that now stand between those with certain disabilities and a satisfying life is understandable and activism to remove barriers and get needed support is justifiable and urgent.

However, it seems to me that some of the arguments intended to further that goal can be, as I suggested earlier, inadequate and counterproductive. Downplaying in every context the suffering that can be caused by disability itself as Saxton and Asch do, is, I think, an example. Thus Saxton, at one point, seems to claim that *all* suffering is social: "the 'suffering' we may experience is a result of not enough human caring, acceptance, and respect" (page. 308).

SUFFERING

I do not doubt that a great deal of the suffering caused by disease and disability does arise from that source. Perhaps all the suffering felt by some people is of this sort—people with minimal or cosmetic problems, or those who have been able to tailor their desires to their circumstances. But in other cases, even were every conceivable aid available, the disease or disability itself would remain and be itself the cause of limit or pain. Neither immense human caring nor the most sophisticated gadgetry will restore freedom of movement to the paraplegic, for example. And it is not only such major disability that can cause misery: I have both observed and felt it in connections that might well be dismissed as minor by those who are not experiencing them. In my own case, for example, my inability to see adequately at a crucial period in my development as a dancer was in part responsible for the failure to progress enough to make a career worthwhile. Yet that was a goal toward which I had worked since I was a small child, and for which both I and my parents had made major sacrifices.[27] Although I was able to make another satisfying life for myself, not everybody who has this kind of experience is so lucky.

That the degree of suffering may not be directly correlated with the apparent severity of disability may be taken as a reason for giving up on the idea of avoiding the birth of children at risk for serious health problems. After all, discussion of this issue always focuses on the most severe diseases and disabilities, assumes that these are the ones that cause the most suffering, and usually ends with what is taken as the trump question: where do we draw the line? But my guess is that it is true that the most severe disabilities do often cause great suffering; it is just that more minor ones can also do so more often than most of us suppose, and not just because the environment is so harsh. That seems to me to be good reason for being concerned about both kinds rather than grounds for throwing up our hands.

Of course it is necessary to draw some lines, since everybody carries deleterious genes, and hardly any of us are free of at least minor inadequacies in health functioning. Common sense would suggest some preliminary guidelines, however. Being a carrier, for example, is no problem unless the relevant gene is dominant and carries with it the threat of serious problems, or is recessive but your mate also carries it. Likewise decisions about what constitutes a major threat will depend to a considerable extent on the environment a child can reasonably be expected to live in. Demanding certainty in these judgments would be irrational, but that does not mean that we should ignore the probabilities. Different people obviously have different intuitions about such matters, but that does not mean that we should give up on attempting to achieve some consensus through discussion and debate.

Concern about the broader context of reproduction raises important questions here about the morality of creating children who will face other kinds of hardships. What, for instance, of those who by their very existence as females, or African Americans, can be expected to live especially difficult lives? It would be tempting to say that there is nothing intrinsically undesirable about such characteristics: whatever special difficulties such persons face are purely a social matter, and hence that my thesis about refraining from reproduction would not hold here. Unfortunately, however, that answer will not do. For my argument ultimately depends more upon the degree and inevitability of the suffering than its source. So, where we can be certain about these things, there is at least a prima facie case against reproduction in these cases, too.[28] If we want to reproduce in a situation of this sort, we need to ask ourselves whether we truly have the welfare of our possible offspring at heart, or are we merely gratifying a desire of our own. Dealing with situations of this kind in the detail they deserve is impossible here, but it does seem reasonable to point out one consequence of the purely social nature of the problem, namely that we might in general be both less certain of the drawbacks and that there is more possibility of unexpected social progress.

Before going any further here, it is important to note two points. First, discussion about what we owe others tends to stick with the minimum; second, what might be an appropriate moral framework for thinking about the present might not be adequate for thinking about the future.

Thinking in terms of the moral minimum seems both to keep us on the firmest moral ground and is consistent with the moral atmosphere we are most used to. It also closely resembles the legal definitions and principles that parallel our moral thinking, structures intended to facilitate legal decision-making. Such legal premises are in part, too, a legacy of the narrow classical liberalism that still colors our perceptions of what a good society should look like. Thus we tend quite naturally here to fall into talking in terms of "minimally bearable lives," rather than satisfying or even downright happy ones. And, while we may feel quite sure that it is wrong to bring into existence those whose lives will be truly miserable, there is a great deal more uneasiness about the judgment that we ought on moral grounds to refrain from bringing to existence those who, despite much legitimate dissatisfaction, can be expected to prefer life to the alternative.

This intellectual groove is seriously problematic, I believe, even for the garden-variety moral decisions that face us every day; however, it clearly fails to guide us in an intelligent and compassionate way when decisions affecting future people are at stake. If individuals can harm each other only by worsening their condition, then by definition, we cannot harm future people if avoiding the harm also means that a particular person will not be brought to existence.[29] According to your moral perspective, it becomes either supererogatory—or morally suspect.[30] In either case it undermines not only the kind of reproductive concerns discussed here, but also denies any moral urgency to more general attempts to improve the quality of future people's lives.[31] But it's not clear why we should accept a moral approach with such consequences. In particular, a few moments' reflection on the benefits many of us enjoy as a result of the efforts of previous generations should reinforce my point.[32]

There are, of course, other obstacles to the project of protecting future people from serious physical problems. We as yet know very little about genetic traits. Furthermore, there may be insuperable moral objections to the kind of research necessary to find out more, or to the procedures necessary to utilize that knowledge.[33] Still worse, it might turn out that some genes are inextricably linked with others that it may be important to keep in the gene pool; others may confer, like a single copy of the gene for sickle cell anemia, a benefit. However, none of these problems entail that we should not, other things being equal, do what we can here to avoid creating people with serious health problems. I think that ordinary decency would therefore suggest that we at least make the effort to investigate our genetic history and, if necessary, attempt to avoid transmitting serious conditions.

Arguing against this position, Saxton denies that the fact that disabled individuals suffer and even commit suicide is a reason to prevent their births: after all, she argues, non-disabled people commit suicide too. That non-disabled people also commit suicide is irrelevant, however. A good society does what it can to prevent or alleviate suffering on the part of its members. That there are many and diverse causes of such suffering isn't a good reason to ignore any particular one. Her attitude toward some kinds of suffering seems oddly cavalier, almost as though it is good for us.

This question of morally appropriate challenges never seems far in the background here. Much of the writing about disability emphasizes the advantages of such challenge. For instance, Denise Karuth, in her moving and informative essay, "If I Were a Car, I Would Be a Lemon," writes that "the process of learning to live with a disability presents an opportunity to develop competencies in judgment, problem solving, and compassion that few of life's other experiences can equal" (p. 25). Perhaps. But as I read what it takes to manage her lot of blindness and MS—only some of which could be alleviated by maximal social support—I am skeptical about whether the lessons learned justify the suffering they require. Since wise and compassionate folk exist who have not had such difficulties, it would surely be good to reduce the number who do to a minimum; the experiences of those who suffer from health catastrophes after birth will surely suffice.[34]

There may well be compensations for some disabilities. In *Seeing Voices,* Oliver Sacks takes us on a "journey into the world of the deaf." American Sign Language, it turns out, is a powerful and elegant means of communication, one that might in the future help communication not only with deaf persons, but with chimps, babies and those who speak languages other than our own. The world would clearly be a poorer place without ASL; now that it is here, it can enrich the lives of both those who are hearing-impaired and those who are not. It seems nonetheless doubtful that many deaf persons would refuse new ears.[35]

A somewhat different, but related, cluster of worries about preventing the birth of disabled individuals centers on issues of control. Asch (1989) asks what will happen when women who abort fetuses with problems they do not think they can cope with, have other children who "develop characteristics [they] dislike or find overwhelming" (p. 320). She goes on to suggest that such women may not recognize or may refuse to accept that childbearing should be undertaken only if "we are willing to face what we cannot control and to seek resources in themselves and the world to master it" (p. 320). Now it may very well be that some women who knowingly choose to avoid bringing a child with a disability into the world have an unrealistic view of childrearing, as do, no doubt, many who go ahead. But the solution in both these cases is early and universal education to pierce the rosy haze pronatalism still wraps around babies and having babies.[36] There is no reason to slight or belittle the judgment of those who attempt to avoid foreseeable problems, nor to prejudge their ability to cope with unexpected ones.

It would be all too easy here to fall in line with the backlash's rejection of women's barely won right to control our bodies and lives. It is only lately that women have begun to be able to exert such control, and we should be wary of suggestions that there is something wrong with it—especially since it is still mostly women who are expected to sacrifice their other plans to care for others, and this without much support.[37] In any case, it is one thing to have to cope with difficulties that couldn't have been avoided; it is quite another when they could have been.[38] Given that difference, it in no way follows (or is even empirically likely) that by attempting to prevent the birth of children with disabilities we encourage the kind of self-indulgence that refuses to come to terms with the demands of life.

Despite the importance of questions about the social costs of certain decisions about reproduction, the main focus here still needs to be on what happens to children, not the attitudes of others. Thus I am deeply troubled by Saxton's comment that she would "like to welcome any child born to me. I believe that I have the emotional, financial, and other resources to effectively care for a child. I know I can be a good mother and my husband a good father to any child" (p. 310). Would that her warmth and generosity were more common! But although these traits would help children deal with their problems, wouldn't it be better to try to avoid the serious and foreseeable burdens in the first place?

EXISTING AND POSSIBLE PERSONS

As I write these last paragraphs, I can hear in my mind's ear the angry reaction build: she wants to kill us off—she's talking about getting rid of persons who have a right to life just to get rid of their problems. That would be true if what were at issue was killing those with serious health problems; that would of course also be a ludicrous misunderstanding of my position, comparable to the reception of Peter Singer's views in Austria.[39]

One of the most common themes in writing on this topic is the distressing possibility that if we attempt to avoid the birth of children with disease or disability, we will harm those who already exist. At the most practical level, some believe that acting so as to avoid such births will lead us to reduce the social resources now allocated to the disabled. At a more theoretical level, the judgment that life is better without such problems is taken as an insult to those now facing them.[40]

The first worry would be legitimate if the only reason for attempting to prevent such births is the kind of aesthetic preference for perfection to which I objected earlier, an outlook that does indeed fail to see any morally significant difference between existing and possible persons. But I mean to make, maintain, and rely on this difference.

It *is* unreasonable, in a world of limited resources and great need, to be required to allocate resources for those who didn't have to need them. The obvious rejoinder is to point to the waste and corruption now apparent in the distribution of resources. Unfortunately, that does not make those resources available for human welfare. Even were such waste eradicated, it is quite likely that, given the overall world situation, every spare dime would be needed to avert the suffering of already existing persons. Isn't it immoral to knowingly act so as to increase the demands on these resources, resources that could otherwise be used for projects such as feeding the starving or averting environmental disaster? Isn't attempting to avoid the birth of those who are likely to require extra resources, other things being equal, on a par with other attempts to share resources more equally? But from none of this does it follow that we should reduce the concern for those who already exist: on the contrary, it is in part *their* welfare that dictates such careful use of resources. This is not to say, as I suggested earlier, that any and all measures should be used to achieve the goal I am recommending, for some may themselves be wasteful of resources or have other morally dubious consequences. Whereas it may be wrong to refuse to undergo relatively noninvasive testing when there is evidence that you are at risk of passing some serious problem on to your child,[41] it does not follow that you ought to be taking every conceivable step to avoid that outcome. Nor am I recommending anything like legally sanctioned invasions of women's bodies for prenatal testing or therapy.[42]

Asch (1989) warns of more subtle harm to the living from attempts to avoid the birth of disabled children. She asks whether "we want to send the message to all such people now living that there should be 'no more of your kind' in the future (p. 319)." This interpretation draws its force from the possibility that what is being said is that although you are a perfectly nice person, because of your imperfections and neediness, you still aren't worth the trouble and we don't want to repeat you. And that would be a devastating thing to hear. If this interpretation were correct, it would also reflect very badly on the speaker: one would hardly know where to start in on such a crude, instrumental view of human life.[43]

But I would dispute Asch's view that by attempting to avoid the birth of individuals with serious impairments that we either intend or in fact send such a message to the living, wanting a world where fewer suffer implies doing what we can to alleviate the difficulties of those who now exist as well as doing what we can to relieve future people of them. This is an entirely different justification for the position in question, one that ought to be reassuring, not threatening. Too, it is surely important here once again to resist the identification of disability and the disabled. My disability is not me, no matter how much it may affect my choices.[44] With this point firmly in mind, it should be possible to mentally separate my existence from the existence of my disability. Thus, I could rejoice, for instance, at the goal of eradicating nearsightedness, without taking that aim as an attempt to eradicate *me*, or people like me— even if achieving it means avoiding the birth of certain children.[45] But it's not as if the world is to be cleansed of me or people relevantly like me: of, say, all future brown-eyed woman philosophers.

Contributing to the misunderstandings here is, I think, a fundamental uneasiness about our power to determine who shall be brought into being. Such uneasiness is, I think, an appropriate danger signal: it alerts us to the fact that we are embarking on a new and potentially harmful project. But we need to resist the urge to latch onto apparently plausible limits that may in fact be undesirable.[46]

I believe that such limits show up in the argument at the intersection of the philosopher's case against attempting to prevent the birth of unhealthy babies and the one advanced by disability rights activists. It is the claim that if potential individuals would judge their lives worth living, then bringing them to life is no injury, and thus that there are no grounds for asserting on their behalf that it is wrong to create them.[47]

Derek Parfit is one of the philosophers who has been considering this problem.[48] He supposes that a child will have some defect—say, a withered arm— if she is conceived now; in 3 months, her mother could instead conceive a sound child, since the teratogenic drug that would cause the problem will have passed out of her system. But waiting would mean that the child with a withered arm (let us call her Minnie) would not exist; the child who would be born 3 months later would be someone else. So the price of existence, for Minnie, is a withered arm. Consequently, unless she agrees that non-existence would be preferable to life with a bad arm, she is not wronged.

But this case rests in part on the assumption that a different egg and a different sperm necessarily produce a different person. And, of course, if we define ourselves as the product of a given egg and sperm, then it is indeed trivially true that different ones would not be us. We do know that some genetic rolls of the dice result in vastly different characteristics, but it seems quite likely that many would produce only tiny differences—grayish eyes instead of greenish, the ability to curl your tongue or not, a slightly bigger pancreas. On the other hand, however, nurture clearly plays a significant role in who we are. Not only does it affect our personality, it also affects the expression of physical traits.[49] So a given environment is quite likely to mold even somewhat genetically diverse children into similar patterns. Conversely, different environments help create different people out of those with similar genetic endowments. For example, a friend of mine was born to poor, uneducated Druse villagers, but adopted at birth by Scottish missionaries and is now a professor of literature. Is there any serious sense in which we could say she is the same person she would have been had she never left her original family? On a smaller scale, perhaps, we can be deeply changed by divorce, war, or accident. Thus the idea that the only significant determinant of who we are is the union of a particular egg and sperm seems rather unsatisfactory.

But even suppose that premise where true; does it necessarily have any significance, moral or otherwise? Consider Minnie, the child of the mother who didn't wait. She is quite happy with life, although she would prefer not to have a withered arm. Suppose we suggest to her that she could have been born whole only at the cost of being somebody else?

A rational Minnie would be aware of the odds against *any* of us having our particular genetic and environmental constitution. If mom had failed to ovulate in July, the August-conceived you might have had curly hair instead of straight. If there was a crisis at work and dad was too tired to make love on Friday night, the Saturday morning you might have a talent for running instead of race-walking.... In any case, the rational Minnie, although glad to be alive, would realize that if some other Minnie had been born instead, she herself wouldn't be looking enviously down from heaven saying "Drat, there, but for my mother's misplaced moral concern, would be me."[50]

Furthermore, let us imagine that Minnie's mother *had* waited, and that as a result, sound-bodied Minnie$_2$ was born instead of Minnie. Maybe Minnie$_2$ would have had other problems but let us suppose that all else is equal, so that the only difference between them is that the two Minnies are "different" people—that is, conceived of different eggs and sperm. Even assuming that they are quite different, if Minnie$_2$ had been born instead of Minnie, is there any reason for thinking that she would be any less attached to her particular self than the original Minnie? Is there any reason for her to regret not having been the bad-armed Minnie? In short, if Minnie$_2$ is brought to life, why should she be any less glad to be who she is than Minnie would have been had she existed? Furthermore, wouldn't she be delighted that her mother had been thoughtful and waited? Her delight at being alive is no less than Minnie's would have been and she has two good arms to boot.

In short, if Minnie had been born instead, Minnie$_2$ wouldn't be here to be upset about that—and the converse. The other would just be one of trillion of unconceived possibilities out there. Furthermore, the realization that we ourselves might have been one of

them seems to me to demand some detachment from the conditions that led us to be here. Saxton asks whether she could in good conscience have a medical test that would, if her mother had had access to it, have led to her being aborted. Not only would that reasoning militate against legal abortion in general, but it would demand that we commend fruitful acts of rape or incest. I myself would never have been born had World War II not occurred. Was it therefore a good thing?

The conclusion to be drawn from this thought exercise is surely that there is no good reason to conceive a child at special risk for disability when you could with little effort conceive one at only the usual odds. There are, additionally, good reasons for not doing so, based on the welfare of future persons. Parfit himself cannot, given his premises, find any way out of the dilemma he has described, and concludes that we need to change the focus of our moral concern: "our reasons for acting should become *more impersonal*. Greater impersonality may seem threatening. But it would often be better for everyone" (1984, p. 443). By this he means that we ought to be more willing to judge that the prospect of people living in a harmed state should deter us from bringing it about, even if, according to the usual criteria, no one has been harmed.[51] That conclusion is compatible with a utilitarian approach that seeks greater happiness for each individual, rather than a highly populated world where individual lives are barely worth living.

Although Parfit's conclusion that we should lessen our fixation on individual rights and be more attentive to the overall picture is attractive, I am not quite ready to concede it as the whole story. Can it really be true that we do not wrong a child with serious impairments when we knowingly bring it into the world?[52] There is no space here for a full analysis of the issue, but one promising avenue would be further questioning the extreme abstraction of some of the premises Parfit uses to generate his paradoxes, an abstraction that sometimes beguiles us into accepting implausible assumptions.[53] Reasoning with such bare-boned instruments denies us the context essential for developing livable moral views.

In general, the conjunction of abstract method and focus on harming individuals (as opposed to states of harm) in the way Parfit poses the question is most unfortunate, since it implicitly promotes an unattractive ethic of moral minimalism that could hardly be distinguished from libertarianism. The underlying moral principle here seems to be that it is morally permissible to bring you to life so long as you can be expected to find your life worth living, because you are not thereby harmed (even if you have been born in a harmed state) and it is permissible to do anything that does not harm you.[54] What we owe others is thus reduced to not harming them, and the standard for not having harmed them is set very low. Generalizing these principles to other cases would lead to a great deal of misery. Why couldn't a government refuse to fund polio vaccination programs, for instance, on the grounds that even if a certain percentage of babies become paralyzed, they'll still be glad to be alive? Why pay for good schools when poor ones won't make kids wish they were dead?

PREVENTABLE AND UNPREVENTABLE HARMS

The stopper is supposed to be the morally relevant distinction between preventable harms and unpreventable ones. In this situation, unpreventable harm is one that couldn't have been avoided without precluding your existence. But there is no particular reason for thinking that such a stringent criterion would be required in other cases. For instance, there might be no way for manufacturers to make "satisfactory" profits and reduce occupational hazards, and so the harm to workers would be neither preventable, nor, if their subsequent life still is worth living, a wrong done to them. Moreover, a different (and I think more realistic) view of personal identity, one that views some life experiences as constitutive of who you are, could undermine the crucial stopper effect still more. For if we recognize that some experiences can make you a different person, the impetus for social intervention, especially in children's lives, would be seriously undermined. At risk would be such desirable enterprises as Head Start and early nutrition programs.

However, my worry here goes still deeper. Although facts and logic constrain possible moral theories, they do not by themselves determine the values inherent in them. Thus how we approach ethics reflects our more general attitudes and dispositions. A narrow focus on not harming others, rather than enthusiasm for flourishing and happiness, will therefore both arise from—but also help perpetuate—the relevant attitudes. Yet it is not from such a narrow, almost legalistic conception of morality that flows the kind of generosity that will *of course* do everything to dissolve the effects of disability and disease: it flows, instead, from a utilitarian preoccupation with doing whatever good one can. So to the extent that disability rights activists borrow the morally minimalistic terms of Parfit's dilemma, they implicitly work against their own moral interests.

CONCLUSION

As I suggested earlier, it is good, other things being equal, for desires to be satisfied. It does not follow from this that we should accept desires uncritically, but merely that there is a prima facie case for satisfying them, other things being equal. In the case of the desire for genetically related children, however, other things are often not equal. It has in the past led to a great deal of misery when, for instance, a couple could not produce an appropriate heir, or when an inappropriate ("illegitimate") one was instead produced. Today, the first problem is leading women to try dangerous and expensive reproductive technologies in the search for a genetically related child when they could instead adopt a child in need of a good home. It can also motivate people to risk the health of their future children, even though they could still enjoy the other aspects of having children by sacrificing all or part of the genetic link.

It is true that providing a decent quality of life for each of us would, by itself, go far toward avoiding the birth of children with serious health problems, and is, for this and other reasons, morally obligatory. Since efforts in this direction are not even on the political horizon, and since they will not by themselves make every problematic case go away, how are we to face these issues in the meantime?

Having said that there is a serious strike against bringing certain children to life does not give us much specific guidance, and there is no space here to consider that issue in the detail it deserves.[55] It is well known that a variety of options now exist for those who want to refrain from producing children with their own genetic material. Among them are AID and egg donation, as well as contract pregnancy and adoption. Although AID is widely used and, for the most part regarded as uncontroversial, egg donation and contract pregnancy are not.[56] The last word on these remains to be said; I have argued elsewhere at length that contract pregnancy, if stringently regulated, could be made a morally acceptable alternative to the usual method of childbearing.[57] Adoption, although more morally problematic and practically difficult than is often thought, may also be in many cases a reasonable option.

Unfortunately these compromises have only limited utility for some, most notably the poor. Not only do the poor face more than their share of the kinds of health problems that create risk for babies, but they get less help with them. And the reproductive risk now posed for them by the AIDS epidemic is making their lives still more difficult. Given society's responsibility for so much of their plight, it hardly seems tenable to argue that they are now to forego one of their only sources of satisfaction, reproducing "their own" genetically related children. Yet, that does not protect their children. As John Arras points out in his sensitive paper on the topic, "the reproductive decisions of infected women have serious and problematic ethical implications for their offspring...."[58] The interplay of social and individual responsibility here creates moral problems that cannot be adequately resolved by pointing the finger solely at individuals, even if doing that seems to be the only way to prevent immediate harm. However, the unfair price such individuals pay for stopping it underlines once again our ultimate social responsibility in many of these matters.

Notes

1. Thanks to Joan Callahan and Dorothy Wertz for their helpful comments on this paper.

2. Working for change is the job of political activists. Of course, moral philosophers can be activists, too; in fact, given our positions of moral authority, we may well have a moral duty in this regard.

3. This lengthy preface is intended to emphasize the priority of fighting both for human welfare and especially for women's basic welfare—a priority that may

well seem to disappear in any treatment of a limited and problematic area. (I am not excluding in the scope of my concern here the welfare of other sentient creatures; however, in this paper I will be concentrating on human welfare.)

4. Even if there is no clear constitutional right to procreate, the consequences of failing to act as if there is one would be at present very harmful to women. See my "Are Pregnant Women Fetal Containers?" *Bioethics* 4, 4 (Oct. 1990), 273-91.

5. My position that it is sometimes wrong to reproduce in the usual way does not require any prior showing that there is such a right. For if there is, it doesn't follow that it can always be morally exercised; if there isn't, it is still necessary to lay out the conditions for morally acceptable reproduction.

6. Consider, for example, the recent debate about the nature and justification of the desire for children that is emerging in the feminist debate about artificial reproductive technologies. For further readings see *Reproductive Technologies; Gender, Motherhood and Medicine,* ed. Michelle Stanworth (Minneapolis: University of Minnesota Press, 1987), and *Feminist Perspectives in Medical Ethics,* ed. Helen Bequaert Holmes and Laura M. Purdy (Bloomington: Indiana University Press, 1992).

7. For an examination of other possibilities, see Ruth F. Chadwick, "Having Children: An Introduction," *Ethics, Reproduction and Genetic Control,* ed. Ruth F. Chadwick (London: Croom Helm, 1987), pp. 3-10. The status of the desire for children needs more work; in particular, its sources and consequences need much more thorough scrutiny.

8. See "Genetic Disease: Can Having Children Be Immoral?" *Genetics Now,* ed. John L. Buckley (Washington D.C. : University Press of America, 1978); reprinted in *Biomedical Ethics,* ed. Thomas A. Mappes and Jane S. Zembaty, 3rd ed. (New York: McGraw-Hill, 1991).

9. This last is not entirely unconnected with the others, of course.

10. It may not be possible to reconcile the two if either the population grows too large or if the definition of basic welfare is too inclusive, so that acute conflicts arise between present needs and future ones.

11. See, for example, my "Are Pregnant Women Fetal Containers?"; John D. Arras, "AIDS and Reproduc-

tive Decisions: Having Children in Fear and Trembling," *The Milbank Quarterly* 68, 3 (1990), 353-82; and Noam Zohar, "Prospects for 'Genetic Therapy'— Can a Person Benefit from Being Altered?" and Jeffery P. Kahn, "Genetic Harm: Bitten by the Body That Keeps You?" both in *Bioethics* 5, 4 (October 1991), 275-308.

12. Robert Simon has pointed out to me that there are good reasons for thinking in terms of a more objective criterion than "opportunity for a normal life." They center on the otherwise difficult-to-manage relativistic element in judgments about what is "normal."

13. The main objection has been that HD doesn't require such moral restraint. It is argued that potential parents are usually going ahead without knowing for sure whether they have the disease. If they don't, then their children are not really at risk. Even if they do, there is only a fifty percent chance that each child will be afflicted with the disease. And, even if a child turns out to have the disease, he or she will have between twenty and fifty years of good life. My evaluation of these factors has not changed in the time since I wrote the paper; they seem to me, if anything, to increase the horror of the disease. In particular, the prospect of a short life seems to me especially tragic, not only because of the depression quite likely to be caused by knowledge of it, but because of the loss to all those (like women) whose early lives are often taken up with the demands of others. It takes many women well into middle age to overcome the sexist upbringing that deprives them of the self-confidence to make more choices based on their own interests. Deaths of people in their prime also deprives society of some of its best and wisest members. In case such considerations don't move you, it is always possible to find still more dreadful diseases, like Tay-Sachs, where they don't apply.

14. I argued in an earlier paper that although it would not be reasonable at this point to make prenatal harm a crime, it is still wrong for women to act in ways that are likely to harm their fetuses. Among other things, most of such harm arises because of factors beyond women's control and that could be remedied if society made avoiding it a priority. So unless society does what it can, it is hypocritical and unjust to blame women for causing prenatal harms. ("Are Pregnant Women Fetal Containers?")

15. Two points about my focus here. First, I am uneasy about contributing to the balkanization of progressive political movements that arises from criticizing our allies rather than those with whom we have far more basic disagreements. However, it also seems important to try to develop the strongest positions possible in order to facilitate social change. Second, because I am considering primarily arguments of disability rights writers, the following discussion is centered on the question of disability. It should be understood that concern for painful or limiting disease is not thereby excluded.

16. Marsha Saxton, "Born and Unborn: The Implications of Reproductive Technologies for People with Disabilities," *Test-Tube Women: What Future for Motherhood?* ed. Rita Arditti, Renate Duelli-Klein, and Shelley Minden (London: Pandora, 1984); Adrienne Asch, "Can Aborting 'Imperfect' Children Be Immoral?" *Ethical Issues in Modern Medicine*, ed. John Arras and Nancy Rhoden (Mountain View, CA: Mayfield Press, 1989).

17. Asch writes in support of abortion because of women's right to control their bodies; she also asserts that because newborns are legally persons, it is wrong to deprive them of medical care unless they are dying. She does not discuss the philosophical assumptions underlying these positions (Adrienne Asch, "Real Moral Dilemmas," *Christianity and Crisis* 46, 10 [July 14, 1986], 237-40).

18. My arguments also hold for those who regard the relevant kinds of abortions as no more morally significant than failing to conceive.

19. For a recent, moving discussion, see a series of articles in *The Progressive,* August 1991 (Mary Johnson, "Disabled Americans Push for Access," Laura Hershey, "Exit the Nursing Home," and Joseph P. Shapiro, "I Can Do Things for Myself Now," pp. 21-29). These articles highlight both the ignorance and the bad faith involved in much current practice.

20. The recent (1991-92) recession, which included widespread unemployment, cuts in federal and state welfare programs, and the increasingly serious health insurance crisis, should give pause to those of modest means who assume that they will be able to make sure their children's needs will be met. Furthermore, it is by now generally known that women usually fare poorly after divorce, especially if they have stayed at

home to take care of children. Alimony is now rare, and they must now earn a living (with non-existent or rusty job skills). Since they are usually granted custody of the children, and are given only the inadequate child support offered by most fathers, they must somehow cover childcare expenses, too. With a divorce rate of 50 percent, no married woman can be sure that she will not find herself trapped in such difficult circumstances.

21. Anybody who has tried to raise thoughtful and caring children knows how difficult it is to teach them these values, as well as the hostility they face if they accept them. It does not follow that we should give up on such projects, but we need to be realistic about their toll. Therefore, we should think twice about imposing such burdens on children.

22. This approach to grading values might lead to a *reductio ad absurdum* rejection of any value, even that of life itself, since, after all, not everybody can live.

23. Thanks to Dianne Romain for helping me think more clearly about this issue.

24. For a paper on a closely related example, see Janice G. Raymond, "Fetalists Are Not Feminists: They Are Not the Same," *Made To Order: The Myth of Reproductive and Genetic Progress,* ed. Patricia Spallone and Deborah Lynn Steinberg (Oxford: Pergamon, 1987).

25. If ought implies can, we don't, strictly speaking, have a right to a healthy body. But that is not to say that we ought not to be trying to do the best we can.

26. Asch does make some distinction between problems for which changes in reproductive behavior are appropriate, and lesser ones for which they are not. She asks whether "we wish to abort for disability that will not cause great physical pain or death in early childhood" (Adrienne Asch, "Reproductive Technology and Disability,*" Reproductive Laws for the 1990s*, ed. Sherill Cohen and Nadine Taub [Clifton, N.J.: Humana Press, 1988], pp. 88-89). I would include chronic pain, serious physical or mental limitation, and mental suffering (including the prospect of an early but not imminent death) to the list of conditions to which people shouldn't be subjected.

27. The ease with which some dismiss the pains of others is unnerving; some of this arises no doubt from mere thoughtlessness, lack of experience, or the attempt to "cheer up." It hurts nonetheless. I was struck by a letter to Ann Landers that reads in part:

I, too, have suffered because some people have no idea what living with a handicap is like.

I am 33 years old and have multiple sclerosis. I have been told countless times how lucky I am to be able to park in a special place, work only half days, etc. I try to explain calmly that I'd gladly park anywhere and work all day in exchange for the privilege of good health. Surprisingly, that doesn't make an impression. I've been told, "I could handle that," and "It's no big deal," or "They'll find a cure soon."

... I pray a cure will be found soon, but in the meantime it is a VERY big deal to those of us who have it. Anyone who doubts that can speak to my children. We used to live in Montana and climb mountains. Now my life is completely different. We can't even walk around the zoo because Mom has MS ... (*The Ithaca Journal,* Friday, December 6, 1991).

28. Consider Joel Feinberg's comments on this question: " ... if before the child has been born, we *know* that the conditions for the fulfillment of his most basic interests have already been destroyed, and we permit him nevertheless to be born, we become a party to the violation of his rights. It bears repeating that not all interests of the newborn child should or can qualify for prenatal legal protection, but only those very basic ones whose satisfaction is known to be indispensable to a decent life. The state cannot insure all or even many of its citizens against bad luck in the lottery of life.... On the other hand, to be dealt severe mental retardation, congenital syphilis, blindness, deafness, advanced heroin addiction, permanent paralysis or incontinence, guaranteed malnutrition, and economic deprivation so far below a reasonable minimum as to be inescapably degrading and sordid, is not merely to have 'bad luck'" (*Harm to Others* [Oxford: Oxford University Press, 1984], p. 99).

29. See Feinberg, ch. 1, and ch. 2, section 8.

30. Those who imagine future people waiting in line to be born, where the relevant moral rule presumably ought to be first come, first served, will be most apt to see the effort to prefer the birth of those more likely to live more satisfying lives as morally evil.

31. For example, to the extent that women now have babies because of lack of access to contraception and abortion, or even, more broadly, because of the lack

of satisfying alternative social roles, achieving women's equality will alter who gets born. Derek Parfit also points out the counterintuitive consequences with respect to pollution. See his *Reasons and Persons* (Oxford: Oxford University Press, 1984), pt. IV.

32. For example, good social arrangements could now provide everyone with a kind of security and well-being that was unavailable to anybody just a few generations ago. No longer must we bear child after child only to watch them die, no longer need we fear such diseases as polio or smallpox. Although many scientific advances have proved to be mixed blessings, there is no doubt that many of us now have lives of unprecedented satisfaction and that many more could do so if we cared to make it a social priority.

33. Thus, for example, it may be inappropriate to spend such a large proportion of the science research budget on the human genome project, for it may open up possibilities too dangerous to handle at present. Even if it is successful, there may be good reasons to refrain from instituting the kind of mandatory screening programs that would capitalize most effectively on the knowledge gained by it. They might, for example, involve racism or other harmful stereotyped assumptions.

34. It should not be inferred that what I say here implies that children grow best when everything is made easy for them, and that is not, in any case, a situation we are in danger of providing for most of them. See my book *In Their Best Interest? The Case against Equal Rights for Children* (Ithaca: Cornell University Press, 1992).

One might argue that reducing the number of people with disabilities would weaken the disability rights movement, since advocates tend to have personal links with impaired individuals. That wouldn't be a very appealing objection, since it would be a paradigm case of using people as mere means. It's also dubious from a consequentialist viewpoint, since it will be all that most families can do to cope with their own child's immediate needs. The most promising development would be recruiting energetic workers who are free to devote themselves wholeheartedly to advancing the interests of people with impairments, much as the civil rights movement recruited students.

35. The debate about cochlear implants erupted after this piece was written. Some deaf people have refused cochlear implants that could restore hearing for themselves or their children. They do so in part because they do not see deafness as a disability, and in part because they fear that the deaf community will be impoverished if there are fewer young people entering it. The latter concern is understandable and one would think that it would be possible to ensure that hearing children of the deaf would be taught to sign; it would be better still if signing came to be more universal among hearing people. The claim that deafness is not a disability is less appealing. Resolving this question is a delicate matter, but I would be inclined to defer to John Stuart Mill's test for deciding which of two states of affairs is more desirable, namely, consultation with those who have experienced both. I suspect that such persons would not choose to be deaf. (Edward Dolnick, "Deafness as Culture," *The Atlantic* 272, 3 [September 1993], 37-51; John Stuart Mill, "Utilitarianism," *The Utilitarians* [NY: Dolphin Books, 1961], p. 401.

36. It is sad (and instructive) that anybody who tries to get childless students to think in realistic terms about children is immediately plastered with the reputation of "baby-basher," just as those who attempt to get them to think realistically about women's place in society become "male-bashers."

37. Good parenting is by itself a demanding enterprise, one that is barely compatible under present circumstances with many jobs. Adding special needs to that mix will be, in the case of many women, the straw that breaks the camel's back.

38. Asch agrees that elective abortion should remain a legal option for women, even where she doubts the morality of abortion for disability. However, I fear that her position about the wrongness of most abortions for disability will cause some women to feel that they should not abort in that case, even where they would prefer to do so. That is why I think it is important to address this issue head on. See, for example, her article, "Real Moral Dilemmas," and "Shared Dreams: A Left Perspective on Disability Rights and Reproductive Rights," by Adrienne Asch and Michelle Fine, in Asch and Fine's *Women with Disabilities: Essays in Psychology, Culture , and Politics* (Philadelphia: Temple University Press, 1988).

39. See Helga Kuhse and Peter Singer, "From the Editors," *Bioethics* 5, 4 (October 1991), iv-v, for a brief

account. A major conference at which he was to speak was threatened with disruption, on the grounds that he and others who have argued in favor of euthanasia were "preparing the way for a resurgence of Nazi-style mass killing" (p. iv). Rejecting a proposal to withdraw its invitation to Singer, the conference's organizing committee instead canceled the conference.

40. See, for example, Adrienne Asch, who writes in *Reproductive Laws* apropos of suits for wrongful birth and wrongful life: "claiming that life with disability is worse than no life at all offends self-respecting disabled people and represents the extreme of what is dangerous about testing, diagnosing and suing" (p. 95).

41. If *knowing* that you will most likely come down with something dreadful like Huntington's Disease is too much for you to bear, then how can you impose such risk on your children?

42. See my "Are Pregnant Women Fetal Containers?"

43. The beginning of a proper response would be to deny the moral framework that judges people according to a crude cost-benefit analysis, one that would conclude that some people don't "pay off." A livable moral framework must, on the contrary, concentrate on each person's opportunity to live a satisfying life; it recognizes our interdependence and takes for granted that we will all be helping each other at different times and in different ways. This way of looking at things leaves judgments about whether one's life is worth living to the individuals in question. However, it would not necessarily preclude an effort at avoiding some births for the kinds of reasons proposed here. This effort would be precluded by the response that virtually every possible life is worth living. However, that position might have some trouble showing why, other things being equal, we should not prefer to bring a non-disabled rather than a disabled individual into existence.

44. Certain mental disabilities might be an exception to this claim.

45. Since the advent of effective, comfortable, safe, and cheap contact lenses, simple nearsightedness is no longer a persuasive example for the middle-class in Western industrialized nations. In other circumstances such as non-technological societies where keen eyesight is essential for survival, it could still be a ghastly problem.

46. Our reluctance to deliberately monkey with the future in certain ways (together with our apparently foolhardy willingness to do so in others) seems as yet inadequately explored. Bringing these fears out into the open would probably help us make wiser choices. See, for example, Jonathan Glover, *What Sort of People Should There Be?* (Middlesex, England: Penguin Books, 1984).

47. This argument assumes that the only reason for refraining from bringing someone into existence is that it would wrong them; however, if who we bring to existence is neutral—that is, there is no reason for preferring one possible future person over another—then we could still argue against bringing the unhealthy one into existence on the grounds of unnecessary burden to others, which tips the case against the unhealthy.

48. Derek Parfit, "On Doing the Best for Our Children," in *Ethics and Population,* ed. M. D. Bayles (Cambridge, MA: Schenkman, 1976); see also his *Reasons and Persons* (Oxford: Oxford University Press, 1984), pt. 4.

49. Alison Jaggar points out that athletic girls tend to grow taller than non-athletic ones, since being physically active retards the onset of puberty, when growth slows ("Sex Inequality and Bias in Sex Differences Research," *Science, Morality and Feminist Theory,* ed. Marsha Hanen and Kai Nielsen [*Canadian Journal of Philosophy,* supp. Vol. 13, 1987], p. 34).

50. It is enormously important to recognize the limits of our thought experiments. As we try to think through the implications of various choices, we almost necessarily attribute to the "players" a kind of ghostly existence, as if they were waiting in the wings to be called out on stage. This conception tends to lead us astray, causing us to think inappropriately in terms of discrimination, hard feelings and so forth.

51. This distinction is Feinberg's. (See *Harm to Others*, ch 1, section 1.) Feinberg implicitly agrees with Parfit when he asserts that "It is, of course, possible to be wronged without being harmed ... and it is possible to blame *A* for bringing *B* into existence in an initially harmful condition, but that is still another thing than *A* harming *B*, which as we have seen ... requires worsening a person's prior condition, or at

least making it worse than it would otherwise have been ... " (p. 99).

52. This line of argument seems worth pursuing in part because of how odd it is to have to say that it would be wrong to inflict a given problem on an existing person, but not wrong to bring others to life if having it is the condition of their existence—when there is otherwise no particular good reason for "choosing" them. So if I failed to inoculate my child against, say, a bacterial version of Huntington's disease, I would be considered an irresponsible parent, even though the arguments in favor of conception of a child at risk for it downplay the misery of the disease. The differences in these two cases just seem insufficient to bear the moral weight required of them. That anybody has the disease is what's bad, not who they are or why they have it.

53. Thus, for example, he says that his Wide Average Principle "could imply that, in the best possible history, only two people ever live" (p. 416). He comments that: "most of us find this view too extreme. Most of us believe that there is value in quantity, but that this value has, in any period, an upper limit." Because the whole approach is so abstract, adding yet another abstract principle to counteract the counterintuitive consequence of the first becomes necessary. However, it would not be necessary if we thought seriously about what it would mean to imagine a two-person world. This rumination would, by itself, show that the Wide Average Principle could never imply that a two-person history would be best. And so forth. His descriptions of human interactions remind us uncomfortably of billiard balls.

54. There are also difficult epistemological problems, since different people have different thresholds for suffering. Mistaken guesses about a given situation may reap truly dreadful suffering as the individual comes to the conclusion that her life is not worth living, both on her part and that of those who love her.

55. I discussed some of these, such as the question of risk, in "Genetic Disease: Can Having Children Be Immoral?"

56. For views on these issues see Holmes and Purdy, *Issues in Reproductive Technology I: An Anthology*, ed. Helen Bequaert Holmes (New York: Garland, 1992); and Richard Hull, *Ethical Issues in the New Reproductive Technologies* (Belmont, CA: Wadsworth, 1990).

57. See "Surrogate Mothering: Exploitation or Empowerment?" *Bioethics* 3, 1 (January 1989), 18-34; "Another Look at Contract Pregnancy," *Issues in Reproductive Technology I: An Anthology*, ed. Helen Bequaert Holmes (New York: Garland, 1992).

58. Arras, "AIDS and Reproductive Decisions."

29

DECISIONS REGARDING DISABLED NEWBORNS

Mary B. Mahowald

During the 1980s, both the media and the federal government focused their consideration of infants on a few controversial cases, possibly to the neglect of ethical issues involving other children, and larger social and ethical problems affecting all of us.[1] In this chapter, I broaden the perspective on neonatal dilemmas by providing a brief account of the historical, cultural, and medical contexts in which they arise, and a description of alternative approaches to their resolution. I also discuss cases in which nontreatment of extremely ill, impaired, and low birth weight infants may be morally justified. Although these conditions are often addressed separately, in practice they often occur in the same patient. From an egalitarian perspective, each infant should be treated as an individual, just as older patients are to be treated as individuals. In both situations, the patient represents a unique embodiment of limitations, abilities, possibilities, and relationships.[2]

HISTORICAL AND CURRENT CONTEXT

Facilities and technologies for neonatal intensive care are a relatively recent phenomenon, still comparatively unavailable or inaccessible to the populations of less developed nations. The first treatment center for newborn care in the United States was established early in this century, when infant deaths were primarily associated with infection or malnutrition.[3] At that time, rudimentary incubators provided necessary warmth for preterm infants, and oxygen supplementation was introduced to combat respiratory difficulties due to immature lung development. Progress in survival rates was not devoid of setbacks. For example, by 1954 it was recognized that the high oxygen concentrations that had saved some preterm newborns had also caused blindness. Subsequent curtailment of this treatment was accompanied by a corresponding rise in the rate of infant mortality.[4] Similarly, diethylstilbestrol (DES) was initially

thought by some to be effective in bringing problematic pregnancies to term, but the drug was later implicated in carcinogenic and reproductive problems of the offspring.[5]

Further advances produced sophisticated techniques for prenatal diagnosis and treatment, monitoring neonatal heart rate, blood gases, and chemistries, and microsurgical procedures for newborn anomalies. Neonatology became a major pediatric specialty, spawning a huge and ongoing research effort with impressive clinical results.[6] Techniques introduced during the 1960s facilitated successful treatment of infants weighing less than 1,500 grams. These methods included constant positive airway pressure monitoring, by which oxygen requirements are constantly measured without interruption, and hyperalimentation, a means of providing nutrition to those who cannot tolerate other types of feeding. By 1970, the mortality rate from hyaline membrane disease, a common problem of preterm newborns, had dropped from 60 percent to 20 percent of those affected. By 1978, the survival rate for very early and very small babies had improved to the point where those weighing less than 1,000 grams warranted treatment.[7] Since then, fetal viability has advanced earlier into pregnancy, resulting in smaller and younger survivors of preterm birth and even late abortions. Two new techniques, extracorporeal membrane oxygenation (ECMO) and surfactant therapy have decreased the mortality rates of newborns even further. ECMO has improved the outcome for newborns suffering from four common or highly lethal conditions: meconium aspiration, persistent pulmonary hypertension, beta streptococcal sepsis, and congenital diaphragmatic hernia.[8] Surfactant therapy has been remarkably successful in treatment of lung immaturity in preterm infants.[9]

The majority of very low birth weight babies (less than 1.5 kilograms) who survive sustain no serious permanent compromise to their motor or mental functions. For example, 65 percent of the 781 infants weighing less than 1,500 grams who were admitted to the Neonatal Intensive Care Unit at Rainbow Babies and Childrens Hospital in Cleveland between 1975 and 1978 survived; 80 percent of these had normal neurodevelopmental outcomes.[10] As might be suspected, morbidity increases with decreasing birth weight. From 1982 to 1988 a study at the same institution showed an 18 to 20 percent survival rate for newborns weighing less than 750 grams. Among the survivors, 22 to 50 percent had moderate to severe neurodevelopmental impairment.[11] A multicenter study published in 1991 showed a 34 percent survival for infants weighing 750 grams or less and 66 percent for those from 751 through 1,000 grams.[12] Morbidity factors for survivors in this study include chronic lung disease, severe bowel infection, and brain hemorrhage, all of which may lead to long-term severe impairment. Despite the impressive technological developments, not everyone agrees that all critically ill newborns should be provided with lifesaving or life-prolonging treatment. Infanticide is a long-standing practice with which nontreatment decisions may be compared.

Anthropologists tell us that infanticide has been practiced throughout history in many cultures, including those of the western world.[13] At times, the practice was deemed acceptable because it was undertaken indirectly rather than directly. In other words, infants were not killed outright, but were left to die—often because they were defective, sometimes because they were twins or female or illegitimate. Since abandonment of an infant inevitably leads to death, there is little practical distinction between killing and letting a newborn die. Just as euthanasia is morally problematic, regardless of whether it is characterized as active or passive, so is infanticide, whether characterized as direct or indirect.[14] Refusing to institute respiratory support in a newborn whose lungs are not yet mature may be construed as indirect infanticide. The refusal to provide intravenous nutrition to an infant who is incapable of normal digestion may be construed similarly.[15] The difficulty of maintaining a sharp distinction between direct and indirect termination of life-saving treatment has led Robert Weir to argue that it is sometimes morally justified to terminate an infant's life directly and actively.[16]

Several factors in contemporary American society conspire to exacerbate moral problems regarding infants. One is the emphasis on patient autonomy, which is generally assumed to be captured in the concept of "informed consent." While this concept is obviously inapplicable to newborns, it is sometimes applied to parents who make decisions on behalf of their children. In fact, the distinction between informed consent and proxy or substitute consent is often overlooked, and parents are falsely assumed to provide the former rather than the latter.[17] Legal and moral grounds for requiring informed consent of competent patients are stronger than those for substitute consent. Nonetheless, parental rights regarding their children have generally been perceived as primary, requiring practitioners to respect their decisions even when these involve the refusal of life-prolonging treatment.[18] Since the Baby Doe controversies of the 1980s, this emphasis has shifted to a situation where some physicians see themselves as advocates for infants even if this pits them against parents.[19]

In the past, a variety of treatment options were unavailable for many infants, regardless of whether they were disabled. Reversible life-threatening medical problems, which occur more frequently in permanently impaired newborns than in other infants, are now routinely repaired through surgery. The development of antibiotic therapy, feeding techniques, and fluid exchange procedures has greatly increased the actual number of disabled children who survive to adulthood. Moreover, while greater numbers of preterm infants now survive to live normal lives, some pay for their survival with iatrogenically induced permanent disabilities. There is thus an inevitable connection between very low birth weight babies and disabled infants.[20]

Two conflicting social phenomena make neonatal ethical dilemmas even more prevalent and complicated. One is the "premium baby" mentality that has resulted from the trend toward reduced family size, as well as the availability of contraceptive measures and abortion, discussed in earlier chapters. Allowing severely compromised infants to die is consistent with this mentality. In contrast, the "right to life" ideology and movement affirm the primacy of fetal interests over those of other individuals. Not surprisingly, "right to life" activists have joined the government and organizations representing the disabled in arguing that infants should not be denied treatment on the basis of their disabilities.[21] Either of these positions is supportable by an egalitarian perspective. Which position weighs more than the other depends on whether survival of a severely disabled newborn is of greater value than parental autonomy, or whether the obligation to respect parental autonomy overrides that of beneficence toward their infant. The cases considered next are well-known illustrations of this dilemma.

THE DOE BABIES

In the spring of 1982, an infant afflicted with Down syndrome and esophageal atresia was born at Bloomington Hospital in Indiana. Surgical repair is usually undertaken to correct the latter problem, but the former condition, with its concomitant mental retardation, is not correctable. For individuals with Down syndrome, the degree of mental retardation is not predictable at birth. The obstetrician informed the mother that she might choose between two "medical options" regarding her newborn: (1) consent to the surgery necessary for survival, or (2) decline that consent and request that the baby not be fed so as not to prolong his dying. The parents chose the latter course. Hospital personnel respected their choice, and local and state courts reviewed and approved their decision. Local attorneys attempted to reverse the decision through appeal to the U. S. Supreme Court. When the child died while the attorneys were en route to Washington for a special hearing of the court, the case became moot.[22]

Although his parents had him baptized, presumably giving him a name, the public came to know this infant as "Baby Doe." During his six days of life, he became uniquely but anonymously famous because of media coverage and public reaction to it. As a resident of Bloomington at the time, I knew several of the principals associated with the case (the obstetrician, the pediatrician, the lawyer for the parents, the priest who baptized the baby, and the pathologist who performed the autopsy), but never learned the identity of the infant or his parents. To their credit, the press respected the family's privacy.

Following the infant's death, the government notified all federally supported institutions caring for infants that funding would be denied if they discriminated against the disabled, as had allegedly occurred with Baby Doe. In March of 1983, the Department of Health and Human Services issued a ruling that required all such institutions to post signs citing both the government statute prohibiting discrimination against the disabled and a phone number to use in reporting suspected violations of the statute.[23] This ruling was overturned one month later by U.S. District Judge Gerhard A. Gesell, who described it as conceived in "haste and inexperience," and "based on inadequate consideration of the regulation's consequences."[24]

The second Baby Doe was born in Port Jefferson, New York, in fall of 1983, this one distinguished from the other by being called "Jane Doe." Like her predecessor, she too became a subject of public controversy within her first days of life. Unlike him, her name (Keri-Lynn) was eventually revealed by the media, and the child survived despite her parents' initial refusal of treatment.

Baby Jane Doe was born with spina bifida (an open spine), hydrocephalus (excess fluid on the brain), and microcephaly (reduced brain size), conditions predictive of paralysis in her lower extremities, incontinence, and retardation. According to reports published during her first weeks of life, surgical intervention might allow the child to survive for approximately twenty years; without the surgery she was likely to die within two years. A physician who counseled the father told him that his daughter was so neurologically compromised that she "would never experience joy, never experience sorrow."[25] When both parents declined consent for the surgery, their decision was reviewed and approved at local and state levels, and supported by their priest counselor. Lawrence Washburn, an attorney from New Jersey, brought the case to the attention of federal authorities, who attempted unsuccessfully to obtain the medical records. As with the Bloomington case, the government considered nontreatment of Baby Jane Doe to be a violation of the 1973 statute prohibiting discrimination against the handicapped.[26]

Litigation relevant to the second Baby Doe case led to a denial of the government's right to require the surrender of medical records in order to investigate treatment decisions regarding disabled infants.

During the summer of 1984, the government's Baby Doe regulations were permanently enjoined by the U.S. District Court in New York. However, in fall of the same year Congress passed legislation requiring state child protection agencies to intervene in cases where severely disabled infants are refused "medically indicated treatment." Exceptions to this requirement are situations where "the infant is irreversibly comatose or the treatment would be futile and inhumane or would only prolong dying."[27] According to Betty W. Levin, pediatric professionals tend to overestimate the degree of interventions required by this legislation.[28]

Conflicting position regarding the role of government in "Baby Doe" cases reflect different constituencies: medical organizations, associations for the disabled, the Department of Health and Human Services, and the President's Commission for the Study of Ethical Problems in Medicine and Biomedical and Behavioral Research (hereafter, President's Commission). However, the documents in which these positions are articulated all invoke the same criterion, namely, the best interests of infants.[29] While disagreement continues about interpretation of, and procedures for implementing, the "best interest" criterion,[30] broader agreement may be reached through an examination of its meaning. Before addressing this, however, I wish to deal with an equally controversial question relevant to guideline 4: who should decide the fate of severely disabled newborns?

WHO SHOULD DECIDE?

"Informed consent" is often seen as a sine qua non of justification for medical interventions.[31] Competent adults may legally decline even lifesaving therapy by removing themselves from hospital treatment programs against medical advice. Exceptions have been based on the patient's responsibilities to others, or the claim that hospital personnel are not obliged to violate their own professional standards or commitments.[32] Since newborns are incapable of providing informed consent, their parents usually act as proxy or surrogate decision makers in their behalf. The right of parents to act as proxies may be overruled, however, if their decision opposes their child's best interest. For example, if a Jehovah's Witness parent declines a blood transfusion essential to the life of

his child, hospital authorities will obtain a court order allowing hospital personnel to intervene in the child's behalf. Thus, the parents' right to decide about their infant's treatment is legally less binding than their right to decide about their own treatments.

The distinction between informed and proxy consent is also significant from a moral point of view. It suggests that a priority of decision makers be observed, based on the degree to which each decision maker is related to the infant. Typically, the child's parents hold first place. However, the child's caretakers are also related to the child through their professional commitment, as well as the personal and contractual relationships they maintain with the infant and family.

Despite the legal and moral requirement of informed or proxy consent, long standing practice assigns the role of principal decision maker of medical dilemmas to the physician.[33] The justification for this priority is sometimes comparable to the argument presented by the cardinal in Dostoyevsky's story of "The Grand Inquisitor."[34] By assuming control of people's lives, the cardinal claimed that his church had gradually removed the burden of freedom that Christ brought to the world. Similarly, the physician or the health care team may accept sole responsibility for difficult decisions in order to spare families the anguish and unnecessary guilt that often occurs in such situations. Despite its plausibility and appeal, this paternalistic reasoning has several crucial flaws. One is the failure to acknowledge that a sense of guilt may be experienced regardless of how a decision is made. If this is true, it is more helpful to focus on the moral justification for a decision to prolong or discontinue treatment—that is, the intent to do what is best for the patient. Both families and practitioners may need explicit reassurance that relinquishing the hold on another's life is sometimes the most loving and caring alternative available.

Another flaw in arguments favoring decisions made solely by physicians (or parents) is the fact that responsibility for decision making is inevitably shared by all of the autonomous participants in a dilemma. Even if an attending physician writes an order or parents indicate their wishes, others choose to implement, ignore, or challenge those decisions. At times, a practitioner does not consider her actions to be a matter of choice; rather, she may simply be following the order of the attending physician or supervisor. At other times, a practitioner may subtly, perhaps even inadvertently, interpret an "order" in a manner that compromises its intent. For example, in a situation where a physician has instructed staff to resuscitate a critically ill patient if necessary, a nurse or resident who disagrees with that decision may respond with deliberate slowness to a signal that the patient has suffered cardiac arrest.

In many cases regarding neonates, there is neither ambiguity nor controversy about what constitutes morally appropriate behavior. For example, the vast majority of pediatricians and pediatric surgeons agree that an anencephalic newborn who is afflicted with intestinal atresia should not have corrective surgery for the latter condition.[35] The invasiveness of surgery cannot be justified on the basis of benefit to the patient because the infant is already dying. In cases where agreement has been reached about moral aspects of treatment or nontreatment, it is probably neither necessary nor helpful to extend the decision base beyond the delivery room or nursery. In fact, involving others in the decision process increases the possibility of violating confidentiality for family privacy.

Moreover, treatment deferral sometimes involves a real risk of harming the patient. Possibly the most common example of such a situation involves intubation of very small (e.g., less than 650 grams) or very early (e.g., less than 24 weeks gestation) preterm newborns. Without intubation, the infant cannot survive. At such times, whoever is competent to provide the treatment is justified in making the decision on the patient's behalf. Subsequently, however, and in most chronic cases, there is time for discussion and broader input, which ought to be obtained in cases where ambiguity or disagreement continues. Since most decisions to terminate lifesaving treatment are irrevocable, treatment should continue until the conflict is resolved.

Why should there be broader input? Mainly because neither health care practitioners nor parents have any special moral expertise, and the possibility of arriving at well-reasoned moral decisions is increased by the collaborative efforts of reasonable people. Those who maintain a distance from the situation can sometimes provide a more objective perspective, which may complement and supplement the view of those whose involvement in the situation may preclude a totally rational analysis. Extending the decision base in unclear or controversial cases may also be reassuring to those closest to the patient because it represents one more attempt at responsible resolution of a difficult dilemma.

A decision base may be extended beyond the physician or parents through consultation with other clinicians, the entire health care team, a hospital-based review committee, or recourse to the courts. In the interests of maintaining confidentiality and family privacy, it is preferable to use the least public forum in which ambiguity or disagreement may be resolved. The widespread endorsement of the health care team's effectiveness in providing basic health care suggests that it might also be effective in dealing with medically related moral problems.[36] Hospital-based review committees are a newer phenomenon whose efficacy deserves to be tested.[37] Recourse to the courts is a particularly troublesome means of extending the decision base for ethical dilemmas. The legal system introduces an adversarial dimension into a set of relationships that should ideally be based on trust, openness, and consensus. Litigation threatens, and sometimes severs, those relationships, thwarting the therapeutic purpose of the practitioner-patient alliance. There are times when legal recourse may be the only way of resolving ambiguity and disagreement—for example, in cases involving blood transfusions for children of Jehovah's Witnesses. But court decisions are not necessarily morally correct. In the case of Bloomington's Baby Doe, for example, there is widespread agreement that the court's concurrence with the parents' decision to decline treatment was morally unjustified.[38]

Recent government attempts to impose investigative procedures on federally funded facilities that care for newborns seem to be intrusions on the right of privacy and the confidentiality of the physician-patient relationship, and may even be harmful to the patients affected. After investigating many anonymous reports of suspected neglect of impaired newborns, the Department of Health and Human Services concluded that appropriate medical, legal, and moral decisions had already been made in the vast majority of cases. In cases at Vanderbilt University in Nashville, Tennessee, and Strong Memorial Hospital in Rochester,

New York, however, it was reported that the government investigation obstructed care of the infants who had allegedly been neglected as well as other patients. The time required for personnel to respond to the queries of investigators could only be purchased at the price of time spent in caring for patients.[39]

In January, 1984, the Department of Health and Human Services strongly encouraged the formation of hospital ethics review committees to consider cases of suspected neglect of disabled infants through denial of treatment.[40] In addition to health care professionals from various disciplines, it was recommended that representatives of the disabled also serve on these committees. In general, the government's encouragement of the committee review mechanism supported the recommendation of the President's Commission.[41] The American Academy of Pediatrics also recommended the formation of local review committees and suggested appropriate procedures and principles.[42] However, the Commission had proposed the local review mechanism as an alternative to federal investigative procedures, arguing that the latter was unlikely to promote the best interests of infants and might actually impede the achievement of that purpose.

The continuing legal controversy surrounding "Baby Doe" cases evoked fairly widespread interest in the use of hospital review committees to address difficult cases. The extent of this interest and the influence of committees on practice remain to be seen.[43] Regardless of how decisions are made, however, we must also deal with the substantive issue of criteria for ethical decisions regarding disabled neonates. These reflect egalitarian considerations and traditional principles of biomedical ethics. An emphasis on the best interests of others also reflects an ethic of care for them.

PROLONGING LIFE IN OTHERS' INTERESTS
Since life is commonly perceived as a great gift, it may credibly be maintained that loss of life is always negative for the patient, and therefore the loss can only (possibly) be justified on the basis of others' interests. Indeed, in certain cases, the interests of others may be primarily served through the prolongation of an infant's life. Consider, for example, the fact that fees paid to neonatologists, hospitals, and hospital

personnel are partly dependent on the patient population, which is incremented through preservation of lives, no matter what their quality. So long as infants survive, the possibility of obtaining new knowledge through experimental therapies and further clinical data also continues. Beyond these results, there are more subtle rewards that accrue to clinicians who succeed in prolonging infants' lives. First is the feeling of accomplishment borne of the experience of doing rather than just letting go. Most doctors, after all, are activists, more inclined to cure than sustained caring. As one neonatologist put it, "It is easier for me to live with the consequences of something I've done than it is to worry about something I have not done which might have given better results."[44] Second is a perceived consistency between the end of health care and the prolongation of life. Conversely, for some clinicians the death of any patient evokes a sense of professional failure.[45] And third, effective ties build up between clinicians and child (as well as between parents and child, and clinicians and parents), sometimes reaching a point where the emotional needs of the concerned adults obfuscate their recognition of the infant's interests. A nurse thus made a pertinent and poignant comment concerning an infant whose life had been prolonged for two years, despite a preponderance of anguish to him with no expectation of ultimate relief or survival: "We have been doing this for ourselves rather than for him."[46]

Legally it may well be in the interests of clinicians and parents to prolong the life of an infant. Although malpractice suits may be pressed for prolonging life, suits are more likely when treatment has been withdrawn.[47] Even in that case, however, the probability of a successful suit is very slim so long as "letting die" (passive euthanasia) is distinguished from active euthanasia. It is also possible that efforts to prolong the lives of severely disabled infants serve the interests of politicians or political parties. Support for the Reagan administration was surely enhanced in some quarters by the steps it took to prevent a "Baby Doe" situation from recurring.

While motives for prolonging life are sometimes mixed, it may still be maintained that the prolongation is always in the infant's interests. This position is justified if life is assumed to be an absolute value, separable from any quality of life consideration. The assumption has often been associated with an essentially religious perspective, such as that of the Roman Catholic Church in its teaching regarding abortion. Yet religious reasons may also be given, from that tradition as well as from others, for the contrary view, namely, that life is an important but relative value.[48] Christian Science argues against any kind of medical intervention as impeding the natural course of God's plan among human beings.[49] Jehovah's Witnesses argue more selectively against blood transfusions, allowing that deaths which occur through loss of blood fulfill God's will.[50] If faith in divine omniscience and omnipotence is assumed, it may in fact be blasphemous to maintain that human beings can either prolong or shorten life. If faith in an afterlife is affirmed, death may sometimes be construed as preferable to life on earth.

Several nonreligious factors also support an assertion of the absolute value of an infant's life. One may be described as "the uncertainty principle," which applies to infancy more than to other periods of (extrauterine) human existence. While neonatology has achieved wondrous things in recent years, and programs for facilitating maximum development of disabled children have yielded impressive results, it remains impossible to predict with certainty what the subjective or objective future experience of a particular newborn will be.[51] Most clinicians have in their reservoir of experience recollections of minor and major "miracles," that is, cases whose happy outcome was totally unexpected in light of the facts known at the time and the technology available. I think, for example, of an infant born with heart defects so grave that none similarly afflicted had ever been known to survive, whose recovery after surgery changed the mortality rate applicable to others. However, in this particular case, the issue was mainly a choice between probable death and an extremely slim chance of survival with neurological normalcy (or relative normalcy), rather than a choice between death and survival at a level of extreme neurological compromise.

Another relevant feature of newborn status or the status of children in general is the obvious contrast between them and adults with regard to the span of life already lived and that anticipated. The "right to life" is sometimes more compelling when asserted on behalf of those who have scarcely lived, which partly explains why children's deaths seem more tragic than those of the elderly. In some respects, new life signifies the fullness of hope, which may be dashed through death. On the other hand, in the case of a neonate, there has been little time and opportunity to build the affective ties that make death so painful for a loved one's survivors.

If the interests of the infant are primary, I do not believe that features peculiar to infants provide adequate justification for the preservation of any and every newborn's life. Nonetheless, these features do argue persuasively for a conservative approach to the irreversible decision to terminate or not initiate life-prolonging treatment. By "conservative" approach I mean one that seeks to prolong life if there is some real, although small, chance that the continuation is in the infant's own interests. Where there is high probability that this will not be the case, then the same criterion argues against prolonging life. To the extent that prolongation is likely to increase suffering for the child, a decision not to prolong life through technological support may be morally mandatory. It reflects our realization that those that can suffer should not be caused to suffer (guideline 3), and that individuals should not be treated as other than who or what they are (guideline 5). Just as the right to die may be construed as part of an adult's right to life, the same claim may be made with regard to infants. To deny this right to children is to practice what Richard McCormick has called a "racism of the adult world."[52]

AN INFANT'S RIGHT TO DIE

While the priority of the infant's interests suggests that decisions to prolong life will be made much more frequently than decisions to the contrary, that priority also suggests the relevance of "quality of life" considerations. Three types of cases are relevant in this regard. The first and simplest type is where therapy is futile because the underlying condition is irremediably fatal, and therapy would in no way reduce pain to the infant. In other words, survival beyond a few hours or days or weeks is not expected, no matter what is done or not done. Anencephaly, a condition where the infant's brain has failed to develop, is a commonly accepted example of this situation. Even those who claim "quality of life" factors are irrelevant agree that the life of an anencephalic infant need not be prolonged.

The second type of case is less simple: one where repeated, intrusive, painful interventions would prolong the infant's life, possibly for years, but continued life is of dubious benefit to the child. In such a situation, efforts to preserve life are likely to result in a preponderance of negative experiences for the infant without realistic expectation of improvement. The prolongation itself can only occur through multiple medical and surgical intrusions that are sometimes iatrogenic, and generally interfere with the natural course of the body's function. Not infrequently, despite use of analgesics and anesthesia, the interventions are also painful.

Consider, for example, an infant with the chromosomal abnormality trisomy 13, which involves profound mental retardation and frequent seizures for the 18 percent who survive beyond the first year of life.[53] Often, these infants face immediate life-threatening problems such as severe heart defects. Correction of these and concomitant problems requires multiple surgeries, medical and orthopedic interventions, and permanent hospitalization. To prolong life through invasive procedures might serve the interests of parents and clinicians, but can scarcely be judged to serve those of the infants themselves. The decision to let such an infant die is usually based on the fallible judgment that prolonging life will cause the child a preponderance of suffering.

The third type of case is more problematic than the preceding: one where the required therapy is not itself a source of pain, but neither is it curative, and the life thus prolonged is probably devoid of any qualitative satisfaction for the infant. Consider, for instance, a newborn who has had a Grade IV cranial hemorrhage (bleeding into the cerebral tissues) with uncontrollable seizures, whose intestines have necrotized. The child can only be fed through parenteral hyperalimentation, a process by which predigested food is infused into the body. The combination of the hemorrhage and seizures indicates high probability that the child might survive but only at a vegetative level of existence, that is, without any cognitive function or capacity for social interchange. Although such a child might survive for years, it is doubtful that his survival is in anyone's interest, including his own. Unless life is an end in itself, rather than a necessary condition for the actualization of human values and potential, maintaining life in these circumstances may be exploiting the child, that is, using him as a means of furthering others' ends.

A claim that infants' interests include the right to die may be based on a conception of life that is not merely quantitative.[54] Life is then perceived as a crucial but relative value, extremely significant as the basis of all other human values, but not absolute. This view necessarily involves the notion that quality of life factors are essential to any full affirmation of the value of human life. However, which factors are relevant, and how they are relevant, remains problematic.

Decisions made in behalf of incompetent or unconscious adults may enlighten us with regard to infants. Either of two approaches is generally followed with adults: (1) the decision is based on the patient's history, that is, an understanding of the patient's desires or values as applicable to such a situation (as expressed, for example, in a living will or other form of advance directive), or (2) utilization of the "reasonable person" standard, that is, determination of treatment and nontreatment on the basis of what any competent, conscious person would reasonably choose in similar circumstances. Obviously the first approach is inapplicable to newborns, but the second seems appropriate even though infants may not be described as "reasonable persons."[55] If, for example, a reasonable person would decline surgery that could in no way benefit her, and might in fact prolong a predominantly painful existence, why might we not invoke this criterion to justify a similar decision for an infant? In all three types of cases, that criterion would apply. Thus, in situations where (1) therapy is futile, (2) where it would prolong a life of predominant anguish, or (3) where the patient has suffered irreparable neurological devastation, the decision not to prolong life beyond its natural limits is reasonable, and should be respected as such. To reject the applicability of this standard to infants or children suggests complicity in what we have already described as adult racism. It thus stands opposed to an egalitarian perspective.

GIVING PRIORITY TO INFANTS' INTERESTS

Where individuals attempt to observe the priority of infants' interests, the nuances of particular cases may be interpreted in light of certain distinctions. For example, natural law theology has long invoked the distinction between "ordinary" and "extraordinary" treatment, claiming that the former is obligatory while the latter is not. Ordinary and extraordinary treatment is explained as relative to the unique circumstances of the case, including the accessibility of necessary technology and therapy.[56] Thus, what might count as extraordinary treatment of a cancer-ridden elderly patient who has indicated a desire to die may be ordinary in dealing with a newborn, whether seriously ill or not. Similarly, a distinction between optimal and maximal care is pertinent: maximal care means prolonging life no matter what the cost to the patient; optimal care means prolonging life only to the extent that the prolongation is in the patient's interests.[57] Maximal care may (inadvertently) serve the interests of others—for example, students who can gain more clinical experience by continuing care for the dying; it may simultaneously impede optimal care for the patient. An obligation to provide optimal care implies that others' interests do not constitute a sufficient criterion for refusal of treatment, while those interests may be relevant in applying the ordinary versus extraordinary distinction.

Clinical interpretations that have served as guides for individuals addressing problematic cases include a distinction between "coercing" and "helping" someone to live, and between "doing to" and "doing for" a patient.[58] Roughly, "coercing " and "doing to" constitute unjustifiable intrusions, while "helping" and "doing for" are justifiable because they are oriented toward the patient's own interests. Determination of where the distinctions apply remains difficult, and may never be made with absolute certainty, but some cases involve a very high expectation that survival will mean prolonged and unmitigated misery for a particular patient, child or adult. An example of coercing someone to live might be a situation where a patient experiencing the terminal stage of an incurable cancer has suffered kidney failure that is treatable by dialysis. Performing corrective cardiac surgery on an infant with an incurable and fatal genetic abnormality may be another. In such cases, the right to die, as part of the right to life, seems an undeniable component of patient rights.

Another relevant distinction is between "defensive" and patient-centered medicine. Increasingly and unfortunately, "defensive medicine" (that is, medicine practiced to avoid legal entanglements) has motivated clinicians to prolong lives in cases where there is persuasive evidence that this is not in the best interests of the patient. In 1983, James Strain, as president of the American Academy of Pediatrics, wrote that today's pediatricians have a different view from those interviewed for a 1977 national survey that disclosed that the majority would acquiesce to parental refusal of lifesaving surgery for seriously disabled infants.[59] At this point in time, he alleged, physicians would not accede to the refusal. A 1988 survey of pediatricians in Massachusetts by I. David Todres confirmed Strain's thesis.[60] Todres found that physicians were less inclined to give priority to parents' wishes and more inclined to treat disabled infants than they were ten years earlier. Unfortunately, some erroneously believe they are legally obliged to treat disabled infants more aggressively than others. In the interest of "defensive medicine," disabled newborns are then subjected to the discrimination of overtreatment.

Medical as well as moral decisions continually need to be reassessed in light of the changing condition of the patient. Thus a decision to prolong life may be reversed because a patient's condition has so gravely deteriorated that the prognosis is one of overwhelming misery for him. For example, extremely premature or very low birth weight babies who have been kept alive through intubation immediately after birth may fail to develop independent respiratory function, and suffer further internal malfunction such as renal failure and cerebral hemorrhage. As already suggested, such instances, which are increasing in our neonatal intensive care units, argue that a distinction between a very ill and impaired infant is not a clear one; in fact, illnesses that can be cured may induce permanent and profound disabilities through the very process by which the infant's life is prolonged.[61]

Similarly, decisions not to prolong life need to be continually reassessed in light of the infant's progress. Because clinical judgments are fallible, certain patients may outlive (both qualitatively and quantitatively) a decision not to provide lifesaving treatment in their behalf. Where that occurs, a decision to terminate or not to initiate treatment needs to be reviewed, and aggressive treatment instituted, continuing so long as there is reasonable expectation that the infant's interests will thus be served. The fact that mistakes in judgment occur in ethical as well as clinical dilemmas in no way argues that the judgments themselves are wrong or right in the context of what was known at the time. Only in the long run do such results justifiably exert an influence on subsequent decisions. They do so then because of the knowledge built up over time, providing the rational basis for a general way of acting.

BABY DOE REVISITED

The decision to allow Bloomington's Baby Doe to die could not be justified on the basis of the priority criterion discussed here. In light of what we know about children with Down syndrome, it is more likely that this infant's interests would be best served by overriding the parents' refusal of lifesaving treatment for him. The therapy was not futile, the prognosis was not one of neurological devastation, and the predominant future experiences of the child might well have been positive for him. Moreover, while the parents preferred not to raise the child, adoption was a viable option. In fact, a number of couples, two of whom already had children with Down syndrome, offered to adopt Baby Doe before he died. This is a significant factor because actual promotion of infants' interests depends on the attitudes and resources of those who might (or might not) care for them, including government agencies. If a challenge to parental preference for withholding treatment does not address ways by which ongoing care will be provided, the challenge itself may pose a threat to the child's best interests.

In contrast to the Bloomington situation, the case of Baby Jane Doe was one where the priority of the infant's interests may have justified refusal of treatment. *If* the reported facts were correct (e.g., the prognosis that the child "would never experience joy, never experience sorrow"),[62] the option here was between intervention that would allow an extended period of life in a neurologically devastated state; and nonintervention that would permit gradual deterioration, with death occurring sometime during infancy. Obviously, the degree of uncertainty regarding these possibilities was a critical factor. Whether the child's medical problems and condition predict-

ed a predominantly negative experience for her was crucial in determining the applicability of the criterion. However, if there were a high probability that this was so, the priority of the child's interests would be observed by foregoing medical interventions. In other words, the infant's right to life in such circumstances might best be respected by supporting her right to die. The parents' decision to respect that right was apparently motivated by a desire to place the interests of their child before their own: their ethic of care reasoned that love (especially parental love) occasionally means letting go of the one loved.

If the facts reported are correct, then the main difference between these cases is the probability that the future experience of one child would be predominantly positive for him, and the other child's future experience would probably be predominantly negative for her. Because of their differing prognoses, one infant's right to life had priority, and the other's right to die had priority. From an egalitarian perspective that respects differences among individual infants, each deserves to be treated differently.

Notes

1. "Nondiscrimination on the Basis of Handicaps; Procedures and Guidelines Relating to Health Care for Handicapped Infants," *Federal Register* (Jan. 12, 1984) 49: 1622-54: "Big Brother Doe," *Wall Street Journal* (Oct. 31, 1983), 20; "Baby Jane's Big Brothers," *New York Times* (Nov. 4, 1983), 28; and Mary B. Mahowald and Jerome Paulson, "The Baby Does: Two Different Situations," *The Cleveland Plain Dealer* (Dec. 31, 1983), 9-A.

2. Much of the material in this chapter is adapted from two of my earlier articles: "Ethical Decisions in Neonatal Intensive Care," in *Human Values in Critical Care Medicine,* ed. Stuart Youngner (Philadelphia: Praeger Publishers, 1986), and "In the Interest of Infants," *Philosophy in Context* 14, no. 9 (1984): 9-18.

3. William H. Tooley and Roderick H. Phibbs, "Neonatal Intensive Care: The State of the Art," in *Ethics of Newborn Intensive Care,* ed. Albert R. Jonsen and Michael J. Garland (San Francisco: Health Policy Program, University of California, 1976), 11-15.

4. Tooley and Phibbs, 11-15.

5. Barbara C. Tilley, "Assessment of Risks from DES," in *The Custom-Made Child?* ed. Helen B. Holmes, Betty B. Hoskins, and Michael Gross (Clifton, New Jersey: Humana Press, 1981), 29-39. Concerning ineffectiveness of the therapy, see W. J. Dieckmann, M. D. Davis, L. M. Rynkiewiez, et al., "Does Administration of Diethylstilbestrol During Pregnancy Have Therapeutic Value?" *American Journal of Obstetrics and Gynecology* 66, no. 5 (Nov. 1953): 1062-81. Concerning cancer and reproductive complications in offspring, see Arthur L. Herbst and Diane Anderson, "Clear Cell Adenocarcinoma of the Vagina and Cervix Secondary to Intrauterine Exposure to Diethylstilbestrol," *Seminars in Surgical Oncology* 6 (1990): 343-46; and Raymond H. Kaufman, Kenneth Noller, Ervin Adam, et al., "Upper Genital Tract Abnormalities and Pregnancy Outcome in Diethylstilbestrol-Exposed Progeny," *American Journal of Obstetrics and Gynecology,* 148, no. 7 (April 1, 1984): 973-82.

6. Marshall H. Klaus and Avroy Fanaroff, *Care of the High-Risk Neonate* (Philadelphia: W. B. Saunders, 1973), xi.

7. Mildred T. Stahlman, "Neonatal Intensive Care: Success or Failure," *Journal of Pediatrics* 105 (1984): 162-67.

8. Jay Goldsmith and Robert Arensman, "Predicting the Failure of Mechanical Ventilation: New Therapeutic Options," *Neonatal Intensive Care* 3 (1990): 40-47. Data supporting success rates in treatment of all four conditions are available through the Extracorporeal Life Support Registry, University of Michigan, 1991.

9. Richard Martin, "Neonatal Surfactant Therapy—Where Do We Go from Here?" *Journal of Pediatrics* 118, no. 4 (April 1991): 555-56; and T. Allen Merritt, Mikko Hallman, Charles Berry, et al., "Randomized, Placebo-Controlled Trial of Human Surfactant Given at Birth Versus Rescue Administration in Very Low Birth Weight Infants with Lung Immaturity," *Journal of Pediatrics* 118, no. 4 (April 1991): 581-94.

10. Maureen Hack, B. Caron, Ann Rivers, and Avroy Fanaroff, "The Very Low Birth Weight Infant: The Broader Spectrum of Morbidity during Infancy and Early Childhood," *Journal of Developmental and Behavioral Pediatrics* 4, no. 4 (Dec. 1983): 243-49.

11. Maureen Hack, Ann Rivers, and Avroy Fanaroff, "Outcomes of Extremely Low Birth Weight Infants between 1982 and 1988," *New England Journal of Medicine* 321, no 24 (Dec 14, 1989): 1642-47.

12. See Maureen Hack, Jeffery D. Horbar, Michael H. Malloy, et al., "Very Low Birth Weight Outcomes of the National Institute of Child Health and Human Development Neonatal Network," *Pediatrics,* 87, no. 5 (May 1991): 587-97.

13. Laila Williamson, "Infanticide: An Anthropological Analysis," in *Infanticide and the Value of Life,* ed. Marvin Kohl (Buffalo, New York: Prometheus Books, 1978), 61-75.

14. James Rachels, "Active and Passive Euthanasia," *New England Journal of Medicine* 292, no. 2 (Jan. 9, 1975): 78-80.

15. John J. Paris and Anne B. Fletcher, "Infant Doe Regulations and the Absolute Requirement to Use Nourishment and Fluids for the Dying Infant," *Law, Medicine and Health Care* 11 (1983): 210-13.

16. Robert Weir, *Selective Nontreatment of Handicapped Infants: Moral Dilemmas in Neonatal Medicine* (New York: Oxford University Press, 1984), 215-21.

17. Anthony Shaw, "Dilemmas of 'Informed Consent' in Children," *New England Journal of Medicine* 289, no 17 (Oct. 25, 1973): 885-90.

18. President's Commission for the Study of Ethical Problems in Medicine and Biomedical and Behavioral Research, *Making Health Care Decisions,* vol. 3, Appendices: Studies on the Foundations of Informed Consent (Washington D.C.: U.S. Government Printing Office, 1982), 175-245.

19. Gina Kolata, "Parents of Tiny Infants Find Care Choices Are Not Theirs," *New York Times* (Sept. 30, 1991), 1 and A11.

20. Hack, Rivers, and Fanaroff, 243-49.

21. H.E. Ehrhardt, "Abortion and Euthanasia: Common Problems—the Termination of Developing and Expiring Life," *Human Life Review* 1 (1975): 12-31.

22. See articles in *The Herald-Telephone,* Bloomington, Indiana, April 23 and May 1-3, 1982, and *The Criterion,* Indianapolis, Indiana, April 23, 1982. Also see Weir, 128-29.

23. U.S. Department of Health and Human Services, "Interim Final Rule 45 CFR Part 84, Nondiscrimination on the Basis of a Handicap," *Federal Register* 48 (March 7, 1983), 9630-32.

24. Barbara J. Culliton, "Baby Doe Regs Thrown Out by Court," *Science* 220 (April 29, 1983):479-80.

25. It should be noted that the reported facts and media coverage of this case have been disputed, and the infant fared better than had been anticipated. In time, the parents consented to surgery for treatment of the hydrocephalus, her spinal lesion closed naturally, and her parents took her home from the hospital the following spring. See Steven Baer, "The Half-told Story of Baby Jane Doe," *Columbia Journalism Review* (Nov./Dec., 1984), 35-38; and "Baby Doe at Age 1: A Joy and Burden," *New York Times* (Oct. 14, 1984), Sect. 1, 56.

26. See note 1.

27. U.S. Department of Health and Human Services, "Child Abuse and Neglect Prevention and Treatment Program; Final Rule," *Federal Register* 50 (Jan. 11, 1985), 1487-92.

28. Betty W. Levin, "Consensus and Controversy in the Treatment of Catastrophically Ill Newborns," in *Which Babies Shall Live?* (Clifton, New Jersey: Humana Press, 1985), 169-205.

29. See President's Commission for the Study of Ethical Problems in Medicine and Biomedical and Behavioral Research, *Deciding to Forego Life-Sustaining Treatment, A Report of the Ethical, Medical, and Legal Issues in Treatment Decisions* (Washington, D. C.: Government Printing Office, March 1983), 214-22; James Strain, "The American Academy of Pediatrics' Comments on the 'Baby Doe II' Regulations," *New England Journal of Medicine* 309, no. 7 (Aug. 18, 1983): 443-44; and *Handicapped Americans Report (July 14, 1983),6.*

30. That neonatologists' interpretations of the best interest standard are widely divergent is evident in statements attributed to them by Elisabeth Rosenthal in "As More Tiny Infants Live, Choices and Burden Grow," *New York Times* (Sept. 29, 1991), 1. John Arras has addressed the limitations of this standard in his "Toward an Ethic of Ambiguity," *Hastings Center Report* 14, no. 2 (April 1984): 30-31.

31. See, for example, Paul Ramsey, *The Patient as Person* (New Haven, Connecticut: Yale University Press, 1970), 1-11; see also note 18.

32. Bernard M. Dickens, "Legally Informed Consent," in *Contemporary Issues in Biomedical Ethics,* ed. John W. Davis, Barry Hoffmaster, and Sarah Shorten (Clifton, New Jersey: Humana Press, 1978), 199-204.

33. David Thomasma, "Beyond Medical Paternalism and Patient Autonomy: A Model of Physician-Patient Relationship," *Annals of Internal Medicine* 98 (Feb. 1983): 243-48; and Thomas S. Szasz and Marc H. Hollender, "The Basic Models of the Doctor-Patient Relationship," *Archives of Internal Medicine* 97 (1956): 585-92.

34. Fyador Dostoyevsky, "The Grand Inquisitor," in *The Brothers Karamazov* (New York: Modern Library, 1950), 255-74.

35. Anthony Shaw, Judson G. Randolph, and Barbara B. Manard, "Ethical Issues in Pediatric Surgery: A National Survey of Pediatricians and Pediatric Surgeons," *Pediatrics* 60 (1977):590

36. Lawrence A. Rosini, Mary C. Howell, David Todres and John J. Dorman, "Group Meetings in a Pediatric Intensive Care Unit," *Pediatrics* 53 (1974): 371-74.

37. Richard A. McCormick, "Ethics Committees: Promise or Peril?" *Law, Medicine and Health Care* 12 (1984): 150-55; ; and Mary B. Mahowald, "Hospital Ethics Committees: Diverse and Problematic" *Newsletter on Philosophy and Medicine (American Philosophical Association)* 88, no. 2 (March 1989): 88-94, reprinted in HEC *Forum* 1 (1989): 237-46 and in *Bioethics News* 2 (1990): 4-13.

38. Alan R. Fleischman and Thomas Murray, "Ethics Committees for Infants Doe?" *Hastings Center Report* 13, no. 6 (Dec. 1983): 5-9.

39. James Strain, "The American Academy of Pediatrics' Comments on the 'Baby Doe II' Regulations," *New England Journal of Medicine* 309, no. 7 (Aug. 18, 1983): 443-44.

40. U.S. Department of Health and Human Services, "Nondiscrimination on the Basis of Handicap: Procedures and Guidelines Relating to Health Care for Handicapped Infants," *Federal Register* 49 (Jan. 12, 1984), 1651.

41. President's Commission for the Study of Ethical Problems in Medicine and Biomedical and Behavioral Research, 227.

42. American Academy of Pediatrics, *Guidelines for Infant Bioethics Committees* (Evanston, Illinois: American Academy of Pediatrics, 1984).

43. See Mary B. Mahowald, "Hospital Ethics Committees: Diverse and Problematic," 88-94. I have attempted to evaluate infant ethics committees in "Baby Doe Committees: A Critical Evaluation," *Cur-*

rent Controversies in Perinatal Care 15, no. 4 (Dec. 1988), 789-800.

44. Joan E. Hoggman, "Withholding Treatment from Seriously Ill Newborns: A Neonatologist's View," in *Legal and Ethical Aspects of Treating Critically and Terminally Ill Patients,* ed. A. Edward Doudera, J.D., and J. Douglas Peters, J.D. (Ann Arbor, Michigan: AUPHA Press, 1982), 243. Note, however, that living more *easily* with the consequences of something one has done is not equivalent to moral justification for doing it.

45. See August Kasper, "The Doctor and Death," in *Moral Problems in Medicine,* ed. Samuel Gorowitz, Andrew L. Jameton, Ruth Macklin, John M. O'Connor, Eugene V. Perrin, Beverly Page St. Clair, and Susan Sherwin (Englewood Cliffs, New Jersey: Prentice Hall, Inc., 1976), 69-72.

46. Brenda Miller, at a health care team meeting, Pediatric Intensive Care Unit, Rainbow Babies and Childrens Hospital, Cleveland, Ohio, September 27, 1983.

47. See Susan Schmidt, "Wrongful Life,*" Journal of the American Medical Association* 250, no. 16 (Oct. 28, 1983): 2209-10: "Of all the birth-related legal theories, wrongful life, and action filed on behalf of the infant born with a genetic or other congenital birth defect, has met with the most disapproval."

48. For example, Richard McCormick, "To Save or Let Die," *Journal of the American Medical Association* 229, no. 2 (July 8, 1974): 174-45.

49. *Academic American Encyclopedia*, vol. 4 (Danbury, Connecticut: Grolier Press, 1983), 412.

50. *Academic American Encyclopedia* vol. 11, 394.

51. See Carson Strong, "The Tiniest Newborns," *Hastings Center Report* 13, no. 1 (Feb. 1983): 14-19.

52. Richard McCormick, "Experimental Subjects—Who Should They Be?" *Journal of the American Medical Association* 235, no. 20 (May 17, 1976): 2197.

53. Kenneth Lyons Jones, *Smith's Recognizable Patterns of Human Malformation,* 4th ed. (Philadelphia: W. B. Saunders, 1988), 20-21.

54. See Hans Jonas, "The Right to Die," *Hastings Center Report* 8, no. 4 (Aug. 1978): 36: "Fully understood, it [i.e., the right to life] also includes the right to death."

55. Norman Fost applies this standard to infants under the aegis of "ideal observer theory" in "Ethical Issues in the Treatment of Critically Ill Newborns," *Pediatric Annals* 10, no.10 (Oct. 1981): 21. Jonathan Glover has a similar suggestion for dealing with infants. He claims that the best substitute for asking whether they wish to go on living (since they cannot register their own preferences) is "to ask whether we ourselves would find such a life preferable to death." See Jonathan Glover, *Causing Death and Saving Lives* (New York: Penguin, 1977), 161.

56. See Gerald Kelly, *Medico-Moral Problems* (St. Louis, Missouri: The Catholic Hospital Association, 1958), 129. For an excellent critique of this distinction, see James Rachels, *The End of Life* (New York: Oxford University Press, 1986), 96-100.

57. My formulation here is different from that of David Smith, who identifies "maximal" with "extraordinary," and "optimal" with "ordinary." See David H. Smith, "On Letting Some Babies Die," *Hastings Center Studies* 2, no. 2 (May 1974): 44. I return to the concept of "optimal care" in Chapter 15.

58. These are distinctions employed by pediatricians with whom I have worked: the first by Donald Schussler, M.D., the second by Jeffery Blumer, M.D., Ph.D., both working in the Division of Critical Care, Rainbow Babies and Childrens's Hospital, Cleveland, Ohio, during the 1980's.

59. James Strain, "The Decision to Forego Life-Sustaining Treatment for Seriously Ill Newborns," *Pediatrics* 72, no. 4 (Oct. 1983): 572. Strain was comparing the pediatricians of 1983 with those interviewed for studies published in 1977 based on data obtained several years earlier. See, for example, Shaw, Randolph, and Manard, 588; and I. David Todres, Diane Krane, Mary C. Howell, et al., "Pediatricians' Attitudes Affecting Decision-Making in Defective Newborns," *Pediatrics* 6, no. 2 (Aug. 1977), 197-201.

60. Kolata, 1, A11; and I. David Todres, Jeanne Guillemin, Michael A. Grodin, and Dick Batten, "Life-Saving Therapy for Newborn: A Questionnaire Survey in the State of Massachusetts," *Pediatrics* 81, no. 5 (May 1988):643.

61. See Note 7.

62. My analysis here is crucially dependent on the accuracy of the reported facts and of the prognosis associated with them. As indicated in note 25, both were disputed in subsequent accounts of the case.

30

CHOOSING CHILDREN'S SEX: CHALLENGES TO FEMINIST ETHICS

Helen Bequaert Holmes

If the person is from a month old up to five years old, your valuation shall be for a male five shekels of silver, and for a female your valuation shall be three shekels of silver.

—Leviticus 27:6.

WHEN THE STORK
DELIVERS A BOY
OUR WHOLE
DARN FACTORY
JUMPS FOR JOY
BURMA SHAVE

—1963 Burma-Shave roadside rhyme.

IT'S A BOY!

—Great Moments 1992 Michelob Beer television commercial.

From prehistory through the twentieth century, the preference has been for males—as tiny newborns, as teenage athletes, as senators, whatever. Females may be preferred for one or another specific purpose, such as gestating fetuses or changing diapers or caring for the senile, but not in general. Those who *simply* prefer females or who genuinely have no preference are in the minority.

Choosing the sex of a future child, or choosing *not* to choose, is no longer a hypothetical issue. Wherever "Western" medicine is practiced, pregnant upper-and middle-class women receive ultrasound scans of their fetuses and are told the sex unless they assertively preempt the message by begging nurse, doctor, or technician to keep the secret. For unplanned pregnancies— and for some planned ones—the idea must flit through each woman's head: shall sex influence my choice to abort?

Unless targeted killing of female fetuses occurs, the normal secondary sex ratio—the ratio at birth—in human populations is 50 females to 53 males.[1] Unless female infanticide or neglect occurs, this reaches 50:50 in the early teens: boys are more vulnerable to childhood diseases and accidents. In the United States, by the age of marriage this ratio has skewed to 52 females for every 50 males; as people age, the ratio becomes more skewed —for example, to 50:20 at age 85.[2] In an extensive study of human sex ratios, Guttentag and Secord found that throughout history in various geographical locations, sex ratios have been highly skewed—from losses in war, mass migrations of men, or such cultural practices as child neglect and infanticide. Their review of the effects of various ratios on peoples' lives shows that, in general— although there are many exceptions—women seem to benefit most when sex ratios are close to 50:50. When their proportion is lower, women may be confined to traditional gender roles and excluded from high-status positions; when their proportion is higher, misogyny increases, and women are likely to be exploited in sexual relationships and have difficulty in finding committed male partners.[3] Although I have deliberately oversimplified here to argue *for* the 50:50 society, a biased sex ratio might indeed *benefit* women, given certain power relationships between the sexes in a given society. Mary Anne Warren, author of the first major book on sex selection, presents a thorough and thoughtful analysis of the nuanced implications of Guttentag and Secord's discussion.[4]

In what follows, I plan to show how the case of choosing a child's sex raises perplexing questions about legitimate use of autonomy and can get us into hot water as we attempt to apply feminist theory and feminist ethics to reproductive medicine. First, I shall select and examine some arguments supporting sex selection and then some arguments opposing it. My aim here is not to be comprehensive nor to survey the considerable literature on the ethical issues, but merely to introduce themes for in-depth analysis later.[5] For further background, I'll summarize the state of the art—what is technically possible now in sex detection and sex determination. Then I shall describe how certain aspects of the technology foster commercialization of sex selection by "hoaxers, incompetents, madmen, and cranks, as well as scientists."[6] After discussing the special case of sex-linked diseases and the feminist issues they raise, I turn to four challenges to feminist ethics for which sex selection is an ideal exemplar. I conclude by outlining difficulties that hinder the formulation of effective and just policies on sex selection, policies that can foster feminist goals.

Sex selection has been called a "paradigm, a type case, for policy decisions about genetic engineering in general."[7] Further, it is perhaps the best type case for applying feminist ethics to *all* reproductive technologies, not just to genetic engineering. One commonly used type case, infertility "treatment" (artificial insemination, in vitro fertilization [IVF], etc.) applies to only one-tenth of the population; another, prenatal diagnosis of genetic anomalies, is relevant in even fewer pregnancies. However, since *every* fetus is "at risk" for sex, every pregnancy is at risk for sex selection. Furthermore, sex selection is no pipe dream: some techniques—not, of course, the hoaxes—are now completely effective.

In my arguments I make no moral distinction between preconception and post-conception sex selection. If a couple wishes to choose the sex of their child but does not do so because it involves abortion, the *desire*, in my view, is the moral issue. Potential consumers of sex selection technologies, however, are likely to make a strong distinction between preconception and postconception methods. The reasons someone does not abort a fetus of the "wrong" sex may be practical, political, social, or moral: for example, cost, refusal of a doctor to cooperate, fear of objections from friends or relatives, religious dictum, bonding already with that fetus, a state law, a belief that elective abortion is immoral. Commercial methods that purport to select sex are more likely to succeed in attracting the public when they use *preconception* sex selection methods and preempt the variety of reasons people have for not selecting sex via abortion.

ARGUMENTS FOR SEX SELECTION

Several reasons have been advanced for letting people choose their children's sex. First, of course, is freedom of choice—we should have the right to do anything we wish as long as it doesn't harm other people. This includes using the advances of technology to exercise our freedom—for example, taking the Concorde to Paris to visit the Louvre or selecting the sex composition of our family. According to Bill Allen, a prospective father interviewed on the 1981 *Hard Choices* "Boy or Girl?" TV program, "Why shouldn't we have the right ... to do that sort of [family] planning?"[8]

Of course, such a person would not select sex unless he or she believed that it would increase happiness—for one or both parents and for the selected child. Warren considers in depth the happiness aspect of the free choice argument, pointing out the dangers inherent in unrealistic expectations of one's child. Yet she concludes, "Getting what one wants is not a guarantee of happiness, but it is usually a good deal more conducive to happiness than *not* getting what one wants."[9]

Acquiring a "balanced family" is yet another facet of the happiness and free choice argument. One nonsexist justification for trying to achieve such a family is that children would grow up without sex bias, that girls would learn to get along with boys and vice versa. Balance (for whatever reason) is very important to upper- and middle-class parents in North America. In her analysis of 2505 letters written by couples wishing to have sperm separation for selection, Nan Chico found that 86 percent of the writers gave balance (not necessarily using that term) as an important reason for applying.[10] (And how many of us have said when visiting a new baby, "How nice to have one of each!") The search for balance is a key reason why parents can be victims of unproved sex selection schemes and the motivation for most sex selection case studies in textbooks: "Mr. and Mrs. X have three daughters; Mrs. X discovers that she is pregnant...."

Christine Overall, whose book is a feminist analysis of reproductive technologies, argues persuasively for another nonsexist and morally acceptable reason to prefer a child of a certain sex. Putting a strong emphasis on experience, she claims that sex preferences in "the lived experience of close human relationships" are not necessarily sexist.

[F]undamental differences between the experiences of the sexes are not just the result of socialization, but they are not just biological either, since they are constituted by our *awareness* of the capacities unique to our sex.

If one's sex is central to one's own identity, then ... the sex of other persons will be significant in ... relationships involving strong friendship, love and/ or sexual intimacy...[11]

According to Overall, a lesbian's preference for intimate relations with another woman is not sexist. She continues, "One would be seeking a child of a specific sex because of the anticipated rewards and pleasures to be gained through a parenting relationship with a younger human being who is either like oneself or different from oneself in ... sexual identity." Yet she then questions whether this reason is *"sufficient* to justify the practice of sex preselection."[12]

A step beyond *permitting* sex selection is *advocating* it. For example, some physicians favor its use to avoid sex-linked diseases.[13] Even those authors who generally denounce sex selection may sanction it for families at risk of any such disease.[14] Prima facie, this seems to be a straightforward argument for sex selection because sex-linked diseases are relatively common, usually afflict only males, and are often devastating or lethal in their effects. Yet a feminist ethics sees a nuanced mesh of complications in what seems to be a clear argument—so important that I discuss the mesh separately below.

Population control is yet another reason proposed for choosing sex, that is, for choosing males. John Postgate claimed in 1973 that overpopulation is "the only really important problem facing humanity today."[15] The argument that selecting males can ameliorate overpopulation is mathematically sound: equations used in population ecology show clearly that rates of population growth decrease when the proportion of females in a population drops. The population control movement has long advocated male selection: Ehrlich in his 1968 *Population Bomb;* Postgate, who in 1973 urged stopping "multiplication in ... unenlightened communities"; Luce, who in 1978 proposed "the manchild pill"; and, recently and cautiously, Kuhse and Singer.[16]

Feminists might claim that if sex choice were practiced universally, then all girls who exist would be

wanted as girls. Many women suffer because they've been unwanted—in a family, in a job, in a classroom—simply because of their sex. So why not spare the next generation this pain? We have no way to measure how much or how little suffering would be prevented by knowing that one was wanted only for one's sex (and hence to play some sex role), wanted to be a little sister for a firstborn male, or wanted to balance a family. And, as a perceptive Spelman College student once pointed out to me, what her father expected of a boy would have made life very difficult for his son, and she thus was better off as an obviously unwanted girl.

However, wantedness or unwantedness in an affluent American family is trivial compared to the neglect, abuse, and even death suffered by girls in such countries as India, China, and Korea.[17] Therefore logic might dictate that feminists concerned about women worldwide should aggressively advocate the development of cheap, safe, and effective means of male sex selection--a much stronger stance than simply considering the process morally permissible. This blends into another feminist argument for sex selection—mere survival of adult women. Mothers who have only daughters in India and China, for example, undergo ostracism, are at risk for suicide, and often face beatings, divorce, or fatal "accidents."[18]

An assertively feminist reason for selecting children's sex is to use it as a strategy for resistance to patriarchy. Warren argues that some feminists might choose to have sons to raise them to be nonsexist; others might raise daughters in order not to contribute to the ruling sex class or to establish all-female communities. Although, in her view, these uses of sex selection are ways in which women may resist male domination, sex selection in itself will not be sufficient to overthrow that domination. Warren argues that these tactics are not "a substitute for any of the substantive goals of feminism," and "to the extent that these goals are met, interest in selecting sex will decline."[19]

ARGUMENTS AGAINST SEX SELECTION
Few doubt that if sex selection were cheap and effective, many more males than females would be born. From this Amitai Etzioni postulated dire consequences: more crime, less culture and churchgoing, "the rougher features of a frontier town."[20] If fewer

men can marry, this is likely to have a negative impact on their health and longevity.[21]

Sex selection literature often emphasizes the desire of most prospective parents for a firstborn male. Are girls handicapped if they are not first-borns? Most authors who take an anti-selection stance argue that they are. However, after surveying the literature, Warren adopts the opposite view. Strongly influenced by the conclusions of Ernst and Angst, who in 1983 reviewed the results of some 1500 studies, Warren states, "Nearly all of the reports of birth-order effects are due to errors in the design of the studies and the analysis of the data.... [I]t would seem that virtually any outcome can be 'explained' in terms of birth order, but that no particular outcome can ever be predicted."[22]

Another argument counteracts the population control advocates: use of sex selection for such a purpose is not only morally suspect, but might have the opposite effect—it might actually *increase* population. First on the moral question here, Warren and I have each pointed out the pernicious misogyny, racism, and classism of eliminating females to control populations.[23] If a cheap chemical to put in drinking water, a pill or an injection were developed, its use might be required for under-developed countries, say, to get World Bank loans or to become "most favored nation" trading partner of the United States. Second, there is the mathematical argument that selecting males might lead to higher population because a shortage of women is likely to change other numbers in the population equation as well. For example, the fact that women were few might cause governments to decree (or might cause customs to arise among the people for) an earlier age for first childbearing, shorter intervals between children, or prohibition of the lesbian lifestyle—all of which would tend to increase population.

Many feminists and their sympathizers argue vehemently that any sex selection is sexist: "one of the most stupendously sexist acts in which it is possible to engage"[24]; that it moves us into the "realm of previc-timization ... women being destroyed and sacrificed before even being born"[25]; that "a preference for one sex over the other, for its own sake, is simply sexism.... [M]any of the most common instrumental rea-

sons [for desiring a child of a particular sex] probably mask an irrational sexism"[26]; or "[A]ny argument for sex selection cannot overcome the unfair and sexist bias of a choice to select the sex of a child."[27]

A variant of the sexism allegation is that exercising sex selection, even if one has nonsexist reasons, reinforces sexism. Consider Overall's response to Warren's arguments that selecting a boy "may be motivated by an unselfish desire to ensure that the child will have the best possible life" and that "poor people have the right to seek to better their economic status by having sons rather than daughters."[28] Warren concludes that these actions and desires may be a result of sexism in society, but are not inherently sexist. Overall, however, holds that such reasons represent "complicity with the patriarchal system," and that choosing sons for these reasons is "still a way of saying yes ... to patriarchal power and the oppression of women."[29]

Many authors believe that sex selection is nothing more than eugenics and base their strongest objections on this. Sex selection clearly fits the definition, "the striving to increase wanted traits in the population."[30] According to Ruth Hubbard, "Eugenics died down in the 1930s ... partly because it didn't work .... We now have a whole series of techniques that *will* do the job. Sex preselection is one of them."[31] Another facet to the discussion is a slippery slope variant: if sex has nothing to do with disease, will we set precedents for attempts to select other non-disease characteristics that many people already include in visualizing their perfect children?[32] Still another consideration is that sex selection may be the entrée into a game of *personal* eugenics. Previously, we worried about evil dictators imposing eugenics on large populations; now parents may impose it on their children.[33]

Before we ferret out the feminist dilemmas sparked by these arguments and discuss some perplexing questions of public policy, let's take a close look at what currently is technically feasible.

THE STATE OF THE ART

Fetal Sex Detection in the Uterus

With access to modern medical technology, prospective parents almost invariably learn the sex of their fetus. Routine ultrasound in the second trimester can identify sex correctly about 90 percent of the time.[34] Visualization is difficult in obese women and in breech presentations; accuracy depends on the skill of the sonogram readers and the quality of the equipment. Recent improvements in ultrasonography include putting the transducer up the vagina instead of on the abdomen, which has increased the accuracy of ascertainment to about 95 percent.[35] Therefore, except for the possibility of false results (and sonographers usually honestly report any uncertainty about the sex), all couples in Western Europe, North America, and Australasia can, at least in theory, act on a sex preference by requesting abortion.

Two other prenatal diagnostic technologies—chorionic villus sampling (CVS) and amniocentesis—are routinely prescribed to screen for defective fetuses in women over 35. Sex detection is usually incidental in these cases—but the accuracy here is essentially 100 percent (except when vials get mixed or mislabelled).[36] Results from CVS can be reported during the first trimester, and a few centers also do "early amnio," which can give results early in the second trimester before quickening.[37] If one plans to abort for sex, such early data can minimize emotional problems (which often occur after quickening or when the pregnancy shows) or political problems (in locations where second-trimester abortion is not permitted).

To be done properly, ultrasound, amniocentesis, and CVS require costly equipment and skilled technicians; they are done with the pregnant women's knowledge; all three are inconvenient; the latter two are unpleasant and worrisome.[38] Therefore, a 1989 breakthrough in finding fetal cells circulating in women's blood is significant. Because very few fetal blood cells cross the placenta, sophisticated technologies are required to find them, to concentrate them, and then to determine whether they really come from the fetus.[39] These techniques, which have been hailed as potential noninvasive methods of detecting fetal abnormalities, are still quite crude. However, once they get refined, fetal sex might be detected without a woman's knowledge after a mere needle stick; furthermore, in the current poor state of the art, sex is the trait experimenters must use in working out each technique. (And they must take care not to be fooled by male cells still circulating in

the blood from a previous pregnancy!) Every pregnant woman's fetus has a sex; so any pregnant woman could be recruited for *any* experiment involving sifting through blood for those elusive cells.

Sex Detection in the Test Tube Embryo

Called "preimplantation diagnosis" or "embryo biopsy," analysis of the chromosomes in a cell removed from an early "test tube" embryo has been touted as a marvelous way to prevent the birth of defective infants *without* using abortion.[40] Some mothers of children with cystic fibrosis (CF) would like this method to be perfected so that, by using IVF, they could have an embryo implanted that is free of CF. This would let them avoid the message that abortion of a CF fetus otherwise would give to their living CF child.[41] The techniques take considerable skill, and many bugs must still be worked out. For example, the covering of the early embryo—the zona—must be dissected away for a cell to be removed. The removed cell, of course, is destroyed in the testing, but the remaining cells should be able to form a complete baby with no missing parts.[42] Another caution, however, is the poor success of IVF. Only 16 to 18 percent of transferred embryos result in a "take-home baby,"[43] although with *fertile* couples the percentage might be higher.

But here again, as in the technologies already mentioned, the easiest trait to detect is sex and so the early experiments on preimplantation diagnosis are in sex detection. Most researchers do recruit experimental subjects who are indeed at risk for offspring with sex-linked diseases, and many such women are very eager to participate.[44] Yet, confidence in this method is so low that usually the sex of each implanted fetus is checked later by CVS and by repeated ultrasonography.[45]

Sex Determination before Conception

A logical way to specify sex would be to separate sperm in a semen sample so that either those with X-chromosomes or those with Y-chromosomes are the only ones contacting an egg.[46] A clinic's laboratory might separate the sperm, or an at-home method might use a device or take advantage of some aspect of the female reproductive cycle. Since the 1960s many have played with both at-home and laboratory methods and produced theories for separating or favoring one or another sperm type—imaginative and ingenious theories. But none works. Any proposed theory gets nourished by the fact that the actual 52:50 ratio is really quite good as gambling odds go.

a) *At-home methods*. Folk methods from previous centuries have reappeared disguised in twentieth century medical language. One involves specifying the prospective mother's diet: in modern lingo, minerals in her diet might affect the cervical mucus, the inner surface of the fallopian tubes, or the egg surface and thus allow only one kind of sperm to pass through the cervix, travel up the fallopian tube, or penetrate the egg, as the case may be.[47] But only the diet theorists themselves publish the data to "prove" their theories; there are no independent confirmations. One critic has pointed out that the high calcium in the "girl diet" puts women at risk of kidney problems or excessive nervousness, while the "boy diet" with high salt and very low calcium is especially risky, since it may lead to edema and hypertension.[48]

Other hardy perennials are douches (alkaline for boy; acidic for girl), positions for intercourse (from the rear for boy; missionary for girl); female orgasm (before male orgasm for boy; not at all for girl); frequency of coitus (more for boys).[49] Not all folk methods agree with each other—they are notably discrepant about when, in a woman's cycle, to time intercourse (a really hardy perennial).

Let us scrutinize two conflicting timing theories. According to the Shettles theory, which has been presented to the U. S. public in popular magazines and in three editions of a book written by Landrum Shettles with David Rorvik (1970, 1984, 1989), the Y-bearing sperm are smaller, travel faster up the fallopian tube, and reach the ovary before the X-sperm. If a Y-bearing sperm reaches an egg just as it poofs out of the ovary, it will fertilize the egg and determine a boy; if the Y-sperm have to wait, the somewhat tougher X-sperm will arrive on the scene. For data, Shettles claims to have observed microscopically two different sizes of sperm, with the smaller ones moving more quickly. He also claims that couples who use his method do indeed have boys if they time intercourse close to the moment of ovulation, and girls if intercourse occurs two or three days before ovulation.[50]

However, independent researchers have not corroborated these results; in fact, studies designed to test his results and other studies in which time of fertilization can be correlated with sex of a baby at birth seem to *refute* rather than support Shettles's hypothesis.[51]

In 1977, Elizabeth Whelan proposed a competing theory in her book *Boy or Girl?* She advocated intercourse close to ovulation to obtain a girl and based her theory on reports in the medical literature by Guerrero and by Harlap.[52] Those two researchers' results are suspect, however, because Guerrero's clients were ones who failed at the rhythm method of contraception and Harlap asked mothers to recollect the time of intercourse nine months later, that is, after each baby was born.[53]

In the 1970s and 1980s, disciples who believed in a timing theory used thermal and mucus methods to time ovulation; now, with the advent of ovulation test kits, ovulation can be timed better—but that can't correct a faulty theory.

If any timing theory really worked, selecting sex could be done without telling friends, family, or professionals, and would avoid the intricacies of abortion. Although a partner's cooperation would be useful, it could be controlled by the woman without his knowing by feigning "headaches" or lust, or by appropriate use of the diaphragm. It would be cheap: one could copy instructions from a library book and use the cervical mucus test (free), a basal body temperature thermometer ($6-$10), or an ovulation detection kit ($15-20).

b) *Laboratory sperm separation*. Separation techniques that have survived into the '90s are the sephadex method, which allegedly concentrates X-bearing sperm, and the albumen swim-up, which allegedly concentrates Y-bearing sperm. Ronald Ericsson has several patents on the latter, known as the "Ericsson Method." In each technique, the treated sperm sample is then used in artificial insemination. Advocates of each method claim up to 85 percent success.[54] Several challengers, however, have used one or another technique to detect Y chromosomes in sperm from the separated semen and demonstrated that the methods do not work—that is, they do not enrich above 50 percent.[55]

Although advocates argue that the proof is in the babies, no independent investigators have assessed the sex of those babies. According to Renee Martin, a physician skilled in detecting Y chromosomes, "Some studies ... have relied on clients to inform the clinic of the baby's sex. This practice could easily bias the results as couples who had a child of the desired sex ... might be more likely to report their success."[56] Furthermore, clients using any sex-selective methods are required to sign a consent form that states that they know the method is not foolproof and agree to accept (not abort) the fetus whatever its sex. This means that clients who have ultrasound or amniocentesis (routinely or for the purpose of learning sex) and find out that the technique did not work must sneak off somewhere else for an abortion if they decide to renounce the consent form. They certainly will not report the sex of their conceptus, and clinic directors are unlikely to chase down such clients because they know that artificial insemination, even with nonmanipulated semen samples, often fails.

c) *Hormone stimulation.* When prescribing fertility drugs to subfertile women became standard medical practice in the late 1970s and early 1980s, practitioners began to notice a slight preponderance of female offspring.[57] Clomiphene citrate (Clomid), especially, seems to have this effect. Paul Zarutskie and his colleagues, after reviewing the published reports in this area, conclude that statistically the percentage of females does indeed increase, but so little that the use of these drugs is of little practical importance for an individual couple.[58]

Physicians, thus, have played with a variety of methods which seem to change the secondary sex ratio a little when used by their proponents. This nebulous situation has stimulated several reputable physicians to try the shotgun approach. Sharon Jaffe and her colleagues at the Columbia University College of Physicians and Surgeons and Mark Geier and his colleagues in Bethesda, Maryland, use intrauterine insemination with husband's sperm after sperm separation, timing in the cycle, *and* Clomid. The Columbia team tries for both males and females, using the Ericsson method; for female selection, they use Clomid and a sperm fraction allegedly *not* enriched for Y-sperm. For boy babies, their results are no better than chance alone; for girls, they report 78.6 percent success.[59] Geier's team separates with sephadex and tries only for females, reporting 80

percent success.[60] The latter report so far has prompted two criticisms: one challenges their statistics; the other suggests that they may not have included all births, and that Clomid or intrauterine insemination, but not the sephadex technique, might have been responsible.[61]

SEX SELECTION ENTREPRENEURS

In 1968, Etzioni predicted, "If a simple and safe method of sex control were available, there would probably be no difficulty in finding the investors to promote it because there is a mass-market potential."[62] He did not say "effective." Now we have simple, safe, ineffective methods and we find that his "promotion" prediction has come true. Two factors should nourish the business in sex selection in the United States: (1) Most couples want a "balanced" family; (2) any method tried, even an ineffective one, has a 52:50 success chance—excellent odds. In fact, because of those odds, and because couples who "fail" rarely tell, some entrepreneurs fool even themselves—that is, they honestly believe in what they are doing.

Colorado entrepreneur Robert Marsik, after personal "success" in using Shettles's method to get a daughter to balance the son he already had, founded a company to capitalize on that method. In 1986 his ProCare Industries Ltd started selling Gender Choice, in pink and blue kits, for $49.95. Each kit contained a douche powder, several disposable thermometers to detect the moment of ovulation, and instructions. Later in 1986, however, the Food and Drug Administration told Pro-Care to halt distribution of Gender Choice until documents on its efficacy were submitted. Arguing that the kit was not a medical device, Pro-Care removed the douche powder, modified the instructions to say that not all members of the scientific community agreed with the theory, and offered a money-back guarantee. Although pro-Care's 1986 sales were $1.1 million, sales dropped in 1987 when the FDA labelled the product a "gross deception on the consumer." Product returns in 1987 and 1988 were greater than sales, so Pro-Care filed for bankruptcy in 1988.[63]

Another entrepreneurship was developed by Ronald Ericsson in the 1970s when he franchised the albumin swim-up method of enriching for Y-sperm described above. His Gametrics Limited sells the method to clinics, which charge customers various rates, usually about $500 per insemination attempt. Since almost any manipulation of semen lowers sperm count, and since artificial insemination has a poor success rate even with a good count, the method takes many inseminations (not a very pleasant experience) and thus can be quite expensive. In 1987 Gametrics Limited reported a success rate of 86 percent boys.[64] Ever since 1975, the "Ericsson Method" has inspired some researchers in the gynecology community to test sperm samples "enriched" via albumin gradients; as described above, all studies outside the Gametrics Limited circle find no enrichment of Y-sperm. Nevertheless, the franchise continues to open clinics, including, recently, one in London.[65]

The situation with physician John Stephens is quite different—first, because his method *is* effective, and second, because it involves selective abortion. In 1984 Stephens incorporated his California Prenatal Diagnosis institute to do ultrasound for identifying fetal sex and named it Koala Labs with the "Service Mark" FASA (Fetal Anatomic Sex Assignment). He promises accurate sex assignment of females at 14 weeks and males at 12 weeks.[66] Although he advertised widely, especially in San Francisco periodicals aimed at South Asians, critics objected to the obvious sex selection, and by 1988 his business was not going well. Presumably, also, some potential customers were getting routine ultrasound covered by their health insurance. In 1990, Stephens set up another Koala Labs in northern Washington; in 1991 he was granted United States Patent # 4, 986, 274 on FASA. He now advertises this $500 service across the border in Canada via direct-mail flyers in the Punjabi language and in *The Link*, an Indo-Canadian community newspaper in Vancouver. "Indo-Canadian women have taken up the fight against Stephens; we are still waiting for other groups of women to take up this fight with us."[67]

SEX-LINKED DISEASE AS A FEMINIST ISSUE

The problem of how to alleviate, to "cure," or to prevent sex-linked disease ought to be of concern to feminists. Each sex-linked disease is caused by a defective gene or an aberration on an X-chromosome, but not on a Y-chromosome because that tiny entity carries only a very few of the X-chromosome genes. It is therefore more accurate to call such diseases "X-linked." In females, usually the corresponding "good" gene on one X-chromosome can cover up (be dominant to) any defective gene on the other X, but males (with only one X) have no such protection. Since these deleterious genes are rare in the population, the chance that a female will be affected (have two of them) is very low; thus, these diseases appear mostly in males. Abortion of male fetuses would thus eliminate all full-blown cases of these diseases, but not the disease genes, since these would persist in the carrier females.

Some 400 X-linked diseases have been described. Some are so mild as to be hardly considered diseases: colorblindness is one example. Hemophilia is the most well known; nowadays men with that disease usually survive to reproduce. Fragile-X mental retardation, Duchenne muscular dystrophy, and Lesch-Nyhan syndrome are the most common serious X-linked diseases.[68]

If he is able to reproduce, a male with an X-linked disease can never pass such a gene to his sons because he gives his sons only his Y-chromosome; yet, *all* his daughters will become (usually symptomless) carriers of the bad gene. A female carrying such a gene will give it to *half* her sons, who will then have the disease, and to half her daughters, who will then become carriers. Thus, any male child with such a disease received it from his mother, not his father.

X-linked diseases raise serious questions for feminists. The first, of course, is unjustified blame and guilt, because all boys with the disease get it from their mothers. If the family understands the genetics, a woman with one or more such sons may be blamed by others or burden herself with self-blame. Even if she aborts all males and has only daughters, she may feel guilt for having given a carrier daughter the same problems she has faced. Because the inheritance pattern is complicated, many families do not understand it, even when it is clearly and carefully explained. Despite the common belief that knowledge is power and, therefore, that obtaining knowledge is empowering, in the case of X-linked disease knowledge may well *disempower* women.

The burden of caring for children with these diseases is extreme. For hemophilia, parents need to give blood factor VII injections.[69] In Lesch-Nyhan disease, the baby boy first shows uncontrollable writhing; then spasms of the limbs prevent walking; a few years later bizarre self-mutilation and aggressive behavior start and get progressively worse until the child dies, usually in his teens.[70] In Duchenne-type muscular dystrophy, the boy's muscles progressively degenerate--every year it gets worse until he dies, again usually as a teenager.[71]

Fragile-X syndrome—the most common cause of severe mental retardation in boys—is especially pernicious in its implications for women. It occurs in one in every 2,500 live births. Its gene was just located in 1991 and found to be a "repeated sequence" of three DNA bases. Everyone has from 6 to 2000 repeats. The more repeats, the more serious the retardation. Children with mild cases may be symptomless or show slight to severe learning disabilities; children at the other extreme are profoundly retarded. Furthermore, this X-linked disease is atypical in that girls can also be affected (also in varying degrees). But the repeated sequence behaves peculiarly through the generations. In male testes the number of repetitions usually decreases, but in female ovaries it increases. Therefore, men usually beget daughters with less retardation, whereas women—if they pass on that particular X-chromosome—are likely to produce both sons and daughters with greater retardation.[72]

Let's consider the view that sex selection is in principle unacceptable yet nonetheless acceptable (and even recommended) for preventing the birth of a male who might have an X-linked disease. First, note that half the males aborted will *not* have the disease; next note that all girls born from a carrier mother have a 50:50 chance of being carriers. In solving a problem of health expenses in the present, one creates girls who must in the future endure the psychological problems of being carriers. Of course, many researchers are confident that reasonably soon we shall be able to detect each X-linked gene itself; *then* we can select both healthy boys and noncarrier girls. But note that the "Sophie's Choice" for women, already bad, becomes worse as each such gene is found. A carrier would then be forced to choose whether to abort (or not to have implanted) a daughter *genetically like herself.* (I use the term

"choose" loosely here—in all likelihood the clinic would automatically make the appointment for abortion, but she might well carry guilt for years believing that she had complied too easily.) The Sophie's Choice is even more painful in women who carry fragile-X, because the degree of retardation in both boys and girls cannot be predicted. This lose-lose situation well illustrates Tabitha Powledge's claim that sex selection may be a paradigm for policy decisions about genetic engineering in general,[73] a very cogent example of the problems that can arise for women as a result of increasing genetic knowledge. As potential mothers, we are at risk of living not only as Sophies, but also as Cassandras.

SEX SELECTION AND FOUR TYPE CASES FOR FEMINIST ETHICS

As I discuss these issues, I may seem sometimes to favor one position over another. Instead, I mean to illuminate the richness of the feminist debate. All women cited here are sincerely concerned about alleviating women's oppression; all have valid, helpful contributions to make. To reach any solution, diverse views must be taken into account—not by a masculine practice of compromise, but by a synthesis in which the whole is better than its parts, a synthesis that combines and reinforces women-enhancing strategies.

Compensatory Justice

Should women be given preferential treatment because it is owed to them due to past discriminatory practices? Or would such treatment be instead "reverse discrimination" or "turning the tables" and mean that the "girls" then simply play by the rules that the "boys" used previously? I shall not cite any of the voluminous literature on this topic, but shall instead apply this dilemma to sex selection.

The issue is this: if a cheap and effective method of sex preselection were available, general preferences in the population mean that it would usually be used to select boys in general and boys to be first-born. Is the appropriate feminist response then to use the technology selectively to choose *girls*, in order to compensate for its use by others? This tactic might reflect a deliberate plan to raise strong feminists. Or is the appropriate feminist response to beget boys in order to bring them up to be nurturing, nonviolent persons necessary for human survival on our planet?[74]

This issue stirred up lively discussion in 1979 at the first feminist workshop on reproductive technologies even though, ironically, essentially everyone—of whatever view—was against the development of sex selection technologies. Tabitha Powledge sparked the issue by stating that she "would *of course* object to the use of this technology selectively against males.... The work of the past ten years ... will have gone for nothing if all we want to do is take revenge and reverse the oppression."[75] Janice Raymond responded that any turning-the-tables argument is "utterly ahistorical" and "shifts the focus off the fact that anti-feminism and woman-hating is all around us."[76] Diana Axelsen countered with the question, "[G]iven a social context that encourages both men and women to prefer male children, ... is the right answer really women wanting daughters rather than both parents deciding ... [to] educate their girl and boy children to have a feminist, humane outlook?"[77]

Supporting Axelsen and Powledge, Betty Hoskins raised the discussion to another level. In a "world and social context with women-generated values," she would hope to stop "that patriarchal, hierarchal 'I'm better than, because I'm this kind or that kind.'" She argued that we should not "continue to participate in a male model of rank ordering, better-worse dichotomies."[78] The metaquestion here for feminists, then, is whether we should utilize *any* patriarchal tactics in struggling for a world free of oppression. And in particular, should we refrain from ordering, prioritizing, and using either-or dualisms? Should we not strive for win-win solutions, rather than win-lose (or as so often happens in medical ethics casebook crises, lose-lose) solutions?

Autonomy and Rights

Sex selection is a perplexing autonomy issue. Should not each woman have the right to control her body and to have no interference with any aspect of reproduction, including choosing the sex of her children? Women have fought long and hard for reproductive rights, and all segments of North American society have adopted rights language. A major "principle" of mainstream medical ethics is

autonomy. Genetic counselors are trained in their lessons in nondirective counseling to respect clients' autonomy. A study in 1988 showed that, when asked their response to a hypothetical ethical dilemma in which a couple with four daughters wanted amniocentesis to make sure that their next child would be a son, 62 percent of medical geneticists in the United States (35 percent women) would "either perform prenatal diagnosis for this couple ... or would refer them to someone who would."[79] Women geneticists were twice as likely as men to comply with the request. A study in 1991, in which 199 master's-degree genetic counselors (93.5 percent women) responded to that same dilemma, found that 82 percent of them would perform or refer for sex selection. Many counselors "reasoned that the patient has a right to choose and felt it their duty to respect patient autonomy."[80] These responses illustrate women's strong belief that reproductive autonomy is sacrosanct. Another illustration is the issue of surrogate motherhood: many women think that any woman should have the right to *be* a surrogate and to hire a surrogate.

Many feminist scholars, however, have raised concerns about emphasizing rights. Some point out that the concept of "rights" is masculinist and patriarchal. For example,

[I]n our assertion of rights we play a masculinist game .... "Rights" language seems to assume that society is a collection of atomic particles in which any given individual's happiness or utility is viewed as mutually disinterested from another's, that communities or love relationships are not ethically relevant in deciding what action ought to be taken. Rights language is fundamentally adversarial and negative.... Humans come into being related to one another, not as disinterested egoists, and thus duties and responsibilities are more fundamental notions than rights.[81]

Furthermore, rights discourse can be nonproductive and indeterminate:

[Rights language] fails to resolve moral disputes conclusively .... When a dilemma is stated as a conflict between rights, a hierarchical judgment is required to decide whose rights ought to prevail.[82]

Alison Jaggar describes this feminist concern with the

> core intuition of autonomy ...[of] the self as the ultimate authority in matters of morality or truth .... On the one hand, [contemporary feminists] ... have insisted that women are as autonomous in the moral and intellectual senses as men ... and they have also demanded political, social and economic autonomy of women .... On the other hand, however, some feminists have questioned traditional interpretations of autonomy as masculine fantasies. For instance, they have explored some of the ways in which "choice" is socialized and "consent" manipulated. In addition, they have ... suggested that freeing ourselves from particular attachments might [not result in] a truly moral response.[83]

Moreover, feminist ethics ought to focus on reducing oppression.[84] We can argue that any practice that increases the oppression of women is wrong and reason then that other factors, such as autonomy and reproductive rights, which are important to women, lose their prerogative if they increase oppression. Powledge claims that "we can ignore" reproductive freedom "when it works against" the ultimate goal of social justice. "Therefore we should embargo sex choice in any form because it abrogates the principle that people (in this case the sexes) should be regarded as equally valuable."[85]

Individual Survival vs. the Status of Women

Around the world women are expected to do most of the "shitwork," the basics necessary to keep people clean, healthy, fed, and clothed. Collectively, women are absolutely necessary for patriarchal society; individually, one or more devoted, sacrificing woman is almost always behind any "successful" man. Despite this (because of this?), women are devalued. Despite this (because of this?), men "prefer" sons.

A woman's valuation is lowered if she produces daughters and raised if she produces sons. Of course, the amount of value change is heavily culture-dependent. In the United States, her value changes little; in fact, her production of a daughter to balance a family might increase her value. In India, daughter production lowers a woman's value so much that she become expendable—her in-laws may demand more

dowry from her parents, force a divorce, even kill her. Sex selection, therefore, can be life-saving. If such women can select sons, they "make correct moral choices, using flawless utilitarian reasoning, [for] they maximize their own and their family's happiness and minimize the suffering of little girls."[86]

However, the process is circular. Each act of son-preference, while increasing the value of a particular mother, further devalues women as a class. It ingrains sex selection into the society's mores, making it more necessary in the future. In northwest India, the part of India with the strongest son-preference and the largest sex ratio imbalance, entrepreneurs introduced amniocentesis for sex selection in the mid-1970s. It became very popular.[87] This use of amniocentesis in northwest India caused the practice to spread to other areas of India and to ethnic groups which had had much less son-preference.

The feminist dilemma is now to balance the survival—the very life—of individual women against the increasing societal devaluation of women caused by those women's individual "choices." Or how can we make a lose-lose situation into a win-win one?

The Strange Bedfellows Problem

Strong stances taken by feminists against reproductive technologies often find us advocating the same policies as those proposed by conservative religious groups. If we are against surrogate motherhood, the marketing of infertility "treatments," and abortion for sex selection, we find that the Vatican agrees with us. However, we reach these conclusions by a path of concern for relationships and for alleviating the oppression of women, a path of giving women full status as persons, a path that does not define women solely as reproductive vessels, whereas the Vatican follows the different path of concern for the fetus as an innocent with the fully human right to life.[88] But the "bedfellow" might say to us, "If you won't abort an innocent fetus because of its sex, how can you approve aborting a fetus because it comes from rape or incest or will be the fifth child in an impoverished family?"

Still another aspect of this problem is the banning of research. Some right-wing groups impose bans against the funding of politically charged areas of research, such as fetal tissue transplants or simple methods of abortions ... and sex detection. Yet, the ethos of science and "enlightened" thought contends that it is wrong to set any restrictions to the search for truth. The feminist analysis of science, however, has regularly pointed out that the *choice of what to study,* that is, what piece of "truth" one searches for, is not disinterested, but politically and socially determined.[89] Thus, for entirely different political and social reasons, right-wing groups and feminists may both happen to say "nay" to certain lines of research. For example, feminist Tabitha Powledge is against funding any research on sex detection techniques.[90] If humans are not wise enough to make proper use of results from certain lines of research, perhaps that research ought not be done. Sex detection may well fall into that category. I believe that we must face up squarely to any bedfellow problems in four ways. First, and most important, should be the emphasis on our *values* and the reasoning from those values. Second, the policies for action we propose must be different: some of those are discussed below. Third, it is possible that good-hearted, well-intentioned people from entirely different mindsets may reach the same conclusion because each taps into a common moral force or transcendent virtue without being aware of it. Fourth, we should make use of any commonalities to raise a bedfellow's consciousness: to achieve a humane, feminist world, such conservatives must be converted, and we have an opening here with a joint concern. At bioethics conferences I have sometimes complimented speakers on their remarks and then continued by showing that their views can be reframed to include concern about the oppression of women.

PUBLIC POLICY FOR SEX SELECTION

Regulation

Most authors who contend that selecting children's sex is morally wrong maintain just as strongly that legal prohibition of it would also be wrong.[91] Sex selective abortion is, however, illegal in Great Britain under the 1967 British Abortion Act[92] and in Pennsylvania under the part of that state's 1989 antiabortion law that was not brought to the Supreme Court.[93] Despite her strong anti-selection view quoted above, Powledge uses slippery slope arguments to claim that prohibition would "begin to delineate acceptable and

unacceptable reasons to have an abortion" and would "provide an opening wedge for legal regulation of reproduction in general."[94] Wertz and Fletcher maintain that any such laws would be "a step backward" and "pose real dangers to civil liberties."[95]

Further, according to Wertz and Fletcher, prohibition would not work. "[F]ew would-be murderers tell gun-shop owners that they intend to shoot people and few prospective parents tell doctors that their real reason for having prenatal diagnosis is to discover fetal sex."[96] Certainly the experience in Maharastra state in India shows the difficulties of enforcement. Passed on May 10, 1988, the Regulation of Use of Prenatal Diagnostic Techniques Act banned the use of medical technologies for prenatal sex determination in Maharastra. The Act forbids advertising, spells out procedures for complaints, and specific punishments. But it has not been implemented, and the government would not take action in a test case against a clinic that advertised its sex selection services.[97]

According to Warren, not only will it be impossible to prohibit sex selection, but prohibition might "aggravate the very ills which it was designed to prevent." She classifies sex selection (if indeed it is wrong) as a "victimless crime," along with several other "crimes," such as gambling, prostitution, and production of pornography. For these, Warren and others believe prohibition would have far worse consequences than "legal toleration with regulation."[98] Among the extremely bad consequences are lucrative markets for crime syndicates, encouragement of police and judicial corruption, and the creation of systems of informers.

I agree with Warren about the importance of avoiding these consequences, but doubt they are likely to follow from prohibition of sex selection because the financial incentives are far below those, say, in prostitution and pornography. But I firmly disagree in calling sex selection "victimless." Indeed, I believe that prostitution and pornography are called victimless only because society fails to recognize exploitation of women and children as victimization. Similarly, society does not recognize that lowering the status of all women—not just those directly involved—is a form of victimization. The victims of sex selection are many: selected children, their siblings, unselected children, and finally all women in society. Stereotypes about the sexes became more firmly ingrained with each complicit action taken.

As for legal toleration with regulation, I am uncertain whether "regulation" would be a lesser burden on women or more enforceable than outright prohibition. (Presumably the United States Food and Drug Administration already has regulation meant to protect us against ineffective or unproven selection schemes, as discussed above in the Gender Choice case.) Powledge suggests that we ought not to include "any form of sex choice in the ... medical procedures supported out of tax funds" and we ought to "tax it, perhaps heavily."[99] Some pro-selection authors have concocted extremely cumbersome, to say the least, schemes for regulation should sex-ratio imbalances arise (their only concern). For example, Singer and Wells suggest that sex selection be done only by registered practitioners who would have waiting lists for couples who want a child of the sex being chosen too frequently.[100] Or regulation could be positive, according to suggestions such as Bayles's that "incentives, such as extra tax deductions, ... be offered for having children of a particular sex, or for having them first."[101]

Withholding Information about Sex

Wertz and Fletcher have suggested that information about sex is nonmedical and usually clinically irrelevant: legally, medical practitioners are not required to give it out. These authors are quick to point out that imbalance in information is a power issue for feminists, but they suggest that information about sex could "reside in the laboratory" so that her doctor knows no more than a pregnant woman. However, a direct request for information about sex would be honored.[102] Lynda Birke and her colleagues argue that withholding information about the sex of a fetus is dangerous and paternalistic, but then come to essentially the Wertz/Fletcher position when they "favour better counselling of women" before women choose to have prenatal diagnosis "to help them decide ... precisely what information about the results they wish to be given."[103] They argue for "informed refusal," a concept Barbara Katz Rothman also advocates. The women whom Rothman interviewed, however, found it extremely difficult to tell a genetic counselor that they did *not* wish to be told certain information.[104]

Wait and See

A good many feminists and nonfeminists see nothing problematic about sex selection. They suggest waiting to find out whether there are problems and then turn to regulation—to them, problems would be imbalances to the human sex ratio that turn out to have deleterious consequences. In 1983 Fletcher's view was, "Prior to having evidence that [social harm from effects of sex choice] exists, however, there is no reason to prevent an extension of freedom and fairness to the first decisions about sex choice.... The mills of a democratic society ... are probably sufficient to grind and resolve the problems."[105]

Warren's wait-and-see policy suggests research on and monitoring of the consequences of using sex selection throughout the world. "If evidence that it *is* detrimental [to women] emerges, we will need to publicize this fact.... [W]e will have to argue for self-regulatory practices by those providing sex-selection services."[106]

Some male scholars have predicted that, if a girl shortage should occur, this would affect parents strongly, first leading to an excess of girls, but the oscillations would eventually damp out, with an eventual return to a balanced sex ratio. One such scholar, Keyfitz, says that selection technology therefore "could be a major force for sex equality.... [Women] will become more desirable in marriage."[107] Rothman and Holmes have each pointed out the absurdity of both the damping off and the sex equality claims. Rothman asks, "In a real woman shortage, would nonsexual and nonreproducing women be tolerated?"[108]

Moral Exhortation. To Powledge, one acceptable method of trying to stop sex selection is moral exhortation. "We must say over and over again to friends and neighbors, in the pages of magazines and newspapers, ... that this technology, even if available, should simply not be used."[109]

Although Warren recommends regulation (if necessary), most of her policy recommendations fit under the moral exhortation category, that is, persuading prospective parents not to use sex-selection services and urging providers to self-regulate. Wertz and Fletcher also suggest that state medical societies—because they control licensure—should discourage private doctors from using prenatal diagnosis merely for sex selection.[110]

But in the long run, the only way to stop sex selection, should cheap and easy methods become available, is to eliminate sexism. According to Warren, to "eliminate the cultural and economic bases of son-preference ... will require nothing less than the elimination of patriarchy itself."[111] An extremely difficult task, especially with the current conservative backlash against feminism! Warren proffers numerous recommendations on how to snip away at patriarchy: each may seem insignificant, but each is clearly morally right in itself—and what other course have we to follow? Among her suggestions are the repeal of laws that property be inherited through the male line, equal education for females, the elimination of sexist discrimination in hiring and promotion, and improving women's wages.

In a humane, feminist utopia, no one would wish to select children's sex. Suppose they gave a sex selection clinic and nobody came?

Notes

1. Barry Bean, "Pregenitive Sex Ratio among Functioning Sperm Cells," *American Journal of Human Genetics*, 47 (1990): 351. The standard way to express sex ratio is to put the male figure *first* per 100 females. I deliberately reverse the convention, putting females first, and also cut 100 in half to jibe with the more common expression "50:50." In putting females first, I become a "militant feminist," according to Ronald Wells. See his *Human Sex Determination* (Tharwa, Australia: Riverlea, 1990), 25.

2. *A Profile of Older Americans—1986*, American Association of Retired Persons, Washington, D.C.

3. Marcia Guttentag and Paul F. Secord, *Too Many Women? The Sex Ratio Question* (Beverly Hills: Sage, 1983), 190.

4. Mary Anne Warren, *Gendercide: The Implications of Sex Selection* (Totowa, NJ: Rowman and Allanheld, 1985), 132-138.

5. For additional ethical arguments, some supporting, some opposing, sex selection, and a competent, detailed analysis, see Warren, *Gendercide*, chs. 4-8. See also ch. 2 in Christine Overall, *Ethics and Human Reproduction: A Feminist Analysis* (Boston: Allen & Unwin, 1987) 17-39, and two essays in *Biomedical Ethics Reviews 1985*: Helen Bequaert Holmes, "Sex Preselection: Eugenics for Everyone," 39-71; and Mary Anne Warren, "The Ethics of Sex Preselection," 73-89. Other issues are raised in three interdisciplinary collections: Janice Raymond, section ed., "Sex Preselection," in Helen Bequaert Holmes, Betty B. Hoskins, and Michael Gross, eds., *The Custom-Made Child? Women-Centered Perspectives* (Clifton, NJ: Humana, 1981), 177-224; Neil G. Bennett, ed., *Sex Selection of Children* (New York: Academic Press, 1983); and Gena Corea et al., eds., *Man-Made Women: How New Reproductive Technologies Affect Women* (Bloomington: Indiana University press, 1987).

6. William H. James, "Timing of Fertilization and the Sex Ratio of Offspring," in Bennett, *Sex Selection*, 73. James has published over 20 papers analyzing the timing of intercourse.

7. Tabitha M. Powledge, "Toward a Moral Policy for Sex Choice," in Bennett, *Sex Selection*, 208.

8. PBS, "Boy or Girl? Should the Choice Be Ours?" *Hard Choices* (1981 TV series).

9. Warren, *Gendercide*, 173.

10. Nan Paulsen Chico, "Confronting the Dilemmas of Reproductive Choice: The Process of Sex Preselection" (Ph.D. diss., University of California at San Francisco, 1989).

11. Overall, *Ethics and Human Reproduction*, 26.

12. Overall, *Ethics and Human Reproduction*, 27, 28.

13. See, for example, Landrum B. Shettles and David M. Rorvik, *How to Choose the Sex of Your Baby* (New York: Doubleday, 1989), 21; John C. Hobbins, "Determination of Fetal Sex in Early Pregnancy," *New England Journal of Medicine* 309 (1983): 979-980.

14. See, for example, Michael D. Bayles, *Reproductive Ethics* (Englewood Cliffs, NJ: Prentice-Hall, 1984), 351; Dorothy C. Wertz and John C. Fletcher, "Sex Selection Through Prenatal Diagnosis: A Feminist Critique," in Helen Bequaert Holmes and Laura M. Purdy, eds, *Feminist Perspectives in Medical Ethics* (Bloomington: Indiana University Press, 1992), 251n.

15. John Postgate, "Bat's Chance in Hell," *New Scientist* 5 April 1973:12-16. See also Peter Singer and Deane Wells, *Making Babies: The New Science and Ethics of Conception* (New York: Scribner's, 1985), 153.

16. Paul Ehrlich, *The Population Bomb* (New York: Ballantine, 1968); Postgate, "Bat's Chance," 14; Clare

Boothe Luce, "Next: Pills to Make Most Babies Male," *Washington Star* 9 July 1978: C1, C4; Singer and Wells, *Making Babies*, 154; Helga Kuhse and Peter Singer, "From the Editors," *Bioethics* 7(4) (1993), iv.

17. Warren, *Gendercide*, 15-16, 36, 175-176; Elizabeth Moen, "Sex Selective Abortion: Prospects in China and India," *Issues in Reproductive and Genetic Engineering: Journal of International Feminist Analysis* 4(3) (1991): 231-249; Irene Sege, "The Grim Mystery of World's Missing Women," *Boston Globe*, 3 Feb. 1992:23, 25; S.H. Venkatramani, "Female Infanticide: Born to Die," *India Today* 15 June 1986:10-17; Madhu Kishwar, "The Continuing Deficit of Women in India and the Impact of Amniocentesis," in Corea et al., *Man-Made Women*, 30-37; Kusum, "The Use of Pre-Natal Diagnostic Techniques for Sex Selection: The Indian Scene," *Bioethics* 7 (2/3) (1993): 150-152, 163.

18. Venkatramani, "Born to Die," 16-17; Kishwar, "Continuing Deficit," 30.

19. Warren, *Gendercide*, 176.

20. Amitai Etzioni, "Sex Control, Science, and Society," *Science* 161 (1968):1107; Powledge, "Moral Policy," 204-205; Warren, *Gendercide*, 109. In ch. 5 of *Gendercide*, Warren discusses detailed evidence from the biology of hormones and from anthropological studies of gentle and violent cultures and questions the hypothesis that a higher proportion of males will result in more aggression.

21. Jessie Bernard, *The Future of Marriage* (London: Souvenir Press, 1973), 19, 24.

22. Warren, *Gendercide*, 141. See Cécile Ernst and Jules Angst, *Birth Order: Its Influence on Personality* (New York: Springer-Verlag, 1983).

23. Warren, *Gendercide*, 163ff; Holmes, "Eugenics," 57-59.

24. Powledge, "Moral Policy," 196.

25. Janice G. Raymond, "Introduction," in Holmes et al., *The Custom-Made Child?* 177.

26. Bayles, *Reproductive Ethics*, 34-35.

27. John C. Fletcher, "Is Sex Selection Ethical?" *Research Ethics: Progress in Clinical and Biological Research* 128 (1983):347.

28. Warren, *Gendercide*, 83, 86.

29. Overall, *Ethics and Human Reproduction*, 22.

30. K.M. Ludmerer, "Eugenics: History," *Encyclopedia of Bioethics* (New York: Macmillan, 1978), 457-461.

31. Ruth Hubbard in Emily Culpepper, moderator, "Sex Preselection Discussion," in Holmes et al., *The Custom-Made Child?* 224.

32. Wertz and Fletcher, "Feminist Critique," 245; also cited in Matt Ridley, "A Boy or a Girl: Is It Possible to Load the Dice?" *Smithsonian* June 1993: 122.

33. Holmes, "Eugenics," 39; Powledge, "Moral Policy," 211. Anne Waldschmidt calls this "grassroots eugenics" in her "Against Selection of Human Life—People with Disabilities Oppose Genetic Counselling, *Issues in Reproductive and Genetic Engineering* 5(2) (1992): 164-166.

34. William J. Watson, "Early-Second-Trimester Fetal Sex Determination with Ultrasound," *Journal of Reproductive Medicine* 35 (1990): 247-249; B.R. Elajalde et al., "Visualization of the Fetal Genitalia," *Journal of Ultrasound in Medicine* 4(1985):633-639.

35. M. Bronshtein et al., "Early Determination of Fetal Sex Using Transvaginal Sonography," *Journal of Clinical Ultrasound* 18 (1990): 302-326; I.E. Timor-Tritsch, D. Farine, and M.G. Rosen, "A Close Look at Early Embryonic Development with the High-Frequency Transvaginal Transducer," *American Journal of Obstetrics and Gynecology* 159 (1988): 676-681; Karen M. Ferroni and Avis Vincensi, "Ultrasound Frontiers: Transvaginal and Doppler Sonography," *Genetic Resource* 6(1) (1991):12-14.

36. David H. Ledbetter et al., "Cytogenetic Results of Chorionic Villus Sampling: High Success Rate and Diagnostic Accuracy in the United States Collaborative Study," *American Journal of Obstetrics and Gynecology* 162 (1990):495-501.

37. Wayne A. Miller and Barbara Thayer, "Early Amniocentesis," *Genetic Resource* 6(1) (1991): 10-11; D.E. Rooney et al., "Early Amniocentesis: A Cytogenetic Evaluation," *British Medical Journal* 299 (1989):25; C.A. Penso and F.D. Frigoletto, "Early Amniocentesis," *Seminars in Perinatology*, 14 (1990):465-470.

38. Barbara Katz Rothman, *The Tentative Pregnancy* (New York: Viking Penguin, 1986), 87-92; Powledge, "Moral Policy," 201.

39. Diana W. Bianchi et al., "Isolation of Fetal DNA from Nucleated Erythrocytes in Maternal Blood," *Proceedings of the National Academy of Sciences, USA* 87 (1990): 3279-3283; Frank Lesser and Ian Anderson, "'Safe' Test May Spot Fetal Abnormalities," *New Scientist* 11 August 1990:32; U.W. Mueller et al., "Isola-

tion of Fetal Trophoblast Cells from Peripheral Blood of Pregnant Women," *Lancet* 336 (1990):197-200; Y-M.D. Lo et al., "Prenatal Sex Determination by DNA Amplification from Maternal Peripheral Blood," *Lancet* 9 Dec. 1989:1363-1365. For a discussion of related social and ethical issues, see Rothman, *Tentative Pregnancy,* 79-82.

40. A. Dokras et al., "Trophectoderm Biopsy in Human Blastocysts," *Human Reproduction* 5(7) (1990):821-825; John D. West et al., "Sexing Whole Human Pre-Embryos by In-situ Hybridization with a Y-Chromosome Specific DNA Probe," *Human Reproduction,* 3(8) (1988):1010-1019; A. H. Handyside et al., "Biopsy of Human Preimplantation Embryos and Sexing by DNA Amplification," *Lancet* 18 Feb. 1989:347-349; A.H. Handyside et al., "Pregnancies from Biopsied Human Preimplantation Embryos Sexed by Y-Specific DNA Amplification," *Nature* 344 (1990):768-770; Gail Vines, "Early Embryo Sex Test Forewarns of Disease," *New Scientist,* 25 Feb. 1989:25.

41. Dorothy C. Wertz, "How Parents of Affected Children View Selective Abortion," in Helen Bequaert Holmes, ed., *Issues in Reproductive Technology I: An Anthology* (New York: Garland, 1992), 182.

42. K. Hardy et al., "Human Implantation Development *in vitro* Is Not Adversely Affected by Biopsy at the 8-Cell Stage," *Human Reproduction,* 5 (1990):708-714.

43. Medical Research International, "In Vitro Fertilization-Embryo Transfer (IVF-ET) in the United States: 1990 Results from the National IVF-ET Registry," *Fertility and Sterility* 57(1) (1992):17.

44. Judy Berlfein, "The Earliest Warning," *Discover* Feb. 1992:14.

45. Handyside, "Pregnancies from," 770.

46. In humans, sex is determined when the sperm merges with the egg. Each human egg contains 23 chromosomes, one of these an X-chromosome. Each human sperm also contains 23 chromosomes, but one of these is either an X or a Y. In normal fertilization, the chromosome count is brought to 46 and either a female (XX) or a male (XY) progeny is conceived.

47. Sally Langendoen and William Proctor, *The Preconception Gender Diet* (New York: M. Evans, 1982); J. Stolkowski and J. Lorrain, "Preconceptual Selection of Fetal Sex," *International Journal of Gynaecology and Obstetrics* 18 (1980): 440-443; Sandra Ann Carson, "Sex Selection: The Ultimate in Family Planning," *Fertility and Sterility* 50 (1988):16.

48. Shettles and Rorvik, *How to Choose,* 105-107; Jonathan Hewitt, "Preconceptional Sex Selection," *British Journal of Hospital Medicine* 37 (1987):154.

49. See, for example, Carson, "Sex Selection," 17; Ridley, "A Boy or a Girl," 113-114, 118-119; Wells, *Human Sex Determination,* ch. 11. For explanations in medical lingo, see Ridley, 118-119, and Wells, 171.

50. Shettles and Rorvik, *How to Choose,* 64, 72-74; Landrum B. Shettles, letter to the editor, *Fertility and Sterility* 29 (1978):386.

51. For tests of Shettles's theory, see John T. France et al., "A Prospective Study of the Preselection of the Sex of Offspring by Timing Intercourse Relative to Ovulation," *Fertility and Sterility* 41 (1984):894-900, and B.W. Simcock, "Sons and Daughters—A Sex Preselection Study," *Medical Journal of Australia* 142 (1985);541-542. For evaluation of such studies, see Paul W. Zarutskie et al., "The Clinical Relevance of Sex Selection Techniques," *Fertility and Sterility* 52 (1989):891-905, especially table 3, p. 896. For discussion of various timing theories, especially before 1970, see James, "Timing of Fertilization," 74-80, 91-92, and William H. James, "Timing of Fertilization and Sex Ratio of Offspring—A Review," *Annals of Human Biology* 3 (1976): 549-556.

52. Elizabeth M. Whelan, *Boy or Girl? The Sex Selection Technique That Makes All Others Obsolete* (New York: Bobbs-Merrill, 1977); Rodrigo Guerrero, "Association of the Type and Time of Insemination within the Menstrual Cycle with the Human Sex Ratio at Birth," *New England Journal of Medicine* 291 (1974) 1056-1059; Susan Harlap, "Gender of Infants Conceived on Different Days of the Menstrual Cycle." *New England Journal of Medicine* 300 (1979): 1445-1448.

53. James, "Timing of Fertilization," in Bennett, 78-79.

54. For both methods, see W.L.G. Quinlivan et al., "Separation Of Human X and Y Spermatozoa by Albumin Gradients and Sephadex Chromatography," *Fertiliy and Sterility* 37 (1982):104; for the Sephadex method, see Stephen L. Corson et al., "Sex Selection by Sperm Separation and Insemination," *Fertility and Sterility* 42 (1984):756; for the albumin method, see Ferdinand J. Beernink and Ronald J. Ericsson, "Male Sex Preselection through Sperm Isolation," *Fertility and Sterility* 38(4) (1982):493-495.

55. For example, see Brigitte F. Brandriff et al., "Sex Chromosome Ratios Determined by Karyotypic Analysis in Albumin-Isolated Human Sperm," *Fertility and Sterility* 46 (1986):678-685; Sharon B. Jaffe et al., "A Controlled Study for Gender Selection," *Fertility and Sterility* 56(2)(1991):254-258; and Teresa A. Beckett, Renee H. Martin, and David I. Hoar, "Assessment of the Sephadex Technique for Selection of X-bearing Human Sperm by Analysis of Sperm Chromosomes, Deoxyribonucleic Acid and Y-Bodies," *Fertility and Sterility* 52 (1989):829-835; Gail Vines, "Old Wives' Tales 'as Good as Sperm Sorting'," *New Scientist* 30 January 1993:4.

56. Renee H. Martin, "Reply of the Author," letter, *Fertility and Sterility* 53 (6)(1990):1112. See also Carson, "Sex Selection," 17-18.

57. For example, see E. Caspi et al., "The Outcome of Pregnancy after Gonadotropin Therapy," *British Journal of Obstetrics and Gynaecology* 83 (1976):976; William H. James, "Gonadotropin and the Human Secondary Sex Ratio," *British Medical Journal* 281 (1980):711; and William H. James, "The Sex Ratio of Infants Born after Hormonal Induction of Ovulation," *British Journal of Obstetrics and Gynaecology* 92 (1985):299.

58. Zarutskie et al., "Clinical Relevance," table 5, p. 898 and discussion, pp. 894-895.

59. Jaffe et al., "A Controlled Study" 251-256.

60. Mark R. Geier, John L. Young, and Dagmar Kessler, "Too Much or Too Little Science in Sex Selection Techniques," letter, *Fertility and Sterility* 53 (6) (1990):1112.

61. Paul G. McDonough, "Editorial Comment," *Fertility and Sterility*, 53 (6) (1990)1113; Martin, "Reply," 1112-1113.

62. Etzioni, "Sex Control," 1108.

63. Christine Russell, "Boy or Girl? FDA Says the Outcome Isn't as Simple as Home Kit Implies," *Washington Post* 28 Jan. 1986; "Deception Charged on Choosing Sex of Babies," *New York Times* 1 Feb. 1987:26; L. Wayne Hicks, "Gender Choice Saga Ends with Liquidation of Assets," *Denver Business Journal* 26 March 1990:1, 23.

64. Gametrics Limited Memorandum #3 (in-house publication), Alzada, Montana, October 1987.

65. Vines, "Old Wives' Tales," 4; Kuhse and Singer, "From the Editors," iii.

66. John D. Stephens, "Morality of Induced Abortion and Freedom of Choice," *American Journal of Obstetrics and Gynecology* 159 (1988):218; John D. Stephens, "Fetal Anatomic Sex Assignment by Ultrasonography during Early Pregnancy," patent no. 4, 986,274, 22 Jan. 1991; "It's a Girl!" advertisement in *India Currents* June 1988.

67. Sunera Thobani, "More Than Sexist ...," *Healthsharing*, Spring 1991:10, 13.

68. Arthur P. Mange and Elaine Johansen Mange, *Genetics: Human Aspects,* 2nd ed. (Sunderland, MA: Sinauer, 1990), 18-21, 36, 322, 514-515.

69. Mange and Mange, *Genetics: Human Aspects,* 514-515.

70. Mange and Mange, *Genetics:Human Aspects,* 322; W.N. Kelley and J.B. Wyngaarden, "Clinical Syndromes Associated with Hypoxanthine-Guanine Phosphoribosyltransferase Deficiency," in J.B. Stanbury et al., eds., *Metabolic Basis of Inherited Disease* (New York: McGraw-Hill, 1983), 1115-1143.

71. Mange and Mange, *Genetics: Human Aspects,* 36; A. E.H. Emery, *Duchenne Muscular Dystrophy*, Oxford Monographs in Medical Genetics 15 (New York: Oxford University Press, 1987).

72. "Retardation Gene Found; Prenatal Test Now Expected," *Washington Post* 16 June 1991:17; G.R. Sutherland et al., "Hereditary Unstable DNA: A New Explanation for Some Old Genetic Questions?" *Lancet* 338 (1991):289.

73. Powledge, "Moral Policy," 208.

74. Warren, *Gendercide*, 175-176.

75. Tabitha M. Powledge, "Unnatural Selection: On Choosing Children's Sex," in Holmes et al., *Custom-Made Child?,* 199.

76. Janice G. Raymond, "Sex Preselection: A Response," in Holmes et al., *Custom-Made Child?,* 210.

77. Culpepper, "Discussion," 221.

78. Culpepper, "Discussion," 220.

79. Wertz and Fletcher, "Feminist Critique," 250n; Dorothy C. Wertz and John C. Fletcher, "Fatal Knowledge? Prenatal Diagnosis and Sex Selection," *Hastings Center Report* 19(3) (1989):21.

80. Deborah F. Pencarinha et al., "Ethical Issues in Genetic Counseling: A Comparison of an M.S. Genetic Counselor and a Medical Geneticist Perspective," *Journal of Genetic Counseling* 1 (1) (1992):24.

81. Helen Bequaert Holmes and Susan Rae Peterson, "Rights Over One's Own Body: A Woman-Affirming

Health Care Policy," *Human Rights Quarterly* 3(2) (1981):73. See also Susan Sherwin, "A Feminist Approach to Ethics," *Resources for Feminist Research RFR/DRF* 16(3) (1987):25-26.

82. Holmes and Peterson, "Rights Over Body," 74.

83. Alison M. Jaggar, "Feminist Ethics: Some Issues for the Nineties," *Journal of Social Philosophy* 20 (1990):100.

84. Susan Sherwin, *No Longer Patient: Feminist Ethics and Health Care* (Philadelphia: Temple University Press, 1992), 54-57, 75.

85. Powledge, "Moral Policy," 206.

86. Holmes, "Eugenics," 60; see also Kusum, "Indian Scene," 163-164.

87. Kusum, "Indian Scene," 152-153.

88. For personal experiences with the strange bedfellows phenomenon and an excellent analysis of the paths, values, and goals involved, see Barbara Katz Rothman, *Recreating Motherhood: Ideology and Technology in a Patriarchal Society* (New York: W.W. Norton, 1989), 240-245.

89. See, for example, Sue V. Rosser, "Re-visioning Clinical Research: Gender and the Ethics of Experimental Design," in Helen Bequaert Holmes and Laura M. Purdy, eds., *Feminist Perspectives in Medical Ethics* (Bloomington: Indiana University Press), 128-129; also in *Hypatia* 4(2) (1989):126-127; see also the reference lists in these.

90. Powledge, "Moral Policy," 209.

91. Helen Bequaert Holmes, review of *Gendercide,* by Mary Anne Warren, *Bioethics* 1 (1) (1987):109; Powledge, "Moral Policy," 207; Powledge, "Unnatural Selection," 197; Wertz and Fletcher, "Feminist Critique," 248; Wertz and Fletcher, "Fatal Knowledge," 26.

92. Lynda Birke, Susan Himmelweit, and Gail Vines, *Tomorrow's Child: Reproductive Technologies in the 90s* (London: Virago, 1990), 248.

93. Charlotte Allen, "Boys Only," *New Republic* 9 March 1992:16.

94. Powledge, "Unnatural Selection," 197.

95. Wertz and Fletcher, "Feminist Critique," 248; see also Wertz and Fletcher, "Fatal Knowledge," 26.

96. Wertz and Fletcher, "Feminist Critique," 248.

97. Radhakrishna Rao, "Sex Selection Continues in Maharastra," *Nature* 343 (1990):497; see also Kusum, "Indian Scene," 153-154, 159-162.

98. Warren, *Gendercide,* 186.

99. Powledge, "Moral Policy," 210-211. The Canadian Royal Commission on New Reproductive Technologies does indeed recommend that no tax monies be used to support any sex choice in clinics or research into methods (ch. 28 in *Proceed with Care* [Ottawa: Canada Communications Group, 1993]). Elsewhere Owen Jones proposes a countercycle earmarked excise tax (CEET) in which sex selecting procedures or products would be taxed and the taxes used to fund advertising programs that combat sex stereotyping or publicize adverse consequences of sex selection. Owen D. Jones, "Sex Selection: Regulating Technology Enabling the Predetermination of a Child's Gender," *Harvard Journal of Law and Technology* 6 (1992):1-62.

100. Singer and Wells, *Making Babies,* 154; also quoted in Warren, *Gendercide,* 168.

101. Bayles, *Reproductive Ethics,* 37.

102. Wertz and Fletcher, "Feminist Critique," 248-249; Wertz and Fletcher, "Fatal Knowledge," 27.

103. Birke et al., *Tomorrow's Child,* 292

104. Rothman, *Tentative Pregnancy,* 255-256.

105. John C. Fletcher, "Ethics and Public Policy: Should Sex Choice Be Discouraged?" in Bennett, *Sex Selection,* 248.

106. Warren, *Gendercide,* 194. Teresa Marteau of Guy's Hospital in London also recommends monitoring. See Gail Vines, "The Hidden Cost of Sex Selection," *New Scientist* 1 May 1993:13.

107. Nathan Keyfitz, "Foreword," in Bennett, *Sex Selection,* xii; see also Charles F. Westoff and Ronald R. Rindfuss, "Sex Preselection in the United States: Some Implications," *Science* 184 (1974):636. Both are cited in Holmes, "Eugenics," 52.

108. Rothman, *Tentative Pregnancy,* 136; Holmes, "Eugenics," 52. See also Gail Vines, "Killing Girls and Aborting Female Fetuses," *New Scientist* 1 May 1993:13.

109. Powledge, "Unnatural Selection," 198.

110. Wertz and Fletcher, "Feminist Critique," 248; Wertz and Fletcher, "Fatal Knowledge," 26.

111. Warren, *Gendercide,* 195.

CHAPTER SEVEN

DEATH, DYING,
AND EUTHANASIA

31.
EUTHANASIA: THE FUNDAMENTAL ISSUES

Margaret P. Battin

Because it arouses questions about the morality of killing, the effectiveness of consent, the duties of physicians, and equity in the distribution of resources, euthanasia is one of the most acute and uncomfortable contemporary problems in medical ethics. It is not a new problem; euthanasia has been discussed—and practiced—in both Eastern and Western cultures from the earliest historical times to the present. But because of medicine's new technological capacities to extend life, the problem is much more pressing than it has been in the past, and both the discussion and practice of euthanasia are more widespread. Despite this, much of contemporary Western culture remains strongly opposed to euthanasia: doctors ought not kill people, its public voices maintain, and ought not let them die if it is possible to save life.

I believe that this opposition to euthanasia is in serious moral error—on grounds of mercy, autonomy, and justice. I shall argue for the rightness of granting a person a humane, merciful death, if he or she wants it, even when this can be achieved only by a direct and deliberate killing. But I think there are dangers here. Consequently, I shall also suggest that there is a safer way to discharge our moral duties than relying on physician-initiated euthanasia, one that nevertheless will satisfy those moral demands upon which the case for euthanasia rests.

THE CASE FOR EUTHANASIA, PART I: MERCY

The case for euthanasia rests on three fundamental moral principles: mercy, autonomy, and justice.

The principle of mercy asserts that *where possible, one ought to relieve the pain or suffering of another person, when it does not contravene that person's wishes, where one can do so without undue costs to oneself, where one will not violate other moral obligations, where the pain or suffering itself is not necessary for the sufferer's attainment of some overriding good, and where the pain or suffering can*

be relieved without precluding the sufferer's attainment of some overriding good.[1] (This principle might best be called the principle of medical mercy, to distinguish it from principles concerning mercy in judicial contexts.)[2] Stated in this relatively weak form, and limited by these provisos, the principle of (medical) mercy is not controversial, though the point I wish to argue here certainly is: contexts that require mercy sometimes require euthanasia as a way of granting mercy—both by direct killing and by letting die.

Although philosophers do not agree on whether moral agents have positive duties of beneficence, including duties to those in pain, members of the medical world are not reticent about asserting them. "Relief of pain is the least disputed and most universal of the moral obligations of the physician," writes one doctor. "Few things a doctor does are more important than relieving pain," says another.[3] These are not simply assertions that the physician ought "do no harm," as the Hippocratic Oath is traditionally interpreted, but assertions of positive obligation. It might be argued that the physician's duty of mercy derives from a special contractual or fiduciary relationship with the patient, but I think that this is in error: rather, the duty of (medical) mercy is generally binding on all moral agents,[4] and it is only by virtue of their more frequent exposure to pain and their specialized training in its treatment that this duty falls more heavily on physicians and nurses than on others. Hence, though we may call it the principle of *medical* mercy, it asserts an obligation that we all have.

This principle of mercy establishes two component duties:

1. the duty not to cause further pain or suffering; and
2. the duty to act to end pain or suffering already occurring.

Under the first of these, for a physician or other caregiver to extend mercy to a suffering patient may mean to refrain from procedures that cause further suffering—provided, of course, that the treatment offers the patient no overriding benefits. So, for instance, the physician must refrain from ordering painful tests, therapies, or surgical procedures when they cannot alleviate suffering or contribute to a patient's improvement or cure. Perhaps the most familiar contemporary medical example is the treatment of burn victims when survival is unprecedented;[5] if with the treatments or without them the patient's chance of survival is nil, mercy requires the physician not to impose the debridement treatments, which are excruciatingly painful, when they can provide the patient no benefit at all.

Although it is increasingly difficult to determine when survival is unprecedented in burn victims, other practices that the principles of mercy would rule out remain common. For instance, repeated cardiac resuscitation is sometimes performed even though a patient's survival is highly unlikely; although patients in arrest are unconscious at the time of resuscitation, it can be a brutal procedure, and if the patient regains consciousness, its aftermath can involve considerable pain. (On the contrary, of course, attempts at resuscitation would indeed be permitted under the principle of mercy if there were some chance of survival with good recovery, as in hypothermia or electrocution.) Patients are sometimes subjected to continued unproductive, painful treatment to complete a research protocol, to train student physicians, to protect the physician or hospital from legal action, or to appease the emotional needs of family members; although in some specific cases such practices may be justified on other grounds, in general they are prohibited by the principle of mercy. Of course, whether a painful test or therapy will actually contribute to some overriding good for the patient is not always clear. Nevertheless, the principle of mercy directs that where such procedures can reasonably be expected to impose suffering on the patient without overriding benefits for him or her, they ought not be done.

In many such cases, the patient will die whether or not the treatments are performed. In some cases, however, the principle of mercy may also demand withholding treatment that could extend the patient's life if the treatment is itself painful or discomforting and there is very little or no possibility that it will provide life that is pain-free or offers the possibility of other important goods. For instance, to provide respiratory support for a patient in the final, irreversible stages of a deteriorative disease may extend his or her life but will mean permanent dependence and incapacitation; though some patients may take continuing existence to make possible other important goods, for some patients continued treatment means the pointless imposition of continuing pain. "Death," whispered Abe Perlmutter, the Florida patient with amyotrophic lateral sclerosis–"Lou Gehrig's Disease"—who pursued through the courts his wish to have the tracheotomy tube connecting him to a respirator removed, "can't be any worse than what I'm going through now."[6] In such cases, the principle of mercy demands that the "treatments" no longer be imposed, and that the patient be allowed to die.

But the principle of mercy may also demand "letting die" in a still stronger sense. Under its second component, the principle asserts a duty to act to end suffering that is already occurring. Medicine already honors this duty through its various techniques of pain management, including physiological means such as narcotics, nerve blocks, acupuncture, and neurosurgery, and psychotherapeutic means such as self-hypnosis, conditioning, and good old-fashioned comforting care. But there are some difficult cases in which pain or suffering is severe but cannot be effectively controlled, at least as long as the patient remains sentient at all. Classical examples include tumors of the throat (where agonizing discomfort is not just a matter of pain but of inability to swallow); "air hunger," or acute shortness of breath; tumors of the brain or bone; and so on. Severe nausea, vomiting, and exhaustion may increase the patient's misery. In these cases, continuing life—or, at least, continuing consciousness—may mean continuing pain. Consequently, mercy's demand for euthanasia takes hold here: mercy demands that the pain, even if with it the life, be brought to an end.

Ending the pain, though with it the life, may be accomplished through what is usually called "passive euthanasia": withholding or withdrawing treatment that could prolong life. In the most indirect of these cases, the patient is simply not given treatment that might extend his or her life—say, radiation therapy in advanced cancer. In the more direct cases, lifesaving treatment is deliberately withheld in the face of an immediate, lethal threat—for instance, antibiotics are withheld from a cancer patient when an overwhelming infection develops; either the cancer or the infection will kill the patient, but the infection does so sooner and in a much gentler way. In all of the passive euthanasia cases, properly so called, the patient's life could be extended; it is mercy that demands that he or she be "allowed to die."

But the second component of the principle of mercy may also demand the easing of pain by means more direct than mere allowing to die; it may require *killing*. This is usually called "active euthanasia," and despite borderline cases (for instance, removing a respirator or a lifesaving IV), it can in general be conceptually distinguished from passive euthanasia. In passive euthanasia, treatment is withheld that could support failing bodily functions, either in warding off external threats or in performing its own processes; active euthanasia, in contrast, involves the direct interruption of ongoing bodily processes that otherwise would have been adequate to sustain life. However, although it may be possible to draw a conceptual distinction between passive and active euthanasia, this provides no warrant for the ubiquitous view that killing is morally worse than letting die.[7] Nor does it support the view that withdrawing treatment is worse than withholding it. If the patient's condition is so tragic that continuing life brings only pain, and there is no other way to relieve the pain than by death, then the more merciful act is not one that merely removes support for bodily processes and waits for eventual death to ensue; rather, it is one that brings the pain—and the patient's life—to an end *now*. If there are grounds on which it is merciful not to prolong life, then there are also grounds on which it is merciful to terminate it at once. The easy overdose, the lethal injection (successors to the hemlock used for this purpose by non-Hippocratic physicians in ancient Greece[8]), are what mercy demands when no other means will bring relief.

But, it may be objected, the cases I have mentioned to illustrate intolerable pain are classical ones;

such cases are controllable now. Pain is a thing of the medical past, and euthanasia is no longer necessary, though it once may have been, to relieve pain. Given modern medical technology and recent remarkable advances in pain management, the sufferings of the mortally wounded and dying can be relieved by less dramatic means. For instance, many once-feared or painful diseases—tetanus, rabies, leprosy, tuberculosis—are now preventable or treatable. Improvements in battlefield first aid and transport of the wounded have been so great that the military coup de grace is now officially obsolete. We no longer speak of "mortal agony" and "death throes" as the probable last scenes of life. Particularly impressive are the huge advances under the hospice program in the amelioration of both the physical and emotional pain of terminal illness,[9] and our culture-wide fears of pain in terminal cancer are no longer justified: cancer pain, when it occurs, can now be controlled in virtually all cases. We can now end the pain without also ending the life.

This is a powerful objection, and one very frequently heard in medical circles. Nevertheless, it does not succeed. It is flatly incorrect to say that all pain, including pain in terminal illness, is or can be controlled. Some people still die in unspeakable agony. With superlative care, many kinds of pain can indeed be reduced in many patients, and adequate control of pain in terminal illness is often quite easy to achieve. Nevertheless, complete, universal, fully reliable pain control is a myth. Pain is not yet a "thing of the past," nor are many associated kinds of physical distress. Some kinds of conditions, such as difficulty in swallowing, are still difficult to relieve without introducing other discomforting limitations. Some kinds of pain are resistant to medication, as in elevated intracranial pressure or bone metastases and fractures. For some patients, narcotic drugs are dysphoric. Pain and distress may be increased by nausea, vomiting, itching, constipation, dry mouth, abscesses and decubitus ulcers that do not heal, weakness, breathing difficulties, and offensive smells. Severe respiratory insufficiency may mean—as Joanne Lynn describes it—"a singularly terrifying and agonizing final few hours."[10] Even a patient receiving the most advanced and sympathetic medical attention may still experience episodes of pain, perhaps alternating with unconsciousness, as his or her condition deteriorates and the physician attempts to adjust schedules and dosages of pain medication. Many dying patients, including half of all terminal cancer patients, have little or no pain,[11] but there are still cases in which pain management is difficult and erratic. Finally, there are cases in which pain control is theoretically possible but for various extraneous reasons does not occur. Some deaths take place in remote locations where there are no pain-relieving resources. Some patients are unable to communicate the nature or extent of their pain. And some institutions and institutional personnel who have the capacity to control pain do not do so, whether from inattention, malevolence, fears of addiction, or divergent priorities in resources.

In all these cases, of course, the patient can be sedated into unconsciousness; this does indeed end the pain. But in respect of the patient's experience, this is tantamount to causing death: the patient has no further conscious experience and thus can achieve no goods, experience no significant communication, satisfy no goals. Furthermore, adequate sedation, by depressing respiratory function, may hasten death. Thus, although it is always technically possible to achieve relief from pain, at least when the appropriate resources are available, the price may be functionally and practically equivalent, at least from the patient's point of view, to death. And this, of course, is just what the issue of euthanasia is about.

Of course, to see what the issue is about is not yet to reach its resolution, or to explain why attitudes about this issue are so starkly divergent. Rather, we must examine the logic of the argument for euthanasia and observe in particular how the principle of mercy functions in the overall case. The canon "One ought to act to end suffering," the second of the abstract duties generated by the principle of mercy, can be traced to the more general principle of beneficence. But its application in a given case also involves a minor premise that is ostensive in character: it points to an alleged case of suffering. This person is suffering, the applied argument from mercy holds, in a way that lays claim on us for help in relieving that pain.

It may be difficult to appreciate the force of this argument if its character is not adequately recognized. By asserting the abstract duty of mercy and pointing to specific occasions of pain, the argument generates the conclusion that we ought not let these cases of pain occur: not only ought we to prevent them from occurring if we can, but also we ought to bring them to an end if they do. In practice, most arguments for euthanasia on grounds of mercy are pursued by the graphic evocation of cases: the tortures suffered by victims of awful diseases.

But this argument strategy is problematic. The evocation of cases may be very powerful, but it is also subject to a certain unreliability. After all, pain is, in general, not well remembered by those not currently suffering it, and though bystanders may be capable of very great sympathy, no person can actually feel another's pain. Suffering that does not involve pain may be even harder for the bystander to assess. Conversely, however, bystanders sometimes seem to suffer more than the patient: pain, particularly in those for whom one has strong emotional attachments, is notoriously difficult to watch. Furthermore, sensitivity on the part of others to pain and suffering is very much subject to individual differences in experience with pain, beliefs concerning the purpose of suffering and pain, fears about pain, and physical sensitivity to painful stimuli. Yet there is no objective way to establish how seriously the ostensive premise of the argument from mercy should be taken in any specific case, or how one should respond. Clearly, such a premise can be taken too seriously—so that concern for another's pain or suffering outweighs all other considerations—or one can be far too cavalier about the facts. To break a promise to a patient—say, not to intubate him—because you perceive that he is in pain may be to overreact to his suffering. However, it is morally repugnant to stand by and watch another person suffer when one could prevent it; it is a moral failing, too, to be insensitive, when there is no overriding reason for doing so, to the fact that another person is in pain.

The principle of mercy holds that suffering ought to be relieved—unless, among other provisos, the suffering itself will give rise to some overriding benefit or unless the attainment of some benefit would be precluded by relieving the pain. But it might be argued that life itself is a benefit, always an overriding one. Certainly life is usually a benefit, one that we prize. But unless we accept certain metaphysical assumptions, such as "life is a gift from God," we must recognize that life is a benefit because of the experiences and interests associated with it. For the most part, we prize these, but when they are unrelievedly negative, life is not a benefit after all. Philippa Foot treats this as a conceptual point: "Ordinary human lives, even very hard lives, contain a minimum of basic goods, but when these are absent the idea of life is no longer linked to that of good."[12] Such basic goods, she explains, include not being forced to work far beyond one's capacity; having the support of a family or community, being able to more or less satisfy one's hunger, having hopes for the future; and being able to lie down to rest at night. When these goods are missing, she asserts, the connection between *life* and *good* is broken, and we cannot count it as a benefit to the person whose life it is that his or her life is preserved.

These basic goods may all be severely compromised or entirely absent in the severely ill or dying patient. He or she may be isolated from family or community, perhaps by virtue of institutionalization or for various other reasons; he or she may be unable to eat, to have hopes for the future, or even to sleep undisturbed at night. Yet even for someone lacking all of what Foot considers to be basic goods, the experiences associated with life may not be unrelievedly negative. We must be very cautious in asserting of someone, even someone in the most abysmal-seeming conditions of the severely ill or dying, that life is no longer a benefit, since the way in which particular experiences, interests, and "basic goods" are valued may vary widely from one person to the next. Whether a given set of experiences constitutes a life that is a benefit to the person whose life it is, is not a matter for *objective* determination, though there may be very good external clues to the way in which that person is in fact valuing them; it is, in the end, very much a function of subjective preference and choice. For some persons, life may be of value even in the grimmest conditions, for others, not. The crucial point is this: when a suffering person is conscious enough to have any experience at all, whether that experience counts as a benefit overriding the suffering or not is relative to

that person and can be decided ultimately only by him or her.[13]

If this is so, then we can no longer assume that the cases in which euthanasia is indicated on grounds of mercy are infrequent or rare. It is true that contemporary pain-management techniques do make possible the control of pain to a considerable degree. But unless pain and discomforting symptoms are eliminated altogether without loss of function, the underlying problem for the principle of mercy remains: how does *this* patient value life, how does he or she weigh death against pain? We are accustomed to assume that only patients suffering extreme, irremediable pain could be candidates for euthanasia at all and do not consider whether some patients might choose death in preference to comparatively moderate chronic pain, even when the condition is not a terminal one. Of course, a patient's perceptions of pain are extremely subject to stress, anxiety, fear, exhaustion, and other factors, but even though these perceptions may vary, the underlying weighing still demands respect. This is not just a matter of differing sensitivities to pain, but of differing values as well: for some patients, severe pain may be accepted with resignation or even pious joy, whereas for others mild or moderate discomfort is simply not worth enduring. Yet, without appeal to religious beliefs about the spiritual value of suffering, we have no objective way to determine how much pain a person *ought* to stand. Consequently, we cannot assume that euthanasia is justified, if at all, in only the most severe cases. Thus, the issue of euthanasia looms larger, rather than smaller, in the contemporary medical world.

That we cannot objectively determine whether life is a benefit to a person or whether pain outweighs its value might seem to undermine all possibility of appeal to the principle of mercy. But I think it does not. Rather, it shows simply that the issue is more complex, and that we must recognize that the principle of mercy itself demands recognition of a second fundamental principle relevant in euthanasia cases: the principle of autonomy. If the sufferer is the best judge of the relative values of that suffering and other benefits to him- or herself, then his or her own choices in the matter of mercy ought to be respected. To impose "mercy" on someone who insists that despite his or her suffering life is still valuable to him or her would hardly be mercy; to withhold mercy from someone who pleads for it, on the basis that his or her life could still be worthwhile for him or her, is insensitive and cruel. Thus, the principle of mercy is conceptually tied to that of autonomy, at least insofar as what guarantees the best application of the principle—and hence, what guarantees the proper response to the ostensive premise in the argument from mercy—is respect for the patient's own wishes concerning the relief of his or her suffering or pain.

To this issue we now turn.

THE CASE FOR EUTHANASIA, PART II: AUTONOMY

The second principle supporting euthanasia is that of (patient) autonomy: *one ought to respect a competent person's choices, where one can do so without undue costs to oneself, where doing so will not violate other moral obligations, and where these choices do not threaten harm to other persons or parties.* This principle of autonomy, though limited by these provisos, grounds a person's right to have his or her own choices respected in determining the course of medical treatment, including those relevant to euthanasia: whether the patient wishes treatment that will extend life, though perhaps also suffering, or whether he or she wants the suffering relieved, either by being killed or by being allowed to die. It would of course also require respect for the choices of the person whose condition is chronic but not terminal, the person who is disabled though not dying, and the person not yet suffering at all, but facing senility or old age. Indeed, the principle of autonomy would require respect for self-determination in the matter of life and death in any condition at all, provided that the choice is freely and rationally made and does not harm others or violate other moral rules. Thus, the principle of autonomy would protect a much wider range of life-and-death acts than those we call euthanasia, as well as those performed for reasons of mercy.

Support for patient autonomy in matters of life and death is partially reflected in U.S. law, in which a patient's right to passive voluntary euthanasia (though it is not called by this name) is established in a long series of cases. In 1914, in the case of *Schloendorff v. New York Hospital*,[14] Justice Cardo-

zo asserted that "every human being of adult years and sound mind has a right to determine what shall be done with his own body" and held that the plaintiff, who had been treated against his will, had the right to refuse treatment; more recent cases, including *Yetter,*[15] *Perlmutter,*[16] and *Bartling,*[17] establish that the competent adult has the right to refuse medical treatment, on religious or personal grounds, even if it means he or she will die. (Exceptions include some persons with dependents and persons who suffer from communicable diseases that pose a risk to the public at large.) Furthermore, the patient has the right to refuse a component of a course of treatment, even though he or she consents to others; this is established in the Jehovah's Witnesses cases in which patients refused blood transfusions but accepted surgery and other care. In many states, the law also recognizes passive voluntary euthanasia of the no longer competent adult who has signed a refusal-of-treatment document while still competent; such documents, called "natural death directives" or living wills, protect the physician from legal action for failure to treat if he or she follows the patient's antecedent request to be allowed to die. Additionally, the durable power of attorney permits a person to designate a relative, friend, or other person to make treatment decisions on his or her behalf after he or she is no longer competent; these may include decisions to refuse life-sustaining treatment. Many hospitals have adopted policies permitting the writing of orders not to resuscitate, or "no-code" orders, which stipulate that no attempt is to be made to revive a patient following a cardiorespiratory arrest. These policies typically are stated to require that such orders be issued only with the concurrence of the patient, if competent, or the patient's family or legal guardian. In theory, at least, living wills, no-code orders, durable powers of attorney, and similar devices are designed to protect the patient's voluntary choice to refuse life-prolonging treatment.

These legal mechanisms for refusal of treatment all protect individual autonomy in matters of euthanasia: the right to choose to live or to die. But it is crucial to see that they all protect only passive euthanasia, not any more active form. The Natural Death Act of California, like similar legislation in other states, expressly states that "nothing in this

[Act] shall be construed to condone, authorize, or approve mercy killing."[18] Likewise, the living will directs only the withholding or cessation of treatment, in the absence of which the patient will die.[19] A durable power of attorney permits the same choices on behalf of the patient by a designated second party. These legal mechanisms are sometimes said to protect the "right to die," but it is important to see that this is only the right to be *allowed* to die, not to be helped to die or to have death actively brought about. However, we have already seen that allowing to die is sometimes less merciful than direct, humane killing: the principle of mercy demands the right to be killed, as well as to be allowed to die. Thus, the protections offered by the legal mechanisms now available may be seen as truncated conclusions from the principle of patient autonomy that supports them; this principle should protect not only the patient's choice of refusal of treatment but also a choice of a more active means of death.

It is often objected that autonomy in euthanasia choices should not be recognized in practice, whether or not it is accepted in principle, because such choices are often erroneously made. One version of this argument points to physician error. Physicians make mistakes, it holds, and since medicine in any case is not a rigorous science, predictions of oncoming, painful death with no possibility of cure are never wholly reliable. People diagnosed as dying rapidly of inexorable cancers have survived, cancer-free, for dozens of years; people in cardiac failure or long-term irreversible coma have revived and regained full health. Although some of this can be attributed simply to physician error, we must also guard against the more pernicious phenomenon of the "hanging of crepe," in which the physician (usually not intentionally) delivers a prognosis dimmer than is actually warranted by the facts. If the patient succumbs, the physician cannot be blamed, since that is what was predicted; but if the patient survives, the physician is credited with the cure.[20] Other factors interfering with the accuracy of a diagnosis or prognosis include impatience on the part of a physician with a patient who is not doing well, difficulties in accurately estimating future complications, ignorance of a treatment or cure that is about to be discovered or is on the way, and a host of additional factors arising when the physician is emotionally involved, inexperienced, uninformed, or incompetent.[21]

A second argument pointing to the possibility of erroneous choice on the part of the patient asserts the very great likelihood of impairment of the patient's mental processes when seriously ill. Impairing factors include depression, anxiety, pain, fear, intimidation by authoritarian physicians or institutions, and drugs used in medical treatment that affect mental status. Perhaps a person in good health would be capable of calm, objective judgments even in such serious matters as euthanasia, so this view holds, but the person as patient is not. Depression, extremely common in terminal illness, is a particular culprit: it tends to narrow one's view of the possibilities still open; it may make recovery look impossible, it may screen off the possibilities, even without recovery, of significant human relationships and important human experience in the time that is left.[22] A choice of euthanasia in terminal illness, this view holds, probably reflects largely the gloominess of the depression, not the gravity of the underlying disease or any genuine intention to die.

If this is so, ought not the euthanasia request of a patient be ignored for his or her own sake? According to a limited paternalist view (sometimes called "soft" or "weak" paternalism), intervention in a person's choices for his or her own sake is justified if the person's thinking is impaired. Under this principle, not every euthanasia request should be honored; such requests should be construed, rather, as pleas for more sensitive physical and emotional care.

It is no doubt true that many requests to die are pleas for better care or improved conditions of life. But this still does not establish that all euthanasia requests should be ignored, because the principle of paternalism licenses intervention in a person's choices just *for his or her own good*. Sometimes the choice of euthanasia, though made in an impaired, irrational way, may seem to serve the person's own good better than remaining alive. Thus, since the paternalist, in intervening, must act for the sake of the person in whose liberty he or she interferes, the paternalist must take into account not only the costs for the person of failing to interfere with a euthanasia decision when euthanasia was not warranted (the cost is death, when death was not in this person's interests) but also the costs for that person of interfering in a decision that was warranted (the cost is continuing life—and continuing suffering—when death would have been the better choice).[23] The likelihood of these two undesirable outcomes must then be weighed. To claim that "there's always hope" or to insist that "the diagnosis could be wrong" in a morally responsible way, one must weigh not only the cost of unnecessary death to the patient but also the costs to the patient of dying in agony if the diagnosis is right and the cure does not materialize. But cases in which the diagnosis is right and the cure does not materialize are, unfortunately, much more frequent than cases in which the cure arrives or the diagnosis is wrong. The "there's always hope" argument, used to dissuade a person from choosing euthanasia, is morally irresponsible unless there is some quite good reason to think there actually *is* hope. Of course, the "diagnosis could be wrong" argument against euthanasia is a good one in areas or specialities in which diagnoses are frequently inaccurate (the chief of one neurology service admitted that on initial diagnoses "we get it right about 50 percent of the time"), or where there is a systematic bias in favor of unduly grim prognoses—but it is not a good argument against euthanasia in general. Similarly, "a miracle cure may be developed tomorrow" is also almost always irresponsible. The paternalist who attempts to interfere with a patient's choice of euthanasia must weigh the enormous suffering of those to whom unrealistic hopes are held out against the benefits to those very few whose lives are saved in this way.

As with limited paternalism, extended "strong" or "hard" paternalism—permitting intervention not merely to counteract impairment but also to avoid great harm—provides a special case when applied to euthanasia situations. The hard paternalist may be tempted to argue that because death is the greatest of harms, euthanasia choices must always be thwarted. But the initial premise of this argument is precisely what is at issue in the euthanasia dispute itself, as we've seen: is death the worst of harms that can befall a person, or is unrelieved, hopeless suffering a still worse harm? The principle of mercy obliges us to relive suffering when it does not serve some overriding good; but the principle itself cannot tell us whether sheer existence—life—is an overriding good. In the absence of an objectively valid answer, we must appeal to the individual's own preferences and values. Which is the greater evil—death or pain? Some persons may adopt religious answers to this question, others may devise their own; but the answer always is tied to the person whose life it is, and cannot be supplied in any objective way. Hence, unless he or she can discover what the suffering person's preferences and values are, the hard paternalist cannot determine whether intervening to prolong life or to terminate it will count as acting for that person's sake.

Of course, there are limits to such a claim. When there is no evidence of suffering or pain, mental or physical, and no evidence of factors like depression, psychoactive drugs, or affect-altering disease that might impair cognitive functioning, an external observer usually can accurately determine whether life is a benefit: unless the person has an overriding commitment to a principle or cause that requires sacrifice of that life, life *is* a benefit to him or her. (But such a person, of course, is probably not a patient.) Conversely, when there is every evidence of pain and little or no evidence of factors that might outweigh the pain, such as cognitive capacities that might give rise to other valuable experience, then an external observer generally can also accurately determine the value of this person's life: it is a disbenefit, a burden, to him or her. (Given pain and complete cognitive incapacity, such a person is almost always a patient.) It is when both pain and cognitive capacities are found that the person-relative character of the value of life becomes most apparent, and most demanding of respect.

Thus, if we view the spectrum of persons from fully healthy through severely ill to decerebrate or brain dead, we may assert that the principle of autonomy operates most strongly at the middle of this range. The more severe a person's pain and suffering, when his or her condition is not so diminished as to preclude cognitive capacities altogether, the stronger the respect we must accord his or her own view of whether life is a benefit or not. At both ends of the scale, however, paternalistic considerations come into play: if the person is healthy and without pain, we will interfere to keep him or her alive (preventing, for instance, suicide attempts); if his or her life means *only* pain, we act for the person's sake by causing him or her to die (as we should for certain severely defective neonates who cannot survive, but are in continuous pain). But when the patient retains cognitive capacities, the greater is his or her suffering, and the more his or her choices concerning it deserve our respect. When the choice that is faced is death or pain, it is the patient who must choose which is worse.

We saw earlier that in euthanasia issues the principle of mercy is conceptually tied to the principle of autonomy, at least for its exercise; we now see that the principle of autonomy is dependent on the principle of mercy in certain sorts of cases. It is *not* dependent in this way, however, in those cases most likely to generate euthanasia requests. That someone voluntarily and knowingly requests release from what he or she experiences as misery is sufficient, other things being equal, for the request to be honored; although this request is rooted in the patient's desire for mercy, we cannot insist on independent, objective evidence that mercy would in fact be served, or that death is better than pain. We can demand such evidence to protect a perfectly healthy person, and we can summon it to end the sufferings of someone who can no longer choose; but we cannot demand it or use it for the seriously ill person in pain. To claim that an incessantly pain-racked but conscious person cannot make a rational choice in matters of life and death is to misconstrue the point: he or she, better than anyone else, can make such a choice, based on intimate acquaintance with pain and his or her own beliefs and fears about death. If the patient wishes to live, despite such suffering, he or she must be allowed to do so; or the patient must be granted help if he or she wishes to die.

But this introduces a further problem. The principle of autonomy, when there are no countervailing considerations on paternalistic grounds or on grounds of harm to others, supports the practice of voluntary euthanasia and, in fact, any form of rational, voluntary suicide. We already recognize a patient's right to refuse any or all medical treatment and hence correlative duties of noninterference on the part of the physician to refrain from treating the patient against his or her will. But does the patient's right of self-determination also give rise to any positive obligation on the part of the physician or other bystander to actively produce death? Pope John Paul II asserts that "no one may ask to be killed";[24] Peter Williams argues that a person does not have a right to be killed even though to kill him might be humane.[25] But I think that both the Pope and Williams are wrong. Although we usually recognize only that the principle of autonomy generates rights to noninterference, in some circumstances a right of self-determination does generate claims to assistance or to the provision of goods.

We typically acknowledge this in cases of handicap or disability. For instance, the right of a person to seek an education ordinarily generates on the part of others only an obligation not to interfere with his or her attendance at the university, provided the person meets its standards; but the same right on the part of a person with a severe physical handicap may generate an obligation on the part of others to provide transportation, assist in acquiring textbooks, or provide interpretive services. The infant, incapable of earning or acquiring its own nourishment, has a right to be fed. There is a good deal of philosophic dispute about such claims, and public policies vary from one administration and court to the next. But if, in a situation of handicap or disability, a right to self-determination can generate claim rights (rights to be aided) as well as noninterference rights, the consequences for euthanasia practices are far-reaching indeed. Some singularly sympathetic cases—like that of Elizabeth Bouvier, who is almost completely paralyzed by cerebral palsy—have brought this issue to public attention. But notice that in euthanasia situations, *most* persons are handicapped with respect to producing for themselves an easy, "good," merciful death. The handicaps are occasionally physical, but most often involve lack of knowledge of how to bring this about and lack of access to means for so doing. If a patient chooses to refuse treatment and so die, he or she still may not know what components of the treatment to refuse in order to produce an easy rather than painful death; if the person chooses death by active means, he or she may not know what drugs or other methods would be appropriate, in what dosages, and in any case he or she may be unable to obtain them. Yet full autonomy is not achieved until one can both choose and act upon one's choices. It is here, in these cases of "handicap" that afflict many or most patients, that rights to self-determination may generate obligations on the part of physicians (provided, perhaps, that they do not have principled objections to participation in such activities themselves[26]). The physician's obligation is not only to respect the patient's choices but also to make it possible for the patient to act upon those choices. This means supplying the knowledge and equipment to enable the person to stay alive, if he or she so chooses; this is an obligation physicians now recognize. But it may also mean providing the knowledge, equipment, and help to enable the patient to die, if that is his or her choice; this is the other part of the physician's obligation, not yet recognized by the medical profession or the law in the United States.[27]

This is not to say that any doctor should be forced to kill any person who asks that: other contravening considerations—particularly that of ascertaining that the request is autonomous and not the product of coerced or irrational choice, and that of controlling abuses by unscrupulous physicians, relatives, or patients—would quickly override. Nor would the physician have an obligation to assist in "euthanasia" for someone not severely ill. But when the physician is sufficiently familiar with the patient to know the seriousness of the condition and the earnestness of the patient's request, when the patient is sufficiently helpless, and when there are no adequate objections on grounds of personal scruples or social welfare, then the principle of autonomy—like the principle of mercy—imposes on the physician the obligation to help the patient in achieving an easy, painless death.

THE CASE FOR EUTHANASIA, PART III: JUSTICE

Although the term euthanasia originates from Greek roots meaning "good death," especially the avoidance of suffering, in recent years use of the term has been extended to cover cases in which the patient is neither suffering nor capable of choosing to die. Ruth Russell, for instance, includes among cases of euthanasia the ending of "a meaningless existence."[28] For Tom Beauchamp and Arnold Davidson, euthanasia can be the termination of an irreversibly comatose state.[29] Termination of the lives of the brain dead, the permanently comatose, and those

who are, as Paul Ramsey puts it, "irretrievably inaccessible to human care"[30] is justified, it is argued, under the principle of justice: euthanasia permits fairer distribution of medical resources in a society that lacks sufficient resources to provide maximum care for all. Once this principle is invoked, however, it may seem that it also applies in cases in which the patient is still competent: to permit earlier, easier dying will be favored not only on grounds of mercy and autonomy but on grounds of justice as well.

Drawing on the principle of mercy advanced earlier, we may assert that each person, by virtue of his or her medical illness, injury, disability, or other medical abnormality that causes pain or suffering, has a claim on whatever medical resources might be effective in the full treatment of his or her condition: because we have an obligation (subject to the provisos mentioned previously) to relieve the person's suffering, he or she has a correlative claim (subject to corresponding provisos) to whatever medical treatment can be used. But since there are not enough resources to supply full treatment for every condition for every person, and since the resources typically cannot be subdivided in a way that makes equal apportionment of them possible (half an operation will do you no good), full treatment can be devoted only to some conditions, or only to some persons. In a scarcity situation, not all competing claims can be satisfied, and a principle of distributive justice must be invoked to adjudicate among them.

Various principles can be proposed for allocating medical resources: to those in greatest medical need, to those for whom restoration of function would be most complete; to those who can pay; to those whose societal contributions are or have been greatest; to those who have been most deprived of medical care in the past; to those whose conditions are not self-induced (this might rule out people suffering from smokers' diseases, conditions exacerbated by obesity, suicide attempts, and perhaps venereal diseases and high-risk sports injuries); or to those who are the winners in a coin toss, lottery, or other system of random selection. Alternatively, treatment could be allocated on the basis of the medical condition involved; to end-stage kidney patients, for instance, but not to those with deteriorative heart disease. But, unless we expand the size of the resources pool, treatment will still be denied to some, *whatever* distributive principle is adopted. Hence, whatever the principle (except perhaps one that allocates all available resources simply to staving off death for the last few minutes in every medical condition), some of those denied treatment will die sooner than otherwise would be the case. But this, it can be argued, would be unjust, since it would impose earlier death on some persons on the basis of characteristics that are not legitimate grounds for death—ability to pay, and so on. Rather, it is often argued, if treatment is to be denied to some people with the result that they will die, it is better to deny it just to those people who are (loosely speaking) medically unsalvageable and will die soon anyway: the terminally ill, the extremely aged, and the seriously defective neonate. The practices of euthanasia in accord with this principle—which can be called the salvageability principle—is justified, this argument then concludes, by the demands of justice in a scarcity situation.

Of course, to deny treatment to a dying patient on grounds of justice cannot properly be called euthanasia in the traditional sense, since it is not done for the sake of the patient or to provide a "good death." A congressional decision not to fund artificial heart research or not to provide Medicaid/Medicare payments for heart transplants can hardly be called euthanasia for those heart patients who will die. However, as we saw at the outset of this section, policies involving withholding treatment are frequently called euthanasia when practiced on the permanently comatose, the brain dead, the profoundly retarded, or others in nonsapient states. Despite the abuse of the term under the Nazi regime, our linguistic usage is again undergoing rapid change, and it is apparent that we are coming to use the term euthanasia not just for pain-sparing deaths but for resource-conserving deaths as well. It is in this newer sense that we can consider whether justice requires the practice of euthanasia in certain kinds of scarcity situations.

The argument from justice, though not always put forward in a coherent, comprehensive way, is often initiated with a recitation of facts. The hospital bill [in 1985] for a 500 gram newborn with serious deficits, it is said, may run somewhere between $60,000 and 80,000, or even more than $100,000;

this does not by any means guarantee that the infant will survive or live a normal life. The cost of a coronary bypass, a procedure frequently employed even when it does not extend life expectancy (though it greatly increases the quality of life) is somewhere around $30,000. The bill for a series of bone marrow transplants may run to $80,000, even though the transplants may not succeed in staving off death. According to a study published late in 1981, the average intensive care unit bill (total hospital charges, plus ancillary charges) was $7,112—for patients who survived.[31] But for patients who died, the bill was more than double, a staggering $15,874. A vast proportion of medical costs are incurred during the final year of life (this includes unsalvageable neonates as well as adults), most of it in the last few weeks or days. Justice, under the distributive principle articulated previously, demands that the dying be allowed to die, and these resources be given instead to other, salvageable competitors for full health care.

This is not to suggest that the dying should be denied palliative and comfort care: indeed, if their claims to therapeutic treatment diminish, the principle of mercy demands that their claims to palliative care increase. Nor is it to suggest that the dying "do not deserve" medical care that could prolong their lives. *All* parties in the distribution have prima facie claims to care, under the principle of justice, but the claims of the dying are weakest.

This argument from justice is usually employed only to justify the denial of treatment, that is, to justify passive euthanasia, but similar considerations also favor active euthanasia. Passive euthanasia is often practiced upon unsalvageable patients by withholding treatment if a medical crisis occurs: for instance, no-code orders are issued, or pneumonias are not treated, or electrolyte imbalances not corrected if they occur. If justice demands that, despite the prima facie claims of these patients, the resources allocated to their care are better assigned somewhere else, then we must notice that *passive* euthanasia does not provide the most just redistribution of these resources. To "allow" the patient to die may still involve enormous expenditures of money, scarce supplies, or caregiver time. This is most evident in cases of "irretrievably inaccessible" patients, for whom no considerations of mercy or autonomy override the demands of justice in weighing claims. The cost [in 1985] of maintaining a coma patient in a nursing home without heroic treatment is somewhere around $15,000 a year; the cost for a profoundly retarded resident of a state institution is more than $20,000. Whole-brain dead patients may survive on life supports in hospital settings from several hours to a few days or more; upper-brain dead patients may live for years. The total cost of maintaining a permanently comatose woman, who was injured in a riding accident in 1956 at age twenty-seven and died eighteen years later, has been estimated at just over $6,000,000; this care provided her with not a single moment of conscious life.[32] The record survival for a coma patient is 37 years and 111 days.[33] The argument from justice demands that these patients, since their claims for care are so weak as to have virtually no force at all, be killed, not simply allowed to die.

OBJECTION TO THE ARGUMENT FROM JUSTICE: THE SLIPPERY SLOPE

But if justice, under the salvageability principle considered here, licenses the killing of permanently comatose patients, will it not also license the killing of still-conscious, still-competent dying patients, perhaps still salvageable, close or not so close to death? What extensions of the scope of this principle might be made, should resources become still more scarce? These concerns introduce the "wedge" or "slippery slope" argument, which holds that although some acts of euthanasia may be morally permissible (say, on grounds of mercy or autonomy), to allow them to occur will set a logical precedent for, or will causally result in, consequences that are morally repugnant.[34] Just as Hitler's 1938 "euthanasia" program for mentally defective, senile, and terminally ill Aryans paved the way for the establishment of the extermination camps several years later, it is argued, so permissive euthanasia policies invite irreversible descent down that slippery slope that leads to mass murder. Indeed, to permit even the most humane euthanasia may do more than set a precedent: by accustoming doctors to ending life, by supplying death technology, by changing the expectations of family members or other guardians of those who become candidates for death, and by changing the expectations of patients themselves, the practice of euthanasia even in humane cases may lead to moral holocaust.

As it is usually posed, the form of the argument that points to the Nazi experience does not succeed: the forces that brought the mass extermination camps into being were not *caused* by the earlier euthanasia program, and, other things being equal, the extermination camps for Jews would no doubt have been established had there been no euthanasia program at all. To argue that permitting euthanasia now will lead to death camps like Hitler's is to overlook the many other political, social, and psychological factors of the Nazi period. Yet the wedge argument cannot be simply discarded; the factors operating to favor the slide from morally warranted euthanasia to murder are probably much stronger than we realize. They are best seen, I think, as misunderstandings or corruptions of the very principles that favor euthanasia: mercy, autonomy, and perhaps most prominently, justice.

A contemporary version of the wedge argument holds that to permit euthanasia at all—including cases justified on grounds of mercy, autonomy, or justice—will in the presence of strong financial incentives lead to circumstances in which people are killed who are not suffering or who do not wish to die. Furthermore, to permit some doctors to allow their patients to die or to kill them would invite cavalier attitudes concerning the lives of the patients and, in addition to financial incentives, ordinary greed, insensitivity, hastiness, and self-interest, would cause some doctors to let their patients die—or kill them—when there was no moral warrant for doing so.[35] Doctors treating difficult or unresponding patients would find an easy way out. Medical blunders could be more easily covered up, and doctors might use euthanasia as a way of avoiding criticism in cases that were medically difficult to treat. Particularly important, perhaps, are societal and political pressures, most evident in cost-containment policies, to which doctors might respond. After all, to permit earlier, less expensive death would ease the enormous pressure on third-party insurers, hospitals, and the Medicaid/Medicare system: euthanasia is less expensive than continuing medical care. The diagnosis-related group reimbursement system would particularly favor this since a hospital profits most from the patient who remains hospitalized for the shortest amount of time, but loses money on the one who remains longer than what is average for the DRG. Although passive euthanasia is cheaper than continuing life-prolonging treatment, active euthanasia is cheaper still: killing is the least expensive, most resource-conserving treatment of intractable disease.

Is there any reason to think such practices would actually occur? The reasons are closer to hand than one might imagine. Rather than predicting the future, we need simply look to our present practices for evidence that violations of the moral limits to euthanasia can occur. It is tempting to reply to a wedge argument against any social practice that we will always be able to draw a moral line when the time comes, but the clear evidence in the case of euthanasia is that we are not managing to do so now.

First, contemporary euthanasia practices sometimes involve violations of the principle of mercy. These violations are of two forms, neither conspicuous because neither involves evident physical cruelty. Nevertheless, both are cases of euthanasia that the principle of mercy does not endorse. First, there are cases in which the rhetoric of euthanasia, with its concept of painless, easy death, is used though considerations of mercy cannot possibly apply: these are the cases of the permanently comatose or brain dead. Since these persons do not suffer, euthanasia as the granting of mercy cannot be practiced upon them, and we mislead ourselves if we claim that they are "better off" dead. Second, there are cases in which the principle of mercy is violated when more than enough relief is given to those who do suffer. The principle of mercy demands euthanasia *only* when no other means of relieving pain will suffice. Yet we fail to acknowledge that the continuous, very heavy use of narcotizing drugs can be functionally equivalent to mercy killing itself: when used in a sustained way, without drug-free, conscious intervals or careful titration against alertness, such therapy effectively ends the patient's sentient life: his or her existence as a person ends when the drugging begins.[36] Of course, it may sometimes be difficult to obtain adequate and effective narcotics; nevertheless, because we do not recognize such drugging as equivalent in some respects to *active* euthanasia, we may be incautious and hasty in its use.

Contemporary euthanasia practices sometimes also involve violations of the principle of autonomy. It is true that much euthanasia, both passive and active, occurs at the request or with the consent of the individual who dies; passive euthanasia practices are provided for in natural death legislation and the use of durable powers of attorney and living wills. But we are also beginning to see the widespread development of hospital policies concerning nonresuscitation, and more frequent, routine physician exercise of this practice. It may even be fair to speak of a widespread consensus that in certain cases, nonresuscitation is the appropriate response. Official policies require that the patient—if competent—or his or her legal guardian be consulted before nonresuscitation orders are written. But such directives are by no means always followed. In Salt Lake City recently (though the story is universal), a physician reminded the granddaughter of an alert, competent eighty-nine-year-old nursing home patient, "You can always have 'do not resuscitate' orders written into her record." ("Why don't you ask her if that's what she wants?" was the granddaughter's reply.) A cardiologist at a major university says, in contrast, that he would not make such a suggestion to the family—because he "wouldn't want to put them through that"; this physician writes no-code orders on his own, without consulting either patient or family. In some places, no-code orders are written in pencil, so that they can be erased from records if desired; or circumlocutions not intelligible to laypersons ("consult primary physician before initiating treatment") are used.

Most significant among our current euthanasia practices may be the violations of justice. The argument from justice, as discussed so far, favors permitting euthanasia on the grounds that denial of treatment is morally permissible in certain specific cases: those in which the claims of a dying individual to medical resources are overridden by the claims of others in medical need. However, we often see the use of distributive policies that deny treatment to some but do not involve either the weighing of claims between the dying and others or the assurance that resources conserved would in fact be redistributed in accord with justice. The congressional decisions concerning artificial and transplant heart care may be one kind of example; arbitrary age minimums and ceilings for transplants, pacemakers, and dialysis, when they are not medically appropriate, may be another. Yet distributive justice concerns the point at which a dying person's right to medical treatment is outweighed by the claims of others; and the salvageability principle considered here does not hold that dying deprives one altogether of rights to medical care. In a situation of dire scarcity, such as urgent organ transplants, denying a transplant to one person usually means granting a transplant to someone else; if without it each person would die, the distributive principle of salvageability considered here holds that the person more likely to survive and benefit from the procedure has the stronger claim. But many distributive policies do not involve this kind of direct weighing of claims or assurances of reallocation, and much denial of treatment is done simply for thrift. *Thrift,* however, is not the same as *justice in distribution.* To deny treatment to the dying to "conserve resources" to "save money" is not to show that the claims of the dying are overridden by stronger claims on the part of someone else, or a group of persons, to whom such resources would in fact be redistributed; yet it is this point that is essential in preserving the principle of justice as applied to euthanasia.

In all these areas, then, there is evidence of "euthanasia" practices not justified by moral principle. Given these facts, the wedge argument and its objection to permitting euthanasia may loom larger. The wedge argument forecasts a slide down the slippery slope from morally permissible practices to impermissible ones; but even if we accept its model, there is no reason to assume that we are still at the top of this slope. Indeed, the evidence available suggests that we are already slipping. We already engage in "euthanasia" practices not justified on grounds of mercy, autonomy, or justice, and there is no reason to think that such abuses will not become still more widespread.

Nevertheless, I do not agree with the conclusion of the slippery slope argument: that because permissible euthanasia practices would lead (or are leading) to impermissible ones, we ought not allow them at all. We should not cease no-coding; mercy demands it. We should not restrict refusal of treatment or insist that all who can conceivably benefit be given as much treatment as possible; respect for autonomy requires that the patient be permitted to determine what is done to him or her. We should not resist legislative protections for passive euthanasia, like living wills and natural death laws, or oppose legislation permitting voluntary active euthanasia: justice, mercy, and autonomy all demand that euthanasia—both passive and active—be legally protected. Although the wedge argument is a serious one, prohibiting euthanasia is not the appropriate conclusion.

Most advocates of the wedge argument overlook a crucial feature of the structure of the argument itself. The wedge argument is teleological in character: it points to the bad consequence of permitting a morally acceptable type of action (call it A), namely, that morally unacceptable type (B) occurs. But users of the wedge argument err in failing to recognize that B's occurrence is not the sole outcome of A; A and B are *distinct* actions, each with its own set of consequences. Thus, in deciding whether to permit A, one must reckon in the bad consequences of the occurrence of B, but must also reckon in the other, possibly good consequences of A. Or, if one is deciding to prohibit A, the reckoning will include the (good) effects of avoiding B, but must also include the other (bad) effects of not having A occur. The wedge argument against euthanasia usually takes the form of an appeal to the welfare or rights of those who would become victims of later, unjustified practices. Usually, however, when the conclusion is offered that euthanasia therefore ought not be permitted, no account is taken of the welfare or rights of those who are to be denied the benefits of this practice. Hence, even if the causal claims advanced in the wedge argument are true and we are not able to hold the line or avoid the slide, they still do not establish the conclusion. Rather, the argument sets up a conflict. Either we ignore the welfare and abridge the rights of persons for whom euthanasia would clearly be morally permissible in order to protect those who would be the victims of corrupt euthanasia practices, or we ignore the potential victims in order to extend mercy and respect for autonomy to those who are the current victims of euthanasia prohibitions.

Thus, this conflict itself reveals an issue of justice still more fundamental than the distributive problems with which I began. The wedge argument assumes, without adequate justification, that the rights of those who may become the victims of abuses of a practice outweigh the rights of those who become victims if a practice is prohibited to whose benefits they are morally entitled and urgently need.

To protect those who might wrongly be killed or allowed to die might seem a stronger obligation than to satisfy the wishes of those who desire release from pain, analogous perhaps to the principle in law that "better ten guilty men go free than one be unjustly convicted."[37] However, the situation is not in fact analogous and does not favor protecting those who might wrongly be killed. To let ten guilty men go free in the interests of protecting one innocent man is not to impose harm on the ten guilty men. But to require the person who chooses to die to stay alive in order to protect those who might unwillingly be killed sometime in the future is to impose an extreme harm—intolerable suffering—on that person, which he or she must bear for the sake of others. Furthermore, since, as I have argued, the question of which is worse, suffering or death, is person-relative, we have no independent, objective basis for protecting the class of persons who might be killed at the expense of those who would suffer intolerable pain; perhaps our protecting ought to be done the other way around. Thus, I return to the recurrent problem throughout this discussion: which is the worse of two evils, death or pain? Since there are no prior agreements or claims that are relevant here, justice requires that rights to avoid the worse of the two evils be honored first, before others come into play. This, however, may be an obligation that, because it is person-relative and hence resistant to policy construction, we do not know how to meet.

JUSTICE AND REALISTIC DESIRE

Is there a workable solution to the problem that euthanasia poses? Certainly we can make some progress by attending to the violations of principle we have discovered. First, we must improve the conditions of dying; mercy will not demand euthanasia, nor the autonomous person choose it, when the conditions of dying are humane. Cicely Saunders, the founder of St. Christopher's Hospice in England and an ardent opponent of euthanasia, is perfectly right when she says of euthanasia, "one should be working to see that it is not needed."[38] Second, we need to improve the quality of the mercy we extend by attending to the element of autonomy in it: we must learn to respond to suffering in a way that takes account of the patient's own wishes and tolerances for pain, so that we give neither too little relief nor too much. Third, we must broaden our respect of autonomy in matters of dying by recognizing that the patient may choose active as well as passive means of coming to die—or none at all. It is crucial that the dying person receive full information about the consequences of accepting treatment or refusing it, so that he or she can rationally choose the way of dying—or staying alive—most in accord with his or her own values.[39] After all, a "good death" must always be a death that counts as good *for the patient*. For some it is the least painful, for others it is the quickest, for others one that permits final communication with family, and for still others the one that can be delayed the longest possible time. In this most personal of matters, a person's choice deserves the greatest respect.

But attention to mercy and autonomy does not yet seem to solve the problem of justice: the problems of whose rights are to be honored, and who is to be denied care. I mentioned earlier that all the workable distributive principles we might adopt would have the effect of forcing death on some persons who do not want it—those who cannot pay, those who have made no societal contributions, etc. Even the most plausible of these principles—the salvageability principle—would force earlier death upon the already dying, some of whom may wish to die but some of whom, under their own conception of the relative disvalue of suffering and death, want to continue as long as they possibly can. Thus, I think that the salvageability principle too is in error. Rather, we should favor a distributive principle that would allocate medical resources to those who *want* treatment, where "wanting" is interpreted as "realistic desire." This is to say, realistic desire ought to be considered both a necessary and a sufficient condition for providing treatment for those who are seriously ill.

To desire medical treatment in a realistic, reasonable, or rational way, the patient must not only actually have or be about to contract the condition for which treatment is proposed but also must understand the treatment's intended purposes, its possible side effects, the probability of success or failure, and the possible end condition to which the treatment would lead. For, say, an appendectomy, the patient must not only have appendicitis but also must understand at least roughly the nature of the procedure, what could go wrong, the approximate likelihood of success, and the end condition: relief of the acute pain in the abdomen, avoidance of death, and a small scar on the side. In most cases of acute appendicitis, an appendectomy will be the object of realistic desire. In a few cases, however, it is not, such as when the patient believes on religious grounds that the end condition of accepting medical treatment or a blood transfusion includes eventual damnation. Although religious cases are comparatively rare, there are many cases in which the principle of realistic desire would require substantial changes in our current distribution of medical care. Life-prolonging care given to the permanently comatose, decerebrate, profoundly brain damaged, and others who lack cognitive function is not, even in the case of antecedently executed directives, realistically desired, since such patients cannot want it, they are not entitled to life-prolonging care. Not even supportive care—such as feeding or routine hygiene—should be supplied, since this too cannot be realistically desired, patients in these extreme conditions should be allowed—or perhaps caused—to die.

Withholding care from permanently comatose patients may not seem morally problematic. But in a serious illness in which a cure cannot be guaranteed yet the patient remains competent, the problem becomes much more complex. Do patients with cancer of the larynx, for instance, *want* surgical treatment that, while providing a better-than-half chance of survival three years later, entails the permanent destruction of the normal voice? Most do, but, according to one study, at least 20 percent do not.[40] In such situations, the new distributive principle articulated here apportions treatment solely on the basis of a patient's desires, not on characteristics such as age or social worth. Most patients will receive appendectomies; four-fifths will have surgery on the larynx; permanently comatose patients will receive no care at all.

Would a distributive principle of realistic desire be effective in a scarcity situation? Although one's initial impression may be to the contrary, I believe that it would. It is crucial to remember that medical treatment is not like any ordinary consumer good; getting more of it does not entail that your advantages are increased. (Indeed, in an ideal lifetime, the amount of therapeutic medical treatment a person realistically wants is zero; this is the mark of the perfectly healthy life.) The treatments that are less likely to be realistically desired are, generally speaking, precisely those likely to occur at the end of life—the heroic, last-ditch, odds-against measures, undertaken because nothing else has worked. The chances are that the procedures will be painful, that they will introduce new limitations, and that they will not succeed. And the chance is also that these treatments will be extremely expensive. It is not possible to tell whether the savings in treatment costs under such a distributive policy would make it possible to provide full treatment for all who do want it, but there is no reason to *assume* that such savings would not: we need only recall the huge financial costs for nonsurvivors in an intensive care unit, for severely defective, unsalvageable neonates, or for permanently comatose patients in a nursing home or institution. A vast proportion of medical costs, as stated before, occurs in the last year of life. Most of this can be described as "needed" treatment. No doubt much of this is also "wanted" treatment, but much of it is not.

If use of the distributive principle of realistic desire should prove inadequate to solve the scarcity problem, then an additional distributive principle would need to be adopted to resolve conflicting claims among competitors who all realistically desire treatment: the salvageability principle, denying treatment to those who will die soon anyway, might then be brought into play. But those who will die soon may nevertheless want every moment of life they can possibly get, and it is unacceptable to adopt a distributive principle that has the effect of depriving some persons of wanted life before there is clear need to do so.

Of course, a distributive principle of realistic desire must have built into it paternalistic proxy procedures for providing medical care for incompetents of a variety of sorts, including infants and children, unconscious accident victims, the mentally ill, and the retarded. But I believe that these procedures should *not* include persons who are capable of realistic desire in the matter of terminal care but who have failed to consider and articulate their desires. Rather, it is becoming apparent that the individual has an obligation, increasingly evident as advances in medical technology both exacerbate the scarcity situation and offer heroic life-prolonging treatment that may not be desired, to stipulate in advance which modes of treatment he or she will accept and which he or she will decline, insofar as the patient's probable future can be foreseen. Only about one death in ten is wholly unexpected, and most result from prolonged, chronic illnesses.[41] Thus, most deaths can be predicted, within a fairly limited range of possibilities, before the event, and the course of the dying in certain general ways anticipated. What, most basically, the patient is obliged to do is indicate, as fully as possible, which he or she takes to be worse in situations that can be foreseen: pain or death. From this basic choice the treatment alternatives appropriate to the patient's condition can be deduced. By failing to exercise this obligation, the individual may force others—his or her physician, family members, or the courts—to make what are often morally precarious euthanasia decisions for him or her, perhaps on the basis of self-interest, societal pressure, or distributive principles for which there is no moral warrant. Because the patient has rights to medical treatment that he or she realistically desires and because it is the corresponding obligation of others to distribute treatment in accord with these desires, it is in turn the obligation of the patient to make his or her desires known whenever it is possible to do so.

However, it is particularly important to notice that continuous sedation is *not* an option the patient may choose, nor is it a defensible general solution to the problem of euthanasia. The patient's autonomous requests must still conform to the demands of justice, particularly as specified for medical situations by the principle of realistic desire. It is true that continuous sedation may satisfy both the principles of mercy and autonomy, but because there is no ongoing experience or sentient end state to which the treatment leads, the patient cannot realistically desire the treatment that would maintain him or her. Of course, there may be many cases in which the patient's condition is potentially reversible or the sedation can be interrupted to permit further personal experience, and in these circumstances sedation may indeed be realistically preferred to either pain or death (given the difficulty of accurately predicting circumstances in which continuous sedation will be permanently required without any hope of intervening lucidity, such cases may be the rule rather than the exception); in these cases the patient retains his or her claim to care. There may also be certain special situations in which the needs of, say, family members or transplant recipients outweigh the claims of other patients competing for resources, so that justice will permit maintaining a patient in continuous sedation on the same basis as it might in rare cases permit maintaining a patient who is permanently comatose. But when such conditions do not obtain, even the patient who articulates his or her choices in advance is not entitled to request *permanent* sedation, since the principle of realistic desire prohibits him or her, like the proverbial dog in the manger, from laying claim to resources he or she cannot possibly enjoy. Nor may physicians turn to continuous sedation as a way of avoiding difficult moral dilemmas in terminal care (except, of course, in the frequent situations in which they think that their predictions may be wrong); they are bound to honor the choices of a patient made in accord with the principle of realistic desire, but this principle does not permit such a choice. At least in any scarcity situation, the patient must choose either death or periodically sentient life, though this may involve pain; he or she cannot morally choose to be maintained in a permanently sedated or unconscious state when that means depriving someone else of care.

CONCLUSION: EUTHANASIA AND SUICIDE

It may be objected that requiring the patient to choose between death and life, insofar as the patient must antecedently consider treatment decisions that affect the circumstances and timing of his or her own demise, is equivalent to requiring the patient's consideration of suicide. In a sense, it is; but this is also the more general solution to the euthanasia problem. Although euthanasia is indeed warranted on grounds of mercy, autonomy, and justice, these principles can be more effectively and safely honored by permitting suicide, perhaps assisted by the physician who has care of the patient or a family member under the advice of the physicians,[42] and supplemented by nonvoluntary euthanasia *only* when the patient is permanently comatose or otherwise irretrievably inaccessible. Not only do practical reasons like avoiding greed and manipulation on the part of physicians or the institutions controlling them speak for preferring physician-assisted suicide to physician-initiated euthanasia, but there are conceptual reasons as well. The conditions that distinguish morally permissible euthanasia from impermissible murder all involve matters that the patient, not the physician, is in a privileged position to know. To extend mercy, the physician must know how the patient weighs suffering against death, and at what point *for the patient* death becomes the lesser of two evils. To respect the patient's autonomy, the physician must know what his or her preferences are, given the alternatives available, in the matter of dying. And to exercise justice, the physician must know what treatment the patient realistically desires. Perhaps the physician who is painstakingly careful in listening to an articulate and self-aware patient may discover these things, but he or she cannot have the patient's knowledge. Consequently, since the risk of misinterpretation is great and the possibility of manipulation or coercion high, the physician should not be the one to *initiate* the choice. Rather, he or she must be prepared to assist the patient who chooses death, just as he or she is prepared to assist the patient who chooses continuing life. In physician-assisted suicide, it is the person whose death is in question who is responsible for the death; he or she originates and chooses this course of action, rather than having death chosen for him or her. Of course, to permit suicide in these situations may seem to increase the risk of encouraging ill-considered suicide among emotionally disturbed or mentally ill persons, but here the physician serves as a check: in the role of assistant to the suicide, the physician will refuse to assist whenever in his or her professional perception the circumstances clearly do not warrant such an act (such as in cases in which there is neither pain nor approaching death, but not in those exhibiting one or both). This is by no means a foolproof policy; the physician will no doubt often influence the patient. But this intrusion is still a far cry from having the physician decide when or why euthanasia is appropriate and initiate the act.

Furthermore, physician-assisted suicide is less subject to the erection of policy requirements than are euthanasia practices. The choices of patients about whether and how to die will vary widely; but then, there is no reason why they should not. These choices are influenced by an enormous range of individual values, past experiences, and moral and religious beliefs. Euthanasia policies developed by physicians or medical institutions may overlook individual differences in patients' wishes by establishing routine, common procedures for dealing with terminal illness, and in this way invite the continuing slide down the slippery slope. We must be prepared to permit and perform mercy killing when the patient desires it and when there is no other way to avoid the sufferings of death. But we do not want doctors to assume the responsibility for such killings, or to appeal to standardized, court-approved procedures, made under economic constraints, for determining when such killings are appropriate. Rather, mercy killing must ideally always be mercy killing of the patient by him- or herself, in which the patient is entitled to the assistance of the physician he or she has chosen. When proxy procedures are required, we must be sure that they approximate as nearly as possible what the person's own decision would have been. It is crucial to exercise mercy; it is essential to respect autonomy, and though we must submit to the demands of justice, we can hope to do so at no one's expense. It is extremely important to avoid any further slide down the involuntary thrift-euthanasia slope. Recognition of physician-aided suicide, as distinguished from physician-directed euthanasia, comes closest to satisfying all of these moral demands.

After all, we must not forget that we already practice euthanasia on quite a wide scale, but we do not always practice it in a morally defensible way. We practice passive euthanasia by withholding and withdrawing treatment, and we practice active quasi-euthanasia by using sedation sufficient to terminate the personal existence of a human being. Some of this is in accord with the principles of mercy, autonomy, and justice, but much of it is not. What grows dimmer in contemporary practice is the sense that euthanasia, as "good death," must be good *for the person whose death it is*; we are losing any sense that mercy must play a major role or that the patient's choice is crucial in determining whether that death counts as good. Already we are beginning to count resource-conserving deaths under this term. Paul Ramsey remarks that "it is better if you do not know the Greek language or the root meaning of the word";[43]—but, of course, knowing these things permits us to see the shifts in our use of the term, shifts that are perhaps symptomatic of the slide already under way down the slippery slope. Our very language invites us to overlook distinctions that we ought to make. The concept of euthanasia has come to include letting patients die and killings that are not required by mercy, autonomy, or justice, but are simply the product of thrift in medical affairs. Yet at the same time our discomfort with this fact leads us to claim, at least officially, that we reject any practice of euthanasia at all, though of course this is not true. In this way, the increasing distortion of the term itself leads us to overlook a double moral fault: often, we practice "euthanasia" when we should not, and very often, we fail to practice euthanasia when we should.

Author's Note

I'd like to thank Arthur G. Lipmand, Pharm.D., and Howard Wilcox, M.D., as well as my collegues in philosophy, Bruce Landesman and Leslie Francis, for comments on earlier drafts of this chapter.

Notes

1. Perhaps the principle of (medical) mercy is stronger than this and asserts a duty to relieve the suffering of others even at some substantial cost to oneself, or in violation of others of these provisos. The quite weak form of the principle, as I have stated it here, requires, for instance, that one ought not stand idly by (all other things being equal) when one could easily help an injured person but does not require feats of physical or financial heroism or self-sacrifice. This is not to say that I think a stronger version of the duty to relieve suffering (as defended, for instance, by Susan James, "The Duty to Relieve Suffering," *Ethics* [October 1982] 93:4-21), could not be supported, but that the stronger version is not necessary for the case I am making here: a prima facie duty to participate in both passive and active euthanasia, at least in a more permissive legal climate, is entailed even by the very weak form of the principle of mercy.

   Incidentally, although much of the medical literature distinguishes between pain and suffering, I have not chosen to do so here: it would raise difficult mind/body problems, and in any case the two are clearly intertwined. I grant, however, that the principle of (medical) mercy would meet still broader assent if phrased to require the relieving of physical pain alone.

2. It is important not to confuse the principle of (medical) mercy with a principle permitting or requiring judicial mercy. In judicial and political contexts, such as pardons or amnesties, the individual on whom penalties have been or are about to be imposed may have no claim to benevolent treatment, and the issue concerns whether mercy may or should be granted. Many authors treat judicial mercy as a work of individual supererogation, not a requirement or duty, and some suggest that it is morally forbidden: one ought not excuse a person guilty of a crime. However, we are concerned here not with judicial mercy, but rather with mercy as it arises primarily in medical contexts: injuries, illnesses, disabilities, degenerative processes, and genetic defect or disease. Unlike pain or suffering inflicted in judicial contexts, in the medical context these are not warranted by the past actions of the suffering individual, but are usually of natural or accidental origin and in most cases are beyond the individual's control: pain and suffering are something that happen to him or her, not something the patient has earned. The principle of medical mercy is usually taken to apply even in cases in which a medical condition is caused or exacerbated by the individual's voluntary behavior, as in smokers' diseases or injuries from attempted suicide. It is consistent to hold that mercy is supererogatory (or perhaps morally forbid-

den) in judicial or political contexts, but also that it is required in medical ones.

3. Edmund D. Pellegrino, M.D., "The Clinical Ethics of Pain Management in the Terminally Ill," *Hospital Formulary* 17 (November 1982): 1495-96; and Marcia Angell, "The Quality of Mercy," *New England Journal of Medicine* 306 (January 1982): 98-99.

4. For instance, I take it to be a moral duty, and not merely a nice thing to do, to help a child remove a painful splinter from a finger when the child cannot do so alone and when this can be done without undue costs to oneself. (I assume that the splinter case satisfies the other provisos of the principle of medical mercy.) Similarly, I take it to be a moral duty to stop the bleeding of a person who has been wounded or to pull someone from a fire, though in very many of the cases in which such circumstances arise (wars, accidents) this duty is abrogated because we cannot do so without risks to ourselves. The duty of medical mercy is not simply equivalent to either nonmaleficence or beneficence, though perhaps derived from them, since the former is understood as a duty to refrain from causing harm and the latter to do good in a positive sense; the duty of medical mercy requires one to counteract harms one did not cause, though it may not require conferring additional positive benefits.

5. See Sharon H. Imbus and Bruce E. Zawacki, "Autonomy for Burned Patients When Survival Is Unprecedented," *New England Journal of Medicine* 297 (August 11, 1977): 309-311.

6. See Mary Voboril, *Miami Herald*, Saturday, July 1, 1978, see also note 17.

7. An extensive discussion of the conceptual and moral distinctions between killing and letting die begins with Jonathan Bennett, "Whatever the Consequences," *Analysis* 26 (1966):83-97, and, after the American Medical Association's stand prohibiting mercy killing but permitting cessation of treatment, continues in James Rachels's "Active and Passive Euthanasia," *New England Journal of Medicine* 292 (January 9, 1975): 78-80, and many subsequent papers.

8. See Ludwig Edelstein, "The Hippocratic Oath," in *Ancient Medicine: Selected Papers of Ludwig Edelstein,* ed. Owsei Temkin and C. Lilian Temkin (Baltimore: The Johns Hopkins University Press, 1967), esp. 9-15, on the Greek physician's role in euthanasia.

9. Hospice, founded and directed by Cicely Saunders, is a movement devoted to the development of institutions for providing palliative but medically nonaggressive care for terminal patients. In addition to its extraordinary contribution in developing methods of prophylactic pain control, according to which analgesics are administered on a scheduled basis in advance of experienced pain, Hospice has also emphasized attention to the emotional needs of the patient's family. An account of the theory and methodology of Hospice can be found in various publications by Saunders, including "Terminal Care in Medical Oncology," in *Medical Oncology*, ed. K.D. Bagshawe (Oxford: Blackwell, 1975), 563-576.

10. Joanne Lynn, M.D., "Supportive Care for Dying Patients: An Introduction for Health Care Professionals," Appendix B of the President's Commission for the Study of Ethical Problems in Medicine and Biomedical and Behavioral Research, *Deciding to Forego Life-Sustaining Treatment* (Washington, D.C.: Government Printing Office, 1983), 295.

11. Robert G. Twycross, "Voluntary Euthanasia," in *Suicide and Euthanasia: The Rights of Personhood,* ed. Samuel E. Wallace and Albin Eser (Knoxville: The University of Tennessee Press, 1981), 89.

12. Phillippa Foot, "Euthanasia," *Philosophy & Public Affairs* 6 (Winter 1977): 95.

13. To discover what one's own views are, try the following thought experiment. Imagine that you have been captured by a gang of ruthless and superlatively clever criminals, whom you know with certainty will never be caught or change their minds. They plan either to execute you now, or to torture you unremittingly for the next twenty years and then put you to death. Which would be worse? Does your view change if the length of the torture period is reduced to twenty days or twenty minutes, and if so, why? How severe does the torture need to be?

14. 211 N.Y. 127, 129; 105 N.E. 92, 93 (1914).

15. *In re Yetter*, 62 Pa. D. & C. 2d 619 (1973).

16. *Satz v. Perlmutter,* 362 S. 2d 160 (Fla. App. 1978), affirmed by Florida Supreme Court 379 So. 2d 359 (1980).

17. *Bartling v. Superior Court,* 2 Civ. No. B007907 (Calif. App. 1984).

18. California Health & Safety Code, Sections 7195-7196.

19. The living will and durable power of attorney forms valid in different states are distributed by Choice in Dying, 200 Varig Street, New York, NY 10014. Copies are also available from hospitals and attorneys.

20. M. Siegler, "Pascal's Wager and the Hanging of Crepe," *The New England Journal of Medicine* 293 (1975): 853-857.

21. See also a study of other factors associated with differences in prognosis and treatment decisions: R. Pearlman, T. Inui, and W. Carter, "Variability in Physician Bioethical Decision-Making," *Annals of Internal Medicine* 97 (September 1982): 420-425.

22. The effects of depression on the choice concerning whether to live or die are described by Richard B. Brandt, "The Morality and Rationality of Suicide," in *A Handbook for the Study of Suicide,* ed. Seymour Perlin (New York: Oxford University Press, 1975), 61-76, and reprinted in part in M. Pabst Battin and David J. Mayo, eds., *Suicide: The Philosophical Issues* (New York: St. Martin's Press, 1980), 117-132.

23. I've considered elsewhere the symmetrical argument that if death is in some circumstances actually better than life, the paternalist should be prepared to override a patient's choice of life. See M. Pabst Battin, *Ethical Issues in Suicide* (Englewood Cliffs, N. J.: Prentice-Hall, 1982), 160-175.

24. Vatican Congregation for the Doctrine of the Faith, "Declaration on Euthanasia," June 26, 1980; see Section II, "Euthanasia."

25. Peter C. Williams, "Rights and the Alleged Right of Innocents to Be Killed," *Ethics* 87 (1976-77): 383-394.

26. This proviso may appear to resemble similar provisos exempting physicians, nurses, and other caregivers who have principled objections to participating in abortions. But I am much less certain that weight should be given to the scruples of physicians in euthanasia cases, at least at the time of need. As I will suggest in the final section of this chapter, the patient has an obligation to make his or her wishes concerning euthanasia known in advance in a foreseeable decline; if the physician objects, it is his or her duty to excuse himself or herself from the case and from the care of the patient altogether *before* the patient's deteriorating condition prevents or makes it difficult to transfer to another physician; the doctor cannot simply voice his or her objections when the patient finally reaches the point of requesting help in dying. The physician should of course object if, for instance, he or she believes that the patient is acting on faulty information; but the physician ought not introduce a principled objection to participation in euthanasia in general at this late date.

27. To this end, the British and Scottish voluntary euthanasia societies have published booklets of explicit information concerning methods of suicide for distribution to their members; the Dutch voluntary euthanasia society has published a handbook intended specifically for physicians, and voluntary physician-assisted euthanasia is legally tolerated in Holland. In the United States, Hemlock, a society advocating legalization of voluntary euthanasia and assisted suicide, also makes available similar information.

28. O. Ruth Russell, *Freedom to Die: Moral and Legal Aspects of Euthanasia,* rev. ed. (New York: Human Sciences Press, 1977), 19.

29. Tom L. Beauchamp and Arnold I. Davidson, "The Definition of Euthanasia," *The Journal of Medicine and Philosophy* 4 (September 1979): 301.

30. Paul Ramsey, *The Patient as Person* (New Haven: Yale University Press, 1970), 161.

31. Allan S. Detsky et al., "Prognosis, Survival, and the Expenditure of Hospital Resources for Patients in an Intensive-Care Unit," *The New England Journal of Medicine* 305 (September 17, 1981): 667-672; figures from Table 1.

32. This case, originally presented in the *Illinois Medical Journal* and reprinted in *Connecticut Medicine* with commentary from medical, ethical, and legal experts, is summarized in *Concern for Dying* 8 (Summer 1982): 3. This patient did receive treatment for intervening infections, pneumonia, dermatitis, and convulsions, and for the ten days before her death was maintained on oxygen, respiratory therapy, and antibiotics.

33. President's Commission for the Study of Ethical Problems in Medicine and Biomedical and Behavioral Research, *Defining Death: Medical, Legal, and Ethical Issues in the Determination of Death* (Washington, D.C.: Government Printing Office, 1981), 18, citing the *Guinness Book of World Records* regarding the case of Elaine Esposito.

34. See the useful discussion of the form of the wedge argument in Tom L. Beauchamp and James F. Childress, *Principles of Biomedical Ethics* (New York: Oxford University Press, 1979). 109-117. I am concerned primarily with the second, empirical form of the argument here, but disagree with the conclusions Beauchamp and Childress reach.

35. As one physician has pointed out, objecting to the wedge argument's contention that greed would bring doctors to kill their patients, there is "not much financial incentive with a dead patient." In fact, greed may work the other way around: doctors strive to keep their patients alive, whatever the physical or financial costs to the patients, because their income is derived from services provided. As another physician has pointed out, however, not all patients are profitable, and the physician who has enough profitable ones will find that killing off the unprofitable ones further improves the bottom line. Needless to say, greed in any of these varieties will violate the principles of mercy, autonomy, and justice.

36. See the position of Pope Pius XII on the use of painkillers in "The Prolongation of Life," an address to an international congress of anesthesiologists, reprinted in Dennis J. Horan and David Mall, eds., *Death, Dying, and Euthanasia* (Frederick, Md.: University Publications of America, 1980), 281-287. The view of Pius XII is reemphasized by Pope John Paul II (see note 24). Although both permit the use of painkillers that shorten life, provided they are intended to relieve pain, not intended to produce death, both also warn against the casual use of painkillers that cause unconsciousness, since, in the words of the latter, "a person not only has to be able to satisfy his or her moral duties and family obligations; he or she also has to prepare himself or herself with full consciousness for meeting Christ" (Section III). Advanced pain-management techniques may be able to reduce the problem, but in practice the excessive use of painkillers remains common.

37. See the discussion of this analogy in John D. Arras, "The Right to Die on the Slippery Slope," *Social Theory and Practice* 8 (Fall 1982): 301 ff.

38. Cicely Saunders, "The Moment of Truth: Care of the Dying Person," in *Confrontations of Death: A Book of Readings and a Suggested Method of Instruction,* ed. Francis G. Scott and Ruth M. Brewer (Corvalis,

Ore.: A Continuing Education Book, 1971), 119, quoted in Paul Ramsey, *Ethics at the Edges of Life* (New Haven: Yale University Press, 1978), 152. Dame Saunders is the founder and medical director of St. Christopher's Hospice near London, which has provided the stimulus and model for the contemporary hospice movement.

39. See chapter 1 of this book [*Least Worth Death: Essays on the End of Life* (Philadelphia: Temple University Press, 1994)].

40. Barbara J. McNeil, Ralph Weichselbaum, and Stephen G. Pauker, "Speech and Survival: Tradeoffs between Quality and Quantity of Life in Laryngeal Cancer," *New England Journal of Medicine* 305 (October 22, 1981): 982-987. The study, however, was performed with healthy volunteers, not actual patients. See Correspondence, *New England Journal of Medicine* 306 (February 25, 1982): 482-483, for other criticisms of this study, including evidence that rehabilitation of speech may be quite satisfactory.

41. See Courtney S. Campbell, "'Aid-in-Dying' and the Taking of Human Life," *Journal of Medical Ethics* 18 (1992): 128-134, for an estimate that 76-84 percent of deaths are caused by chronic conditions.

42. It is sometimes argued that physician assistance in a patient's suicide would violate the Hippocratic Oath. It is true that the oath, in its original form, does contain an explicit injunction that the physician shall not give a lethal potion to a patient who requests it, nor make a suggestion to that effect (to do so was apparently common Greek medical practice at the time). But the oath in its original form also contains explicit prohibitions of the physician's accepting fees for teaching medicine, and of performing surgery—even on gallstones. These latter prohibitions are not retained in modern reformulations of the oath, and I see no reason why the provision against giving lethal potions to patients who request it should be. What is central to the oath and cannot be deleted without altering its essential character is the requirement that the physician shall come "for the benefit of the sick." Under the argument advanced here, physician assistance in patient suicide may in some cases indeed be for the benefit of the patient. What the oath would continue to prohibit is physician assistance in a suicide for the physician's own gain or to serve other institutional or societal ends.

43. Ramsey, *The Patient as Person*, 145.

32.
WHEN SELF-DETERMINATION RUNS AMOK

Daniel Callahan

The euthanasia debate is not just another moral debate, one in a long list of arguments in our pluralistic society. It is profoundly emblematic of three important turning points in Western thought. The first is that of the legitimate conditions under which one person can kill another. The first is that of the legitimate conditions under which one person can kill another. The acceptance of voluntary active euthanasia would morally sanction what can only be called "consenting adult killing." By that term I mean the killing of one person by another in the name of their mutual right to be a killer and killed if they freely agree to play those roles. This turn flies in the face of a longstanding effort to limit the circumstances under which one person can take the life of another, from efforts to control the free flow of guns and arms, to abolish capital punishment, and to more tightly control warfare. Euthanasia would add a whole new category of killing to a society that already has too many excuses to indulge itself in that way.

The second turning point lies in the meaning and limits of self-determination. The acceptance of euthanasia would sanction a view of autonomy holding that individuals may, in the name of their own private, idiosyncratic view of the good life, call upon others, including such institutions as medicine, to help them pursue that life, even at the risk of harm to the common good. This works against the idea that the meaning and scope of our own right to lead our own lives must be conditioned by, and be compatible with, the good of the community, which is more than an aggregate of self-directing individuals.

The third turning point is to be found in the claim being made upon medicine: it should be prepared to make its skills available to individuals to help them achieve their private vision of the good life. This puts medicine in the business of promoting the individualistic pursuit of general human happiness and well-being. It would overturn the traditional belief that medicine should limit its domain to promoting and preserving human health, redirecting it instead to the relief of that suffering which stems from life itself, not merely from a sick body.

I believe that, at each of these three turning points, proponents of euthanasia push us in the wrong direction. Arguments in favor of euthanasia fall into four general categories, which I will take up in turn: (1) the moral claim of individual self-determination and well-being; (2) the moral irrelevance of the difference between killing and allowing to die; (3) the supposed paucity of evidence to show likely harmful consequences of legalized euthanasia; and (4) the compatibility of euthanasia and medical practice.

SELF-DETERMINATION

Central to most arguments for euthanasia is the principle of self-determination. People are presumed to have an interest in deciding for themselves, according to their own beliefs about what makes life good, how they will conduct their lives. That is an important value, but the question in the euthanasia context is, What does it mean and how far should it extend? If it were a question of suicide, where a person takes her own life without assistance from another, that principle might be pertinent, at least for debate. But euthanasia is not that limited a matter. The self-determination in that case can only be effected by the moral and physical assistance of another. Euthanasia is thus no longer a matter only of self-determination, but of a mutual, social decision between two people, the one to be killed and the other to do the killing.

How are we to make the moral move from my right of self-determination to some doctor's right to kill me—from *my* right to *his* right? Where does the doctor's moral warrant to kill come from? Ought doctors to be able to kill anyone they want as long as permission is given by competent persons? Is our right to life just like a piece of property, to be given away or alienated if the price (happiness, relief of suffering) is right? And then to be destroyed with our permission once alienated?

In answer to all those questions, I will say this: I have yet to hear a plausible argument why it should be permissible for us to put this kind of power in the hands of another, whether a doctor or anyone else. The idea that we can waive our right to life, and then give to another the power to take that life, requires a justification yet to be provided by anyone.

Slavery was long ago outlawed on the ground that one person should not have the right to own another, even with the other's permission. Why? Because it is a fundamental moral wrong for one person to give over his life and fate to another, whatever the good consequences, and no less a wrong for another person to have that kind of total, final power, Like slavery, dueling was long ago banned on similar grounds: even free, competent individuals should not have the power to kill each other, whatever their motives whatever the circumstances. Consenting adult killing, like consenting adult slavery or degradation, is a strange route to human dignity.

There is another problem as well. IF doctors, once sanctioned to carry out euthanasia, are to be themselves responsible moral agents—not simply hired hands with lethal injections at the ready—then they must have their own *independent* moral grounds to kill those who request such services. What do I mean? As those who favor euthanasia are quick to point out, some people want it because their life has become so burdensome it no longer seems worth living.

The doctor will have a difficulty at this point. The degree and intensity to which people suffer from their diseases and their dying, and whether they find life more of a burden than a benefit, has very little directly to do with the nature or extent of their actual physical nature or extent of their actual physical condition. Three people can have the same condition, but only one will find the suffering unbearable. People suffer, but suffering is as much a function of the values of individuals as it is of the physical causes of that suffering. Inevitably in that circumstance, the doctor will in effect be treating the patient's values. To be responsible, the doctor would have to share those values. The doctor would have to decide, on her own, whether the patient's life was "no longer worth living."

But how could a doctor possibly know that or make such a judgment? Just because the patient said so? I raise this question because, while in Holland at [a] euthanasia conference ... the doctors present agreed that there is no objective way of measuring or judging the claims of patients that their suffering is unbearable. And if it is difficult to measure suffering, how much more difficult to determine the value of a patient's statement that her life is not worth living?

However one might want to answer such questions, the very need to ask them, to inquire into the physician's responsibility and grounds for medical and moral judgment, points out the social nature of the decision. Euthanasia is not a private matter of self-determination. It is an act that requires two people to make it possible, and a complicit society to make it acceptable.

KILLING AND ALLOWING TO DIE

Against common opinion, the argument is sometimes made that there is no moral difference between stopping life-sustaining treatment and more active forms of killing, such as lethal injection. Instead I would contend that the notion that there is no morally significant difference between omission and commission is just wrong. Consider in its broad implications what the eradication of the distinction implies: that death from disease has been banished, leaving only the actions of physicians in terminating treatment as the cause of death. Biology, which used to bring about death, has apparently been displaced by human agency. Doctors have finally, I suppose, thus genuinely become gods, now doing what nature and the deities once did.

What is the mistake here? It lies in confusing causality and culpability, and in failing to note the way in which human societies have overlaid natural causes with moral rules and interpretations. Causality (by which I mean the direct physical causes of death) and culpability (by which I mean our attribution of moral responsibility to human actions) are confused under three circumstances.

They are confused, first, when the action of a physician in stopping treatment of a patient with an underlying lethal disease is construed as *causing* death. On the contrary, the physician's omission can only bring about death on the condition that the patient's disease will kill him in the absence of treatment. We may hold the physician morally responsible for the death, if we have morally judged such actions wrongful omissions. But it confuses reality and moral judgment to see an omitted action as having the same causal status as one that directly kills. A lethal injection will kill both a healthy person and a sick person. A physician's omitted treatment will have no effect on a healthy person. Turn off the machine on me, a healthy person, and nothing will happen. It will only, in contrast, bring the life of a sick person to an end because of an underlying fatal disease.

Causality and culpability are confused, second, when we fail to note that judgments of moral responsibility and culpability are human constructs. By that I mean that we human beings, after moral reflection, have decided to call some actions right or wrong, and to devise moral rules to deal with them. When physicians could do nothing to stop death, they were not held responsible for it. When, with medical progress, they began to have some power over death—but only its timing and circumstances, not its ultimate inevitability—moral rules were devised to set forth their obligations. Natural causes of death were not thereby banished. They were, instead, overlaid with a medical ethics designed to determine moral culpability in deploying medical power.

To confuse the judgments of this ethics with the physical causes of death—which is the connotation of the word *kill*—is to confuse nature and human action. People will, one way or another, die of some disease; death will have dominion over all of us. To say that a doctor "kills" a patient by allowing this to happen should only be understood as a moral judgment about the licitness of his omission, nothing more. We can, as a fashion of speech only, talk about a doctor *killing* a patient by omitting treatment he should have provided. It is a fashion of speech precisely because it is the underlying disease that brings death when treatment is omitted; that is it s cause, not the physician's omission. It is a misuse of the work *killing* to use it when a doctor stops a treatment he believes will no longer benefit that patient—when, that is, he steps aside to allow an eventually inevitable death to occur now rather than later. The only deaths that human beings invented are those

that come from direct killing—when, with a lethal injection, we both cause death and are morally responsible for it. In the case of omissions, we do not cause death even if we may be judged morally responsible for it.

This difference between causality and culpability also helps us see why a doctor who has omitted a treatment he should have provided has "killed" that patient while another doctor—performing precisely the same act of omission on another patient in different circumstances—does not kill her, but only allows her to die. The difference is that we have come, by moral convention and conviction, to classify unauthorized or illegitimate omissions as acts of "killing." We call them "killing" in the expanded sense of the term: a culpable action that permits the real cause of death, the underlying disease, to proceed to its lethal conclusion. By contrast, the doctor who, at the patient's request, omits or terminates unwanted treatment does not kill at all. Her underlying disease, not his action, is the physical cause of death; and we have agreed to consider actions of that kind to be morally licit. He thus can truly be said to have "allowed" her to die.

If we fail to maintain the distinction between killing and allowing to die, moreover, there are some disturbing possibilities. The first would be to confirm many physicians in their already too powerful belief that, when patients die, or when physicians stop treatment because of the futility of continuing it, they are somehow both morally and physically responsible for the deaths that follow. That notion needs to be abolished, not strengthened. It needlessly and wrongly burdens the physician, to whom should not be attributed the powers of the gods. The second possibility would be that, in every case where a doctor judges medical treatment no longer effective in prolonging life, a quick and direct killing of the patient would be seen as the next, most reasonable step, on grounds of both humaneness and economics. I do not see how that logic could easily be rejected.

CALCULATING THE CONSEQUENCES

When concerns about the adverse social consequences of permitting euthanasia are raised, its advocates tend to dismiss them as unfounded and overly speculative. On the contrary, recent data about the Dutch experience suggests that such concerns are right on target. From my own discussions in Holland, and from the articles on that subject in this issue and elsewhere, I believe we can now fully see most of the *likely* consequences of legal euthanasia.

Three consequences seem almost certain, in this or any other country: the inevitability of some abuse of the law; the difficulty of precisely writing, and then enforcing, the law; and the inherent slipperiness of the moral reasons for legalizing euthanasia in the first place.

Why is abuse inevitable? One reason is that almost all laws on delicate, controversial matters are to some extent abused. This happens because not everyone will agree with the law as written and will bend it, or ignore it, if they can get away with it. From explicit admissions to me by Dutch proponents of euthanasia, and from the corroborating information provided by the Remmelink Report and the outside studies of Carlos Gomez and John Keown, I am convinced that in the Netherlands there are a substantial number of cases of nonvoluntary euthanasia, that is, euthanasia undertaken without the explicit permission of the person being killed. The other reason abuse is inevitable is that the law is likely to have a low enforcement priority in the criminal justice system. Like other laws of similar status, unless there is an unrelenting and harsh willingness to pursue abuse, violations will ordinarily be tolerated. The worst thing to me about my experience in Holland was the casual, seemingly indifferent attitude toward abuse. I think that would happen everywhere.

Why would it be hard to precisely write, and then enforce, the law? The Dutch speak about the requirement of "unbearable" suffering, but admit that such a term is just about indefinable, a highly subjective matter admitting of no objective standards. A requirement for outside opinion is nice, but it is easy to find complaisant colleagues. A requirement that a medical condition be "terminal" will run aground on the notorious difficulties of knowing when an illness is actually terminal.

Apart from those technical problems there is a more profound worry. I see no way, even in principle, to write or enforce a meaningful law that can guarantee effective procedural safeguards. The rea-

son is obvious yet almost always overlooked. The euthanasia transaction will ordinarily take place within the boundaries of the private and confidential doctor-patient relationship. No one can possibly know what takes place in that context unless the doctor chooses to reveal it. In Holland, less than 10 percent of the physicians report their acts of euthanasia and do so with almost complete legal impunity. There is no reason why the situation should be any better elsewhere. Doctors will have their own reasons for keeping euthanasia secret, and some patients will have no less a motive for wanting it concealed.

I would mention, finally, that the moral logic of the motives for euthanasia contain within them the ingredients of abuse. The two standard motives for euthanasia and assisted suicide are said to be our right of self-determination, and our claim upon the mercy of others, especially doctors, to relieve our suffering. These two motives are typically spliced together and presented as a single justification. Yet if they are considered independently—and there is no inherent reason why they must be linked—they reveal serious problems. It is said that a competent, adult person should have a right to euthanasia for the relief of suffering. But why must the person be suffering? Does not that stipulation already compromise the principle of self-determination? How can self-determination have any limits? Whatever the person's motives may be, why are they not sufficient?

Consider next the person who is suffering but not competent, who is perhaps demented or mentally retarded. The standard argument would deny euthanasia to that person. But why? If a person is suffering but not competent, then it would seem grossly unfair to deny relief solely on the grounds of incompetence. Are the incompetent less entitled to relief from suffering than the competent? Will it only be affluent, middle-class people, mentally fit and savvy about working the medical system, who can qualify? Do the incompetent suffer less because of their incompetence?

Considered from these angles, there are no good moral reasons to limit euthanasia once the principle of taking life for that purpose has been legitimated. If we really believe in self-determination, then any competent person should have a right to be killed by a doctor for any reason that suits him. If we believe in the relief of suffering, then it seems cruel and capricious to deny it to the incompetent. There is, in short, no reasonable or logical stopping point once the turn has been made down the road to euthanasia, which could soon turn into a convenient and commodious expressway.

EUTHANASIA AND MEDICAL PRACTICE

A fourth kind of argument one often hears both in the Netherlands and in this country is that euthanasia and assisted suicide are perfectly compatible with the aims of medicine. I would note at the very outset that a physician who participates in another person's suicide already abuses medicine. Apart from depression (the main statistical cause of suicide), people commit suicide, because they find life empty, oppressive, or meaningless. Their judgment is a judgment about the value of continued life, not only about health (even if they are sick). Are doctors now to be given the right to make judgments about the kinds of life worth living and to give their blessing to suicide for those they judge wanting? What conceivable competence, technical or moral, could doctors claim to play such a role? Are we to medicalize suicide, turning judgments about its worth and value into one more clinical issue? Yes, those are rhetorical questions.

Yet they bring us to the core of the problem of euthanasia and medicine. The great temptation of modern medicine, not always resisted, is to move beyond the promotion and preservation of health into the boundless realm of general human happiness and wellbeing. The root problem of illness and mortality is both medical and philosophical or religious. "Why must I die?" can be asked as a technical, biological question or as a question about the meaning of life. When medicine tries to respond to the latter, which it is always under pressure to do, it moves beyond its proper role.

It is not medicine's place to lift from us the burden of that suffering which turns on the meaning we assign to the decay of the body and its eventual death. It is not medicine's place to determine when lives are not worth living or when the burden of life is too great to be borne. Doctors have no conceivable way of evaluating such claims on the part of patients, and they should have no right to act in response to them. Medicine should try to relive human suffering, but only that suffering which is brought on by illness and dying as biological phenomena, not that suffering which comes from anguish or despair at the human condition.

Doctors ought to relieve those forms of suffering that medically accompany serious illness and the threat of death. They should relive pain, do what they can to allay anxiety and uncertainty, and be a comforting presence. As sensitive human beings, doctors should be prepared to respond to patients who ask why they must die, or die in pain. But here the doctor and the patient are at the same level. The doctor may have no better an answer to those old questions than anyone else; and certainly no special insight from his training as a physician. It would be terrible for physicians to forget this, and to think that in a swift, lethal injection, medicine has found its own answer to the riddle of life. It would be a false answer, given by the wrong people. It would be no less a false answer for patients. They should neither ask medicine to put its own vocation at risk to serve their private interest, nor think that the answer to suffering is to be killed by another. The problem is precisely that, too often in human history, killing has seemed the quick, efficient way to put aside that which burdens us. It rarely helps, and too often simply adds to one evil still another. That is what I believe euthanasia would accomplish. It is self-determination run amok.

33.
VOLUNTARY EUTHANASIA AND PHYSICIAN-ASSISTED SUICIDE: BEYOND CONTROL?

John Keown

The "slippery slope" argument is, to many policy makers, the central issue in the euthanasia debate. Of major importance in assessing the validity of that argument is the experience of the Netherlands, where euthanasia and physician-assisted suicide have, since 1984, been officially approved and widely practised. Does the Dutch experience confirm or confute the slippery slope argument? This paper offers a concise answer. But first we need to address three preliminary questions: "What is 'euthanasia'?"; "What is the 'slippery slope' argument?" and "What are the Dutch guidelines?"

WHAT IS "EUTHANASIA"?

A standard definition, from Stedman's *Medical Dictionary*, is "[t]he intentional putting to death of a person with an incurable or painful disease." Similarly, this paper's definition is the *intentional shortening of a patient's life, by act or omission, as part of his or her medical care.* Euthanasia is "active" when performed by an act and "passive" if carried out by the withholding or withdrawal of treatment. We are, in either case, concerned with cases of *intentional* killing, that is, where it is the doctor's *purpose* to kill. Consequently, the administration of drugs to alleviate pain, even if they will, as a foreseen but unintended side-effect, hasten death, is *not* euthanasia. Nor is the withholding or withdrawal of life-sustaining treatment on the ground that it is futile or too burdensome, even though the patient will foreseeably die earlier than would otherwise have been the case.

Euthanasia is "voluntary" when it is carried out at the patient's request; "non-voluntary" when the patient is incapable of making a request; and "involuntary" when a competent patient is killed without request. Oddly, the Dutch use "euthanasia" to mean only *active, voluntary euthanasia*.

Closely related to euthanasia is physician-assisted suicide (PAS), in which a doctor assists a patient to commit suicide. The current tactic by campaigners for relaxation of the law to focus on PAS rather than euthanasia should not be allowed to obscure the fact that decriminalization of PAS raises essentially the same issues as the decriminalization of euthanasia. For several reasons, it would be a mistake to think that the two can be distinguished for the purposes of formulating law and public policy. In the Netherlands, both are permitted.

WHAT IS THE "SLIPPERY SLOPE" ARGUMENT?

This argument has two independent yet related forms: the "practical" and the "logical." In its "practical" form the argument asserts that even if a line can in principle be drawn between voluntary and non-voluntary euthanasia, a slide from one to the other is inevitable because *in practice* the safeguards to prevent it cannot be made effective.

The "logical" form of the argument, less familiar but no less important, holds that no line can *in principle* be drawn between voluntary and non-voluntary euthanasia because the principle which seeks to justify the former also justifies the latter. What is that principle? It is not, as is often claimed by campaigners for voluntary euthanasia, respect for personal autonomy. For no responsible doctor would kill a patient just because the patient requested it any more than the doctor would remove an organ just because the patient requested it. The patient's request merely triggers the *doctor's* judgment that death would (or would not) be a "benefit" for the patient. In other words, the patient proposes, but the doctor disposes. So, when all the rhetoric about patient autonomy is stripped away, the underlying principle which seeks to justify even voluntary euthanasia is that *doctors can make a judgment that certain patients are better off dead.* And, if such a judgment can be made in relation to a competent patient, *there is no reason in logic why it cannot be made in relation to an incompetent patient.* Again, if death can be a benefit for competent patients, it can also be a benefit for incompetent patients in the same situation. How can the incompetent logically be denied that benefit simply because they are incapable of asking for it?

Does the Dutch experience confirm or confute the "slippery slope" argument in either of its forms? Let us first outline the Dutch guidelines.

WHAT ARE THE DUTCH GUIDELINES?
In 1984 the Dutch Supreme Court held that a doctor, if acting in accordance with "responsible medical opinion," may lawfully perform euthanasia or assist suicide. In the same year guidelines were issued by the Royal Dutch Medical Association (KNMG). Since that time, the lives of thousands of Dutch patients have been intentionally shortened by their doctors. The guidelines were summarized in 1989 by Mrs. Borst-Eilers, now Minister of Health, as follows:

1. The request for euthanasia must come only from the patient and must be entirely free and voluntary.
2. The patient's request must be well-considered, durable and persistent.
3. The patient must be experiencing intolerable (not necessarily physical) suffering, with no prospect of improvement.
4. Euthanasia must be a last resort. Other alternatives to alleviate the patient's suffering must have been considered and found wanting.
5. Euthanasia must be performed by a physician.
6. The physician must consult with an independent physician colleague who has experience in this field.

Following an arrangement between the Ministry of Justice and the KNMG in 1990, the doctor should not fill in the death certificate but should call in the local medical examiner who will interview the doctor and report to the public prosecutor. Only if it appears that the guidelines have not been followed is the prosecutor likely to order further investigation.

SLIDING DOWN THE SLIPPERY SLOPE?
Have the Dutch confirmed or confuted the "slippery slope" argument in either of its forms? Defenders of the Dutch experience have argued that there neither has been nor could be a slide down the slope. They have urged that the guidelines are sufficiently "strict" and "precise" to prevent such a slide and that the growing body of empirical evidence confirms that contention. However, as can be illustrated by a brief critique of the guidelines, a summary of the empirical data and a number of recent developments in the Netherlands, these claims are unpersuasive.

1. The guidelines—a critique
Far from being "precise" and "strict," the guidelines are, as even a cursory reading may suggest, vague and lax. First, it is unclear what the guidelines are: the Supreme Court has never laid down a definitive list. Indeed, it is now doubtful whether consultation, and even a request by the patient, are essential. Secondly, even if it were clear that the six guidelines were definitive, those guidelines are themselves far from transparent. A hypothetical case highlights their elasticity.

During my first research trip to Holland in 1989, I interviewed a general practitioner who is widely respected in Holland as a leading practitioner of euthanasia. Testing his interpretation of the guidelines, I put to him the hypothetical case of a patient who requested euthanasia because he felt a nuisance to his relatives who wanted him dead so they could enjoy his estate. When asked whether he would rule out such a case, the doctor replied:

> I ... think in the end I wouldn't, because that kind of influence—these children wanting the money now—is the same kind of power from the past that ... shaped us all. The same thing goes for religion ... education ... the kind of family he was raised in, all kinds of influences from the past that we can't put aside.

If a leading practitioner can interpret the guidelines requiring a "free and voluntary" request and "intolerable suffering" as possibly extending to such a case, little more need be said about their supposed precision. Nor are they "strict." The only checks on a doctor's decision making are consultation with a colleague and an interview with the local medical examiner. But consultation may not even be legally required and, even if it is, it is arguably satisfied by a telephone conversation with a compliant (or even a non-compliant) colleague. Although revised guidelines issued in September 1995 by the KNMG explain that consultation means discussion with an independent colleague who has examined the patient, the very fact that this has had to be spelled out is revealing.

Nor can the interview with the local medical examiner act as an effective check. For one thing, it is left to the doctor to call in the medical examiner and to provide the relevant information. Small wonder that one experienced prosecutor (who supports euthanasia) complained to me that the medical examiner (who is a doctor) does not have the necessary investigative expertise, conducts an inquiry which is "just a chat between doctors and no inquiry at all" and that the reporting procedure requires prosecutors to lower their professional standards below the "absolute minimum." That so many, not least journalists, should uncritically describe the guidelines as "strict" is, therefore, remarkable.

2. The empirical data—a summary

In 1990 the Dutch government appointed a Commission, under the Chairmanship of Professor Remmelink, the Attorney-General, to report on the practice of euthanasia in Holland. The Commission asked PJ van der Maas, Professor of Public Health and Social Medicine at the Erasmus University, Rotterdam, to carry out a survey to produce qualitative and quantitative data relating not only to "euthanasia" but to all medical decisions affecting the end of life. The Commission's Report and the van der Maas Survey were published in Dutch in September 1991. One year later, the survey was published in English. Readers interested in a comprehensive analysis of the empirical evidence are referred to my 1995 book *Euthanasia Examined: Ethical, Clinical and Legal Perspectives.* For present purposes it suffices to make just three points which illuminate the reality, extent and speed of the Dutch descent down the "slippery slope."

i. The incidence of euthanasia

First, the Survey states that in 1990, the year studied, there were 2300 cases of euthanasia and 400 cases of assisted suicide, around 2.1 percent of all deaths. But even this total is an underestimate, largely because of the narrow Dutch definition of "euthanasia" as *active, voluntary euthanasia.*

When killing *without explicit request* and killing by *deliberate omission* are included the total rises steeply to 10,558 cases in which it was the doctor's primary purpose (more graphically but less accurately called "explicit" purpose in the survey) to shorten life. (It bears repetition that we are not counting as passive euthanasia cases in which doctors omitted treatment merely foreseeing that death would be hastened but *only* those in which they said that their primary purpose in omitting to treat was to hasten death.) In short, over one in 12 deaths from all causes in 1990 was intentionally accelerated by a doctor.

ii. Non-voluntary euthanasia

Although the guidelines require an explicit request by the patient, many of the patients killed in 1990 had made no such request. The survey stated that over 1000 patients were euthanised without an explicit request. *Even on the survey's own interpretation of its figures, therefore, 27 percent of patients (1000 of 3700) were killed without an explicit request.* That figure is disturbing enough. On the definition of euthanasia used in this paper, the figure is even larger: out of a total of 10,558 cases of euthanasia, there was no explicit request in 52 percent (5450) of cases.

The reaction of the Remmelink Commission to the 1000 cases was scarcely less remarkable than the statistic itself. While criticizing the killing of those patients among the 1000 who were competent, the Commission condoned the killing of the vast majority of those who were not. It observed that "active intervention" was usually "inevitable" because of the patients' "death agony." Not only is the Commission's attempted defence factually shaky, but it amounts to little more than an unsubstantiated assertion that euthanasia without request, a practice in clear violation of the guidelines, is acceptable.

iii. Reporting

How many cases of euthanasia and assisted suicide were reported by doctors to the local medical examiner? Before the survey, a leading defender of Dutch euthanasia had claimed that, if the situation in Holland was unique, it was perhaps in "the wish of physicians to subject their actions to public scrutiny." However, the survey revealed that in *over 70 percent* of the cases doctors failed to report and instead filled in the death certificate as death by "natural causes." In so doing, they not only breached an important guideline but also committed the offence of falsifying a death certificate. Even in relation to those cases that are reported, it must be doubted, in view of the lax system of investigation, whether the authorities can realistically hope to detect the doctor who, either through negligence or worse, has ignored the guidelines.

3. Recent Developments

If further evidence of the Dutch descent down the slipper slope were needed, it has been amply provided by developments in Holland over the past few years. We shall mention just three.

i. Reporting non-voluntary euthanasia

The growing condonation of non-voluntary euthanasia in the Netherlands is reflected not only by the views of the Remmelink Commission and of leading Dutch experts, but also in legislation. In 1993, implementing a recommendation of the Commission, Parliament enacted legislation, not to decriminalize euthanasia but to set out in statutory form the report the doctor should file with the local medical examiner. This form explicitly provides for the reporting of non-voluntary euthanasia.

ii. Euthanasia for mental grief and for infant disability

In 1994 the Supreme Court held that a doctor could lawfully assist a patient to commit suicide even if the patient was not somatically ill, let alone terminally ill. The case involved the prosecution of a psychiatrist for assisting the suicide of a 50-year old woman. The woman told him she wanted to die not because of physical illness but because of her grief at the loss of her two sons.

This case came in for particular criticism by members of the House of Lords Select Committee on Medical Ethics, which was set up by the British Government to examine the euthanasia question and

which reported in 1994 (Report of the House of Lords Select Committee on Medical Ethics). Lord Walton, its Chairman, commented that those members of the Committee who had comprised a delegation to Holland had returned "feeling uncomfortable, especially in the light of evidence indicating that non-voluntary euthanasia ... was commonly performed." His Lordship added that they were "particularly uncomfortable" about this case.

Such criticism has not, however, halted the Dutch slide. In 1995 the Court of Appeal held that the administration of a lethal injection to a disabled baby at the request of its parents—a clear case of non-voluntary euthanasia—was lawful.

iii. The second van der Maas survey

In 1996, a second comprehensive survey by Professor van der Maas was published. This survey showed that the practice of euthanasia had improved little since 1990. The survey (even using the narrow Dutch definition of euthanasia) disclosed that the total number of cases of euthanasia and assisted suicide had risen by a third from 2700 to 3600; that almost 60 percent had not been reported; and that the number of cases of euthanasia without request was still running at 900 cases. As with the first survey, closer analysis actually reveals a significantly higher number of cases in which doctors intended to hasten death, both by act and omission, and with or without request.

CONCLUSION

Policy makers need fact, not fantasy; reason not rhetoric; informed research not opinion polls of the uninformed. The Dutch experience repays close study, not only because it provides hard data about the reality of euthanasia in practice and enables policy makers to cut through the media-generated emotional hype which clouds the euthanasia debate, but also because it clearly confirms the validity of the slippery slope argument in *both* its forms, practical and logical.

The growing body of objective academic research confirms that, within a decade, the so-called "strict" safeguards against the slide have proved largely ineffectual and that non-voluntary euthanasia is now widely practised and increasingly condoned. The exclusive emphasis on the need for a free and explicit request by the patient, which characterized the campaign to secure acceptance of voluntary euthanasia in the 1980s has, at least since the early 1990s, given way to an extension of euthanasia to the incompetent on the basis that they would be better off dead. In September 1995 the KNMG issued revised guidelines, but these do not even attempt to prohibit non-voluntary euthanasia.

The Dutch experience, albeit of major significance, is by no means the only source meriting the attention of those concerned with the formulation of legal, social and health policy. For in recent years euthanasia has been *exhaustively* considered by several distinguished and independent bodies.

In 1994 the House of Lords Select Committee on Medical Ethics and the New York State Task Force on Life and the Law, in reports which command the attention of anyone seriously interested in the euthanasia debate, *unanimously* rejected the decriminalization of active euthanasia and recommended instead improvements in the quality and availability of palliative care. The following year, so too did a majority of the Special Committee of the Canadian Senate. And in 1997 the Parliament of Australia repealed the euthanasia legislation which had been enacted in its Northern Territory. Similarly unpersuaded by the case for relaxation of the law have been the Supreme Courts of Canada and of the US. Although not all the expert bodies or courts have been unanimous, the degree of consensus that decriminalization of voluntary euthanasia would be counter-productive—a consensus shared even by those members with no objection to voluntary euthanasia in principle—is striking. And recognition of the validity of the slippery slope argument, and its illustration by the Dutch experience, has played a significant role in shaping that consen-

sus. The Dutch experience confirms that the decriminalization of voluntary euthanasia or physician-assisted suicide, far from increasing patient autonomy and reducing suffering, places even greater power in the hands of doctors and undermines the impetus for improved palliative care, care which is so sadly lacking in the Netherlands.

That voluntary euthanasia should resist effective regulation is unsurprising. As Dan Callahan and Margot White have convincingly argued in a comprehensive review of legislative proposals, effective regulation is destined to be frustrated by several factors, not least the inherent confidentiality of the doctor/patient relationship. Nor, even if the logical slippery slope argument were left to one side, is it easy to see how campaigners for voluntary euthanasia could come up with proposals that would ensure effective regulation. Relying largely on self-regulation by the profession, the Dutch approach has proved ineffective. But it does not follow that stricter external regulation would prove any more effective. For if doctors are unwilling to comply even with minimal Dutch requirements such as consultation and reporting, they are hardly likely to observe more onerous requirements. Proponents of voluntary euthanasia are, therefore, locked in a regulatory "Catch 22"situation: the more the hand of regulation tries to exert control, the more inevitably slips through its fingers.

Using slogans about "autonomy" and "dignity," it is easy to make the case for voluntary euthanasia seem attractive. When, however, that case is subjected to the sort of close examination which policy makers need to make, it quickly collapses, not least because voluntary euthanasia is in theory, and that has shown itself to be in practice, quite beyond control.

34

GENDER, FEMINISM, AND DEATH: PHYSICIAN-ASSISTED SUICIDE AND EUTHANASIA

Susan M. Wolf

The debate in the United States over whether to legitimate physician-assisted suicide and active euthanasia has reached new levels of intensity. Oregon has become the first state to legalize physician-assisted suicide, and there have been campaigns, ballot measures, bills, and litigation in other states in attempts to legalize one or both practices.[1] Scholars and others increasingly urge either outright legalization or some other form of legitimation, through recognition of an affirmative defense of "mercy killing" to a homicide prosecution or other means.[2]

Yet the debate over whether to legitimate physician-assisted suicide and euthanasia (by which I mean active euthanasia, as opposed to the termination of life-sustaining treatment)[3] is most often about a patient who does not exist—a patient with no gender, race, or insurance status. This is the same generic patient featured in most bioethics debates. Little discussion has focused on how differences between patients might alter the equation.

Even though the debate has largely ignored this question, there is ample reason to suspect that gender, among other factors, deserves analysis. The cases prominent in the American debate mostly feature women patients. This occurs against a backdrop of a long history of cultural images revering women's sacrifice and self-sacrifice. Moreover, dimensions of health status and health care that may affect a patient's vulnerability to considering physician-assisted suicide and euthanasia—including depression, poor pain relief, and difficulty obtaining good health care—differentially plague women. And suicide patterns themselves show a strong gender effect: women less often complete suicide, but more often attempt it.[4] These and other factors raise the question of whether the dynamics surrounding physician-assisted suicide and euthanasia may vary by gender.

Indeed, it would be surprising if gender had no influence. Women in America still live in a society marred by sexism, a society that particularly disvalues women with illness, disability, or merely advanced age. It would be hard to explain if health care, suicide, and fundamental dimensions of American society showed marked differences by gender, but gender suddenly dropped out of the equation when people became desperate enough to seek a physician's help in ending their lives.

What sort of gender effects might we expect? There are four different possibilities. First, we might anticipate a higher incidence of women than men dying by physician-assisted suicide and euthanasia in this country. This is an empirical claim that we cannot yet test; we currently lack good data in the face of the illegality of the practices in most states[5] and the condemnation of the organized medical profession.[6] The best data we do have are from the Netherlands and are inconclusive. As I discuss below, the Dutch data show that women predominate among patients dying through euthanasia or administration of drugs for pain relief, but not by much. In the smaller categories of physician-assisted suicide and "life-terminating events without request," however, men predominate. And men predominate too in making requests rejected by physicians. It is hard to say what this means for the United States. The Netherlands differs in a number of relevant respects, with universal health care and a more homogeneous society. But the Dutch data suggest that gender differences in the United States will not necessarily translate into higher numbers of women dying. At least one author speculates that there may in fact be a sexist tendency to discount and refuse women's requests.[7]

There may, however, be a second gender effect. Gender differences may translate into women seeking physician-assisted suicide and euthanasia for somewhat different reasons than men. Problems we know to be correlated with gender—difficulty getting good medical care generally, poor pain relief, a higher incidence of depression, and a higher rate of poverty—may figure more prominently in women's motivation. Society's persisting sexism may figure as well. And the long history of valorizing women's self-sacrifice may be expressed in women's requesting assisted suicide or euthanasia.

The well-recognized gender differences in suicide statistics also suggest that women's requests for physician-assisted suicide and euthanasia may more often than men's requests be an effort to change an oppressive situation rather than a literal request for death. Thus some suicidologists interpret men's predominance among suicide "completers" and women's among suicide "attempters" to mean that women more often engage in suicidal behavior with a goal other than "completion."[8] The relationship between suicide and the practices of physician-assisted suicide and euthanasia itself deserves further study; not all suicides are even motivated by terminal disease or other factors relevant to the latter practices. But the marked gender differences in suicidal behavior are suggestive.

Third, gender differences may also come to the fore in physicians' decisions about whether to grant or refuse requests for assisted suicide or euthanasia. The same historical valorization of women's self-sacrifice and the same background sexism that may affect women's readiness to request may also affect physicians' responses. Physicians may be susceptible to affirming women's negative self-judgments. This might or might not result in physicians agreeing to assist; other gender-related judgments (such as that women are too emotionally labile, or that their choices should not be taken seriously) may intervene.[9] But the point is that gender may affect not just patient but physician.

Finally, gender may affect the broad public debate. The prominent U.S. cases so far and related historical imagery suggest that in debating physician-assisted suicide and euthanasia, many in our culture may envision a woman patient. Although the AIDS epidemic has called attention to physician-assisted suicide and euthanasia in men, the cases that have dominated the news accounts and scholarly journals in the recent renewal of debate have featured women patients. Thus we have reason to be concerned that at least some advocacy for these practices may build on the sense that these stories of women's deaths are somehow "right." If there is a felt correctness to these accounts, that may be playing a hidden and undesirable part in catalyzing support for the practices' legitimation.

Thus we have cause to worry whether the debate about and practice of physician-assisted suicide and euthanasia in this country are gender in a number of respects. Serious attention to gender therefore seems essential. Before we license physicians to kill their patients or to assist patients in killing themselves, we had better understand the dynamic at work in that encounter, why the practice seems so alluring that we should court its dangers, and what dangers are likely to manifest. After all, the consequences of permitting killing or assistance in private encounters are serious, indeed fatal. We had better understand what distinguishes this from other forms of private violence, and other relationships of asymmetrical power that result in the deaths of women. And we had better determine whether tacit assumptions about gender are influencing the enthusiasm for legalization.

Yet even that is not enough. Beyond analysing the way gender figures in our cases, cultural imagery and practice, we must analyse the substantive arguments. For attention to gender, in the last two decades particularly, has yielded a wealth of feminist critiques and theoretical tools that can fruitfully be brought to bear. After all, the debate over physician-assisted suicide and euthanasia revolves around precisely the kind of issues on which feminist work has focused: what it means to talk about rights of self-determination and autonomy; the reconciliation of those rights with physicians' duties of beneficence and caring; and how to place all of this in a context including the strengths and failures of families, professionals, and communities, as well as real differentials of power and resources.

The debate over physician-assisted suicide and euthanasia so starkly raises questions of rights, caring, and context that at this point it would take determination *not* to bring to bear a literature that has been devoted to understanding those notions.

Indeed, the work of Lawrence Kohlberg bears witness to what an obvious candidate this debate is for such analysis.[10] It was Kohlberg's work on moral development, of course, that provoked Carol Gilligan's *In A Different Voice,* criticizing Kohlberg's vision of progressive stages in moral maturation as one that was partial and gender.[11] Gilligan proposed that there were really two different approaches to moral problems, one that emphasized generalized rights and universal principles, and the other that instead emphasized conceptualized caring and the maintenance of particular human relationships. She suggested that although women and men could use both approaches, women tended to use the latter and men the former. Both approaches, however, were important to moral maturity. Though Gilligan's and others' work on the ethics of care has been much debated and criticized, a number of bioethicists and health care professionals have found a particular pertinence to questions of physician caregiving.[12]

Embedded in Kohlberg's work, one finds proof that the euthanasia debate in particular calls for analysis in the very terms that he employs, and that Gilligan then critiques, enlarges, and reformulates. For one of the nine moral dilemmas Kohlberg used to gauge subjects' stage of moral development was a euthanasia problem. "Dilemma IV" features "a woman" with "very bad cancer" and "in terrible pain." Her physician, Dr. Jefferson, knows she has "only about six months to live." Between periods in which she is "delirious and almost crazy with pain," she asks the doctor to kill her with morphine. The question is what he should do.[13]

The euthanasia debate thus demands analysis along the care, rights, and context axes that the Kohlberg-Gilligan debate has identified.[14] Kohlberg himself used this problem to reveal how well respondents were doing in elevating general principles over the idiosyncrasies of relationship and context. It is no stretch, then, to apply the fruits of more than a decade of feminist critique. The problem has a genuine pedigree.

The purpose of this chapter thus is twofold. First, I explore gender's significance for analysing physician-assisted suicide and euthanasia. Thus I examine the prominent cases and cultural images, against the background of cautions recommended by what little

data we have from the Netherlands. Finding indications that gender may well be significant, I investigate what that implies for the debate over physician-assisted suicide and euthanasia. Clearly more research is required. But in the meantime, patients' vulnerability to requesting these fatal interventions because of failures in health care and other background conditions, or because of a desire not to die but to alter circumstances, introduces reasons why we should be reluctant to endorse these practices. Indeed, we should be worried about the role of the physician in these cases, and consider the lessons we have learned from analysing other relationships that result in women's deaths. What we glean from looking at gender should lead us to look at other characteristics historically associated with disadvantage, and thus should prompt a general caution applicable to all patients.

My second purpose is to go beyond analysis of gender itself, to analysis of the arguments offered on whether to condone and legitimate these practices. Here is where I bring to bear the feminist literature on caring, rights, and context. I criticize the usual argument that patients' rights of self-determination dictate legitimation of physician-assisted suicide and euthanasia, on the grounds that this misconstrues the utility of rights talk for resolving this debate, and ignores essential features of the context. I then turn to arguments based on beneficence and caring. It is no accident that the word "mercy" has figured so large in our language about these problems; they do involve questions of compassion and caring. However, a shallow understanding of caring will lead us astray and I go on to elaborate what a deep and conceptualized understanding demands. I argue that physicians should be guided by a notion of "principled caring." Finally, I step back to suggest what a proper integration of rights and caring would look like in this context, how it can be coupled with attention to the fate of women and other historically disadvantaged groups, and what practical steps all of this counsels.

This chapter takes a position. As I have before, I oppose the legitimation of physician-assisted suicide and euthanasia.[15] Yet the most important part of what I do here is urge the necessity of feminist analysis of this issue. Physician-assisted suicide and euthanasia

are difficult problems on which people may disagree. But I hope to persuade that attending to gender and feminist concerns in analysing these problems is no longer optional.

GENDER IN CASES, IMAGES, AND PRACTICE

The tremendous upsurge in American debate over
whether to legitimate physician-assisted suicide and
euthanasia in recent years has been fueled by a series
of cases featuring women. The case that seems to
have begun this series is that of Debbie, published in
1988 by the *Journal of the American Medical Association (JAMA)*.[16] *JAMA* published this now infamous, first-person, and anonymous account by a resident in obstetrics and gynecology of performing
euthanasia. Some subsequently queried whether the
account was fiction. Yet it successfully catalyzed an
enormous response.

The narrator of the piece tells us that Debbie is a
young woman suffering from ovarian cancer. The
resident has no prior relationship with her, but is
called to her bedside late one night while on call and
exhausted. Entering Debbie's room, the resident
finds an older woman with her, but never pauses to
find out who that second woman is and what relational context Debbie acts within. Instead, the resident responds to the patient's clear discomfort and to
her words. Debbie says only one sentence, "Let's get
this over with." It is unclear whether she thinks the
resident is there to draw blood and wants that over
with, or means something else. But on the strength
of that one sentence, the resident retreats to the nursing station, prepares a lethal injection, returns to the
room, and administers it. The story relates this as an
act of mercy under the title "It's Over, Debbie," as if
in caring response to the patient's words.

The lack of relationship to the patient; the failure
to attend to her own history, relationships, and
resources; the failure to explore beyond the patient's
presented words and engage her in conversation; the
sense that the cancer diagnosis plus the patient's
words demand death; and the construal of that
response as an act of mercy are all themes that recur
in the later cases. The equally infamous Dr. Jack
Kevorkian has provided a slew of them.

They begin with Janet Adkins, a 54-year-old Oregon woman diagnosed with Alzheimer's disease.[17]

Again, on the basis of almost no relationship with
Ms. Adkins, on the basis of a diagnosis by exclusion
that Kevorkian could not verify, prompted by a professed desire to die that is a predictable stage in
response to a number of dire diagnoses, Kevorkian
rigs her up to his "Mercitron" machine in a parking
lot outside Detroit in what he presents as an act of
mercy.

Then there is Marjorie Wantz, a 58-year-old
woman without even a diagnosis.[18] Instead, she has
pelvic pain whose source remains undetermined. By
the time Kevorkian reaches Ms. Wantz, he is making
little pretense of focusing on her needs in the context
of a therapeutic relationship. Instead, he tells the
press that he is determined to create a new medical
specialty of "obitiatry." Ms. Wantz is among the first
six potential patients with whom he is conferring.
When Kevorkian presides over her death there is
another woman who dies as well, Sherry Miller.
Miller, 43, has multiple sclerosis. Thus neither
woman is terminal.

The subsequent cases reiterate the basic themes.[19]
And it is not until the ninth "patient" that Kevorkian
finally presides over the death of a man.[20] By this
time, published criticism of the predominance of
women had begun to appear.[21]

Kevorkian's actions might be dismissed as the
bizarre behavior of one man. But the public and
press response has been enormous, attesting to the
power of these accounts. Many people have treated
these cases as important to the debate over physician-assisted suicide and euthanasia. Nor are
Kevorkian's cases so aberrant—they pick up all the
themes that emerge in "Debbie."

But we cannot proceed without analysis of Diane.
This is the respectable version of what Kevorkian
makes strange. I refer to the story published by Dr.
Timothy Quill in the *New England Journal of Medicine,* recounting his assisting the suicide of his
patient Diane.[22] She is a woman in her forties diagnosed with leukemia, who seeks and obtains from
Dr. Quill a prescription for drugs to take her life. Dr.
Quill cures some of the problems with the prior
cases. He does have a real relationship with her, he
knows her history, and he obtains a psychiatric consult on her mental state. He is a caring, empathetic
person. Yet once again we are left wondering about

the broader context of Diane's life—why even the history of other problems that Quill describes has so drastically depleted her resources to deal with this one, and whether there were any alternatives. And we are once again left wondering about the physician's role—why he responded to her as he did, what self-scrutiny he brought to bear on his own urge to comply and how he reconciled this with the arguments that physicians who are moved to so respond should nonetheless resist.[23]

These cases will undoubtedly be joined by others, including cases featuring men, as the debate progresses. Indeed, they already have been. Yet the initial group of cases involving women has somehow played a pivotal role in catalyzing reexamination of two of the most fundamental and long-standing promotions in medicine. These are prohibitions that have been deemed by some constitutive of the physician's role: above all, do no harm; and give no deadly drug, even if asked. The power of this core of cases seems somehow evident.

This collection of early cases involving women cries out for analysis. It cannot be taken as significant evidence predicting that more women may die through physician-assisted suicide and euthanasia; these individual cases are no substitute for systematic data. But to understand what they suggest about the role of gender, we need to place them in context.

The images in these cases have a cultural lineage. We could trace a long history of portrayals of women as victims of sacrifice and self-sacrifice. In Greek tragedy, that ancient source of still reverberating images, "suicide ... [is] a woman's solution."[24] Almost no men die in this way. Specifically, suicide is a wife's solution; it is one of the few acts of autonomy open to her. Wives use suicide in these tragedies often to join their husbands in death. The other form of death specific to women is the sacrifice of young women who are virgins. The person putting such a woman to death must be male.[25] Thus "[i]t is by men that women meet their death, and it is for men, usually, that they kill themselves."[26] Men, in contrast, die by the sword or spear in battle.[27]

The connection between societal gender roles and modes of death persists through history. Howard Kushner writes that "Nineteenth-century European and American fiction is littered with the corpses of ...

women.... [T]he cause was always ... rejection after an illicit love affair.... If women's death by suicide could not be attributed to dishonor, it was invariably tied to women's adopting roles ... assigned to men."[28] "By the mid-nineteenth century characterizations of women's suicides meshed with the ideology described by Barbara Welter as that of 'True Womanhood.... Adherence to the virtues of piety, purity, submissiveness and domesticity" translated into the belief that a 'fallen woman' was a 'fallen angel.'"[29] Even after statistics emerged showing that women completed suicide less often than men, the explanations offered centered on women's supposedly greater willingness to suffer misfortune, their lack of courage, and less arduous social role.[30]

Thus, prevailing values have imbued women's deaths with specific meaning. Indeed, Carol Gilligan builds on images of women's suicides and sacrifice in novels and drama, as well as on her own data, in finding a psychology and even an ethic of self-sacrifice among women. Gilligan finds one of the "conventions of femininity" to be "the moral equation of goodness with self-sacrifice."[31] "[V]irtue for women lies in self-sacrifice...."[32]

Given this history of images and the valorization of women's self-sacrifice, it should come as no surprise that the early cases dominating the debate about self-sacrifice through physician-assisted suicide and euthanasia have been cases of women. In Greek tragedy only women were candidates for sacrifice and self-sacrifice,[33] and to this day self-sacrifice is usually regarded as a feminine not masculine virtue.

This lineage has implications. It means that even while we debate physician-assisted suicide and euthanasia rationally, we may be animated by unacknowledged images that give the practices a certain gender logic and felt correctness. In some deep way it makes sense to us to see these women dying, it seems right. It fits an old piece into a familiar, ancient puzzle. Moreover, these acts seem good; they are born of virtue. We may not recognize that the virtues in question—female sacrifice and self-sacrifice—are ones now widely questioned and deliberately rejected. Instead, our subconscious may harken back to older forms, reembracing those ancient virtues, and thus lauding these women's deaths.

Analysing the early cases against the background of this history also suggests hidden gender dynamics to be discovered by attending to the facts found in the accounts of these cases, or more properly the facts not found. What is most important in these accounts is what is left out, how truncated they are. We see a failure to attend to the patient's context, a readiness on the part of these physicians to facilitate death, a seeming lack of concern over why these women turn to these doctors for deliverance. A clue about why we should be concerned about each of these omissions is telegraphed by data from exit polls on the day Californians defeated a referendum measure to legalize active euthanasia. Those polls showed support for the measure lowest among women, older people, Asians, and African Americans, and highest among younger men with postgraduate education and incomes over $75,000 per year.[34] The *New York Times* analysis was that people from more vulnerable groups were more worried about allowing physicians actively to take life. This may suggest concern not only that physicians may be too ready to take their lives, but also that these patients may be markedly vulnerable to seeking such relief. Why would women, in particular, feel this?

Women are at greater risk for inadequate pain relief.[35] Indeed, fear of pain is one of the reasons most frequently cited by Americans for supporting legislation to legalize euthanasia.[36] Women are also at greater risk for depression.[37] And depression appears to underlie numerous requests for physician-assisted suicide and euthanasia.[38] These factors suggest that women may be differentially driven to consider requesting both practices.

That possibility is further supported by data showing systematic problems for women in relationship to physicians. As an American Medical Association report on gender disparities recounts, women receive more care even for the same illness, but the care is generally worse. Women are less likely to receive dialysis, kidney transplants, cardiac catheterization, and diagnostic testing for lung cancer. The report urges physicians to uproot "social or cultural biases that could affect medical care" and "presumptions about the relative worth of certain social roles."[39]

This all occurs against the background of a deeply flawed health care system that ties health insurance to employment. Men are differentially represented in the ranks of those with private health insurance, women in the ranks of the others—those either on government entitlement programs or uninsured.[40] In the U. S. two-tier health care system, men dominate in the higher-quality tier, women in the lower.

Moreover, women are differentially represented among the ranks of the poor. Many may feel they lack the resources to cope with disability and disease. To cope with Alzheimer's, breast cancer, multiple sclerosis, ALS, and a host of other diseases takes resources. It takes not only the financial resource of health insurance, but also access to stable working relationships with clinicians expert in these conditions, in the psychological issues involved, and in palliative care and pain relief. It may take access to home care, eventually residential care, and rehabilitation services. These are services often hard to get even for those with adequate resources, and almost impossible for those without. And who are those without in this country? Disproportionately they are women, people of color, the elderly, and children.[41]

Women may also be driven to consider physician-assisted suicide or euthanasia out of fear of otherwise burdening their families.[42] The dynamic at work in a family in which an ill member chooses suicide or active euthanasia is worrisome. This worry should increase when it is a woman who seeks to "avoid being a burden," or otherwise solve the problem she feels she poses, by opting for her own sacrifice. The history and persistence of family patterns in this country in which women are expected to adopt self-sacrificing behavior for the sake of the family may pave the way too for the patient's request for death. Women requesting death may also be sometimes seeking something other than death. The dominance of women among those attempting but not completing suicide in this country suggests that women may differentially engage in death-seeking behavior with a goal other than death. Instead, they may be seeking to change their relationships or circumstances.[43] A psychiatrist at Harvard has speculated about why those women among Kevorkian's "patients" who were still capable of killing themselves instead sought Kevorkian's help. After all, suicide has been decriminalized in this country and step-by-step instructions are readily available. The psychiatrist was apparently prompted to speculate by interviewing about twenty physicians who assisted patients' deaths and discovering that two-thirds to three-quarters of the patients had been women. The psychiatrist wondered whether turning to Kevorkian was a way to seek a relationship.[44] The women also found a supposed "expert" to rely upon, someone to whom they could yield control. But then we must wonder what circumstances, what relational context, led them to this point.

What I am suggesting is that there are issues relating to gender left out of the accounts of the early prominent cases of physician-assisted suicide and euthanasia or left unexplored that may well be driving or limiting the choices of these women. I am not suggesting that we should denigrate these choices or regard them as irrational. Rather, it is the opposite, that we should assume these decisions to be rational and grounded in a context. That forces us to attend to the background failures in that context.

Important analogies are offered by domestic violence. Such violence has been increasingly recognized as a widespread problem. It presents some structural similarities to physician-assisted suicide and especially active euthanasia. All three can be fatal. All three are typically acts performed behind closed doors. In the United States, all three are illegal in most jurisdictions, though the record of law enforcement on each is extremely inconsistent. Though men may be the victims and women the perpetrators of all three, in the case of domestic violence there are some conceptions of traditional values and virtues that endorse the notion that a husband may beat his wife. As I have suggested above, there are similarly traditional conceptions of feminine self-sacrifice that might bless a physician's assisting a woman's suicide or performing euthanasia.

Clearly there are limits to the analogy. But my point is that questions of choice and consent have been raised in the analysis of domestic violence against women, much as they have in the case of physician-assisted suicide and active euthanasia. If a woman chooses to remain in a battering relationship, do we regard that as a choice to be respected and reason not to intervene? While choosing to remain is

not consent to battery, what if a woman says that she "deserves" to be beaten—do we take that as reason to condone the battering? The answers that have been developed to these questions are instructive, because they combine respect for the rationality of women's choices with a refusal to go the further step of excusing the batterer. We appreciate now that a woman hesitating to leave a battering relationship may have ample and rational reasons: well-grounded fear for her safety and that of her children, a justified expectation of economic distress, and warranted concern that the legal system will not effectively come to her aid. We further see mental health professionals now uncovering some of the deeper reasons why some women might say at some point they "deserve" violence. Taking all of these insights seriously has led to development of a host of new legal, psychotherapeutic, and other interventions meant to address the actual experiences and concerns that might lead women to "choose" to stay in a violent relationship or "choose" violence against them. Yet none of this condones the choice of the partner to batter or, worse yet, kill the woman. Indeed, the victim's consent, we should recall, is no legal defense to murder.

All of this should suggest that in analysing why women may request physician-assisted suicide and euthanasia, and why indeed the California polls indicate that women may feel more vulnerable to and wary of making that request, we have insights to bring to bear from other realms. Those insights render suspect an analysis that merely asserts women are choosing physician-assisted suicide and active euthanasia, without asking why they make that choice. The analogy to other forms of violence against women behind closed doors demands that we ask why the woman is there, what features of her context brought her there, and why she may feel there is no better place to be. Finally, the analogy counsels us that the patient's consent does not resolve the question of whether the physician acts properly in deliberately taking her life through physician-assisted suicide or active euthanasia. The two people are separate moral and legal agents.[45]

This leads us from consideration of why women patients may feel vulnerable to these practices, to the question of whether physicians may be vulnerable to

regarding women's requests for physician-assisted suicide and euthanasia somewhat differently from men's.
There may indeed be gender-linked reasons for physicians in this country to say "yes" to women seeking
assistance in suicide or active euthanasia. In assessing
whether the patient's life has become "meaningless,"
or a "burden," or otherwise what some might regard as
suitable for extinguishing at her request, it would be
remarkable if the physician's background views did
not come into play on what makes a woman's life
meaningful or how much of a burden on her family is
too much.[46]

Second, there is a dynamic many have written
about operating between the powerful expert physician and the woman surrendering to his care.[47] It is
no accident that bioethics has focused on the problem of physician paternalism. Instead of an egalitarianism or what Susan Sherwin calls "amicalism,"[48]
we see a vertically hierarchical arrangement built on
domination and subordination. When the patient is
female and the doctor male, as is true in most medical encounters, the problem is likely to be exacerbated by the background realities and history of male
dominance and female subjugation in the broader
society. Then a set of psychological dynamics are
likely to make the male physician vulnerable to
acceding to the woman patient's request for active
assistance in dying. These may be a complex combination of rescue fantasies[49] and the desire to annihilate. Robert Burt talks about the pervasiveness of the
ambivalence, quite apart from gender: "Rules governing doctor-patient relations must rest on the
premise that anyone's wish to help a desperately
pained, apparently helpless person is intertwined
with a wish to hurt that person, to obliterate him
from sight."[50] When the physician is from a dominant social group and the patient from a subordinate
one, we should expect the ambivalence to be heightened. When the "help" requested is obliteration, the
temptation to enact both parts of the ambivalence in
a single act may be great.

This brief examination of the vulnerability of
women patients and their physicians to collaboration
on actively ending the women's life in a way reflecting gender roles suggests the need to examine the
woman's context and where her request for death
comes from, the physician's context and where his

accession comes from, and the relationship between
the two. We need to do that in a way that uses rather
than ignores all we know about the issues plaguing
the relations between women and men, especially
suffering women and powerful expert men. The California exit polls may well signal both the attraction
and the fear of enacting the familiar dynamics in a
future in which it is legitimate to pursue that dynamic to the death. It would be implausible to maintain
that medicine is somehow exempt from broader
social dynamics. The question, then, is whether we
want to bless deaths driven by those dynamics.

All of this suggests that physician-assisted suicide
and euthanasia, as well as the debate about them,
may be gender. I have shown ways in which this may
be true even if women do not die in greater numbers.
But exploring gender would be incomplete without
examining what data we have on its relationship to
incidence. As noted above, those data, which are
from the Netherlands, neither support the proposition that more women will die from these practices,
nor provide good reason yet to dismiss the concern.
We simply do not know how these practices may
play out by gender in the United States. There is no
good U. S. data, undoubtedly because these practices
remain generally illegal.[51] And the Dutch data come
from another culture, with a more homogeneous
population, a different health care system providing
universal coverage, and perhaps different gender
dynamics.[52]

The status of physician-assisted suicide and
euthanasia in the Netherlands is complex. Both practices remain criminal, but both are tolerated under a
series of court decisions, guidelines from the Dutch
medical association, and a more recent statute that
carve out a domain in which the practices are accepted. If the patient is competent and contemporaneously requests assisted suicide or euthanasia, the
patient's suffering cannot be relieved in any other
way acceptable to the patient, a second physician
concurs that acceding to the request is appropriate,
and the physician performing the act reports it to
permit monitoring and investigation, then the practices are allowed.

Dutch researchers have been reporting rigorous
empirical research on the practices only in the past
several years.[53] The team led by Dr. Paul van der

Maas and working at governmental request published the first results of their nationwide study in 1991.[54] They found that "medical decisions concerning the end of life (MDEL)" were made in 38 percent of all deaths in the Netherlands, and thus were common. They differentiated five different types of MDELs: non-treatment decisions (which are neither physician-assisted suicide nor active euthanasia) caused 17.5 percent of deaths; administration of opiod drugs for pain and symptomatic relief (which would be considered active euthanasia in the United States if the physician's intent were to end life, rather than simply to relieve pain or symptoms with the foreseeable risk of hastening death) accounted for another 17.5 percent; active euthanasia at the patient's request (excluding the previous category) accounted for 1.8 percent; physician-assisted suicide (in which the patient, not physician, administers the drugs) covered 0.3 percent. Finally there was a category of "life-terminating events without explicit and persistent request" accounting for 0.8 percent. In more than half of these cases, the patient had expressed a desire for euthanasia previously, but was no longer able to communicate by the time a decision had to be made and effectuated.

Women predominated in all of these categories except for the two rarest, but not by a great deal.[55] Thus, the ratio of females to males is 52:48 for euthanasia,[56] the same for death from drugs for pain and symptomatic relief, and 55:45 for non-treatment decisions.[57] This is against a background ratio of 48.52 for all deaths in the Netherlands.[58] However, in the much smaller categories of physician-assisted suicide and "life-terminating events without explicit and persistent request," men predominated by 68:32 and 65:35 respectively.[59] Why would men predominate in these two categories? In the case of physician-assisted suicide, the researchers suggest that we are talking about younger, urbanized males who have adopted a more demanding style as patients[60] and may be seeking control.[61] Perhaps women, in contrast, are more often surrendering to their fate and relinquishing control to the physicians whom they ask to take their lives. Unfortunately, the researchers do not venture an explanation of why males predominate in the category of people who die from "life-terminating events without explicit and

persistent request." This is numerically the smallest category and one that should not occur at all under the Dutch guidelines because these are not contemporaneously competent patients articulating a request. Thus the numbers may be particularly unreliable here, if there is reluctance to report this illicit activity. Finally, the researchers report that more males than females made requests for physician-assisted suicide and euthanasia that physicians refused (55:45).[62]

What can we learn from the Dutch data that is relevant to the United States? There are causes for caution in making the cross-cultural comparison. There may be fewer reasons to expect a gender difference in the Dutch practices of euthanasia and physician-assisted suicide (as we would define these terms, that is, including the administration of drugs for pain relief and palliation, when the physician's purpose is to end life). First, the Netherlands provides universal health care coverage, while the United States's failure to provide universal coverage and tolerance of a two-tier health care system differentially disadvantages women (and other historically oppressed groups), leaving them with fewer means to cope with serious illness and more reason to consider seeking death. Second, the Netherlands presents greater homogeneity in race and ethnicity.[63] Again, this means that the United States presents more opportunities for and history of oppression based on difference. Third, we have to wonder whether elderly women in the United States face more difficulties and thus more reason to consider physician-assisted suicide and euthanasia than those in the Netherlands. A significant number in the United States confront lack of financial resources and difficulties associated with the absence of universal health coverage. Older women in the United States may also find themselves disvalued. "[T]here is evidence that the decision to kill oneself is viewed as most 'understandable' when it is made by an older women."[64] Finally, it is worth speculating whether gender dynamics differ in the Netherlands.

Apart from that speculation, the differences in Dutch demographics and health care would be reasons to expect no gender differential in the Netherlands in the practices we are examining. The fact that we nonetheless see something of a gender difference in the case of most deaths intentionally caused by a physician at the patient's request should heighten our concern about gender differences in the United States. Given the general illegality of euthanasia and physician-assisted suicide currently in this country, decent data would be difficult to gather. Yet there seems to be reason to attend to gender in what studies we can do, and in our analysis of these problems. Studies planned for Oregon, the one American jurisdiction to legalize physician-assisted suicide so far, should surely investigate gender.

Attending to gender in the data available for the Netherlands, in the images animating the American debate, and in the cases yielding those images thus suggests that our customarily gender-neutral arguments about the merits of physician-assisted suicide and euthanasia miss much of the point. Though one can certainly conceive of a gender-neutral practice, that may be far from what we have, at least in the United States, with our history and inequalities.

Equally troubling, our failure thus far to attend to gender in debating these practices may represent more than mere oversight. It may be a product of the same deep-rooted sexism that makes the self-destruction of women in Greek tragedy seem somehow natural and right. Indeed, there is something systematic in our current submerging of gender. The details left out of the usual account of a case of assisted suicide or euthanasia—what failures of relationship, context, and resources have brought the woman to this point; precisely why death seems to her the best remaining option; what elements of self-sacrifice motivate her choice—are exactly the kind of details that might make the workings of gender visible.

They are also the kind of details that might make the workings of race, ethnicity, and insurance status visible as well. The sort of gender analysis that I have pursued here should also provoke us to other analyses of the role played by these other factors. To focus here on just the first of these, there is a long history of racism in medicine in this country as vividly demonstrated by the horrors of the Tuskegee Syphilis Study.[65] We now are seeing new studies showing a correlation between race and access to cardiac procedures, for instance.[66] Although analysis of the meaning of these correlations is in progress, we have ample reason to be concerned, to examine the dynamic at work between patients of color and their physicians, and to be wary of expanding the physician's arsenal so that he or she may directly take the patient's life.

This sort of analysis will have to be detailed and specific, whether exploring gender, race, or another historic basis for subordination. The cultural meaning, history, and medical profession's use of each of those categories is specific, even though we can expect commonalities. The analysis will also have to pay close attention to the intersection, when a patient presents multiple characteristics that have historically occasioned discrimination and disadvantage.[67] How all of these categories function in the context of physician-assisted suicide and euthanasia will bear careful examination.

Probably the category of gender is the one we actually know most about in that context. At least we have the most obvious clues about that category, thanks to the gender nature of the imagery. We would be foolish not to pursue those clues. Indeed, given grounds for concern that physician-assisted suicide and euthanasia may work in different and troubling ways when the patient is a woman, we are compelled to investigate gender.

FEMINISM AND THE ARGUMENTS

Shifting from the images and stories that animate debate and the dynamics operating in practice to analysis of the arguments over physician-assisted suicide and euthanasia takes us further into the concerns of feminist theory. Arguments in favor of these practices have often depended on rights claims. More recently, some authors have grounded their arguments instead on ethical concepts of caring. Yet both argumentative strategies have been flawed in ways that feminist work can illuminate. What is missing is an analysis that integrates notions of physician caring with principled boundaries to physician action, while also attending to the patient's broader context and the community's wider concerns. Such an analysis would pay careful attention to the dangers posed by these practices to the historically most vulnerable populations, including women.

Advocacy of physician-assisted suicide and euthanasia has hinged to a great extent on rights claims. The argument is that the patient has a right of self-determination or autonomy that entitles her to assistance in suicide or euthanasia. The strategy is to extend the argument that self-determination entitles the patient to refuse unwanted life-sustaining treatment by maintaining that the same rationale supports patient entitlement to more active physician assistance in death. Indeed, it is sometimes argued that there is no principled difference between termination of life-sustaining treatment and the more active practices.

The narrowness and mechanical quality of this rights thinking, however, is shown by its application to the stories recounted above. That application suggests that the physicians in these stories are dealing with a simple equation: given an eligible rights bearer and her assertion of the right, the correct result is death. What makes a person an eligible rights bearer? Kevorkian seems to require neither a terminal disease nor thorough evaluation of whether the patient has non-fatal alternatives. Indeed, the Wantz case shows he does not even require a diagnosis. Nor does the Oregon physician-assisted suicide statute require evaluation or exhaustion of non-fatal alternatives; a patient could be driven by untreated pain, and still receive physician-assisted suicide. And what counts as an assertion of the right? For Debbie's doctor, merely "Let's get this over with." Disease plus demand requires death.

Such a rights approach raises a number of problems that feminist theory has illuminated. I should note that overlapping critiques of rights have been offered by Critical Legal Studies,[68] Critical Race Theory,[69] and some communitarian theory.[70] Thus some of these points would be echoed by those critiques.[71] Yet as will be seen, feminist theory offers ways to ground evaluation of rights and rights talk[72] in the experiences of women.

In particular, feminist critiques suggest three different sorts of problems with the rights equation offered to justify physician-assisted suicide and euthanasia. First, it ignores context, both the patient's present context and her history. The prior and surrounding failures in her intimate relationships, in her resources to cope with illness and pain, and even in the adequacy of care being offered by the very same physician fade into invisibility next to the bright light of a rights bearer and her demand. In fact, her choices may be severely constrained. Some of those constraints may even be alterable or removable. Yet attention to those dimensions of decision is discouraged by the absolutism of the equation: either she is an eligible rights bearer or not; either she has asserted her right or not. There is no room for conceding her competence and request, yet querying whether under all the circumstances her choices are so constrained and alternatives so unexplored that acceding to the request may not be the proper course. Stark examples are provided by cases in which pain or symptomatic discomfort drives a person to request assisted suicide or euthanasia, yet the pain or discomfort are treatable. A number of Kevorkian's cases raise the problem as well: Did Janet Adkins ever receive psychological support for the predictable despair and desire to die that follow dire diagnoses such as Alzheimer's? Would the cause of Marjorie Wantz's undiagnosed pelvic pain been ascertainable and even ameliorable at a better health center? In circumstances in which women and others who have traditionally lacked resources and experienced oppression are likely to have fewer options and a tougher time getting good care, mechanical application of the rights equation will authorize their deaths even when less drastic alternatives are or should be available. It will wrongly assume that all face serious illness and disability with the resources of the idealized rights bearer—a person of means untroubled by oppression. The realities of women and others whose circumstances are far from that abstraction's will be ignored.

Second, in ignoring context and relationship, the rights equation extols the vision of a rights bearer as an isolated monad and denigrates actual dependencies. Thus it may be seen as improper to ask what family, social, economic, and medical supports she is or is not getting; this insults her individual self-governance. Nor may it be seen as proper to investigate alternatives to acceding to her request for death; this too dilutes self-rule. Yet feminists have reminded us of the actual embeddedness of persons and the descriptive falseness of a vision of each as an isolated individual.[73] In addition, they have argued normatively that a society comprised of isolated individuals, without the pervasive connections and dependencies that we see, would be undesirable.[74]

Indeed, the very meaning of the patient's request for death is socially constructed; that is the point of the prior section's review of the images animating the debate. If we construe the patient's request as a rights bearer's assertion of a right and deem that sufficient grounds on which the physician may proceed, it is because we choose to regard background failures as irrelevant even if they are differentially motivating the requests of the most vulnerable. We thereby avoid real scrutiny of the social arrangements, governmental failures, and health coverage exclusions that may underlie these requests. We also ignore the fact that these patients may be seeking improved circumstances more than death. We elect a myopia that makes the patient's request and death seem proper. We construct a story that clothes the patient's terrible despair in the glorious mantle of "rights."

Formulaic application of the rights equation in this realm thus exalts an Enlightenment vision of autonomy as self-governance and the exclusion of interfering others. Yet as feminists such as Jennifer Nedelsky have argued, this is not the only vision of autonomy available.[75] She argues that a superior vision of autonomy is to be found by rejecting "the pathological conception of autonomy as boundaries against others," a conception that takes the exclusion of others from one's property as its central symbol. Instead, "if we ask ourselves what actually enables people to be autonomous, the answer is not isolation but relationships ... that provide the support and guidance necessary for the development and experience of autonomy." Nedelsky thus proposes that the best "metaphor for autonomy is not property but childrearing. There we have encapsulated the emergence of autonomy through relationship with others."[76] Martha Minow, too, presents a vision of autonomy that resists the isolation of the self, and instead tries to support the relational context in which the rights bearer is embedded.[77] Neither author counsels abandonment of autonomy and rights. But they propose fundamental revisions that would rule out the mechanical application of a narrow rights equation that would regard disease or disability, coupled with demand, as adequate warrant for death.[78]

In fact, there are substantial problems with grounding advocacy for the specific practices of physician-assisted suicide and euthanasia in a rights analysis, even if one accepts the general importance of rights and self-determination. I have elsewhere argued repeatedly for an absolute or near-absolute moral and legal right to be free of unwanted life-sustaining treatment.[79] Yet the negative right to be free of unwanted bodily invasion does not imply an affirmative right to obtain bodily invasion (or assistance with bodily invasion) for the purpose of ending your own life.

Moreover, the former right is clearly grounded in fundamental entitlements to liberty, bodily privacy, and freedom from unconsented touching; in contrast there is no clear "right" to kill yourself or be killed. Suicide has been widely decriminalized, but decriminalizing an act does not mean that you have a positive right to do it and to command the help of others. Indeed, if a friend were to tell me that she wished to kill herself, I would not be lauded for giving her the tools. In fact, that act of assistance has *not* been decriminalized. That continued condemnation shows that whatever my friend's relation to the act of suicide (a "liberty," "right," or neither), it does not create a right in her sufficient to command or even permit my aid.

There are even less grounds for concluding that there is a right to be killed deliberately on request, that is, for euthanasia. There are reasons why a victim's consent has traditionally been no defense to an accusation of homicide. One reason is suggested by analogy to Mill's famous argument that one cannot consent to one's own enslavement: "The reason for not interfering ... with a person's voluntary acts, is consideration for his liberty.... But by selling himself for a slave, he abdicates his liberty; he foregoes any future use of it...."[80] Similarly, acceding to a patient's request to be killed wipes out the possibility of her future exercise of her liberty. The capacity to command or permit another to take your life deliberately, then, would seem beyond the bounds of those things to which you have a right grounded in notions of liberty. We lack the capacity to bless another's enslavement of us or direct killing of us. How is this compatible then with a right to refuse life-sustaining treatment? That right is not grounded in any so-called "right to die," however frequently the phrase appears in the general press.[81] Instead, it is grounded in rights to be free of unwanted bodily invasion, rights so fundamental that they prevail even when the foreseeable consequence is likely to be death.

Finally, the rights argument in favor of physician-assisted suicide and euthanasia confuses two separate questions: what the patient may do, and what the physician may do. After all, the real question in these debates is not what patients may request or even do. It is not at all infrequent for patients to talk about suicide and request assurance that the physician will help or actively bring on death when the patient wants;[82] that is an expected part of reaction to serious disease and discomfort. The real question is what the doctor may do in response to this predictable occurrence. That question is not answered by talk of what patients may ask; patients may and should be encouraged to reveal everything on their minds. Nor is it answered by the fact that decriminalization of suicide permits the patient to take her own life. The physician and patient are separate moral agents. Those who assert that what a patient may say or do determines the same for the physician, ignore the physician's separate moral and legal agency. They also ignore the fact that she is a professional, bound to act in keeping with a professional role and obligations. They thereby avoid a necessary argument over whether the historic obligations of the physician to "do no harm" and "give no deadly drug even if asked" should be abandoned.[83] Assertion of what the patient may do does not resolve that argument.

The inadequacy of rights arguments to legitimate physician-assisted suicide and euthanasia has led to a different approach, grounded on physicians' duties of beneficence. This might seem to be quite in keeping with feminists' development of an ethics of care.[84] Yet the beneficence argument in the euthanasia context is a strange one, because it asserts that the physician's obligation to relieve suffering permits or even commands her to annihilate the person who is experiencing the suffering. Indeed, at the end of this act of beneficence, no patient is left to experience its supposed benefits. Moreover, this argument ignores widespread agreement that fears of patient addiction in these cases should be discarded, physicians may sedate to unconsciousness, and the principle of double effect permits giving pain relief and palliative

care in doses that risk inducing respiratory depression and thereby hastening death. Given all of that, it is far from clear what patients remain in the category of those whose pain or discomfort can only be relieved by killing them.

Thus this argument that a physician should provide so much "care" that she kills the patient is deeply flawed. A more sophisticated version, however, is offered by Howard Brody.[85] He acknowledges that both the usual rights arguments and traditional beneficence arguments have failed. Thus he claims to find a middle path. He advocates legitimation of physician-assisted suicide and euthanasia "as a compassionate response to one sort of medical failure," namely, medical failure to prolong life, restore function, or provide effective palliation. Even in such cases, he does not advocate the creation of a rule providing outright legalization. Instead, "compassionate and competent medical practice" should serve as a defense in a criminal proceeding.[86] Panels should review the practice case by case; a positive review should discourage prosecution.

There are elements of Brody's proposal that seem quite in keeping with much feminist work: his rejection of a binary either-or analysis, his skepticism that a broad rule will yield a proper resolution, his requirement instead of a case-by-case approach. Moreover, the centrality that he accords to "compassion" again echoes feminist work on an ethics of care. Yet ultimately he offers no real arguments for extending compassion to the point of killing a patient, for altering the traditional boundaries of medical practice, or for ignoring the fears that any legitimation of these practices will start us down a slippery slope leading to bad consequences. Brody's is more the proposal of a procedure—what he calls "not resolution but adjudication," following philosopher Hilary Putnam—than it is a true answer to the moral and legal quandaries.

What Brody's analysis does accomplish, however, is that it suggests that attention to method is a necessary, if not sufficient, part of solving the euthanasia problem. Thus we find that two of the most important current debates in bioethics are linked—the debate over euthanasia and the debate over the proper structure of bioethical analysis and method.[87] The inadequacies of rights arguments to establish patient entitlement to assisted suicide and euthanasia are linked to the inadequacies of a "top-down" or deductive bioethics driven by principles, abstract theories, or rules. They share certain flaws: both seem overly to ignore context and the nuances of cases; their simple abstractions overlook real power differentials in society and historic subordination; and they avoid the fact that these principles, rules, abstractions, and rights are themselves a product of historically oppressive social arrangements. Similarly, the inadequacies of beneficence and compassion arguments are linked to some of the problems with a "bottom-up" or inductive bioethics built on cases, ethnography and detailed description. In both instances it is difficult to see where the normative boundaries lie, and where to get a normative keel for the finely described ship.

What does feminism have to offer these debates? Feminists too have struggled extensively with the question of method, with how to integrate detailed attention to individual cases with rights, justice, and principles. Thus in criticizing Kohlberg and going beyond his vision of moral development, Carol Gilligan argued that human beings should be able to utilize both an ethics of justice and an ethics of care. "To understand how the tension between responsibilities and rights sustains the dialectic of human development is to see the integrity of two disparate modes of experience that are in the end connected.... In the representation of maturity both perspectives converge...."[88] What was less clear was precisely how the two should fit together. And unfortunately for our purposes, Gilligan never took up Kohlberg's mercy killing case to illuminate a care perspective or even more importantly how the two perspectives might properly be interwoven in that case.

That finally, I would suggest, is the question. Here we must look to those feminist scholars who have struggled directly with how the two perspectives might fit. Lawrence Blum has distinguished eight different positions that one might take, and that scholars have taken, on "the relation between impartial morality and morality of care:"[89] (1) acting on care is just acting on complicated moral principles; (2) care is mot moral but personal; (3) care is moral but secondary to principle and generally adds mere refinements or supererogatory opportunities; (4)

principle supplies a superior basis for moral action by ensuring consistency; (5) care morality concerns evaluation of persons while principles concern evaluation of acts; (6) principles set outer boundaries within which care can operate; (7) the preferability of a care perspective in some circumstances must be justified by reasoning from principles; and (8) care and justice must be integrated. Many others have struggled with the relationship between the two perspectives as well.

Despite this complexity, the core insight is forthrightly stated by Owen Flanagan and Kathryn Jackson: "[T]he most defensible specification of the moral domain will include issues of both right and good."[90] Martha Minow and Elizabeth Spelman go further. Exploring the axis of abstraction versus context, they argue against dichotomizing the two and in favor of recognizing their "constant interactions."[91] Indeed, they maintain that a dichotomy misdescribes the workings of context. "[C]ontextualists do not merely address each situation as a unique one with no relevance for the next one.... The basic norm of fairness—treat like cases alike—is fulfilled, not undermined, by attention to what particular traits make one case like, or unlike, another."[92] Similarly, "[w]hen a rule specifies a context, it does not undermine the commitment to universal application to the context specified; it merely identifies the situations to be covered by the rule."[93] If this kind of integration is available, then why do we hear such urgent pleas for attention to context? "[T]he call to context in the late twentieth century reflects a critical argument that prevailing legal and political norms have used the form of abstract, general, and universal prescriptions while neglecting the experiences and needs of women of all races and classes, people of color, and people without wealth."[94]

Here we find the beginning of an answer to our dilemma. It appears that we must attend to both context and abstraction, peering through the lenses of both care and justice. Yet our approach to each will be affected by its mate. Our apprehension and understanding of context or cases inevitably involves categories, while our categories and principles should be refined over time to apply to some contexts and not others.[95] Similarly, our understanding of what caring requires in a particular case will grow in part from our understanding of what sort of case this is and what limits principles set to our expressions of caring; while our principles should be scrutinized and amended according to their impact on real lives, especially the lives of those historically excluded from the process of generating principles.[96]

This last point is crucial and a distinctive feminist contribution to the debate over abstraction versus context, or in bioethics, principles versus cases. Various voices in the bioethics debate over method—be they advocating casuistry, specified principlism, principlism itself, or some other position—present various solutions to the question of how cases and principles or other higher-order abstractions should interconnect. Feminist writers too have substantive solutions to offer, as I have suggested. But feminists also urge something that the mainstream writers on bioethics method have overlooked altogether, namely the need to use cases and context to reveal the systematic biases such as sexism and racism built into the principles or other abstractions themselves. Those biases will rarely be explicit in a principle. Instead, we will frequently have to look at how the principle operates in actual cases, what it presupposes (such as wealth or life options), and what it ignores (such as preexisting sexism or racism among the very health care professionals meant to apply it).[97]

What, then, does all of this counsel in application to the debate over physician-assisted suicide and euthanasia? This debate cannot demand a choice between abstract rules or principles and physician caring. Although the debate has sometimes been framed that way, it is difficult to imagine a practice of medicine founded on one to the exclusion of the other. Few would deny that physician beneficence and caring for the individual patient are essential. Indeed, they are constitutive parts of the practice of medicine as it has come to us through the centuries and aims to function today. Yet that caring cannot be unbounded. A physician cannot be free to do whatever caring for or empathy with the patient seems to urge in the moment. Physicians practice a profession with standards and limits, in the context of a democratic polity that itself imposes further limits.[98] These considerations have led the few who have begun to explore an ethics of care for physicians to argue that the notion of care in that context must be carefully

delimited and distinct from the more general caring of a parent for a child (although there are limits, too, on what a caring parent may do).[99] Physicians must pursue what I will call "principled caring."

This notion of principled caring captures the need for limits and standards, whether technically stated as principles or some other form of generalization. Those principles or generalizations will articulate limits and obligations in a provisional way, subject to reconsideration and possible amendment in light of actual cases. Both individual cases and patterns of cases may specifically reveal that generalizations we have embraced are infected by sexism or other bias, either as those generalizations are formulated or as they function in the world. Indeed, given that both medicine and bioethics are cultural practices in a society riddled by such bias and that we have only begun to look carefully for such bias in our bioethical principles and practices, we should expect to find it.

Against this background, arguments for physician-assisted suicide and euthanasia—whether grounded on rights or beneficence—are automatically suspect when they fail to attend to the vulnerability of women and other groups. If our cases, cultural images, and perhaps practice differentially feature the deaths of women, we cannot ignore that. It is one thing to argue for these practices for the patient who is not so vulnerable, the wealthy white male living on Park Avenue in Manhattan who wants to add yet another means of control to his arsenal. It is quite another to suggest that the woman of color with no health care coverage or continuous physician relationship, who is given a dire diagnosis in the city hospital's emergency room, needs then to be offered direct killing.

To institute physician-assisted suicide and euthanasia at this point in this country—in which many millions are denied the resources to cope with serious illness, in which pain relief and palliative care are by all accounts woefully mishandled, and in which we have a long way to go to make proclaimed rights to refuse life-sustaining treatment and to use advance directives working realities in clinical settings—seems, at the very least, to be premature. Were we actually to fix those other problems, we have no idea what demand would remain for these more drastic practices and in what category of patients. We know for example, that the remaining category is likely to include very few, if any, patients in pain, once inappropriate fears of addiction, reluctance to sedate to unconsciousness, and confusion over the principle of double effect are overcome.

Yet against those background conditions, legitimating the practices is more than just premature. It is a danger to women. Those background conditions pose special problems for them. Women in this country are differentially poorer, more likely to be either uninsured or on government entitlement programs, more likely to be alone in their old age, and more susceptible to depression. Those facts alone would spell danger. But when you combine them with the long (indeed, ancient) history of legitimating the sacrifice and self-sacrifice of women, the danger intensifies. That history suggests that a woman requesting assisted suicide or euthanasia is likely to be seen as doing the "right" thing. She will fit into unspoken cultural stereotypes.[100] She may even be valorized for appropriate feminine self-sacrificing behavior, such as sparing her family further burden or the sight of an unaesthetic deterioration. Thus she may be subtly encouraged to seek death. At the least, her physician may have a difficult time seeing past the legitimating stereotypes and valorization to explore what is really going on with this particular patient, why she is so desperate, and what can be done about it. If many more patients in the Netherlands ask about assisted suicide and euthanasia than go through with it,[101] and if such inquiry is a routine part of any patient's responding to a dire diagnosis or improperly managed symptoms and pain, then were the practices to be legitimated in the United States, we would expect to see a large group of patients inquiring. Yet given the differential impact of background conditions in the United States by gender and the legitimating stereotypes of women's deaths, we should also expect to see what has been urged as a neutral practice show marked gender effects.

Is it possible to erect a practice that avoids this? No one has yet explained how. A recent article advocating the legitimation of physician-assisted suicide, for example, acknowledges the need to protect the vulnerable (though it never lists women among them).[102] But none of the seven criteria it proposes to guide the practice involves deeply inquiring into the

patient's life circumstances, whether she is alone, or whether she has health care coverage. Nor do the criteria require the physician to examine whether gender or other stereotypes are figuring in the physician's response to the patient's request. And the article fails to acknowledge the vast inequities and pervasive bias in social institutions that are the background for the whole problem. There is nothing in the piece that requires we remedy or even lessen those problems before these fatal practices begin.

The required interweaving of principles and caring, combined with attention to the heightened vulnerability of women and others, suggests that the right answer to the debate over legitimating these practices is at least "not yet" in this grossly imperfect society and perhaps a flat "no." Beneficence and caring indeed impose positive duties upon physicians, especially with patients who are suffering, despairing, or in pain. Physicians must work with these patients intensively; provide first-rate pain relief, palliative care, and symptomatic relief; and honor patients' exercise of their rights to refuse life-sustaining treatment and use advance directives. Never should the patient's illness, deterioration, or despair occasion physician abandonment. Whatever concerns the patient has should be heard and explored, including thoughts of suicide, or requests for aid or euthanasia.

Such requests should redouble the physician's efforts, prompt consultation with those more expert in pain relief or supportive care, suggest exploration of the details of the patient's circumstance, and a host of other efforts. What such requests should not do is prompt our collective legitimation of the physician's saying "yes" and actively taking the patient's life. The mandates of caring fail to bless killing the person for whom one cares. Any such practice in the United States will inevitably reflect enormous background inequities and persisting societal biases. And there are special reasons to expect gender bias to play a role.

The principles bounding medical practice are not written in stone. They are subject to reconsideration and societal renegotiation over time. Thus the ancient prohibitions against physicians assisting suicide and performing euthanasia do not magically defeat proposals for change. (Nor do mere assertions that "patients want it" mandate change, as I have argued above.)[103] But we ought to have compelling reasons for changing something as serious as the limits on physician killing, and to be rather confident that change will not mire physicians in a practice that is finally untenable.

By situating assisted suicide and euthanasia in a history of women's deaths, by suggesting the social meanings that over time have attached to and justified women's deaths, by revealing the background conditions that may motivate women's requests, and by stating the obvious—that medicine does not somehow sit outside society, exempt from all of this—I have argued that we cannot have that confidence. Moreover, in the real society in which we live, with its actual and for some groups fearful history, there are compelling reasons not to allow doctors to kill. We cannot ignore that such practice would allow what for now remains an elite and predominantly male profession to take the lives of the "other." We cannot explain how we will train the young physician both to care for the patient through difficult straits and to kill. We cannot protect the most vulnerable.

CONCLUSION

Some will find it puzzling that elsewhere we seek to have women's voices heard and moral agency respected, yet here I am urging that physicians not accede to the request for assisted suicide and euthanasia. Indeed, as noted above, I have elsewhere maintained that physicians must honor patients' requests to be free of unwanted life-sustaining treatment. In fact, attention to gender and feminist argument would urge some caution in both realms. As Jay Katz has suggested, any patient request or decision of consequence merits conversation and exploration.[104] And analysis by Steven Miles and Alison August suggests that gender bias may be operating in the realm of the termination of life-sustaining treatment too.[105] Yet finally there is a difference between the two domains. As I have argued above, there is a strong right to be free of unwanted bodily invasion. Indeed, for women, a long history of being harmed specifically through unwanted bodily invasion such as rape presents particularly compelling reasons for honoring a woman's refusal of invasion and effort to maintain bodily intactness. When it

comes to the question of whether women's suicides should be aided, however, or whether women should be actively killed, there is no right to command physician assistance, the dangers of permitting assistance are immense, and the history of women's subordination cuts the other way. Women have historically been seen as fit objects for bodily invasion, self-sacrifice, and death at the hands of others. The task before us is to challenge all three.[106]

Certainly some women, including some feminists, will see this problem differently. That may be especially true of women who feel in control of their lives, are less subject to subordination by age or race or wealth, and seek yet another option to add to their many. I am not arguing that women should lose control of their lives and selves. Instead, I am arguing that when women request to be put to death or ask help in taking their own lives, they become part of a broader social dynamic of which we have properly learned to be extremely wary. These are fatal practices. We can no longer ignore questions of gender or the insights of feminist argument.

Author's Notes

My thanks to Arthur Applbaum, Larry Blum, Alta Charo, Norman Daniels, Johannes J. M. van Delden, Rebecca Dresser, Jorge Garcia, Henk ten Have, Warren Kearney, Elizabeth Kiss, Steven Miles, Christine Mitchell, Remco Oostendorp, Lynn Peterson, Dennis Thompson, and Alan Wertheimer for help at various stages, to the *Texas Journal on Women and the Law* at the University of Texas Law School for the opportunity to elicit comments on an earlier version, and to participants in the University of Minnesota Law School Faculty Workshop for valuable suggestions. Kent Spies and Terrence Dwyer of the University of Minnesota Law School provided important research assistance. Work on this chapter was supported in part by a Fellowship in the Program in Ethics and the Professions at Harvard University.

Notes

1. See, for example, Pamela Carroll, "Proponents of Physician-Assisted Suicide Continuing Efforts," *ACP Observer,* February 1992, p. 29 (describing state ini-

tiatives in Washington, California, Michigan, New Hampshire, and Oregon). Subsequently, Oregon voters made that state the first to legalize physician-assisted suicide. See 1995 Oregon Laws, Ch. 3, I. M. No. 16. But see also Lee V. Oregon, 869 F. Suppl. 1491. (DOOR. 1994), entering an injunction preventing the statute from going into effect. Further legal proceedings will decide the statute's fate. For attempts to legalize physician-assisted suicide through litigation, see Compassion in Dying v. Washington, 850 F. Supp. 1454 (W.D. Wash. 1994), *rev'd,* 49 F. 3d 586 (9th Cir. 1995); Quill v. Koppel, 870 F. Supp. 78 (S. D.N.Y., 1994). See also Hobbins v. Attorney General, 527 N. W. 2d 714 (Mich. 1994).

2. See, for example, Howard Brody "Assisted Death—A Compassionate Response to a Medical Failure," *New England Journal of Medicine* 327 (1992): 1384-88; Timothy E. Quill, Christine K. Cassel, and Diane E. Meier, "Care of the Hopelessly Ill: Proposed Clinical Criteria for Physician-Assisted Suicide," *New England Journal of Medicine* 327 (1992): 1380-84; Guy I. Benrubi, "Euthanasia—The Need for Procedural Safeguards," *New England Journal of Medicine* 326 (1992): 197-99; Christine K. Cassel and Diane E. Meier, "Morals and Moralism in the Debate Over Euthanasia and Assisted Suicide," *New England Journal of Medicine* 323 (1990): 750-52; James Rachels, *The End of Life* (Oxford, England: Oxford University Press, 1986).

3. I restrict the term "euthanasia" to active euthanasia, excluding the termination of life-sustaining treatment, which has sometimes been called "passive euthanasia." Both law and ethics now treat the termination of treatment quite differently from the way they treat active euthanasia, so to use "euthanasia" to refer to both invites confusion. See generally "Report of the Council on Ethical and Judicial Affairs of the American Medical Association," *Issues in Law & Medicine* 10 (1994): 91-97, 92.

4. See Howard I. Kushner, "Women and Suicide in Historical Perspective," in Joyce McCarl Nielsen, ed., *Feminist Research Methods: Exemplary Readings in the Social Sciences* (Boulder, CO: Westview Press, 1990), 193-206, 198-200.

5. See Alan Meisel, *The Right to Die* (New York, NY: John Wiley & Sons, 1989), 62, & *1993 Cumulative Supplement No. 2,* 50-54.

6. See Council on Ethical and Judicial Affairs, *Code of Medical Ethics: Current Opinions with Annotations* (Chicago, Il., American Medical Association, 1994): 50-51; "Report of the Board of Trustees of the American Medical Association," *Issues in Law & Medicine* 10 (1994): 81-90; "Report of the Council on Ethical and Judicial Affairs," *Report of the Council on Ethical and Judicial Affairs of the American Medical Association: Euthanasia* (Chicago, Il. American Medical Association, 1989). There are U.S. data on public opinion and physicians' self-reported practices. See, for example, "Report of the Board of Trustees." But the legal and ethical condemnation of physician-assisted suicide and euthanasia in the United States undoubtedly affect the self-reporting and render this a poor indicator of actual practices.

7. See Nancy S. Jecker, "Physician-Assisted Death in the Netherlands and the United States: Ethical and Cultural Aspects of Health Policy Development," *Journal of the American Geriatrics Society* 42 (1994): 672-78, 676.

8. See generally Howard I. Kushner, "Women and Suicidal Behavior: Epidemiology, Gender, and Lethality in Historical Perspective," in Silvia Sara Canetto and David Lester, eds., *Women And Suicidal Behavior* (New York, NY: Springer, 1995).

9. Compare Jecker, "Physician-Assisted Death," 676, on reasons physicians might differentially refuse women's requests.

10. See Lawrence Kohlberg, *The Philosophy of Moral Development: Moral Stages and the Idea of Justice,* vol. I (San Francisco, CA: Harper & Row, 1981); Lawrence Kohlberg, *The Psychology of Moral Development: The Nature and Validity of Moral Stages,* vol. II (San Francisco, CA: Harper & Row 1984).

11. See Carol Gilligan, *In A Different Voice: Psychological Theory and Women's Development* (Cambridge, MA: Harvard University Press, 1982).

12. Gilligan's work has prompted a large literature, building upon as well as criticizing her insights and methodology. See, for example, the essays collected in Larrabee, ed., *An Ethic of Care.* On attention to the ethics of care in bioethics and on feminist criticism of the ethics of care, see my Introduction to this volume.

13. See Kohlberg, *The Psychology of Moral Development,* 644-47.

14. On the Kohlberg-Gilligan debate, see generally Lawrence A. Blum, "Gilligan and Kohlberg: Implications for Moral Theory" in Larrabee, ed., *An Ethic of Care*, 49-68; Owen Flanagan and Kathryn Jackson, "Justice, Care, and Gender: The Kohlberg-Gilligan Debate Revisited," in Larrabee, ed., *An Ethic of Care*, 69-84; Seyla Benhabib, "The Generalized and the Concrete Other: The Kohlberg-Gilligan Controversy and Feminist Theory," in Seyla Benhabib and Drucilla Cornell, eds., *Feminism as Critique: On the Politics of Gender* (Minneapolis, MN: University of Minnesota Press, 1987), 77-95.

15. See, for example, Susan M. Wolf, "Holding the Line on Euthanasia," *Hastings Center Report* 19 (Jan./Feb. 1989): special supp. 13-15.

16. See "It's Over, Debbie," *Journal of the American Medical Association* 259 (1988): 272.

17. See Timothy Egan, "As Memory and Music Faded, Oregon Woman Chose Death," *New York Times*, June 7, 1990, p.A1, Lisa Belkin, "Doctor Tells of First Death Using His Suicide Device," *New York Times*, June 6, 1990, p. A1.

18. See "Doctor Assists in Two More Suicides in Michigan," *New York Times*, October 24, 1991, p. A1 (Wantz and Miller).

19. See "Death at Kevorkian's Side is Ruled Homicide," *New York Times*, June 6, 1992, p. 10; "Doctor Assists in Another Suicide," *New York Times*, September 27, 1992, p. 32; "Doctor in Michigan Helps a 6th Person To Commit Suicide," *New York Times*, November 24, 1992, p. A10; "2 Commit Suicide, Aided by Michigan Doctor," *New York Times*, December 16, 1992, p. A21.

20. See "Why Dr. Kevorkian Was Called In," *New York Times*, January 25, 1993, p. A16.

21. See B.D. Colen, "Gender Question in Assisted Suicides," *Newsday*, November 25, 1992, p. 17; Ellen Goodman, "Act Now to Stop Dr. Death," *Atlanta Journal and Constitution*, May 27, 1992, p. A11.

22. See Timothy E. Quill, "Death and Dignity—A Case of Individualized Decision Making," *New England Journal of Medicine* 324 (1991): 691-94.

23. On Quill's motivations, see Timothy E. Quill, "The Ambiguity of Clinical Intentions," *New England Journal of Medicine* 329 (1993): 1039-40.

24. Nicole Loraux, *Tragic Ways of Killing a Woman*, Anthony Forster, trans. (Cambridge, MA: Harvard University Press, 1987), 8.

25. *Ibid.*, 12.

26. *Ibid.*, 23.

27. *Ibid.*, 11.

28. Kushner, "Women and Suicidal Behavior," 16-17 (citations omitted).

29. Kushner, "Women and Suicide in Historical Perspective," 195, citing Barbara Welter, "The Cult of True Womanhood: 1820-1860," *American Quarterly* 18 (1966): 151-55.

30. *Ibid.*, 13-19.

31. Gilligan, *In A Different Voice*, 70

32. *Ibid.*, 132.

33. Loraux in *Tragic Ways of Killing a Woman* notes the single exception of Ajax.

34. See Peter Steinfels, "Help for the Helping Hands in Death," *New York Times*, February 14, 1993, sec. 4, pp. 1, 6.

35. See Charles S. Cleeland et al., "Pain and Its Treatment in Outpatients with Metastatic Cancer," *New England Journal of Medicine* 330 (1994): 592-96.

36. See Robert J. Blendon, U.S. Szalay, and R.A. Knox, "Should Physicians Aid Their Patients in Dying?" *Journal of the American Medical Association* 267 (1992): 2658-62.

37. See William Coryell, Jean Endicott, and Martin B. Keller, "Major Depression in a Non-Clinical Sample: Demographic and Clinical Risk Factors for First Onset," *Archives of General Psychiatry* 49 (1992): 117-25.

38. See Susan D. Block and J. Andrew Billings, "Patient Requests to Hasten Death: Evaluation and Management in Terminal Care," *Archives of Internal Medicine* 154 (1994): 2039-47.

39. Council on Ethical and Judicial Affairs, American Medical Association, "Gender Disparities in Clinical Decision Making," *Journal of the American Medical Association* 266 (1991): 559-62, 561-62.

40. See Nancy S. Jecker, "Can an Employer-Based Health Insurance System Be Just?" *Journal of Health Politics, Policy & Law* 18 (1993): 657-73; Employee Benefit Research Institute (EBRI), *Sources of Health Insurance and Characteristics of the Uninsured: Analysis of the March 1992 Current Population Survey*, EBRI Issue Brief No. 133 (Jan. 1993).

41. The patterns of uninsurance and underinsurance are complex. See, for example, Employee Benefit Resources Institute, *Sources of Health Insurance*.

Recall that the poorest and the elderly are covered by Medicaid and Medicare, though they are subject to the gaps and deficiencies in quality of care that plague those programs.

42. Lawrence Schneiderman et al. purport to show that patients already consider burdens to others in making termination of treatment decisions, and—more importantly for this chapter—that men do so more than women. See Lawrence J. Schneiderman et al., "Attitudes of Seriously Ill Patients toward Treatment that Involves High Cost and Burdens on Others," *Journal of Clinical Ethics* 5 (1994): 109-12. But Peter A. Ubel and Robert M. Arnold criticize the methodology and dispute both conclusions in The Euthanasia Debate and Empirical Evidence: Separating Burdens to Others from One's Own Quality of Life," *Journal of Clinical Ethics* 5 (1994): 155-58.

43. See, for example, Kushner, "Women and Suicidal Behavior."

44. See Colen, "Gender Question in Assisted Suicides."

45. Another area in which we do not allow apparent patient consent or request to authorize physician acquiescence is sex between doctor and patient. Even if the patient requests sex, the physician is morally and legally bound to refuse. The considerable consensus that now exists on this, however, has been the result of a difficult uphill battle. See generally Howard Brody, *The Healer's Power* (New Haven, CT: Yale University Press, 1992), 26-27; Nanette Gartrell et al., "Psychiatrist-Patient Sexual Contact: Results of a National Survey, Part 1. Prevalence," *American Journal of Psychiatry* 143 (1986): 1126-31.

46. As noted above, though, Nancy Jecker speculates that a physician's tendency to discount women's choices may also come into play. See Jecker, "Physician-Assisted Death," 676. Compare Silvia Sara Canetto, "Elderly Women and Suicidal Behavior," in Canetto and Lester, eds., "Women and Suicidal Behavior" 215-33, 228, asking whether physicians are more willing to accept women's suicides.

47. See, for example, Susan Sherwin, *No Longer Patient: Feminist Ethics and Health Care* (Philadelphia, PA: Temple University Press, 1992); Barbara Ehrenreich and Deirdre English, *For Her Own Good: 150 Years of the Experts' Advice to Women* (New York, NY: Doubleday, 1978).

48. Sherwin, *No Longer Patient*, 157.

49. Compare Brody "The Rescue Fantasy," in *The Healer's Art*, ch.9.

50. Robert A. Burt, *Taking Care of Strangers* (New York, NY: Free Press, 1979), vi. See also Steven H. Miles, "Physicians and Their Patients' Suicides," *Journal of the American Medical Association* 271 (1994): 1786-88. I discuss the significance of the ambivalence in the euthanasia context in Wolf, "Holding the Line on Euthanasia."

51. In an article advocating the legitimation of physician-assisted suicide, the authors nonetheless note the lack of good data on U.S. Practice: "From 3 to 37 percent of physicians responding to anonymous surveys reported secretly taking active steps to hasten a patient's death, but these survey data were flawed by low response rates and poor design." Quill, Cassel, and Meier, "Care of the Hopelessly Ill," 1381 (footnotes with citations omitted).

52. On relevant differences between the United States and the Netherlands, see Jecker, "Physician-Assisted Death: Report of the Board of Trustees"; Margaret Battin, "Voluntary Euthanasia and the Risks of Abuse: Can We Learn Anything from the Netherlands?" *Law, Medicine & Health Care* 20 (1992): 133-43.

53. There have been two major teams of researchers. The first, conducting research at governmental request, has produced publications including Loes Pijnenborg, Paul J. van der Maas, Johannes J.M. van Delden, and Caspar W.N. Looman, "Life-terminating acts without explicit request of patient," *Lancet* 341 (1993): 1196-99. Paul J. van der Maas, Johannes J.M. van Delden, and Loes Pijnenborg, "Euthanasia and other medical decisions concerning the end of life: An investigation performed upon request of the Commission of Inquiry into the Medical Practice concerning Euthanasia," *Health Policy* 22 (1992): 1-262; and Paul J. van der Maas, Johannes J.M. van Delden, Loes Pijnenborg, and Caspar W.N. Looman, "Euthanasia and other medical decisions concerning the end of life," *Lancet* 338 (1991): 669-74. The second team's publications include G. van der Wal, J.T. van Eijk, H.J. Leenen, and C. Spreeuwenberg, "The use of drugs for euthanasia and assisted suicide in family practice" (Medline translation of Dutch title), *Nederlands Tijdschrift Voor Geneeskunde* 136 (1992): 1299-305; same authors, "Euthanasia and

assisted suicide by physicians in the home situation. 2. Suffering of the patients" (Medline translation of Dutch title), same journal 135 (1991): 1599-603; and same authors, "Euthanasia and assisted suicide by physicians in the home situation. I. Diagnoses, age and sex of patients," same journal 135 (1991): 1593-98. More recently the latter group has published Gerrit van der Wal and Robert J. M. Dillmann, "Euthanasia in the Netherlands," *British Medical Journal* 308 (1994): 1346-49. M.T. Muller et al., "Voluntary Active Euthanasia and Physician-Assisted Suicide in Dutch Nursing Homes. Are the Requirements for Prudent Practice Properly Met?" *Journal of the American Geriatrics Society,* 42 (1994): 624-29. G. van der Wal et al., "Voluntary Active Euthanasia and Physician-Assisted Suicide in Dutch Nursing Homes: Requests and Administrations," *Journal of the American Geriatrics Society* 42 (1994): 620-23.

54. van der Maas et al., "Euthanasia," *Lancet.*

55. Henk ten Have has pointed out to me that women have also predominated in the court cases on physician-assisted suicide and euthanasia in the Netherlands. Personal communication, April 1993. Ideally those judicial opinions will be translated into English or be analyzed by someone bilingual, permitting comparison to the textual analysis of U.S. judicial opinions in Steven Miles and Alison August, "Courts, Gender, and 'the Right to Die,'" *Law, Medicine & Health Care* 18 (1990): 85-95.

56. van der Maas, van Delden, and Pijnenborg, "Euthanasia," *Health Policy,* 50.

57. van der Maas et al., "Euthanasia," *Lancet,* 671.

58. Johannes J.M. van Delden, personal communication, April 2, 1993.

59. Pijnenborg et al., "Life-terminating acts without explicit request of patient"; van der Maas, van Delden, and Pijnenborg, "Euthanasia," *Health Policy*, 50; Johannes J.M. van Delden, personal communication, April, 1993. Note that the 1991 *Lancet* article combines euthanasia, physician-assisted suicide, and "life-terminating events without explicit and persistent request," labeling the combination "euthanasia and related MDEL," and reporting a combined gender ratio of 61:39 with males predominating. See van der Maas et al., "Euthanasia," *Lancet,* 670-71. However, as I indicate in text, when you separate the three subcategories, women predominate for euthanasia.

60. Note that in *Lancet,* the researchers addressed both euthanasia and physician-assisted suicide in stating that, "Euthanasia and assisted suicide were more often found in deaths in relatively young men and in the urbanised western Netherlands, and this may be an indication of a shift towards a more demanding attitude of patients in matters concerning the end of life." van der Maas et al., "Euthanasia," *Lancet,* 673. See also Pijnenborg et al., "Life-terminating acts without explicit request of patient." However, in their subsequent *Health Policy* publication, they reported that euthanasia was *not* more often found in men, though physician-assisted suicide was. van der Maas, van Delden, and Pijnenborg, "Euthanasia," *Heathy Policy,* 50.

61. Johannes J.M. van Delden, personal communication, April 1993.

62. See van der Maas, van Delden, and Pijnenborg, "Euthanasia," *Health Policy,* 52.

63. Compare, for example, "Netherlands: Ethnic Minority Population to Reach One Million by 2000," *Financieele Dagblad,* March 3, 1994 (ethnic minority population will then be 6.6. percent), with U.S. Department of Commerce, Bureau of the Census, *Statistical Abstract of the United States* 1993, 113th ed., 18 (20 percent of the 1990 population was non-white).

64. Canetto, "Elderly Women and Suicidal Behavior," 225-26 (citation omitted). I am grateful to Alta Charo for suggesting I also consider the preponderance of women in American nursing homes. See *Census of the Population, 1990: General Population Characteristics of the United States* (Washington, DC: Government Printing Office, 1992), 48 (1,278,433 women in nursing homes versus 493,609 men). On suicidal behavior, both attempted and completed, in U.S. nursing homes see Nancy J. Osgood, Barbara A. Brant, and Aaron Lipman, *Suicide Among the Elderly in Long-Term Care Facilities* (New York, NY: Greenwood Press, 1991).

65. There is a substantial literature on the Tuskegee study. See, for example, Arthur L. Caplan, "When Evil Intrudes," Harold Edgar, "Outside the Community," Patricia King, "The Dangers of Difference," and James H. Jones, "The Tuskegee Legacy: AIDS and the Black Community," all in "Twenty Years After: The Legacy of the Tuskegee Syphilis Study,"

Hastings Center Report 22 (Nov.-Dec. 1992): 29-40; James H. Jones, *Bad Blood: The Tuskegee Syphilis Experiment* (New York, NY: Free Press, 1981); Allan M. Brandt, "Racism and Research: The Case of the Tuskegee Syphilis Study," *Hastings Center Report* 8 (Dec. 1978): 21-28.

66. See Mark B. Wenneker and Arnold M. Epstein, "Racial Inequalities in the Use of Procedures for Patients with Ischemic Heart Disease in Massachusetts," *Journal of the American Medical Association* 261 (1989): 233-57. See also Robert J. Blendon et al., "Access to Medical Care for Black and White Americans: A Matter of Continuing Concern," *Journal of the American Medical Association* 261 (1989): 278-81, Craig K. Svensson, "Representation of American Blacks in Clinical Trials of New Drugs," *Journal of the American Medical Association* 261 (1989): 263-65.

67. On the intersection of race and gender, for example, see Kimberle Crenshaw, "Demarginalizing the Intersection of Race and Sex: A Black Feminist Critique of Antidiscrimination Doctrine, Feminist Theory and Antiracist Politics," *Chicago Legal Forum* 1989: 139-67. See also Patricia Hill Collins, *Black Feminist Thought: Knowledge, Consciousness, and the Politics of Empowerment* (New York, NY: Routledge, 1991). On the intersection of race and gender in health, see Evelyn C. White, ed., *The Black Women's Health Book: Speaking for Ourselves* (Seattle, WA: Seal Press, 1990).

68. See, for example, Morton J. Horowitz, "Rights," *Harvard Civil Rights-Civil Liberties Law Review* 23 (1988): 393-406; Mark Tushnet, "An Essay on Rights," *Texas Law Review* 62 (1984): 1363-403.

69. Though there is an overlap in the rights critiques of Critical Legal Studies (CLS) and Critical Race Theory, "[t]he CLS critique of rights and rules is the most problematic aspect of the CLS program, and provides few answers for minority scholars and lawyers." Richard Delgado, "The Ethereal Scholar: Does Critical Legal Studies Have What Minorities Want?" *Harvard Civil Rights-Civil Liberties Law Review* 22(1987): 301-22, 304 (footnote omitted). Patricia Williams, indeed, has argued the necessity of rights discourse: "[S]tatements ... about the relative utility of needs over rights discourse overlook that blacks have been describing their needs for generations.... For blacks, describing needs has been a dismal failure...." Patricia J. Williams, *The Alchemy of Race and Rights* (Cambridge, MA: Harvard University Press, 1991), 151.

70. See, for example, Mary Ann Glendon, *Rights Talk: The Impoverishment of Political Discourse* (New York, NY: Free Press, 1991).

71. Margaret Farley has helpfully traced commonalities as well as distinctions between feminist theory and other traditions, noting that it is wrong to demand of any one critical stream that it bear no relation to the others. See Margaret A. Farley "Feminist Theology and Bioethics," in Earl E. Shelp, ed., *Theology and Bioethics: Exploring the Foundations and Frontiers* (Boston, MA: D. Reidel, 1985), 163-85.

72. I take the term "rights talk" from Glendon, *Rights Talk.*

73. See, for example, Jean Grimshaw, *Philosophy and Feminist Thinking* (Minneapolis, MN: University of Minnesota Press, 1986), 175.

74. See, for example, Naomi Scheman, "Individualism and the Objects of Psychology" in Sandra Harding and Merrill B. Hintikka, eds., *Discovering Reality: Feminist Perspectives on Epistemology, Metaphysics, Methodology, and the Philosophy of Science* (Boston, MA: D. Reidel, 1983), 225-44, 240.

75. See Jennifer Nedelsky "Reconceiving Autonomy: Sources, Thoughts and Possibilities," *Yale Journal of Law and Feminism* 1 (1989): 7-36.

76. *Ibid.*, 12-13.

77. See Martha Minow, *Making All the Difference: Inclusion, Exclusion, and American Law* (Ithaca, NY: Cornell University Press, 1990).

78. Another author offering a feminist revision of autonomy and rights is Diana T. Meyers in "The Socialized Individual and Individual Autonomy: An Intersection between Philosophy and Psychology," in Eva Feder Kittay and Diana T. Meyers, eds., *Women And Moral Theory* (Savage, MD: Rowman & Littlefield, 1987), 139-53. See also Elizabeth M. Schneider, "The Dialectic of Rights and Politics: Perspectives from the Women's Movement," *New York University Law Review* 61 (1986): 589-652. There is a large feminist literature presenting a critique of rights, some of it rejecting the utility of such language. See, for example, Catharine MacKinnon, "Feminism, Marxism, Method and the State: Toward Feminist Jurisprudence," *Signs* 8 (1983): 635-58,658 ("Abstract rights will authorize the male experience of the world.").

79. See, for example, Susan M. Wolf, "Nancy Beth Cruzan: In No Voice At All," *Hastings Center Report* 20 (Jan.-Feb. 1990): 38-41, *Guidelines on the Termination of Life-Sustaining Treatment and the Care of the Dying* (Bloomington, IN: Indiana University Press & The Hastings Center, 1987).

80. John Stuart Mill, "On Liberty," in Marshall Cohen, ed., *The Philosophy of John Stuart Mill: Ethical, Political and Religious* (New York, NY: Random House, 1961), 185-319, 304.

81. Leon R. Kass also argues against the existence of a "right to die" in "Is There a Right to Die?" *Hastings Center Report* 23 (Jan.-Feb. 1993): 34-43.

82. The Dutch studies show that even when patients know they can get assisted suicide and euthanasia, three times more patients ask for such assurance from their physicians than actually die that way. See van der Maas et al., "Euthanasia," *Lancet*, 673.

83. On these obligations and their derivation, see Leon R. Kass, "Neither for Love nor Money: Why Doctors Must Not Kill," *The Public Interest* 94 (Winter 1989): 25-46; Tom L. Beauchamp and James F. Childress, *Principles of Biomedical Ethics,* 4th ed. (New York, NY: Oxford University Press, 1994), 189, 226-27.

84. See Leslie Bender, "A Feminist Analysis of Physician-Assisted Dying and Voluntary Active Euthanasia," *Tennessee Law Review* 59 (1992): 519-46, making a "caring" argument in favor of "physician-assisted death."

85. Brody, "Assisted Death."

86. James Rachels offers a like proposal. See Rachels, *The End of Life.*

87. For a summary of the debate over the proper structure of bioethics, see David DeGrazia, "Moving Forward in Bioethical Theory: Theories, Cases, and Specified Principlism," *Journal of Medicine and Philosophy* 17 (1992): 511-40. There have been several different attacks on a bioethics driven by principles, which is usually taken to be exemplified by Beauchamp and Childress, *Principles of Biomedical Ethics.* Clouser and Gert argue for a bioethics that would be even more "top-down" or deductive, proceeding from theory instead of principles. See K. Danner Clouser and Bernard Gert, "A Critique of Principlism," *Journal of Medicine and Philosophy* 15 (1990): 219-36. A different attack is presented by Ronald M. Green, "Method in Bioethics: A Troubled Assessment," *Journal of*

Medicine and Philosophy 15 (1990): 179-97. Hoffmaster argues for an ethnography driven, "bottom-up" or inductive bioethics. Barry Hoffmaster, "The Theory and Practice of Applied Ethics," *Dialogue* XXX (1991): 213-34. Jonsen and Toulmin have urged a revival of casuistry built on case-by-case analysis. Albert R. Jonsen and Stephen Toulmin, *The Abuse of Casuistry: A History of Moral Reasoning*, (Berkeley, CA: University of California Press, 1988). Beauchamp and Childress discuss these challenges at length in the 4th edition of *Principles of Biomedical Ethics.*

88. See Gilligan, *In A Different Voice,* 174. Lawrence Blum points out that Kohlberg himself stated that "the final, most mature stage of moral reasoning involves an 'integration of justice and care that forms a single moral principle,'" but that Kohlberg, too, never spelled out what that integration would be. See Lawrence A. Blum, "Gilligan and Kohlberg: Implications for Moral Theory,*" Ethics* 98 (1988): 472-91, 482-83 (footnote with citation omitted).

89. See Blum, "Gilligan and Kohlberg," 477.

90. Owen Flanagan and Kathryn Jackson, "Justice, Care, and Gender: The Kohlberg-Gilligan Debate Revisited," in Larrabee, ed., *An Ethic of Care,* 69-84, 71.

91. Martha Minow and Elizabeth V. Spelman, "In Context," *Southern California Law Review* 63 (1990): 1597-652, 1625.

92. *Ibid.*, 1629.

93. *Ibid.*, 1630-31.

94. *Ibid.*, 1632-33.

95. There are significant similarities here to Henry Richardson's proposal of "specified principlism." See DeGrazia, "Moving Forward in Bioethical Theory."

96. On the importance of paying attention to who is doing the theorizing and to what end, including in feminist theorizing, see Maria C. Lugones and Elizabeth V. Spelman, "Have We got a Theory for You! Feminist Theory, Cultural Imperialism and the Demand for 'The Woman's Voice,'" *Women's Studies International Forum* 6 (1983): 573-81.

97. I have elsewhere argued that health care institutions should create processes to uncover and combat sexism and racism, among other problems. See Susan M. Wolf, "Toward a Theory of Process," *Law, Medicine & Health Care* 20 (1922): 278-90.

98. On the importance of viewing the medical profession in the context of the democratic polity, see Troyen Bren-

nan, *Just Doctoring: Medical Ethics in the Liberal State* (Berkeley, CA: University of California Press, 1991).

99. See, for example, Howard J. Curzer, "Is Care A Virtue For Health Care Professionals?" *Journal of Medicine and Philosophy* 18 (1993): 51-69. Nancy S. Jecker and Donnie J. Self, "Separating Care and Cure: An Analysis of Historical and Contemporary Images of Nursing and Medicine," *Journal of Medicine and Philosophy* 16 (1991): 285-306.

100. Compare Canetto, "Elderly Women and Suicidal Behavior," finding evidence of this with respect to elderly women electing suicide.

101. See van der Maas, van Delden, and Pijnenborg, "Euthanasia," *Health Policy,* 51-55, 145-46; van der Wal et al., "Voluntary Active Euthanasia and Physician-Assisted Suicide in Dutch Nursing Homes."

102. See Quill, Cassel, and Meier, "Care of the Hopelessly Ill."

103. In these two sentences, I disagree both with Kass's suggestion that the core commitments of medicine are set for all time by the ancient formulation of the doctor's role and with Brock's assertion that the core commitment of medicine is to do whatever the patient wants. See Kass, "Neither for Love Nor Money." Dan Brock, "Voluntary Active Euthanasia," *Hastings Center Report* 22 (Mar.-Apr. 1992): 10-22.

104. See Jay Katz, *The Silent World of Doctor And Patient* (New York, NY: Free Press, 1984), 121-22.

105. See Miles and August, "Gender, Courts, and the 'Right to die.'"

106. While a large literature analyzes the relationship between terminating life-sustaining treatment and the practices of physician-assisted suicide and euthanasia, more recently attention has turned to the relationship between those latter practices and abortion. On the question of whether respect for women's choice of abortion requires legitimation of those practices, see, for example, Seth F. Kreimer, "Does Pro-choice Mean Pro-Kevorkian? An Essay on *Roe, Casey,* And the Right to Die," *American University Law Review* 44 (1995): 803-54. Full analysis of why respect for the choice of abortion does not require legitimation of physician-assisted suicide and euthanasia is beyond the scope of this chapter. However, the courts themselves are beginning to argue the distinction. See Compassion in Dying v. Washington, 49 F. 3d 586 (9th Cir. 1995). On gender specifically, there are strong arguments that gender equity and concern for the fate of women demand respect for the abortion choice, whereas I am arguing that gender concerns cut the other way when it comes to physician-assisted suicide and euthanasia.

35.
FUTILITY AND HOSPITAL POLICY

Tom Tomlinson and Diane Czlonka

Our purpose in this paper is to identify issues relevant to the development of effective and defensible hospital policies supporting physician judgments not to provide futile resuscitation. As we are convinced that such judgments are ethically defensible in principle, our question will be whether that which is defensible in theory can be implemented ethically in practice. We won't, therefore, take the time to provide a comprehensive theoretical defense of futility judgments (we think a successful defense has already been articulated),[1] or to review all of the large number of articles that have been published on this aspect of the debate. Nevertheless, we still need to highlight the most significant elements of the argument over futility, since these will help set some of the criteria by which a hospital futility policy should be judged.

In what follows, we will focus chiefly on issues and policies surrounding futile resuscitation and say little about other treatment interventions, except by implication. Futile resuscitation deserves this special attention because it is the only intervention that requires consent for an order to withhold it; other futile interventions are typically not offered or discussed. Thus, decisions about resuscitation raise the most acute and perhaps the most frequent conflicts between patient or family demands and physician judgments. Certainly, however, there can be similar conflicts regarding other interventions, particularly regarding the withdrawal of an intervention that the physician has come to believe is futile. Much of what we say about problems for futile resuscitation policies may apply as well to policies aimed at futile treatments more generally, but discussion of the particulars will have to wait for another occasion.

THE FUTILITY DEBATE: LESSONS FOR POLICY
There are two fundamental considerations that support hospital authority over futile or grossly harmful interventions: the moral integrity of the health pro-

fessions, and the obligation to enable autonomous choices by patients.

Physicians and nurses have an obligation to help rather than hurt their patients by what they do. If health professionals could never say no to patient or family demands for interventions, they could not have control over the consequences of the procedures they perform. Without this control, physicians and nurses could not fulfill their moral obligation to promote the patient's welfare, an obligation that is fundamental to ethical practice. We in fact recognize the exercise of this moral authority every day, across the whole range of medical interventions. Patients with (or without) angina don't have a right to demand that a surgeon perform a bypass operation despite the risks of death or the likelihood of benefit; why should they have such a right with respect to CPR?

By necessity, judgments by health professionals not to provide particular treatments are value laden. They require assumptions about what counts as a reasonable chance of success, as well as judgments about the proper goals of medicine. The surgeon and not just the patient, gets to decide whether an 80 percent chance of death is too high, and whether a patient's fascination with surgical suites defines an acceptable goal of surgical practice.

The second consideration arguing for physician authority over futile treatment only has the appearance of paradox. The appearance is that limiting the patient's power to demand futile treatments must undermine his autonomy rather than enable it. The appearance is deceiving for two reasons. The first is that autonomy is enabled or enhanced only when there is a real choice being offered between significantly different options. In cases where resuscitation is genuinely futile, the choice between attempting resuscitation or not is a bogus choice, and the offer of it is a deception. Second, the denial of choices is an infringement of the patient's right to autonomy only if the patient has the right to demand the option in question. If the patient's right to autonomy is limited by the rights of others, then limitations of patient choice made on behalf of protecting those other rights are not ethically objectionable. To assert that limiting choices regarding futile treatment is per se a violation of patients' rights of autonomy begs the question, unless the only precept in medicine is "The customer is always right."

There are several common objections leveled against giving physicians this authority over futile or harmful treatment. A review of them will help identify some valid concerns that may need to guide policy.

One of these is that since futility judgements make value-laden assumptions, they should be shaped only by the patient's values. When shaped by the values of the physician or profession, they are an illegitimate infringement of patient autonomy and represent a resurgence of unwarranted paternalism.

As an objection in principle against the exercise of futility judgments this argument is unsuccessful, for the reasons sketched above. In highlighting the value-laden character of these decisions, however, it reminds us that the value assumptions made in cases of futility will have to receive their warrant from somewhere. If the warrant is not found in the patient's right to self-determination, neither can it be found in the individual physician's values. When backed by institutional policy, the refusal to provide futile treatments is made on behalf of professional integrity, not merely individual conscience. Therefore, a futility policy will have to incorporate some means for articulating the professional values at stake and for certifying that they are indeed values for the profession, not values that are ethically optional for individual professionals.

The objection suggests another important concern: that the values employed in futility judgments will be insulated from the values of the wider society the profession is licensed to serve. The futility judgments that result will be at odds with widely understood public convictions about the proper social role of the medical enterprise. This is again a concern that is practical rather than theoretical. Futility policies designed successfully to avoid such a gap between professional and public values and goals will not be objectionable on this score.

Another common objection against physician authority over futile treatment is that it justifies the decision not to discuss resuscitation status with patients or families, and encourages the all-too-common avoidance of uncomfortable conversations about death, dying, and the limits of medicine. This argument is also unsuccessful as a criticism of the ethical justification for permitting futility judgments. There are a number of good reasons supporting an obligation to discuss decisions not to provide futile resuscitation with patients and families, short of reliance upon the patient's right of self-determination.[2] There is no incompatibility between rejecting the patient's right to select futile resuscitation and insisting on the physician's obligation to inform patients about their plan of care, a point apparently missed by some critics of futility judgments. The objection does, however, point to another concern that must be addressed by policy: how to grant authority to physicians to limit futile therapy while encouraging full, honest, and supportive communication.

A third objection made against futility judgments is that the resulting focus on the biomedical aspects of medical interventions will lead to neglect of the worthy social and psychological needs that might be served by biomedically futile interventions. To repeat, a judgment not to provide an intervention always makes implicit assumptions about the proper goals of medicine. The sheer fact that certain needs of patients or families might remain unmet because of a decision not to provide a medical intervention is not a decisive objection against authorizing futility judgments. The truth behind the objection is that a comprehensive justification for not meeting a demand for treatment requires consideration of all the goals that might be served by the intervention, and not just the narrowly biomedical ones. Good futility policies will encourage that breadth of review.

Finally, the argument has been made that unilateral physician authority over futile resuscitation is unnecessary, because in virtually all cases when physicians would think resuscitation futile, patients and families would agree. Authority over futile treatment therefore offers nothing of benefit, only the opportunity for mischief. An equally effective approach to reducing demands for futility treatment is to help physicians to lead better discussions with patients and families about treatment limitation choices.

The difficulty with the objection and the alternative it espouses is that it is extremely difficult for patients and families to make informed, autonomous *choices* about futile resuscitation. When the only way to authorize a DNR order under hospital policy is by the consent of patients or their representatives, discussions about futile resuscitation are inherently misleading offers of bogus choices, increasing the likelihood that a choice will be made in favor of futile treatment. Adamant demands for futile resuscitation are less likely when the goal of discussion is not to have the patient or family made a choice, but rather to gain their understanding and acceptance of the choice already made and presented by the physician against attempting resuscitation. But creating the context for that sort of discussion requires a policy that grants physicians the authority to make such a decision.

There is still a practical lesson here for futility policies: the policy should incorporate a process of negotiation by which patients and families are invited to accept the futility judgment, since indeed most of the time they will, and premature or unnecessary confrontation can be avoided.

This brief discussion of the ethical rationale for futility judgments has suggested several guidelines that should shape defensible futility policies.

- Policy should not empower the solitary judgment of an attending physician, but should require some level of peer review.
- Policy should require validation from a broad spectrum of opinion in cases that may turn on differences between professional and nonprofessional values.
- Policy should require disclosure and discussion of any DNR decisions, and should encourage rather than inhibit discussion around death, dying, and treatment limitations.
- Policy should not define *futility* in a narrow manner that discourages consideration of nonbiomedical goals for medical care.
- Policy should attempt to negotiate patient and family acceptance of futility judgments, without requiring or asking for their consent to a DNR order.

THE PRACTICAL CONTEXT: MORE LESSONS

In addition to the cautions that emerge from an analysis of the ethical arguments surrounding the use of futility judgments, there are also those confusions, difficulties, and unintended side-effects that any policy will generate. Consideration of our two-year experience with application of a futility policy will suggest some further rules of thumb for developing sound futility policy.

The first practical problem with futile CPR judgments is a tendency for caregivers to broaden the scope of *futile* to include interventions other than CPR, or to make inferences from a futility judgment that are not warranted. Once CPR is thought to be futile, physicians may be tempted to withhold scarce resources such as blood products, or expensive diagnostic or treatment interventions such as MRI scanning or renal dialysis, or "marginal" treatments such as admission to an intensive care unit or insertion of a PEG feeding tube. A futile *CPR* policy can in practice slop over into a futile *treatment* policy, without due regard for the relevant clinical differences between CPR and other treatment modalities.

A related difficulty with drawing boundaries between the futility of CPR and the potential appropriateness of other interventions is with communicating that distinction to patients or their surrogates. Success here frequently influences whether the futility judgment will be acceptable to the patient or surrogate decisionmaker. The problem here is similar to one that arises commonly in discussions of CPR, where a fear surfaces among patients and families that if they agree to forgo CPR, that means the medical staff will give up on the patient or not try as hard to ameliorate or stabilize the patient's condition. It becomes necessary to provide explicit reassurance that other interventions will be discussed and evaluated separately, on their own merits.

As we noted above, any policy that authorizes a futility judgment should also require that the attending physician inform the patient or the patient's surrogate that CPR is considered futile and will not be attempted, along with the rationale for that judgment. The objective here is to seek the patient's or family's acceptance of that plan, rather than seek their consent or permission for it.

But this vital theoretical distinction proves to be difficult to embody in practice. There are well-entrenched habits of communication, linked to the consent approach to DNR, that need to be overcome or broadened with a larger repertoire. Even in cases where the physician has made a sound prior determination of futility, when she gets face-to-face with the family, she will often revert to the language of consent by faithfully presenting the dismal facts of prognosis and then asking the family what they would like done. This is, after all, the habitual way in which nontreatment decisions are discussed. It may also seem to be less "threatening" or "confrontational" than directly asserting any claims of medical authority. Such an apparently more benign approach, however, is a trap that gets sprung when the family takes up the invitation to make the decision themselves, and makes "the wrong one" by opting for futile resuscitation. They are understandably angry and confused when the staff responds with aggressive efforts to persuade them to change their mind, which the family readily interprets as an attempt to take back the offer.

The aftermath frequently produces another of the practical difficulties we've found with the application of a futility policy. Frustrated by the family's persistence in making the wrong choice, physicians will turn to the futility policy and the authority it grants to physician judgments as a trump card that is played as an ultimatum. Rather than being used in a manner that facilitates family understanding and acceptance of the futility of CPR, the policy becomes just one more ratchet in an escalating confrontation. Any subsequent ethics consultation that arises becomes doubly difficult, less likely to succeed in winning the family's confidence in the original futility judgment.

Finally, our experience has shown that implementing a futility policy also involves recognizing that the delivery of medical care within a hospital is a public event, and the perception that it is wrong to take the "choice " of attempting futile CPR away from the patient or the surrogate is the equivalent of received moral opinion. Any shift of authority away from the family or patient may bring to the surface questions among hospital staff about whether the futility judgment will be used in an inconsistent and biased way.

A direct expression of the concern we have encountered is the accusation that some vulnerable minority patients will have the futility judgment made unilaterally by a physician, but other more socially powerful or acceptable patients with the same medical condition will be given the choice of CPR.

The practical dangers of futility policies need to be recognized by addressing their causes through several different approaches. These will establish some further parameters for development of a defensible futility policy.

1. The implementation of a futility policy requires a systemwide plan for educating physicians as well as other care providers involved in the clinical setting.

Education should involve not only formal presentations concerning the elements of the policy, but also workshops, simulated interviews, or other formats directed to reforming the consent-based habits of communication just discussed, and to providing effective and honest strategies for communication about death and dying, and not just about the futility judgment itself.

Another focus for these educational efforts must be to help nursing and other care providers understand the ethical rationale and the medical basis for futility judgments. Nurses, therapists, and social workers are often the first line of counselors sought by patients and families as they process their understanding of the medical facts as well as their feelings in circumstances of catastrophic and terminal illness. The staff's understanding of the policy and the basis for its application is important not only to avoid working at cross purposes with attending physicians. It is also necessary to winning the staff's confidence in the fairness of the policy's application to patients. This objective can be well served by the use of interdisciplinary educational activities that not only provide information about the rationale for futility judgments and the conditions under which the judgment may be made, but also offer continuing open dialogue with all who are intimately involved in the care of patients.

2. A futility policy should be embedded within a larger policy and process for making decisions about limitation of treatment, which will include some specific elements.

First, a policy must offer multiple avenues for decisions about limitations of care that do not unduly restrict the freedom of patients, families, and care providers to make such decisions based on considerations of both prior patient preferences and of the patient's best interest. The availability of these avenues will help take the pressure off using the futility policy as an all-purpose treatment limitation tool, and reduce the temptation to draw unwarranted inferences from the DNR decision to other limitations of treatment.

Second, a futility policy will function best in institutions with strong and broadly representative ethics committees involved in providing clinical ethics consultation. Using the committee to affirm or reject support for futility judgments in contested cases can help win staff confidence in the process. For the same reason, ethics consultation or other forms of committee assistance should be available to all caregivers, patients, and families, and not only physicians.

In addition, clinically active members of an ethics committee can provide informal consultation to assist physicians in counseling patients or surrogates about the rationale for the futility judgment, to provide communication strategies for the treatment team, and to help distinguish cases of futile CPR from other circumstances when a DNR order might be justified by a patient's or surrogate's judgment about a particular quality of life.[3]

With these ethical and practical cautions in mind, we can work toward developing a sound futility policy.

DEFINING FUTILITY

When setting out to develop a hospital policy regarding futile treatment, it is tempting to think that the first, essential task is to formulate an explicit operational definition of *futility* that will serve to identify unambiguously those patients to whom the policy should apply. We think that this impulse is mistaken, because it runs afoul of the principles just established.

There are several prominent examples of this approach. Lawrence Schneiderman, Nancy Jecker, and Albert Jonsen propose both a quantitative and a qualitative standard of futility, which set independent thresholds for identifying futile procedures.

Quantitatively, a procedure like CPR is futile if it has less than a 1 percent probability of succeeding, p0.05. Qualitatively, a procedure is futile if it "merely preserves permanent unconsciousness or ... fails to end total dependence on intensive medical care."[4]

Donald Murphy and Thomas Finucane define several categories of patients who should not be provided "futile" CPR.[5] The major rationale for their categories—which range from bedfast patients with metastatic cancer, to patients with dementia requiring long-term care, to patients with coma lasting longer than forty-eight hours—is cost control. Both the predicted likelihood of success and the quality of the supporting evidence offered vary significantly among categories.

Policies that define *futile* by reference to a benchmark probability of success fail our standards in several respects. First, they create the illusion of specificity where none is possible, and warrant superficial medical evaluations. If Mrs. Jones has a diagnosis associated with less than 1 percent chance of survival, then such a policy permits the physician to pigeonhole her case as one of "futile" CPR, without any consideration of her individual clinical circumstances and whether they provide reasons for thinking that she may be an exception to the necessarily crude profile that generated the statistic. It is not difficult, for example, to find studies suggesting that the success rate for CPR in patients with metastatic cancer is close to zero.[6] On the other hand, one can find other studies suggesting that a simple diagnostic category like "cancer" may hide numerous clinical complexities that are relevant to a thorough prognostic evaluation.[7] Accordingly, in our experience few thoughtful and experienced clinicians are satisfied with a medical judgment based simply on any one diagnostic or other medical category.

Of course, one might try to respond to this objection by requiring that the prognosis of a less than 1 percent chance be based on a thorough evaluation of each individual case. But then the judgment of futility will not be wholly based in any quantifiable set of prior cases, since one will not be able to identify the previous 100 cases "just like this one." "Failure to survive in the last 100 cases of metastatic cancer" is then only *relevant to* the judgment of futility of CPR; it is not *definitive of* it.

A second difficulty created by reliance on probabilistic definitions of *futile* is that the probability of success is pegged to a narrowly biomedical goal—the extension of biological life for the patient. Typically, no allowance is made for the possibility that other goals might be served in special, individual circumstances that could justify attempts at resuscitation. An example for our experience was a ninety-year-old man with renal failure, ventilator-dependent adult respiratory distress syndrome, hyperosmolar coma, and other conditions that justified the medical judgment that a CPR attempt would be futile; this patient would not survive to leave the hospital. It was more difficult to say whether a CPR attempt might briefly restore pulse and blood pressure. This limited possibility was a significant one for his family, given their hope that the patient's sister would be able to arrive from out of state before he died. They convinced us to honor their request to attempt resuscitation for the sake of that non-biomedical goal, which would not be at stake in all medically similar cases.

Definitions of *futile* err too much in the other direction when the definition is tied to specific quality-of-life judgments. Such judgments make assumptions about the proper goals of medicine that have not been validated through broad and open public dialogue. Why is it "futile," for instance, to provide resuscitation or other life-prolonging intervention for someone who is permanently unconscious? Assuming the patient is not suffering from other medical conditions that would mitigate against it, resuscitation of such a patient could well be successful at extending the patient's life. Extending a patient's life, even one of such attenuated quality, is most certainly among the traditional goals of medicine. Without the backdrop of such a tradition, there would have been no need to make any ethical or legal arguments on behalf of terminally ill patients' rights to limit life-prolonging treatments. A policy that defines *futile* by reference to permanent unconsciousness, then, departs from this tradition and attempts to change it by fiat. It is a departure, however, that at this stage in our history does not have the clear warrant of broad social agreement. Witness both the Missouri and U.S. Supreme Court reasoning in the *Cruzan* case,[8] the state advance directive statutes that explicitly exclude PVS from among the

conditions within the scope of the act,[9] and court rulings in the Helga Wanglie[10] and Baby K cases,[11] all of which assume that being permanently unconscious is not "as good as dead." These considerations are not philosophical ones, and are not intended as such. Perhaps a case can be made that extended life serves no genuine interest of PVS patients. But until those philosophical arguments have succeeded in expanding public consensus on the question, they are not relevant to the justification of a futility policy, which requires broad public warrant for the values that underlie it. In a democratic polity, the imperialism of moral philosophers is hardly less objectionable than the imperialism of physicians.

The other objection to quality-of-life definitions of *futile* is that they may rely on dangerous generalizations. What is it about "total dependence on intensive medical care" that makes resuscitation in all such cases futile? Of course, *generally* speaking, these patients will be moribund and have overwhelming medical problems, such as multiple organ failure, which in turn make a successful resuscitation highly unlikely. But exceptions are possible. Sometimes, for example, patients are de facto dependent on intensive care because of the lack of alternative settings for the delivery of treatments such as ventilator support. This is once again the danger in definitions of which we complained earlier: reliance on any simple categories of "futile" care encourages superficial evaluations.

Policies such as Murphy's would justify quality-of-life expansions of the meaning of *futile* in the name of cost containment. But first of all, any policy that defines *futile* to mean "not costworthy" has distorted the plain meaning of *futile* beyond all recognition. Of course, any intervention that is futile for achieving any worthy goals whatever is not costworthy by definition. But the inference does not run in the other direction. Many interventions are not costworthy because they consume too many resources *relative to* their benefit, not because they offer no benefits at all. Linking futility with cost containment also fundamentally alters the moral basis for the caregivers' claims of authority over "futile" interventions. That authority would no longer be exercised solely on behalf of professional moral integrity, focused on the obligation to the patient's welfare, but will instead be an exercise of social agency, focused on the welfare of the aggregate of patients. This would in turn poison any efforts at gaining patient or family acceptance of the "futility" judgment. So long as the physician is acting out of professional integrity, she has no apparent motive for misrepresenting the real chances for success. When she's acting as a social agent, she's lost that credibility. A sound futility policy should encourage, rather than obstruct, trust and mutual agreement about the wisdom of foregoing CPR.

PATIENT-CENTERED DEFINITIONS

Some policy proposals attempt to avoid conflict with patient or family wishes by defining *futile* subjectively, including some reference to the patient's expressed goals. On this approach, futility should in some part be judged relative to the patient's values: "Resuscitative efforts should be considered futile if they cannot be expected either to restore cardiac or respiratory function to the patient or to achieve the expressed goals of the informed patient" (AMA Council on Ethical and Judicial Affairs,[12] following John Lantos and colleagues[13]). Nevertheless, "In the unusual circumstance when efforts to resuscitate are judged by the treating physician to be futile, *even if previously requested by the patient*, CPR may be withheld" (emphasis theirs).

These definitions can't have it both ways. One can't give the patient all the power to determine the goals of treatment, and leave the physician any power to refuse a requested intervention. If the intervention is being demanded by the patient, then it necessarily serves one of his goals—satisfaction of his demand. The physician might reason that the patient's demand is motivated by unrealistic expectations, but then he will be making judgments about the patient's values, namely, that because the patient's demand is unrealistic, it is not the duty of the physician to satisfy it. Despite the hope of such definitions, the possibility of conflict with the patient's values is always there when the physician judges what level of probability determines that CPR "cannot be expected" to restore function, or when she judges whether the use of a ventilator counts as "restoring" respiratory function. Faith in any value-free "physiological" concept of futility is misplaced.

A related, widely quoted example comes from the Santa Monica Hospital Medical Center, which defines "futile care" as "any clinical circumstance in which the doctor and his consultants, consistent with the available medical literature, conclude that further treatment (except comfort care) cannot, within a reasonable possibility, cure, ameliorate, improve, or restore a quality of life that would be satisfactory to the patient." The following examples are then given: irreversible coma or persistent vegetative state; terminal illness when the application of life-sustaining procedure would serve only to prolong the moment of death artificially; permanent dependence on ICU care.[14] A disjointed policy like this can provide no unambivalent guidance regarding what will count as "futile" care. On the one hand, the doctor is given the authority to make notoriously value-laden judgments regarding what will count as "reasonable," "cure," "ameliorate," "terminal," and so on; and on the other, the patient is left with complete authority over what quality of life is worth serving. Is life-sustaining care "futile" for those patients who might maintain PVS to be a satisfactory quality of life? Policies like Santa Monica's give us two different answers at once.

All of the considerations we've been urging in this section argue against any attempt to base a futility policy on some concrete definition of *futility*. Any such definition by itself is bound to fail as the basis for defensible judgments of when a physician or hospital can refuse to provide demanded treatment. The defensibility of such judgments must ultimately rest on the existence of a consensus within the profession and between the profession and the public about the proper goals and acceptable means for the moral practice of medicine. A consensus can only be developed, it can't be dictated. Moreover, the test of any consensus on a definition of *futility* is whether the consensus survives the interpretation and application of the definition to contested cases. Is it agreed that CPR is "futile" in all cases of advanced metastatic cancer? We can only see how we respond to the application of this principle to the real people who, one by one, make up those cases to which our policy on futility is to apply.

A workable futility policy, therefore, cannot be a policy that imposes a definition on practice. It must instead be a policy that creates a process for negotiating and developing, case by case, a consensus on the rightful limits of patients' demands for treatment.

PROPOSAL FOR A MODEL POLICY

We would like to conclude with an outline of a model policy, which addresses the principles and problems we have identified as significant aspects of a defensible futility policy.

I. Resuscitation will be attempted for all patients in cardiopulmonary arrest unless:
A. The patient is brain-dead and declared legally dead, as documented in the progress notes in accordance with approved hospital protocol;

This element is important because it sets out the paradigm case of futile resuscitation and offers the basis for analogies to some other situations—for example, other cases of irreversible unconsciousness combined with imminent cardiac death. Of course, some hospitals may have some such principle already incorporated in a brain death policy; but there is an advantage to reiterating it within the context of a futility policy, so that it serves as one clinical anchor for interpreting the meaning of *futility*.

or B. The patient or the patient's qualified representative has requested a Do-Not-Resuscitate order, documented in the progress notes in accordance with approved hospital procedures;

This option assumes that the futility policy is part of a broader policy concerning the right to refuse CPR or other medical treatment, and recognizing the authority of surrogate decision makers. It is especially important that this larger policy encourage communication between physicians and patients or surrogates concerning the overall disease process, treatment and nontreatment alternatives, and prognosis for survival or for an acceptable quality of life. As we've discussed, there must be multiple avenues available for limiting treatment besides appeal to a futility policy, in order to reduce the temptation to expand the concept into an all-purpose justification, as well as to recognize that the patient's authority over *refusals* of treatment is based solely on his or her own values and purposes.

or C. There has been a determination, following the process described in Section II, that attempted resuscitation would be futile or harmful.

II. Futile or harmful attempted resuscitation
A. Attempted resuscitation is futile when it provides no meaningful possibility of extended life or other benefit for the patient. Attempted resuscitation is harmful when the additional suffering or other harm inflicted on the patient is grossly disproportionate to any possibility of benefit.

For reasons that we have explained, no attempt should be made to further specify what *futile* or *harmful* resuscitation refers to. That specification is given within the context of a particular patient's clinical circumstances, and from the perspective of the attending physician's evaluation of the patient's diagnosis and prognosis and the physician's individualized understanding of the patient's values, needs, and preferences. For purposes of policy, any significant possibility of extending life counts as benefit, for reasons discussed earlier. Thus, the PVS patient is not per se a case of futile resuscitation. Moreover, possible benefits to the patient other than extended life require consideration—one of the chief reasons that judgments of futility must be individualized rather than defined a priori.

B. The preliminary judgment of whether attempted resuscitation would be either futile or harmful is made by the attending physician, and confirmed in the progress notes by consultation with an appropriate specialist.

This helps to guard against hasty or controversial medical judgments, and confirms some minimal level of professional consensus about futility of care. It also provides public notice to the community of caregivers, so that they become aware of the determination and its justification in a timely way. This offers an opportunity to ask questions, express disagreement, or seek ethics committee consultation or advice. The authority to initiate the judgment of futility rests entirely with the attending physician, the person with primary ethical and legal responsibility for the patient's welfare.

1. The attending physician will inform the competent patient, or the incompetent patient's representative, that he or she will not attempt resuscitation, and will explain the reasons for the physician's judgment that attempted resuscitation would be either futile or harmful. The physician will seek the patient's or representative's acceptance of this course of action.

The first step is to pursue communication and accommodation, not confrontation. For the reasons mentioned earlier, policy must require that patients or families be informed of the plan of care. In our experience, almost all cases are resolved at this stage. Either everyone comes to agree that resuscitation should not be attempted, or the physician will learn of social, psychological, or medical considerations that lead to a revised judgment.

2. If the patient is incompetent and no legal or natural representative can be identified, the case will be brought to the ethics committee consultation team for disposition under Section D.

Unwarranted or controversial expansions of the futility judgment are most likely for patients who have no family or other concerned persons who might protest. Ethics consultation review is necessary both to protect these vulnerable patients and to maintain institutional control over the way in which the futility concept is being interpreted in practice.

C. If the patient or representative agrees that a futile or harmful resuscitation should not be attempted, then the physician should document the substance of the discussion and its resolution in the medical record. A DNR order may then be put into effect without any formal, signed consent from patient or family.

Other decisions about limitations of treatment will normally require more extensive documentation, including a signed consent from the patient or representative. Relaxing this requirement in cases where there is agreement about the futility of CPR serves to emphasize the difference between seeking acceptance and seeking permission. This in turn reduces the temptation to fall into the habitual language of consent, with its attendant dangers and confusions. As we have mentioned, it will also be necessary to reform habits of communicating by means of education and training, and not just policy.

D. If the patient or family does not agree with the physician's judgment, or if the incompetent patient has no representative, then the attending physician will seek the assistance of the ethics committee con-

sultation team. The purposes of the consultation are: (1) to evaluate the physician's judgment of futility to determine whether it is within the scope of the institutions's policy; and (2) when necessary, to assist with continuing efforts to enhance communication and negotiate mutual understanding.

Required ethics consultation here helps to maintain a relatively narrow conception of futility that is in keeping with the policy's intentions, putting a check on the tendency to expand the notion in unwarranted directions, particularly for vulnerable patients. It can also help to resolve those cases where patient or family disagreement with the physician's futility judgment is the product of misunderstanding or botched communication, rather than fundamental value differences.

E. If ethics consultation confirms the physician's judgment, and family or patient disagreement persists, the medical director will attempt to identify another physician within the hospital willing to assume care, including provision of resuscitation, and will transfer care to that physician. If no such physician can be identified within the hospital, and if transfer would not jeopardize the patient medically, the medical director will attempt to identify another health care facility willing to assume care of the patient, and arrange for transfer.

This step protects the professional and ethical integrity of the attending physician or institution, while accommodating the demands of the patient or family. Push shouldn't come to shove when it can be avoided. It also in effect imposes a requirement to consult with a broader community of professional judgment and values in cases of conflict, rather than overriding patient or family demands merely on the basis of individual or local idiosyncrasies. That broader community will either nullify the original futility judgment or ratify it.

F. If no alternative care provider can be identified, or if the patient or representative refuses to accept the transfer of care, then the case will be presented to the ethics committee, which, in consultation with legal counsel and hospital administration, will determine the course of action to be taken on behalf of the hospital.

This is the second level at which the physician's determination that resuscitation should not be attempted is put to the test of wider community opinion, although here the emphasis will most likely be on the inherently value-laden judgments concerning the "reasonableness" of the chance of success, and the selection of worthy goals of medicine, rather than on the factual basis of the medical prognosis. Since these judgments may be used to justify overriding the demands of families or patients, they require the validation of community discussion and consensus, not the exercise of any one individual's expertise. Obviously, the credibility of the ethics committee's judgment will depend on its makeup, in particular on how well the lay patient population is represented. Moreover, the institutional representatives will help assure that a respectful eye is kept on the potential judgment of wider legal and public opinion.

Options to be considered include:

1. To ratify the physician's and consultation team's judgment that resuscitation should not be attempted because it is futile or harmful, and coordinate further attempts to persuade the patient or representative to agree with that judgment.

2. To ratify the physician's and consultation team's judgment that resuscitation should not be attempted because it is futile or harmful, and enter a DNR order in the progress notes, cosigned by the attending physician, the chairperson of the ethics committee, and appropriate institutional authority, such as a director of medical affairs.

3. To ratify the physician's and consultation team's judgment that resuscitation should not be attempted because it is futile or harmful, and seek custody of the patient through the probate court for the purpose of entering a DNR order.

Which option is chosen will depend on the circumstances; for example, for the incompetent patient with no identifiable representative, option 2 makes sense. For the incompetent patient whose court-appointed guardian is insisting on resuscitation, option 3 may be necessary (one reason the hospital's legal counsel would need to be involved at this stage). These don't exhaust the possibilities, of course. At least one remains:

4. To reject the physician's and consultation team's judgment that resuscitation should not be attempted because it is futile or harmful.

If the attending physician remained adamant in his or her original conviction, this outcome might require the physician to sign off the case. Obviously, in that circumstance, the institution would need to have some provision for transferring care, probably to a physician within the medical administration of the institution.

III. Attending physicians, house staff, or nursing staff who follow a DNR order that has been properly entered in the progress notes in accordance with the above provisions are acting in conformity with hospital policy.

This provides some possible legal protection to physicians and nurses who do not resuscitate a patient under the provisions of the hospital policy. Withholding such protection also puts pressure on the physician whose judgment has not been accepted by the community, and discourages physicians from trying to act in secrecy, or unilaterally beyond the bounds of policy.

GOOD DNR DECISIONS

A hospital futility policy cannot simply endorse the principle that physicians retain authority over futile resuscitation, or be content with a simple operational definition. Consideration of the ethical limits and dangers of futility determinations and of the professional and institutional contexts in which those determinations are made will demand much more than that. Careful procedural safeguards, supplementary policies regarding other limitations of treatment, provision of education and training to caregivers, the availability of effective ethics consultation, and a well-functioning ethics committee are all essential ingredients for an effective and trustworthy policy.

A policy that meets these demands, like the model we have proposed, will be conservative and cautious in conflicts, but liberal and permissive in reviewing agreed-upon plans of care. The best test of the policy's effectiveness will not be in how forcefully it can impose the individual physician's will on patients and families. More important will be how effectively it has reduced these recalcitrant conflicts, by realigning the ethics of resuscitation decisions and infusing more honesty into DNR discussions.

Notes

1. Tom Tomlinson and Howard Brody, "Futility and the Ethics of Resuscitation," *JAMA* 264 (1990): 1276-80.

2. Stuart J. Youngner, "Who Defines Futility?" *JAMA* 260 (1988): 2094-95.

3. Tom Tomlinson and Howard Brody, "Ethics and Communication in DNR Orders," *NEJM* 318 (1988):43-46.

4. Lawrence J. Schneiderman, Nancy S. Jecker, and Albert R. Jonsen, "Medical Futility: Its Meaning and Ethical Implications," *Annals of Internal Medicine* 112 (1990): 949-54, at 952.

5. Donald J. Murphy and Thomas E. Finucane, "New Do-Not-Resuscitate Policies: A First Step in Cost Control," *Archives of Internal Medicine* 153 (1993): 1641-48.

6. Mark H. Ebell, "Prearrest Predictors of Survival Following In-Hospital Cardio-pulmonary Resuscitation: A Meta-Analysis," *Journal of Family Practice* 34 (1992): 551-58.

7. Mark Rosenberg et al., "Results of Cardiopulmonary Resuscitation: Failure to Predict Survival in Two Community Hospitals," *Archives of Internal Medicine* 153 (1993): 1370-75.

8. See George J. Annas, "Nancy Cruzan and the Right to Die," *NEJM* 323 (1990): 670-73; Ronald Dworkin, "The Right to Death," *The New York Review of Books,* 31 January 1991, pp. 14-17.

9. See David Orentlicher, "Advance Medical Directives," *JAMA* 263 (1990): 2365-67.

10. Steven H. Miles, "Informed Demand for 'Non-Beneficial' Medical Treatment," *NEJM* 325 (1991): 512-15.

11. George J. Annas, "Asking the Courts to Set the Standard of Emergency Care: The Case of Baby K," *NEJM* 330 (1994): 1542-45.

12. Council on Ethical and Judicial Affairs, "Guidelines for the Appropriate Use of Do-Not-Resuscitate Orders," *JAMA* 265 (1991): 1868-71.

13. John D. Lantos et al., "The Illusion of Futility in Clinical Practice," *American Journal of Medicine* 87 (1989): 81-84.

14. Santa Monica Hospital Medical Center, "Futile Care Guidelines," supplement, *Medical Ethics Advisor,* October 1993, p. 9.

CHAPTER EIGHT

RESEARCH INVOLVING
HUMAN SUBJECTS

36.
REFRAMING RESEARCH INVOLVING HUMANS

Françoise Baylis, Jocelyn Downie, and Susan Sherwin

In the Spring of 1994, in the wake of a number of research related controversies,[1] a Tri-council working group involving Canada's three major national funding agencies—the Medical Research Council (MRC), the Natural Sciences and Engineering Research Council (NSERC), and the Social Sciences and Humanities Research Council (SSHRC)—was convened at the initiative of the Ministry of Health and the Ministry of Industry and Commerce. The goal was to develop a common set of ethics guidelines (not legislation) that would govern research involving humans in Canada.[2] The task initially set by the Chair, however, was "more circumscribed, namely, to revise the '87 [MRC] guidelines where necessary." (Working Group on Ethics Guidelines for Research with Human Subjects 1994, 7). In the Fall of 1994, the Tri-council Working Group [hereafter, the Working Group] issued a call for input on its task.

Now, whereas many academics believe that they should try to remove themselves from the influence of any special interests in the pursuit of some abstract ideal of "truth," feminists believe that interestedness is more effective in inquiry than disinterestedness, and that knowledge is not incompatible with political and emotional interests. In our view, doing ethics well requires express moral commitments that are clearly visible when addressing ethical issues. Ethics is far more than an intellectual exercise or an application of certain philosophical skills; it is an effort to determine what sorts of behaviours are to be encouraged and what sorts condemned. For us, it also includes a commitment to promoting what is morally right and correcting what is morally wrong. Further, in our view, it is only when ethicists engage in public debate and attend to the implications of their positions in actual policy that they are likely to develop sufficient understanding of the issues in question to decide on morally

appropriate practices.[3] Thus, members of the Network on Feminist Health Care Ethics [hereafter, the Network], rejecting the view that ethical theory and political activism are and must remain distinct activities, chose to respond to the call for input and thereby to engage in the political process initiated by the Working Group (Baylis 1996). While our Network was organized around research activities, we determined that our research agenda required us to take the opportunity offered by the Working Group and to try to influence the guidelines for research involving humans, from a feminist perspective.

In this chapter we document the work of the Network as we participated in the public consultation process in an effort to ensure that the concerns of women and others who are systematically oppressed in society were not overlooked. First, we provide an overview of the theoretical views that informed the Network's participation. Second, we outline a number of specific feminist concerns regarding research involving humans. Third, we summarize and review the Network's various attempts to have an impact on the policy-making process. In conclusion, we focus explicitly on the themes of the book, namely autonomy, agency and politics, and reflect on the substance and process discussed previously.

THEORETICAL FRAMEWORK
Our conception of a feminist approach to the ethical questions associated with research involving humans is rooted in both feminist ethics and feminist epistemology. Feminist ethics informs the view that in addition to the traditional questions about informed consent and respect for persons that bioethicists typically raise, questions of power—i.e., those involving patterns of oppression and of privilege—must also be raised. Feminist ethics begins with at least one clearly defined moral value, namely, a recognition that oppression is morally wrong. Feminist epistemology

informs the view that research is a social activity that is conducted within a community of differently situated individuals that is best accomplished when all participants (including subject-participants and researcher-participants)[4] are clear about their own interests and engaged in forthright negotiations with others to ensure that no one's interests are subordinated to those of more powerful participants.

More specifically, our account is grounded in our understanding that feminist ethics explores questions about political relations as well as interpersonal ones. Unlike traditional (non-feminist) ethics which tends to focus on interactions among individuals (such as between physician and patient or researcher and subject) in isolation from the context in which they are situated, feminist ethics promotes an awareness of the various ways in which people's interpersonal relationships are also structured by larger social patterns; power attaches to people as members of social groups and not merely as a consequence of their own efforts in the world. Feminist ethics is especially concerned with systematic patterns of oppression in a society. This perspective encourages us to consider how expectations are derived from deeply entrenched social patterns that structure social institutions and practices. It also helps us to appreciate how these institutions and practices help to maintain oppressive patterns, for example, by serving some groups' interests at the expense of others. Finally, because it is ultimately committed to challenging and eliminating oppression, feminist ethics asks us to consider how these institutions and practices can be modified to reduce their oppressive impact and increase their liberatory potential.[5]

As such, feminist ethics provides us with a framework for reviewing the norms that govern research involving and affecting women and members of other oppressed groups in a way that invites us to consider how research practices have harmed women and others (individually and collectively). By raising the familiar feminist questions of "whose interests are served?" and "whose interests are harmed?" the ways in which research has historically tended to serve the interests of privileged social groups and to subordinate those of oppressed groups is made visible. Further, feminist ethics' commit-ment to social change encourages us to consider how current research practices might be reformed to better serve the interests of those who have been disadvantaged, so as to improve their health status. Appealing to a concept of social justice that involves not only fair distribution of identifiable and quantifiable benefits and burdens in society, but also fair relations among social groups (see Young 1990), feminists ethics allows us to see the sorts of institutional changes necessary if the conduct of research in our society is to meet the standards of justice that it should.

Feminist epistemology provides us with an analysis that encourages us to challenge the traditional distinction between active researcher-participant and passive object of study. The traditional view is rooted in the belief that accurate scientific observation must be conducted by disinterested parties who study "pure" data that is "free" from the influence of personal interests. Particular interests and desires on the part of either the researcher-participant or the subject-participant are commonly thought to pose a risk of distortion since either or both parties might consciously or unconsciously manipulate the process and thereby skew the research results. Such interest-based distortion is considered to be especially risky in the case of subject-participants because they are typically assumed to be unknowledgeable about the technicalities and requirements of the research process. Hence, if subject-participants have reason to prefer one outcome to another, it is feared that they will modify their behaviour or reports to represent that outcome. It also thought that even highly trained researcher-participants—who are well schooled in the importance of maintaining neutral, dispassionate postures, who appreciate the need to remain open to whatever results appear, and who are thoroughly committed to the necessity of minimizing the effect of their own personal preferences on their observations by erasing the details of their own status in the process of data collection—run the risk of unconsciously contaminating data whenever they have a personal stake in detecting one outcome over others. Hence, for generations scientists have been trained in the ideology of "the scientific method" which requires them to approach their work under norms of objectivity understood to mean that they conduct their research with no preferences as to the outcome(s) that results. This approach encourages them to discount the specificity of their own locations and concerns and it obscures rather than addresses the particular nature of each scientist's distinct agency in the research process.

Feminist epistemologists have been critical of such interpretations of objectivity (Harding 1991). They have argued that researcher-participants are seldom truly indifferent to the outcomes of their studies and that the inevitable personal interests involved are most dangerous when denied rather than made explicit. Science is not a value neutral activity in practice, nor should it aspire to be. The demands of disinterestedness do not promote better science, but rather science that preferentially serves some interests and neglects others while blocking efforts to expose that fact by denying and thereby hiding the interests that are operative. When the determinate interests are those of the dominant group(s) in society, they seem to be both natural and general since they blend seamlessly with the cultural dominance of those groups in all spheres of activity. It is only the particular interests of marginalized groups (i.e., those who are subject to oppression) that appear to be "special interests" which threaten to complicate or contaminate otherwise "pure" scientific methods. Feminist epistemology helps us to understand the importance of challenging the underlying assumptions about the conduct of research in order to ensure that research programs not perpetuate patterns of privilege and oppression, but rather serve to break down such forms of injustice. In such ways, scientific research can help to promote the well-being and autonomy of members of oppressed groups.

SOME FEMINIST CONCERNS REGARDING RESEARCH INVOLVING HUMANS

In this section, we apply the theoretical underpinnings of feminist ethics and epistemology more directly to concrete problems with research involving members of oppressed groups, and in particular women. These issues are discussed with particular (but not exclusive) attention to biomedical and pharmacological research, under the following headings: exclusion and under representation; exploitation; and research priorities.

Exclusion and Under Representation

The exclusion and under representation of women subject-participants is, at this time, the most visible and widely debated issue concerning women in the research process. As Rebecca Dresser notes, women's exclusion is "ubiquitous." For example, using age-standardized morality rates, coronary heart disease is the leading cause of death among North American women (Wilkins and Mark 1992) and yet,

> an NIH-sponsored study showing that heart attacks were reduced when subjects took one aspirin every other day was conducted on men, and the relationship between low cholesterol diets and cardiovascular disease has been almost exclusively studied in men....(Dresser 1992, 24)

Two thirds of the elderly population are women (as on average women live eight years longer than men); and yet, "the first twenty years of a major federal study on health and aging included only men." In fact, until quite recently, issues pertinent to women and aging have been seriously understudied. Women suffer from migraines up to three times as often as men and yet, "the announcement that aspirin can help prevent migraine headaches is based on data from males only." Women are the fastest growing AIDS population and yet, "studies on AIDS treatment frequently omit women." Women, not men, get uterine cancer and yet, "a pilot project on the impact of obesity on breast and uterine cancer [was] conducted ... solely on men."[6] A direct consequence of this sort of exclusion is that the data necessary for making choices regarding prevention and treatment for women are unavailable and must be inferred from data collected about men, even though there are important physiological and psychosocial differences between men and women that make such inferences problematic.

In addition to the problem of complete exclusion, there are the related problems of significant under-representation and the failure to undertake appropriate gender-based analyses of the research data. Many of those who contest the claim that women have been excluded from research fail to appreciate that the issue is not just the inclusion of some women, but the inclusion of women in numbers proportionate to the population expected to benefit from the research results. Of equal concern is the way in which the data are collected and analyzed. In many instances in which women are included in research, the research is not designed to look for anything that is specific to women, or to specific groups of women (e.g., those who are elderly, pregnant, or poor).

In recent years the principle of inclusion and representation has been accepted by North American policy makers. In the United States, the National Institute of Health (NIH) and the Federal Drug Agency (FDA) recently passed guidelines concerning the inclusion and representation of women and minorities in most clinical research studies.[7] And, on September 25, 1996, a policy statement regarding the inclusion and representation of women in clinical trials during drug development was issued by the Drugs Directorate of Health Canada. The policy explicitly requires "the enrollment of a representative number of women into clinical trials for those drugs that are intended to be used specifically by women or in populations that are expected to include women" (Drugs Directorate, Health Canada 1996, 2pp.). Not surprisingly, however, political change has brought political resistance. This resistance is manifested in at least three ways. Some deny the claim that women have been excluded from and underrepresented in research; others deny that the exclusion and underrepresentation of women has harmed women; and others attempt to justify the exclusion and underrepresentation.[8]

The first form of resistance to the principle of required inclusion and representation is evident in the widespread movement among researcher-participants and others to deny that women have ever been (improperly) excluded from or underrepresented in research. This claim is difficult to rebut because data regarding study composition typically are not reported in a manner that would facilitate the requisite analysis.[9] In the United States, at least, this was the finding of the Institute of Medicine Committee on Ethical and Legal Issues Relating to the Inclusion of Women in Clinical Studies (Mastroianni, Faden, and Federman 1994), which had considerable resources at its disposal to address this very issue. The Committee concluded that the full data were unavailable.

It did find, however, examples of federal policies and particular protocols that had the effect of treating female subject-participants differently from male subject-participants. It also found evidence of gender inequity in at least two significant areas of research, namely coronary heart disease and AIDS (Mastroianni, Faden, and Federman 1994). In these areas of study, the exclusion and under representation of women were deemed to be significant because of known important differences between men and women in the disease presentation, progression and response to trial interventions. Whereas in some areas of research it is possible (and appropriate) to extrapolate data from one gender to another (e.g., studies on antibiotics), with cardiovascular and AIDS research the gender-based disparities are such that data from male-only studies cannot be appropriately generalized to females.

The second form of resistance to the principle of required inclusion and representation is the denial of the harm resulting from exclusion and underrepresentation. However, consider, for example, the exclusion of women from many of the studies on cardiovascular disease that have significantly influenced both prevention and treatment—MRFIT, Coronary Drug Project (CPD), Lipid Research Clinic, and the Physician's Health Study (Healy 1991). This exclusion has been harmful to women in at least two ways. First, it has resulted in "insufficient information about preventive strategies, diagnostic testing, responses to medical and surgical therapies, and other aspects of cardiovascular illness in women" (Wenger, Speroff, and Packard 1993). Second, as a result, women have been offered less effective or ineffective interventions. For example, the Physicians's Health Study (a male-only study) found that an aspirin every other day reduced heart attacks. Subsequent data has shown, however, that while aspirin is an effective primary preventative for men, it is not so for women (McAnally, Corn, and Hamilton 1992). Consider also, the exclusion of women from AIDS research. As late as 1991, there were "virtually no published, prospective data on the natural history of HIV infection in women or IVDUs (intravenous drug users)" (Modlin and Saah 1991, 39). Furthermore, "as with the natural history, the literature to date on the clinical management of HIV infection [was] necessarily based almost exclusively on reports involving male patients" (Modlin and Saah, 39). As the disease may manifest itself differently in women than men (Modlin and Saah 1991), there is not doubt that as a result of the male bias in the research, women's health care has been seriously compromised. Clearly, resulting knowledge gaps have limited women's ability to make informed choices about their health care and thus unjustly limited their ability to exercise full autonomy in the affected areas.

A similar male-bias prevails in occupational health research. A recent example is a study by Jack Siemiatycki and colleagues on cancer risks associated with certain occupational exposures (Siemiatycki et al. 1989). When challenged to defend the decision to exclude women from the research, Siemiatycki simply stated "It's a cost-benefit analysis; women don't get many occupational cancers" (Cited in Messing 1995, 231). However, arguably, Siemiatycki's analysis is invalid. Because of the exclusion of women from occupational health research, we simply don't know the incidence of occupational cancers among women. The absence of knowledge that he and others perpetuate through exclusionary studies is harmful to women as it is confused with absence of occupational cancers and then used to justify continued exclusion of women from relevant research. And, lest one think this is an isolated incident in the realm of occupational research, it is worth noting, that 73 percent of all research funded by the Quebec Institute for Research in Occupational Health and Safety during its first six years of operation involved absolutely no women workers (Tremblay 1990).

Further, in the realm of psychological research, we find the now infamous Kohlberg studies on moral development (Kohlberg 1984). As Carol Gilligan demonstrated (to name his most influential critic), Kohlberg's work left invisible an entire supplementary, if not alternative, approach to moral decision-making. As with the other examples discussed above, the harms of the exclusion went beyond invisibility. In this case, they extended to what Kathryn Morgan has characterized as "moral madness" (Morgan 1987).

It is telling that many of the researcher-participants who deny the exclusion and underrepresentation of women from research are among those who object to the provisions aimed at ensuring adequate inclusion and representation. Arguably, this undercuts their denial of such exclusion and underrepresentation. If indeed women have not been excluded or underrepresented from research, and thus special provisions to ensure their appropriate inclusion and representation are unnecessary, then why the vigorous objections to initiatives that presumably would only codify existing practice? If, on the other hand, these initiatives do demand changes in current practice, the objections of researcher-participants would seem to suggest that they do indeed prefer to conduct their studies without the complications that may be created by including women in the subject-participant population. These complications may include dealing with the hormonal changes of the menstrual cycle (and the possible use of exogenous hormones), the need for a larger subject-participant population in order to ensure statistical significance, as well as the tracking of data along more variables.

The final form of resistance to the required inclusion and representation of women involves attempts to justify this exclusion and underrepresentation. For example, it is argued that women can be appropriately excluded from research that examines male-specific conditions. While there is no disagreement with this claim, disagreement arises when the justification for excluding women extends to research on conditions that occur disproportionately in males (e.g., spinal cord injuries), or research using a male population simply for reasons of convenience. Also suspect are claims based on the importance of a homogeneous research population, the need to protect women and fetuses from research harms, and the increased costs associated with the participation of women (see, for example, Baylis 1996).

Consider first the claim that "good science" requires the use of a homogeneous research population. In the realm of the biomedical sciences it is argued, from the perspective of researcher-participants, that "the more alike the [subject-participants], the more any variation can be attributed to the experimental intervention" (Dresser 1992, 25). On this basis it is argued that including women in specific research protocols unnecessarily "complicates" the research. Such "complications" are deemed unnecessary because women and men "have more biolog-ical similarities than differences" (Piantadosi and Wittes 1993, 565). Now, most often when women are excluded from research it is on the basis of stip-ulated inclusion/exclusion criteria. At times, howev-er, they are included in the original subject-partici-pant population and their data is later removed (i.e., not included in the final analysis). One striking example (amongst many) of the scientific elimina-tion of women from a study is the research by Gladys Block and colleagues on cancer among phos-phate-exposed workers in a fertilizer plant. One-hun-dred-and-seventy-three women were included among the 3,400 subject-participants. Their data was eliminated from the research results with the sole comment that "Females accounted for only about 5% of the study population, and were not included in these analyses" (Block et al. 1988, 7298).

There are a number of possible responses to the argument that researchers must keep the sample uni-form. First, even if there are legitimate scientific rea-sons for studying populations that are as "uniform" as possible, it doesn't follow that the homogenous group to be studied should be white males. If women and men "have more biological similarities than dif-ferences" such that it is sufficient to study one gen-der, why assume that "the white male is the normal representative human being?" (Dresser 1992, 28). Second, it is well-documented that, in at least some areas of health care, drug trials for instance, there is good reason to believe that women and men will respond differently to the study intervention. Factors such as body weight, body surface, ratio of lean to adipose tissue can affect optimal doses as can the greater concentration of steroids in men's bodies, the differences in hormones, the use of artificial hor-mones by women (for birth control, control of menopausal symptoms, fertility treatments), etc. Vanessa Merton writes: "Without good science that included the full range of human subjects, patients who depart from the white male norm will not have the advantage of good clinical medicine—medicine that addresses their problems and works safely and effectively for them" (Merton 1994, 276). Focusing on one type of human physiology reduces the gener-alizability of the experimental data and thus reduces the scientific utility of the research. The "best"

approach should surely be linked to the promise of benefit to society (broadly construed).

Consider now the spectre of miscarriages and birth defects. Reference is frequently made to con-cerns about women who are or who could become pregnant while enrolled in clinical trials. This view is problematic in that it is both over-inclusive and under-inclusive. It is over-inclusive because, in the name of potential protection for potentially pregnant women and their fetuses, all women lose opportuni-ties to improve their health and possibly extend their lives. Complete exclusion of women subject-partici-pants is an unnecessarily blunt instrument to accom-plish the goal of fetal protection. This approach is also under-inclusive because it ignores the fact that research participation can carry reproductive risks for men as well as women. For example, it is possi-ble that the research intervention will genetically damage the sperm or, in the alternative, that a new substance will bind to the sperm without affecting motility. If the sperm is able to effectively fertilize an ovum, this could result in birth defects in the off-spring. And yet, the spectre of birth defects is not used to justify a blanket exclusion of men. It should also be noted here that only a very small class of clinical studies are relevant to fetal well-being.

Finally consider the claim of the prohibitive cost of inclusion. One of the main reasons for the power-ful resistance to the principle of inclusion is the fear that inclusion requirements will increase the costs of particular studies and hence make them more diffi-cult to conduct. Unless there are known important gender differences, it is argued that there is no need to assume the additional costs of including women subject-participants. The short response to this is that when there is no anticipated statistical difference between men and women, it is appropriate to include both and inappropriate to exclude either. Such inclu-sion allows for the possibility of recognizing unan-ticipated differences provided that gender is coded for. More importantly, one must recognize that a potential increase in the financial cost of conducting a particular trial is not the only cost associated with the equal participation of men and women in research. As Merton notes, the question that must be asked is "cost to whom?" (Merton 1994, 273). Typi-cally the costs considered are those borne by the researcher-participant (e.g., costs associated with recruiting and retaining a larger subject-participant population and costs associated with tracking and analysing data along more variables), not those borne by the persons whose health may be negatively affected by the absence of relevant health data. While it is likely that a principle of inclusion will involve some additional costs to the researcher-participants, these are legitimate costs to be incurred for the benefit of the subject-participants.

The Risk of Exploitation

It is important not to translate the call for greater research attention towards women and other oppressed groups into a wholesale endorsement of the use of members of oppressed groups as subject-participants in all studies. Clinal trials often expose subject-participants to significant risk, discomfort, or inconvenience without offering any special benefits to either the subject-participants or the groups from which they are recruited. Many shameful events in the history of clinical research testify to the ease with which researcher-participants have exploited the vulnerability of oppressed or devalued members of society for the ultimate benefit of others.

The Nazi studies on concentration camp residents and the Tuskegee syphilis study are two of the most notorious examples in this category (Grodin 1992; Hones 1981). A more contemporary example of exploitation, one involving the exploitation of women, is the contraceptive research in the US on minority populations (e.g., Enovid studies on Puerto Rican and Mexican American women) (Hamilton 1996), and in the Third World (e.g., Norplant studies in Bangladesh, Sri Lanka, the Phillippines, the Dominican Republic, Chile and Nigeria) (Hamilton 1996). There is also the suggestion that experimental AIDS vaccines be tested in high risk populations in the Third World such as prostitutes in Thailand (Hamilton 1996).

While most ethics guidelines recognize the need to take special precautions with certain groups, such as children, prisoners, and very ill patients, none seem to have appreciated that members of oppressed groups also face unacceptable risks of exploitation in a society that values them less highly than members of other groups and so is more inclined to expose

them to risk. To guard against such exploitation, clinical studies which propose to recruit women or members of other oppressed groups should be required to demonstrate that the results produced will be of specific benefit to the individuals or to the group in question (see Sherwin 1992, 159-65).

We recognize that some feminists are wary of this principle as it seems to invite paternalistic approaches to women's participation in research. Their argument against it might run as follows: it allows others to decide whether women should be invited to participate in certain studies; it implies that women are not capable of making such decisions for themselves; there is no reason to assume that women are any less qualified than other competent potential subject-participants to make these decisions independently and no need for special protections to be built in for them as they are for members of groups thought incompetent to make such decisions; moreover, given the historical tendency to exclude women from studies that promise benefits to the participants and to women generally (as discussed above), it is a mistake to build in a principle that serves as a license to disregard our first principle (of inclusion) and allows perpetuation of the historical pattern of exclusion of women from research.

We are sympathetic to this concern but ultimately are not convinced by the argument. We believe it rests on an individualistic view of autonomy that we reject in favour of a more nuanced relational approach (see Sherwin 1998). Specifically, we believe that it is important to keep in mind the role that oppression plays in the choices made by members of oppressed groups as potential subject-participants. Members of oppressed groups experience a far greater risk of exploitation than members of more privileged groups. In our view, the oppression of women is so deeply entrenched in our culture that it often goes unnoticed and women's training in self-sacrifice could mean that many women would be overly compliant with researcher-participant's efforts at recruitment and retention of women subject-participants. Hence, we believe it remains necessary to take steps to ensure that the exploitation of women is not operating in research context.

Two additional but closely related issues must be considered in the context of exploitation: first, the lack of clear distinctions between therapy and innovative practice on the one hand, and research and innovative practice on the other; and second, the resultant lack of norms for innovative practice.[10] Research, unlike innovative practice is governed by regulations and/or guidelines that require peer review (before the initiation of the study or the publication of its results), detailed disclosure of information to prospective subject-participants regarding potential harms and benefits, as well as careful monitoring and the implementation of other precautionary measures to reduce the risk of harm. In contrast, less rigorous controls exist for conventional therapies, and still less for innovative practices.

Historically, many interventions have been developed and offered to women as innovative practices without adequate prior research to establish their safety and efficacy. Consider, for example, contraceptives (Dalkon Shield, early doses of birth control pills), drugs prescribed in pregnancy (DES, thalidomide), and the ever-expanding practices in the area of new reproductive technologies. As a result of the failure to adequately research these "innovations" many women have been seriously harmed. Therapy, research, and innovative practice must be carefully distinguished and innovative practices must be subject to careful scrutiny. Moreover, when dealing with practices offered solely to members of an oppressed group it is especially important to rigorously scrutinize the proposed practices.

Research Priorities: What They Are and Who Sets Them

The research agenda regarding the health needs of women and members of other oppressed groups has historically neglected many important questions. For example, even though the links between poverty and illness are well known, health research often focuses on ways of responding to illness rather than avoiding it in the first place. Also, it is noteworthy that many clinical studies explore expensive, highly technological innovations, even though such treatments will be economically inaccessible to most people in the world. In sharp contrast to the neglect of many of the health needs of women, there has been a substantial body of research directed at gaining control over women's reproduction. In this area, women have received a disproportionately large share of research attention, and, as a result, women must now assume an unfair share of the burden, risks, expenses, and responsibility for managing fertility, because that is where the knowledge base is. The concentration of medical attention on women's reproductive roles not only assumes but also reinforces the conventional view that women are, by nature, to be responsible and available for reproductive activities; it also legitimizes, reinforces, and further entrenches such views and the oppressive attitudes that accompany them.

This unacceptably narrow research focus underscores the importance of moving the control of the research agenda from the hands of an elite group of knowledgeable scientists to a more democratically representative group. In our view, the prevailing norms, according to which research subject-participants are reduced to passive objects of study, is unacceptable. Along with Sandra Harding, and other feminist scholars, we propose that research be pursued as a collegial activity; under this model, subject-participants and researcher-participants collectively negotiate the terms of participation and the goals of the activity (see, for example, Harding 1991). We believe that it is both possible and desirable to conduct scientifically valid research that involves subject-participants in the initial formulation of the research questions to pursue and the method of study, as well as the decision about whether to participate once all the terms of participation have been set. Provided that an effort is made to involve subject-participants with diverse perspectives and experiences, such engagement need not undermine the research endeavour or the validity of the research results. Relational autonomy demands that members of oppressed groups, in particular, be made active participants in the process of determining research priorities and approaches. Restricting a group's involvement to the opportunity to consent to or refuse subject status on a pre-determined project retains the focus on agency alone, and not the more encompassing notion of relational autonomy.

We recognize the moral and epistemological value of efforts aimed at reversing the traditional research pattern in which researcher-participants and those who support their work (funding agencies, publishers, colleagues), who are predominantly drawn from the most privileged sectors of society (white, male, middle class), decide what research projects to pursue and who to recruit to participate in them and on what terms. In place of the traditional pattern we envision a research program that is designed to ensure that the least powerful and most vulnerable participants—those who are, at best, typically afforded only the opportunity to agree or refuse to participate in a set protocol—gain an opportunity to ensure that the research to be pursued is responsible to their interests and needs.

FROM THEORY TO PRACTICE

Our aims, as a Network, were to ensure that the new ethics guidelines governing research with humans give prominence to these feminist values and contain specific proposals to make them operational. This goal required multiple decisions about how best to influence the process and have an impact on the group charged with establishing the new guidelines.

Creating the Space

As noted previously, in the Fall of 1994 the Working Group issued a public memorandum inviting submissions from all interested parties. The initial deadline for submissions was December 15, 1994 and the projected completion date for the new research guidelines was the Spring of 1995. With the call for input, the Working Group released seven questions for consideration and an issues paper outlining 17 sections to be addressed in the revised guidelines.

It was very clear from the beginning that our vision of the appropriate task for the Working Group was much broader than the one it had envisioned for itself. The specific questions asked, the time line set, and private conversations with some members of the Working Group all indicated that initially the Working Group was planning simply to tinker with the existing MRC Guidelines, making minor corrections here and there and broadening the scope of the Guidelines to make them relevant to the other two granting agencies. By defining its mandate as (modestly) revisionary, rather than visionary, it seemed clear that the Working Group planned to avoid addressing many of the deep questions surrounding research involving humans, questions that tend to be invisible to those who do not adopt a feminist perspective.

The changes we sought in the ethics guidelines had to do with fundamental assumptions about research activity; hence, they required significant rethinking of the whole field of research ethics. Addressing our concerns would, therefore, require a longer time frame than initially envisioned and a far more open debate than the Working Group planned. Our first objective, then, was to encourage the Working Group to broaden its mandate and to allow for greater public input into its deliberations; in other words, we began by seeking to change a process the Working Group had tried to impose.

We lobbied for these procedural changes at an open forum the Working Group held in November 1994 at the annual meeting of the Canadian Bioethics Society (CBS). In the discussion period, we called for an extended time frame and more opportunity for public participation in the process. We also raised concerns about: i) the moral framework for the revised guidelines (i.e., despite the generally recognized insufficiency of the principles of autonomy, beneficence, nonmaleficence, and justice,[11] it appeared that these principles might nevertheless be taken as the moral framework for the revised guidelines); ii) the need to attend to the political, social and cultural context of research involving humans (e.g.,"Who determines what counts as research?" and "Who sets the research agenda"), and iii) the need for a broader conception of health and research methods. Happily, this intervention was well-received by those present and our concerns were featured in an official communique sent to the Working Group on behalf of the CBS by its President. There was widespread consensus in the bioethics community that the process should not be rushed and that the Working Group should seek significantly more input from across the country. The deadlines were subsequently relaxed and we had concrete evidence that the process could be changed. Affecting the substance of the report, of course, was a different matter.

The First Official Submission to the Working Group[12]

We determined that the best way for us to influence the Working Group's substantive deliberations was to prepare an official submission that would identify and explain the concerns we thought relevant from the perspective of feminist ethics. More broadly, we thought it important to offer a feminist critique of the way the Working Group had defined its agenda and also to indicate concretely how our concerns could be addressed by modifications to existing guidelines. In the Spring of 1995, the submission was completed and circulated to all members of the Working Group. In addition, subsections of the submission (Parts 1 and 2) were circulated to others, including CBS participants who had indicated an interest in receiving a copy of our final text. Our submission was structured in part in response to the agenda set out by the Working Group in the original memorandum inviting public comment (Working Group 1994) and in part according to our own understanding of how the issues should be framed for the Working Group . By combining our own sense of how to shape the discussion with an openness to responding in the terms invited by the Working Group, we acknowledged the specific context in which we were working for change. This could be seen explicitly in the structure of our submission. Part 1 of our submission briefly spelled out our theoretical perspective and made explicit the breadth of the revisions we sought, and the ethical basis for such a broad approach. In Part 2 of the submission, we turned our attention to the specific questions posed by the Working Group:

1.   Do you use the current Guidelines of one of the Councils in planning and conducting your research? If not, why not? If you do, in what way do you use them?
2.   What needs to be changed to make current Guidelines more useful and relevant?
3.   What difficulties, if any, do you experience in the ethical review of research proposals? How should these difficulties be addressed?
4.   What problems, if any, exist in obtaining informed consent for research?
5.   What issues about the functioning of Research Ethics Boards (REBs) should the Guidelines address?
6.   Have you encountered research-related issues that concern you? Please give examples and how you solved them.
7.   What format for the Guidelines would be most useful for you? Please provide examples.

We did not attempt to answer all of these questions. Rather, we focused narrowly on question 2, the only question we could identify that would capture the broad range of concerns we wanted addressed. We structured our response to include a number of general comments followed by a discussion of specific concerns regarding women in research studies. Three general themes emerged: i) the risk of under representation and exclusion; ii) the risk of exploitation; and iii) the risk of exclusion from the process by which research decisions are made and carried out.

In Part 3 of our submission we considered some of the topics the Working Group had identified as foci for their discussions under the following subheading: I. The Context of Research Involving Humans and Research Ethics;[13] II. Areas of Research Involving Humans;[14] and III. Process Issues.[15] In particular, we expressed very strong reservations about Section 10 on Genetic Research and Section 11 on Embryos and Fetuses.

Finally, in Part 4 of our submission, in an effort to make sure that our theoretical concerns would be translated appropriately into the revised research guidelines, we systematically worked through the existing MRC Guidelines to show how these could be modified to be more attentive to feminist concerns. We identified the site of each of our proposed changes and we offered an explanation/justification of each suggested revision. We thought this level of detail was necessary because we had been given to believe that the Working Group would only be tinkering with the existing MRC Guidelines and we believed that if we actually provided draft text that our suggested revisions were more likely to be understood and adopted. Thus, Parts 1 and 4 represented our efforts to re-frame the discussion from the limited focus proposed by the Working Group; as "bookends," and they framed our responses to both the specific questions posed by the Working Group and those introduced by the Network.

In the months that followed, several members of the Network presented various aspects of our first submission to various audiences including, the Joint Centre for Bioethics at the University of Toronto (Downie 1994), the University of Manitoba (Baylis 1995), the MRC Advisory Council on Women in Clinical Trials (Baylis 1995), the Canadian Bioethics

Society (Downie 1995), and the Canadian Society for Women in Philosophy (Sherwin 1995). In general, the responses to the presentations and to the written submission were enthusiastic and encouraging.

The First Unofficial Submission to a Member of the Working Group[16]

In the Fall of 1995, at the initiative of one member of the Working Group, we were invited to comment on a draft of the subsection on "Populations at risk of exclusion from or exploitation in research." In our report back to the member of the Working Group we made a number of specific suggestions. Following the format dictated by the Working Group, we proposed eight revised guidelines in which we insisted on the importance of: i) including women in clinical trials in adequate number; ii) forbidding research that excluded or under represented women without ethically compelling justification; iii) prohibiting the exploitation of women (especially disadvantaged women); and iv) not using pregnancy or childbearing potential as an automatic exclusion criterion. As regards this last issue, we also attempted to outline some of the relevant considerations in proceeding with research involving pregnant and fertile women.

The Second Official Submission to the Working Group[17]

In March of 1996, the Working Group published a draft *Code of Conduct* and invited public comment. We were pleasantly surprised to find that the document was sensitive to a number of the issues we had raised in our first official submission. In particular, it did include references to inclusion of women and other disadvantages groups (though they did not fully appreciate the complexities of this requirement). As well, we noted that much of our "unofficial submission" to a member of the Working Group was included almost verbatim. The areas in which disagreement remained, however, were quite telling. Most notable was the Working Group's decision to: i) adopt a philosophical framework that relied on the three/four principles approach to bioethics; ii) remain silent on the distinction between therapy, research and innovative practice; iii) allow researcher-participants to require that all women in particular studies be on contraceptives; and iv)

ignore the larger political, social and ethical questions concerning control of the research agenda. These and other concerns were again noted in our second submission to the Working Group.

It seemed that both formal and informal strategies had had some effect, but the limits to our influence around issues of power and control were telling and worrisome.

The Second Unofficial Submission to a Member of the Working Group[18]

After public release of the first draft document, the Working Group was reconstituted. Among other changes, one member was added who did explicitly feminist research. This newly constituted group proceeded to make extensive revisions to the draft Code previously circulated. Once again, at the initiative of a member of the Working Group we were invited to comment on work in progress that overlapped with our area of interest. In an effort to assist this person and to advance the concerns of women we offered a number of suggestions. For example, we indicated that the proposed section on inclusiveness should carefully distinguish between two very different sorts of problems—insufficient inclusion as contrasted with inappropriate inclusion. In discussing the first of these problems we pointed out that the objective is not only to ensure the recruitment of equal numbers of men and women research participants, but also to ensure that there is appropriate subgroup analyses of the data so that one may identify relevant differences. As regards the second issue, we argued that women and other members of disadvantaged groups should not bear an unfair share of the burden of research participation, or be excluded from an appropriate share of the benefits of research.

In addition, we registered a serious concern about several omissions: i) the continued inattention to the differences between research, therapy and innovative practices and the need for more rigorous review of innovative practices offered as therapy when they should be subject to research review; ii) the ongoing silence on the question who controls the research agenda; and iii) the absence of a separate section on women as research participants that would discuss unique issues such as research involving women of childbearing potential, pregnant women, and lactating women.

The External Renew Process[19]

In the final phase of the project, the Working Group invited five scholars to a meeting in Toronto to serve as external reviewers. Each reviewer was provided with a second draft of the *Code*, now titled *Code of Ethical Conduct for Research Involving Humans (February 1997)*. A member of the Network was among the invited reviewers (FB), but not in this capacity. Nonetheless, many of the Network's general concerns were raised in both the written submission and verbal presentation. For example, it was noted that many of the issues repeatedly identified by the Network remained unanswered, such as the failure to address ethical issues that arise in setting the research agenda and the failure to address the need for norms governing innovative practice.

Particular attention was also paid to the section originally titled "Exploitation or Exclusion," and later retitled "Justice and Inclusion in Research." This section, which had been extensively revised between the first and second drafts of the Code, was now so problematic that we despaired of ever making positive changes that would promote social justice for women. This section now included only two prescriptive clauses concerning women, both of which were seriously flawed. The first clause stipulating that women should be included in research allowed that this was only required "when possible and appropriate." Significantly, no such exception qualified the previous prescriptive clause which stipulated the required inclusion of members of social, cultural and racial groups. The other prescriptive clause about women stated that, "presumably fertile women and those who are pregnant or breast-feeding should not be automatically excluded as research participants." And yet, elsewhere in the document, there was implicit tacit permission for researchers to insist on the use of hormonal contraception. Previous objections to this permissive stance in the earlier draft had clearly fallen on deaf ears. Any optimism we might have felt upon seeing the first draft *Code* was dashed by the second draft.

It now appeared that fundamental ethical change was unlikely to emerge from this process despite the clear presence of feminist voices. It seemed clear that other, more powerful voices (both within and without) were influencing the Working Group's deliberations and the broad conceptual shift we had hoped for seemed more elusive than ever.

The Working Group's Final Version of the Code

The final draft of the *Code* was completed and submitted to the three Councils in May 1997 and the final version was released to the public in July.[20] Given our disappointment with both the first and second drafts, we approached the task of reviewing the final version with considerable hesitation. We expected this final version of the *Code* would also fail to effectively address issues relevant to the exploitation and neglect of women in research. We were more than pleasantly surprised. The changes made to produce the final version were little short of extraordinary.

We do not know the cause of the remarkable shift in the approach taken by the Working Group and we do not claim exclusive credit for the positive changes (many others lobbied the Working Group). We do, however, want to carefully document some of the changes that have lead us to believe that the considerable effort devoted on this project was worthwhile.

From the outset, we argued against the moral framework proposed for the revised guidelines namely, the four principles approach to bioethics (autonomy, beneficence, non-maleficence, and justice). We describe other, richer, theoretical approaches that could provide the foundation for the *Code*. While the Working Group remained steadfast in its commitment to the principles approach, the following passage appears in the final version:

> Besides the four basic principles discussed, there are other ways of approaching the ethics of research involving humans.... (13)
>
> Another approach that researchers and REBs will find helpful is in terms of reflecting on relationships of power and socially structured allocations of privilege and status. Feminist researchers and ethicists have been concerned with such relationships and the ways in which they perpetuate disadvantage and inequality. This type of approach to ethics can be extremely illuminating in examining the diverse research agendas of various parties and in dealing with prospective participants who have been systematically disadvantaged. (13-14).

Second, we repeatedly asked the Working Group to address the ethics and politics of who sets the research agenda. Despite earlier indications from members of the Working Group that this issue was beyond their mandate, the final version includes the following:

With this second concern about distributive justice in research [the inappropriate exclusion of women of child-bearing age], it is not nearly as easy to focus on researchers and REBs as it is for the first type of concern (appropriately benefiting and not overburdening research participants). There are multiple agents involved in setting "the research agenda," that is, the general direction of current and future research: attitudes and beliefs of colleagues, availability of funding, technology and infrastructure, and multiple diverse and sometimes conflicting demands by research institutions and society. This is not to deny that individual researchers and REBs have a role to play in the fair distribution of the benefits and burdens of research; rather, it is easier to avoid specific harms in areas under one's own control that to bring about a larger social good (in this case, a fairer distribution of the general benefits of research)

To be effective in setting and maintaining a just research agenda, there must be responsible interaction by all these directing the research project. The Councils have for their part engaged in a variety of endeavours in this area, including this Code, the Report of MRC's Advisory Committee on Women in Clinical Trials, the Programme of Co-Operation on Women's Health, and research projects sponsored by the Councils with populations that are the subject of this Section (e.g., the elderly, children, and women), to name a few. (VI-2)

Finally, our greatest efforts were expended on the problem of exclusion and underrepresentation of women and other oppressed groups in research. The final version of the *Code* acknowledges this problem and takes a strong stance on the inclusion of women and other members of oppressed groups as subject-participant. In a discussion of the social harms and benefits of research, it states:

In recent years, one area of social benefit that has deservedly received increased attention has been the inequitable distribution of the benefits of research to various groups, whether defined by gender, age, illness or social status. If members of particular groups (e.g., women, the elderly or immature children) are excluded as research participants, or are seriously under-represented, then it is quite likely that these groups will not only fail to reap the benefits of research, but they may also suffer from misapplication of outcomes of such research to their unique situations. (17)

Elsewhere, this issue is discussed in greater detail:

Historically, women have been excluded as research participants. The justifications for this exclusion have included fear of damage to the foetus including teratogenicity, the confounding influence of hormonal cycles, and fear of liabilities of research sponsors. Women have also been excluded because of a failure to recognize that certain diseases and conditions might affect men and women differently.

The exclusion of women as research participants also raises serious concerns regarding the generalizability and reliability of the data collected. Research data on, for example, drug dosages, device effects, treatments, cultural norms, moral development, and social behaviour obtained from male-only studies likely will not be generalizable to women. As result, data necessary for the treatment or understanding of women often must be inferred despite important differences which may render such inferences inaccurate. When women, or any group, are excluded from research studies, they may be deprived of the possible benefits that come from participating as research subjects, and may suffer as a result. The inclusion of women in research is essential if men and women are to equally benefit from research. Careful attention to these issues is essential to both justice and the quality of research.

Article 6.3
Researchers and REBs must endeavor to distribute equitably the potential benefits of research. Accordingly, depending on the themes and objectives of the research, researchers and REBs must:
a) select and recruit women from disadvantaged social, ethnic, racial and mentally or physically disabled groups; and
b) ensure that the design of the research reflects appropriately the participation of this group.

While some research is properly focused on particular populations that do not include women or only include very few women, in most studies women should be represented in proportion to their presence in the population affected by the research. In designing and implementing research projects, particular attention also should be paid to the need to include women of colour, women who are members of cultural or religious minorities, and women who are socially or otherwise disadvantaged. (VI-3 VI-4)

On the controversial matter of research involving fertile or pregnant women, the final version states that "No women should be automatically excluded from relevant research." (VI-4)

These excerpts illustrate the remarkable transformation evident between the first, second, and final official versions of the *Code*, and account for the sense of accomplishment experienced by the Network. While some of our concerns were not addressed to our satisfaction, for example, innovative practices are not automatically subject to research review, we believe that with the final version the interests of women in Canada are now better protected and, indeed, promoted than they have been in the past.

REFLECTIONS ON AUTONOMY

Our interactions with the Working Group provided us with an opportunity to put our theorizing about agency and autonomy into practice. As Sherwin argues in Chapter 2, the traditional understanding of autonomy ignores the broader social and political contexts in which nominally autonomous choices are made by others, particularly those who are vulnerable to abuse or exploitation. That is, the conventional understanding of autonomy ignores the oppressive circumstances in which individuals are invited to exercise choice. A richer understanding of autonomy, one that does not merely equate autonomy (self-governance) with agency (the making of "reasonable" choice, i.e., choice that is rational under the circumstances) is needed. This understanding of autonomy which acknowledges the interdependence of individuals and attends to the social relations and political structures that limit self-governance, Sherwin names relational autonomy.

Relational autonomy challenges rather than accepts the prevailing social conditions that limit

choice and effectively perpetuate oppression. Hence our concern, as regards the issue of research involving humans, with ensuring that women and other oppressed groups not be unjustly excluded from, or exploited in, research. We repeatedly demanded of the Working Group that women and members of other oppressed groups be active participants in research both as subject- and researcher-participants so as to ensure that the research agenda and individuals research protocols would not continue to be skewed in favour of the most privileged segments of society. Our aim was to promote women's relational autonomy in all phases of the research process and to draw attention to the connections between research and autonomy-related health practices.

Second, relational autonomy often requires a change in the framework for action by challenging built-in limitations. This accounts for our efforts to maximize the effectiveness of our own voices by pursuing a variety of strategies in addressing the Working Group. We did not accept the limitations on our participation in the policy-making process imposed by the Working Group. Specifically, we resisted the stipulated time frame for the revision of the guidelines, we challenged the proposed mandate of the Working Group and the authority of the Working Group to limit the scope of the discussion, and finally we consciously chose not to limit our efforts to the submission of written documents, as was expected. In addition to preparing official submissions, we gave public lectures on this topic at academic and professional meetings, we initiated and pursued private conversations in the "corridors of power" and, in what might be considered an unusual move, we sought to make the process we were engaged in transparent by publishing the details of our interaction with the Working Group in a peer reviewed journal. All of this activity was conducted not only as an academic endeavour but also as a self-consciously political manoeuvre.

Thus, at the end of this process, we look back and see that the issues of agency and autonomy informed our analysis of the regulation of research involving humans as well as our political action decisions. This conclusion confirms our belief in the value of theoretical reconceptualizations of such concepts as autonomy as well as our belief in the inseparability of ethical theory and political activism. Although we can never know what specific interventions contributed to the improvements between the second and final drafts, we know that change is possible and we leave this project with a renewed sense of optimism about participation in the policy-making process. Attempting to influence the policy-making process from a feminist perspective can be an enormously frustrating and difficult experience, but as we have learned it can also be a rewarding and constructive one.

Notes

1. See, for example: Division of Research Investigations, St. Luc Hospital 1993; Angell and Kassiner 1994; Cowan 1994.

2. Prior to this initiative, NSERC, which has the largest research budget of the three agencies, had not developed its own ethical guidelines for the research that it funded. The other two Councils had had such guidelines since the late 1970s, MRC developed its original guidelines in 1978 (*Medical Research Council of Canada, "MRC Report No. 6, Ethics in Human Experimentation," Ottawa, 1978*) and these were subsequently revised in 1987 (*Medical Research Council of Canada, Guidelines on Research Involving Human Subjects, 1987. Minister of Supply and Services Canada. Ottawa, 1987*). SSHRC adopted its first ethics guidelines in 1979 when it became independent of the Canada Council, at which time the Report of the Consultative Group of Ethics (*Report of the Consultative Group on Ethics, The Canada Council, Ethics, Canada Council, Ottawa, 1977*) was officially endorsed. In 1980, an Ad Hoc Committee on Ethics was established and revised guidelines were published in booklet form in 1981 (*Social Sciences and Humanities Research Council of Canada, "Ethics: Guidelines for Research with Human Subjects," Ottawa, 1981*). The content of these ethics guidelines has since been reordered and reformatted and minor changes have been introduced for clarification. The substance, however, has remained unchanged. The guidelines are reprinted annually in the annexes of the SSHRC applicant guides.

3. In Susan Sherwin, "Theory versus Practice in Ethics: A Feminist Perspective on Justice in Health Care," (1996), the argument is developed as to why efforts to identify concepts and choose morally adequate poli-

cies cannot be complete if ethicists confine themselves to purely philosophical exercises.

4. Where appropriate, we use the expressions "subject-participant" and "researcher-participant" instead of the traditional terms "subject" and "researcher." We do this, despite the somewhat unwieldy nature of these expressions, because of negative connotations associated with the term "subject" which implies passivity, and positive connotations associated with the recognition that *both* researchers and subjects are participants in the research endeavour.

5. See Sherwin (1992) for an elaboration of these claims.

6. All examples are taken from Dresser.

7. The new HIH Guidelines (*"NIH Guidelines on the Inclusion of Women & Minorities as Subjects in Clinical Research" 59 Fed. Reg. 14508 (28 March 1994)*) require the inclusion of women and minorities in all NIH-funded research in numbers that would permit a valid analysis.

8. For a discussion of the recent U.S. backlash against feminist critiques of health research, see Baylis 1996, 235-39.

9. This being said, it is interesting to note that in 1995 an assistant to the MRC Advisory Council on Women and Clinical Trials searched the MRC archives in an effort to address this issue. He was able to retrieve 37 of the 129 MRC-funded clinical trials since 1985. He found that 15 of these proposals made no reference to gender. One specified all male subject-participants (this was a study on knee surgery funded in 1991). Fourteen proposals specified all female subject-participants (all of these studies were about reproduction and breast cancer). Five excluded women of childbearing potential. Only two required proportional gender representation.

10. For a discussion of the differences between research, therapy, and innovative practice, see Baylis 1993, 52-53.

11. See DuBose, Hamel, and O'Connell 1994; Englehardt 1996; Jonsen and Toulain1998; Pellegrino and Thomasma 1998; Sherwin 1992; Singer 1993.

12. Original submission: SSHRC-Supported Strategic Research Network on Feminist Health Care Ethics, Susan Sherwin et al., "Submission to the Tri-Council Working Group on Guidelines for Research with Human Subjects," March 9, 1995. See http://www.dal.ca/law/hli

13. This included sections: 1. The Research Context, 2. Research Ethics, and 3. Applying the Ethics to Research.

14. This included sections 4. Research That Deals with Collectivities, 5. Population Studies/Epidemiology/Health Services Research, 6. Research That Deals with Clinical Problems, 7. Research That Deals with Behavior, 8. Research That Deals with Biomedical and Bioengineering Problems, 9. Research That Deals with Subjects Who Cannot Give Consent, 10. Genetic Research, 11. Research Involving Embryos and Fetuses, and 12. Research Driven by Industrial Needs.

15. This included sections 13. Accountability, 14. Research Ethics Boards (REBs), 15. Monitoring, 16. Processing Private Sector Research, and 17. Educational Issues.

16. These include Jocelyn Downie, "Women in Research Studies: A Feminist View," Joint Center for Bioethics at the University of Toronto, February 1995; Françoise Baylis, "'Confusion Worse Confounded': Revising Canada's Research Guidelines," University of Manitoba, May 1995; Baylis, "Ethical and Social Issues Regarding Research Involving Women," MRC Advisory Council on Women in Clinical Trials, Toronto, May 1995; Downie, "Feminist Analysis of Women and Research," Canadian Bioethics Society, Vancouver, November 1995; and Susan Sherwin, "Translating Values into Facts: Making the Links Between Feminist Ethics and Social Change," Canadian Society for Women in Philosophy, University of Western Ontario, November 1995.

17. Second submission: SSHRC-supported Strategic Research Network on Feminist Health Care Ethics, Susan Sherwin et al, Comments on the Draft Code of Conduct for Research Involving Human Subjects. July 1996. See http:// www. dal.ca/law/hli.

18. Interim unofficial draft of relevant subsection of the research guidelines: Inclusiveness and Integrity in Research Relationships. See http://www.da.ca/law/hli.

19. Tri-Council Working Group. Code of Ethical Conduct for Research Involving Humans. Ottawa: Minister of Supply and Services, Canada, February 1997. See http://www.dal.ca/law/hli.

20. The final *Code* has not yet been released to the public pending review by the three Councils. Revisions may still be made.

References

Angell, Marcia, and Jerome P. Kassirer. 1994. "Setting the Record Straight in the Breast Cancer Trials," *New England Journal of Medicine* 330(20): 1448-49.

Baylis, Françoise. 1993. "Assisted Reproductive Technologies: Informed Choice." In *New Reproductive Technologies,* Royal Commission on New Reproductive Technologies. Ottawa, Ministry of Supplies and Services.

—. 1996. "Women and Health Research: Working for Change." *Journal of Clinical Ethics* 7(3): 229-42.

Block, g., G. Matanoski, R. Seltser, and T. Mitchell. 1988. "Cancer Morbidity and Mortality in Phosphate Workers." *Cancer Research* 48: 7298-303.

Cowan, John Scott. 1994. "Lessons from the Fabrikant File: A Report to the Board of Governors of Concordia University." Paper prepared at Concordia University.

Division of Research Investigations. 1993. "Investigation Report: St. Luc Hospital." Office of Research Integrity, Report no. 91-08, Rockville, Md.

Dresser, Rebecca. 1992. "Wanted: Single, White Male for Medical Research." *Hastings Center Report* 22: 24-29.

Drugs Directorate, Health Canada. 1996. "Inclusion of Women in Clinical Trials During Pregnancy." Ottawa, September 25.

DuBose, E.R., R. Hamel, and L.J. O'Connell. 1994. *A Matter of Principles? Ferment in U.S. Bioethics.* Valley Forge, Pa.: Trinity Press International.

Englehardt, T.H. 1996. *The Foundations of Bioethics*, 2d ed. Oxford: Oxford University Press.

Grodin, M. 1992. *The Nazi Doctors and the Nuremberg Code: Human Rights in Human Experimentation.* New York: Oxford University Press.

Hamilton, J.A. 1996. "Women and Health Policy: On the Inclusion of Females in Clinical Trials." In *Gender and Health: An International Perspective*, ed. Carolyn Sargent and Caroline Brettall. Upper Saddle River, N.J.: Prentice-Hall.

Harding, Sandra. 1991. *Whose Science? Whose Knowledge? Thinking From Women's Lives.* Ithaca, N.Y.: Cornell University Press.

Healey, B. 1991. "The Yentl Syndrome." *New England Journal of Medicine* 325(4): 274-76.

Lohlberg, L. 1984. *Essays on Moral Development.* Vol. 2: *The Psychology of Moral Development: The Nature and Validity of Moral Stages.* San Francisco: Harper and Row.

Jonsen, A.R. and S. Toulmin. 1988. *The Abuse of Casuistry: A History of Reasoning.* Berkeley and Los Angeles: University of California Press.

Mastoianni, Anna C., Ruth Faden, and Daniel Federman, eds. 1994. *Women and Health Research: Ethical and Legal Issues of Including Women in Clinical Studies.* 2 vols. Washington, D.C.: National Academy Press.

McAnally, L.E., C.R. Corn, and S.F. Hamilton. 1992. "Aspirin for the Prevention of Vascular Death in Women." *Annals of Pharmacology* 26: 1530-34.

Merton, Vanessa. 1994. "Review Essay: Women and Health Research." *Journal of Law, Medicine and Ethics* 22(3): 272-79.

Messing, K. 1995. "Don't Use a Wrench to Peel Potatoes: Biological Science Constructed on Male Model Systens Is a Risk to Women Workers' Health." In *Changing Methods: Feminists Transforming Practice*, ed. S. Burt and L. Code. Peterborough, Ont.: Broadview Press.

Modlin, John and Alfred Saah. 1991. "Public Health and Clinical Aspects of HIV Infection and Disease in Women and Children in the United States." In *AIDS, Women and the Next Generation: Towards a Morally Acceptable Public Policy for HIV Testing of Pregnant Women and Newborns*, ed. Ruth Faden, Gail Geller, and Madison Powers. New York: Oxford University Press.

Morgan. 1987. "Women and Moral Madness." In *Science, Morality and Feminist Theory*, ed. Marsha Hanen and Kai Nielsen. *Canadian Journal of Philosophy* 13 (supplementary volume): 201-26.

Pellegrino, E. and D.C. Thomasma. 1988. *For the Patient's Good: The Restoration of Beneficence in Health Care.* New York: Oxford University Press.

Piantodosi, P., and J. Wittles. 1993. "Politically Correct Clinical Trials" (letter to the editor). *Controlled Clinical Trials* 14: 562-67.

Sherwin, Susan. 1992. *No Longer Patient: Feminist Ethics and Health Care.* Philadelphia: Temple University Press.

—. 1996. "Theory versus Practice in Ethics: A Feminist Perspective on Justice in Health Care." In *Philosophical Perspectives on Bioethics*, ed. L.W. Sumner and Joseph Boyle. Toronto: University of Toronto Press.

Siemiatycki, J., R. Dewar, R. Lakhani, L. Nadon, L. Richardson, and M. Ferin. 1989. "Cancer Risks Associated with Ten Organic Dusts: Results from a Case-Control Study in Montreal." *American Journal of Industrial Medicine* 16: 547-67.

Singer, P. 1993. *Practical Ethics*, 2d ed. Cambridge: Cambridge University Press.

Tremblay, Celine. 1990. "Les particularités et les difficultés de l'intervention preventive dans le domaine de la santé et de la securité des femmes en lieu de travail." Paper presented at the 58th Annual Meeting of the Association canadienne-française pour l'avancement des sciences. Université Laval, Quebec City, May 14. Cited in Messing 1995.

Wenger, M.K., L. Speroff, and B. Packard. 1993. "Cardiovascular Health and Disease in Women." *New England Journal of Medicine* 329(4): 247.

Wilkins, K., and E. Mark. 1992. "Potential Years of Life Lost, Canada, 1990." *Chronic Disease in Canada* 13(6): 11-13.

Working Group on Ethics Guidelines for Research with Human Subjects. 1994. Minutes of meeting, Toronto, June 30.

Young, Iris Marion. 1990. *Justice and the Politics of Difference.* Princeton, N.J.: Princeton University Press.

37.
BABY FAE: THE "ANYTHING GOES" SCHOOL OF HUMAN EXPERIMENTATION

George J. Annas

Was Baby Fae a brave medical pioneer whose parents chose the only possible way to save her life, or was she a pathetic sacrificial victim whose dying was exploited and prolonged on the altar of scientific progress? To answer this question we need to examine the historical context of this experiment, together with the actions and expressed motives of the parents and physicians.

In an exclusive interview in *American Medical News* ten days after he had transplanted the heart of a baboon into Baby Fae, Dr. Leonard Bailey described Dr. James D. Hardy as "my silent champion." Speaking of Dr. Hardy's transplant of a chimpanzee heart into a human being in 1964, he said, "He's an idol of mine because he followed through and did what he should have done ... he took a gamble to try to save a human life."[1]

Dr. Hardy, of the University of Mississippi, did the world's first lung transplant on a poor, uneducated, dying patient who was serving a life sentence for murder. John Richard Russell survived the transplant for seventeen days, and died as a result of kidney problems that were expected to kill him in any event. Less than seven months later, in January 1964, Dr. Hardy performed the world's first heart transplant on a human being, using the heart of a chimpanzee. The recipient of the chimpanzee heart, Boyd Rush, did not consent to the procedure. Like Mr. Russell, he was dying and poor. Although not a prisoner, he was particularly vulnerable because he was a deaf-mute. He was brought to the hospital unconscious and never regained consciousness. A search for relatives turned up only a stepsister who was persuaded to sign a consent form authorizing "the insertion of a suitable heart transplant" if this should prove necessary. The form made no mention of a primate heart; in later written reports Dr. Hardy contended that he had discussed the procedure in detail with *relatives,*

although there was only one. Mr. Rush survived two hours with the chimpanzee heart.

Dr. Hardy's justifications for using the chimpanzee heart were the difficulty of obtaining a human heart and the apparent success of Dr. Keith Reemtsma in transplanting chimpanzee kidneys into Jefferson Davis at New Orleans Charity Hospital. Mr. Davis was a forty-three-year-old poor black man who was dying of glomerulonephritis. Davis describes his consent in this transcript of a conversation with his doctors after the operation:

> You told me that's one chance out of a thousand. I said I didn't have no choice .... You told me it gonna be animal kidneys. Well, I ain't had no choice.[2]

The operation took place on November 5, 1963; the patient was doing well on November 18 when he was visited by Dr. Hardy. On December 18 he was released to spend Christmas at home. Two days later he was back in the hospital, and on January 6, 1964, he died.

Whatever else one wants to say about these transplants, it is doubtful that anyone would seriously attempt to justify either the consent procedures or the patient selection procedures. Both experiments took advantage of poor, illiterate, and dying patients for their own research ends. Both seem to have violated the major precepts of the Nuremberg Code regarding voluntary, competent, informed, and understanding consent; sufficient prior animal experimentation; and an *a priori* reason to expect death as a result of the experiment.

The parallels are striking. Like Russell Rush, and Davis, Baby Fae was terminally ill; her dying status was used against her as the primary justification for the experiment. We recognize that children, prisoners, and mental patients are at special risk for exploitation, but the terminally ill are even more so, with their dying status itself used as an excuse to justify otherwise unjustifiable research. Like these previous subjects, Baby Fae was also impoverished; subjects in xenograft experiments have "traditionally" been drawn from this population. Finally, as a newborn, she was even more vulnerable to exploitation. Three issues merit specific discussion: (1) the reasonableness of this experiment on children; (2) the adequacy of IRB review and (3) the quality of the consent.

THE REASONABLENESS OF THE EXPERIMENT

While different accounts have been given, it seems fair to accept the formulation by immunologist Dr. Sandra Nehlsen-Cannarella: "Our hypothesis is that a newborn can, with a combination of its underdeveloped immune system and the aid of the anti-suppressive drug, cyclosporine, accept the heart of a baboon if we can find one with tissue of high enough comparability."[3] Questions that need answers are: Is there sufficient animal evidence to support this "under-developed immune system" hypothesis as reasonable in the human? Does the evidence give any reason to anticipate benefit to the infant? And is there any justification for experimenting on infants before we experiment on adults who can consent for themselves? The answer to all three questions seems to be no.

Only two new relevant scientific developments have occurred since the 1963-64 experiments of Reemtsma and Hardy: better tissue-matching procedures and cyclosporine. Both of these, however, are equally applicable to adults. Only the "underdeveloped immune system" theory, which posits that transplants are more likely to succeed if done in infants with underdeveloped immune systems, is applicable to newborns, and this could be tested equally well with a human heart. Without this type of prior work we are engaged, as one of my physician colleagues puts it, in "dog lab" experiments, using children as means to test a hypothesis rather than as ends in themselves. Without adult testing, there could be no reasonable anticipation of benefit for this child; the best that could be hoped for is that the parents would bury a very young child instead of an infant. There should be no more xenografts on children until they have proven successful on adults.

THE ADEQUACY OF IRB REVIEW

Since the Loma Linda IRB seems to have dealt with these concerns inadequately, we must question whether the IRB mechanism is able to protect human subjects involved in first-of-their-kind organ transplants. The record is not very good. The Utah IRB failed to protect Dr. Barney Clark from being used as a means to promote the artificial heart.[4] Likewise, the Humana Heart Institute IRB seems to have been more interested in promoting its own institutional concerns than in protecting William Schroeder. For example, its consent form requires the subject to sign over all rights he or his heirs or other parties might have in "photographs, slides, films, video tapes, recordings or other materials that may be used in newspaper, magazine articles, television, radio broadcasts, movies or any other media or means of dissemination." Very little is known about the Loma Linda IRB and its process. According to its chairman, Dr. Richard Sheldon, the twenty-three-member IRB first received the protocol in August 1983 and approved it later that year. Dr. Bailey was told to present any changes in it to the IRB when a suitable candidate was available. These were presented and approved by a nine to seven vote, two days before Baby Fae's transplant.

Some general observations about IRBs may explain their failure in these cases. First, IRBs are composed primarily (sometimes almost exclusively) of employees and staff of the research institute itself. When that institute, in addition to its basic research mission, has another common set of beliefs, based on a shared religion like Mormonism or Seventh day Adventism, or a secular belief in the profit motive, there is a disturbing homogeneity in the IRB. This is likely to lead to approval of a project by a researcher who also shares the same belief system.

Second, IRBs are way over their heads in this type of surgical innovation. There is no history of successful IRB review of first-of-their-kind kidney, liver, or heart transplants. Ross Woolley has described the Utah IRB that approved the Barney Clark experiment as a "bunch of folks who get together and stumble around and do our thing." More courteously, Albert Jonsen, professor of ethics at The University of California School of Medicine in San Francisco, described the plight of the same IRB as akin to being "asked to build a Boeing 747 with Wright Brothers parts." Homogeneous IRBs without experience in transplant innovation are no match for surgical "pioneers."

THE CONSENT PROCESS

On day ten after Baby Fae's transplant Dr. Bailey said:

> In the best scenario, Baby Fae will celebrate her 21st birthday without the need for further surgery. That possibility exists.

This was, in fact, never a realistic or reasonable expectation, and raises serious questions both about Dr. Bailey's ability to separate science from emotion, and what exactly he led the parents of Baby Fae to expect. He seemed more honest when he described the experiment as a "tremendous victory" after Baby Fae's death. But this could only mean that the experiment itself was the primary end, and that therapy was never a realistic goal.

As of this writing the Baby Fae consent form remains a Loma Linda Top Secret Document. But the process is much more important than the form, and it has been described by the principals. Minimally, there should have been an independent patient selection committee to screen candidates to ensure that the parents could not easily be taken advantage of, could supply the child with sufficient stable support to make long-term survival possible, were aware of all reasonable alternatives in a timely manner, and were not financially constrained in their decision making.

Baby Fae's parents had a two-and-a-half-year-old son, had been living together for about four years, had never married, and had been separated for the few months prior to Baby Fae's birth. Her mother is a high school dropout who was forced to depend on Aid to Families with Dependent Children at the time of the birth of Baby Fae. Baby Fae's father had three children by a previous marriage and describes himself as a middle-aged adolescent. He was not present at the birth of Baby Fae and did not learn about it until three days later. Both felt guilty about Baby Fae's condition, and wanted to do "anything" that might "save her life."

Dr. Bailey describes the crux of the consent process as a conversation with the parents from about midnight until 7 a.m. on October 20. In Dr. Bailey's words:

> Apparently, the parents had spent three of four hours in debate at home [before admitting the baby] and now, from midnight until well into the next morning, I spent hours talking to them very candidly and very frankly. While Baby Fae was resting in bed, I showed them a film and I gave them a slide show, explaining our research and our belief why a baboon heart might work.

This account, given slightly more than two weeks after the transplant, is in error. Apparently Dr. Bailey is following Dr. Hardy's precedent of exaggerating the number of "relatives" involved in the consent process. What really happened is recounted by the couple in their exclusive interview in *People* magazine. Present at the midnight explanation were not "the parents," but the mother, the grandmother, and a male friend of the mother who was staying at her home at the time of Baby Fae's birth. Baby Fae's father was *not* in attendance, although he says, "I would have been there at the meeting with Dr. Bailey if I'd known it was going to turn into a seven-hour discussion." Nonetheless, even though he missed the explanations about what was going to happen to his daughter, "when it came time to sign the agreements, I was up there."[5]

It is unclear that either of the parents ever read or understood the consent forms, but it is evident that the father was not involved in any meaningful way in the consent process.

LESSONS OF THE CASE

This inadequately reviewed, inappropriately consented to, premature experiment on an impoverished, terminally ill newborn was unjustified. It differs from the xenograft experiments of the early 1960s only in the fact that there was prior review of the proposal by an IRB. But this distinction did not make a difference for Baby Fae. She remained unprotected from ruthless experimentation in which her only role was that of a victim.

Dr. David B. Hinshaw, the Loma Linda spokesman, understood part of the problem. In responding to news reports that the hospital might have taken advantage of a couple in "difficult circumstances to wrest things from them in terms of experimental procedures," he said that if this was true, "The whole basis of medicine in Western civilization is challenged and attacked at its very roots."[6] This is an overstatement. Culpability lies at Loma Linda.

Some will find this indictment too harsh. It may be (although none of us can yet know) that the IRB followed the NIH rules on research involving children to the letter, and that the experiment *could* be fit into the federal regulations by claiming that Baby Fae's terminally ill status was justification for an attempt to save her life. But if the federal regulations cannot prevent this type of gross exploitation of the terminally ill, they must be revised. We may need a "national review board" to deal with such complex matters as artificial hearts, xenographs, genetic engineering, and new reproductive technologies. That Loma Linda might be able to legally "get away with" what they have done demonstrates the need for reform and reassertion of the principles of the Nuremberg Code.

As philosopher Alasdair MacIntyre told a recent graduating class of Boston University School of Medicine, there are two ways to be a bad doctor. One is to break the rules; the other is to follow all the rules to the letter and to assume that by so doing you are being "good." The same can be said of IRBs. We owe experimental subjects more than the cold "letter of the law."

The *Loma Linda University Observer*, the campus newspaper, ran two headline stories on November 13, 1984, two days before Baby Fae's death. The first headline read " ... And the beat goes on for Baby Fae"; the second, which covered an unconnected social event, could have more aptly captioned the Baby Fae story: "'Almost Anything Goes' comes to Loma Linda."

Notes

1. This and later quotes by Dr. Bailey appear in Dennis L. Breo, "Interview with 'Baby Fae's' Surgeon: Therapeutic Intent was Topmost," *American Medical News*, Nov. 16, 1984, p. 1.
2. Material about Dr. Hardy is drawn from Jurgen Thorwald, *The Patients* (New York: Harcourt Brace Jovanovich, 1972).
3. See note 1.
4. George J. Annas, "Consent to the Artificial Heart: The Lion and the Crocodiles," *Hastings Center Report*, April 1983, pp. 20-22.
5. Information and quotes concerning Baby Fae's parents are taken from Eleanor Hoover, "Baby Fae: A Child Loved and Lost," *People,* Dec. 3, 1984, pp. 49-63. The second part of the interview appeared in the Dec. 10 issue.
6. *New York Times*, Nov. 15, 1984, p. A27.

38.
"BEING OLD MAKES YOU DIFFERENT": THE ETHICS OF RESEARCH WITH ELDERLY SUBJECTS

Richard M. Ratzan

In 1963 two researchers and the director of the Department of Medicine at the Jewish Chronic Disease Hospital(JCDH) in Brooklyn injected patients with cells that contained cancerous material.[1] The object of the study was "to test immunological resistance of these patients to cancer"; the result, however, was a well-publicized ethical furor that was influential in establishing the need for more stringent regulation of research involving human subjects.

Many of the issues raised by this case have been broadly debated—problems of informed consent (there was significant doubt that these patients had ever been told that the cells were cancerous) and beneficence (the research was in no way related to the patient's care). However, one important aspect of the case has received less attention: these patients were institutionalized and most were elderly. The general question raised by the case is: do the elderly, simply by virtue of their age, constitute a specially vulnerable group of potential research subjects that requires special protection?

E.W.D. Young sums up the lack of consensus on this question: "While it is true that the aged have special needs, it is not clear that special ethical principles are needed to respond to the moral dilemmas raised by health care and biomedical research in the aged."[2] The lack of consensus is not surprising, partly because there has been little discussion that would even illuminate the issues.

I first became aware of how little attention has been paid to this subject by geriatric specialists, ethicists, and researchers when a quite benign experiment failed to attract any volunteers in the institution for the elderly in which I worked, the Hebrew Home and Hospital in Hartford, Connecticut. An affiliated medical school wanted to measure levels of digoxin, a cardiac drug, in sweat, blood, and urine. After eliminating from a population of 315 residents those

judged to be mentally incompetent, medically unfit, or not already on digoxin, we culled eleven potential volunteers, all of whom refused to participate. A subsequent review of the geriatric literature for a possible clue to our difficulty in securing research subjects produced only five articles that dealt directly with the subject of the ethics of clinical geriatric research;[3] there were no references in the medical ethics literature.

The National Commission for the Protection of Human Subjects of Biomedical and Behavioral Research included the elderly in its *Report and Recommendations in Research Involving Those Institutionalized as Mentally Infirm*[4] (subsequently modified and issued as proposed regulations by the Department of Health, Education and Welfare, now the Department of Health and Human Services),[5] but did not take up the specific problems of elderly research subjects. Yet even a brief look at the changing demography of the elderly in the United States suggests the increasing importance of clinical research in geriatrics, and the seriousness of the inattention to its special ethical questions.

In 1977 there were approximately 20 to 22 million Americans over the age of sixty-five (roughly 10 to 11 percent of the total population), a figure that will probably double in the next fifty years.[6] It is equally important to appreciate the statistics of senile dementia and institutionalization, two closely interrelated conditions that influence clinical geriatric research. Approximately 5 to 10 percent of those over sixty-five, roughly 1.5 million individuals, now suffer from senile dementia; that is, they show symptoms of mental deterioration, such as loss of memory, particularly of recent events; loss of ability to do simple arithmetic problems; and disorientation of time and place.[7] (The terms "senile" and "demented" are often used interchangeably to refer to those affected.) The same percentage of our elderly, including many of these senile persons, are institutionalized for a variety of reasons, not all of them medical and not all of them requiring institutionalization if better community-based supports existed.[8] Since the incidence of senile dementia is much higher (15 to 20 percent) in persons over the age of eighty, the absolute number of senile Americans will obviously increase with the projected increase in this category of the elderly population. Thus, if Census Bureau predictions are correct, in 2025 there will be 55 million Americans over the age of sixty-five; more than 2.5 million will be senile unless an effective therapy or cure is discovered in the interim.[9]

Recognizing that the increasing number of elderly citizens accounts for a disproportionate percentage of our nation's total health care expenditures (11 percent of the population accounting for 30 percent of the bill),[10] the National Institute on Aging, a federal agency, has initiated much of the increased research into age-related diseases in recent years. Yet it is clear that even more research is needed and will be conducted on those diseases, such as senile dementia, which commonly affect the elderly.

TYPES OF RESEARCH

When considering types of clinical geriatric research, three areas are especially problematic: the specificity of the research, the degree of risk with relation to intrusiveness, and dementia research in particular.

Specific Research. Of relevance to geriatric research intended primarily for knowledge rather than therapy is the issue of "specific" research, that is, whether the research is being performed primarily for knowledge about a disease or condition of that specific subject and whether it is necessary to use that subject instead of another noninstitutionalized, or younger, or nonsenile one. For example, is it ethical to ask institutionalized subjects, whether mentally disabled or not, to volunteer for a study of older persons' postinfluenza vaccine serologies when a noninstitutionalized sample would answer the question? Was it ethical for my institution to ask for volunteers for a study designed to establish the correlation (or lack of it) between blood and sweat digoxin levels in adults (not just old adults), when a younger, noninstitutionalized population would have sufficed? Or were

we, like the Jewish Chronic Disease Hospital, using a "wealth of patient material,"[11] conveniently captive due to an "accident of propinquity"?[12]

This question is of paramount importance for senile dementia research. For if research primarily intended for knowledge is not permitted to use institutionalized subjects, it may make such research difficult, leaving unanswered many problems of senile dementia, for example, the correlation between psychological testing and cerebrospinal fluid levels of neurotransmitters, and longitudinal studies of the relationship between arteriosclerosis, hypertension, and senile dementia, to name just a few studies that could not now be interpreted as research intended primarily for therapy for a particular subject.

In its *Report and Recommendations on Those Institutionalized as Mentally Infirm*, the National Commission took a definite stand in favor of patient-specific research. However, its Recommendation (4) permits more-than-minimal-risk research authorized by the proxy of an incompetent, institutionalized patient in the interest of future patients. Hans Jonas, a philosopher, has reminded us that "progress is an optional goal," not worth having if it is at the expense of the loss of society's moral values concerning individual worth.[13] Accordingly, Jonas feels that it is "indefensible" to conduct nonspecific research. However, it is as much an abrogation of competent subjects' autonomy to decide their refusal as it is their acceptance and might be construed by some as paternalism, with all its attendant negative effects.

If we do allow institutionalized elderly subjects to participate in research, specific or otherwise, should there be any limitations? Some have proposed that since institutionalization and/or being mentally disabled is already a burden, such subjects should either not be asked to participate, or if so, only on a proportionate basis. Joseph Goldstein, a legal advocate for the rights of the mentally disabled, says: " ... The institutionalized mentally infirm should not constitute a greater percentage of subjects than they represent in the total community."[14] The National Commission suggested that the equitable way to select subjects institutionalized as mentally disabled would be in such a fashion that "the burdens of research do not fall disproportionately on those who are least able to consent or assent, nor should one group of patients be offered opportunities to participate in research from which they may derive benefits to the unfair exclusion of other equally suitable groups of patients."

Warren Reich, a philosopher, argues, however, that "proportionate or disproportionate use of the elderly in research is not simply calculated arithmetically (e.g., in proportion to the percentage of the aged in the population at large), but rather by an assessment of relevant factors,"[15] which he enumerates in part. However, when we analyze his relevant factors (such as "whether the elderly have the same basic obligation as others to promote health through involvement in research" and "whether other less coerced or less vulnerable categories of potential research subjects are available"), most of them reflect paternalistic thinking. For if we recognize the autonomy of the mentally competent, elderly research subject, these questions become no more relevant, and no more difficult to answer (though no less so either), than they are for any other class of competent research subjects. Once the mentally competent, elderly research subject is treated as an autonomous agent, it becomes reasonable and equitable to apply percentages in recruitment for participation.

The mentally incompetent elderly research subject is a different matter. With respect to these subjects, Reich is certainly correct that simple mathematics will not solve the distribution problem, and that we need more data on current selection policies, the incidence, and the kinds of research that are being performed with aged subjects.

Degree of Risk and Intrusiveness. The National Commission and the proposed regulations define three types of research: that involving not greater than minimal risk (which is defined as "the risk that is normally encountered in the daily lives, or in the routine medical or psychological examination, of normal persons"); greater than minimal risk; and greater than minimal risk but only by "a minor increase."

To define the "minimal risk" of an experiment as the "risk of daily living" may be less true for many elderly subjects, in or out of institutions, than it is for younger subjects for several reasons. First, the elderly tend to reduce the risk of daily living to an absolute minimum. Motor vehicle accidents, power

tool mishaps, exposure to the weather and others' germs—these are daily risks that no longer pertain to many elderly persons who have both consciously and unconsciously minimized their risks while maximizing their comforts. Those who live long enough to become elderly often do so by decreasing the number of risks in their lives, for they know they have little or no control over the magnitude of these risks. For although the risks of daily life for an elderly subject may now be fewer, they are quantitatively greater. A fall can mean a broken hip, permanent disability, and the loss of independence. A cold may lead to pneumonia, a splinter to serious infection.

Second, the desire for maximal comfort often supersedes the fear of dying. For example, it is often difficult to persuade an elderly, critically ill nursing home patient to go to the hospital, leaving a known protective environment of peers, nurses, the familiar begonia on a radiator sill, a favorite aide, and the reliable routine of a final lifestyle—in short, home.

Still another factor is the cognitive difficulty some elderly subjects may have in weighing risks. If the mentally competent writer of this article finds it cognitively taxing to ascertain exactly how much risk is meant when a comparative adjective is used to quantitate a superlative in "greater than minimal risk," how will an eighty-two-year-old with slight but definite senile dementia fare?

For many elderly research subjects, intrusiveness in the form of bodily invasion or psychological trauma has a complex relationship to the actual degree of risk. How this risk is perceived to affect the subject's autonomy and comfort may be more decisive than the real probability of risk or the likely extent of injury. For example, the minimal risk of venesection (taking blood from a vein) was ostensibly the reason the residents of the Hebrew Home refused to participate in the digoxin study. I have no doubt that a drug study, even a potentially dangerous drug study, would have gleaned more volunteers simply because its discomforts would have been less apparent. Similarly, elderly subjects might permit unethical psychological studies that violated their personhood by allowing them to "fail, suffer ridicule, embarrassment, or an increased sense of inadequacy."[16] They might agree to participation not because they do not care, but because the differences in intrusiveness are too subtle, are minimized, or are explained too quickly.

Since they may translate "risk" to mean the risk of discomfort, not death, elderly subjects' interpretation of intrusiveness may appear unreasonable at times. Thus, while the principle that increased risk requires increased protection applies to research involving the elderly subject, it is not sufficient. Respect must also be given the elderly subject's altered value system and perception of risk, whether "accurate" or not. The elderly subject needs as much protection in refusing venesection as in refusing drugs or homologous cancer cell injections. For an elderly subject allowed to choose, the decision to participate or not may center on a harmless needle. He or she must be permitted to say "No" to harmless needles for "irrational" reasons.

Consequently, Recommendation (4) of the National Commission—(Sec. 46.507 of the proposed regulations) permitting greater than minimal risk but not much more—is unacceptable for geriatric research. It would allow such risk if "the anticipated knowledge (i) is of vital importance for the understanding or amelioration of the type of disorder or condition of the subjects, or (ii) may reasonably be expected to benefit the subjects in the future," and as long as the subject consents, or assents. If the subject objects, a guardian's permission or court order is needed. This is a call for progress at the possible expense of the individual, an obligatory sacrifice that society has no right to expect.

Hans Jonas, in writing about self-sacrifice for medical research, draws a clear distinction between moral value and moral obligation: "To have done so [self-sacrifice] would be praise-worthy; not to have done so is not blame-worthy. It cannot be asked of him; if he fails to do so he reneges on no duty."[17] It seems particularly brazen to conscript incompetent elderly patients to serve, at the end of their lives, as "volunteers" under the flag of "anticipated future knowledge."

Since the wording of Recommendation (4) has an "or" between clauses (i) an (ii), any researcher who can show the relevance of an experiment on senile dementia and who can convince an institutional review board (IRB) (not always an effective barrier)[18] need only obtain the permission of a guardian before

subjecting a totally vegetative senile person to more than minimal risk. Whether or not such experimentation affects the subject's condition, such a category of increased risk for nonspecific research is treating an incompetent person as a means. According to the proposed regulations, DHHS is considering four alternatives for subjects incapable of assenting to this category of risk: barring their involvement altogether; adopting the National Commission's recommendations; requiring, in addition, the approval of the legally authorized representative and the court approval by the Secretary; or requiring, in addition to that of the representative and the court, approval by an advocate.[19] If provisions were made for a consent auditor who had to visit the subject and who had veto power, Recommendation (4) might be acceptable.

Senile Dementia Research. The difference of senile dementia research from other types of research is particularly important for any discussion of clinical geriatric research, and is at the heart of many of its ethical quandaries. First, senile dementia of the Alzheimer's type—the most common form among the elderly—is a medically, psychologically, epidemiologically, and financially devastating illness. Second, the research into this disease process—its initial questions; its methodology; and its severe medical, scientific and ethical constraints—has special characteristics. Human subjects must be used at earlier stages of the research process than other types of investigation since there can never be an acceptable animal model. Although the use of toad bladders to understand human kidneys has proven feasible, the study of old, retarded chimps to understand senile dementia never will be. In this, of course, senile dementia is not unique; the study of schizophrenia and other mental disorders is similar and raises equally troublesome problems.

The crux of the problem, of course, is the compelling and unanimously perceived need to *do* research on senile dementia. For if we do no research on senile dementia for "ethical" reasons, we may "be in danger of protecting our patients to the extent that, while nothing bad may happen to them as the result of experimentation, nothing good will happen either."[20] Although there is a consensus for the need for such research, there is yet no ethical consensus how best to perform it.

If we conduct senile dementia research using the National Commission's recommendations, the principles will certainly apply (with the problems mentioned earlier) to older persons institutionalized with senile dementia. They will not apply, however, to older subjects who are mentally disabled but not institutionalized. (The term "mentally infirm" was changed to "mentally disabled" by the regulation writers.) We need more specific guidelines for conducting research using elderly persons as subjects, especially those possibly and definitely senile whether in or outside institutions. These are areas not presently addressed by the National Commission's report or the proposed regulations.

One solution would be to do research on elderly senile subjects of all degrees of disability using no special guidelines (other than those for nonsenile subjects currently published by DHHS). Such is the status of senile dementia research now, and indeed much pharmacological and therapeutic research is currently being reported. Unfortunately, since the present guidelines have such little application to elderly subjects in general and elderly institutionalized subjects in particular, the spectrum of ethical compassion encountered in such research is at least as broad as the spectrum of senile dementia being studied.

Other solutions are to limit senile dementia research to institutionalized, minimally demented subjects (yet how minimal is "minimal"?) and/or noninstitutionalized minimally demented subjects. A good argument can be made for soliciting noninstitutionalized mentally "normal" volunteers over the age of sixty-five for some types of senile dementia research on the grounds that if, when tested, they show the same, albeit earlier, qualitative cognitive deficits seen in senile dementia, then research primarily intended for therapy could be done with truly informed consent; it would probably be more successful than in subjects with far advanced, apparently irreversible disease; and would be sparing of the truly burdened, institutionalized demented person. If any promising drugs or therapies emerge, they can then be tried, according to the National Commissions's recommended guidelines, first on the institutionalized minimally disabled, then on the institutionalized moderately disabled, and so on following Jonas's "descending order" of consent.[21]

If such research is important, and appropriate populations can be identified, can informed consent be obtained? Here lies perhaps the most difficult problem.

INFORMED CONSENT

Although many writers disagree about its function and how—or if—it can be obtained, informed consent is now generally understood to require three conditions. First, the research subject must freely volunteer to participate. Second, the subject must be mentally competent. Third, the subject must be informed of the risks, benefits, discomforts, compensation—in short, all the likely consequences—of the experiment. Although these three conditions are necessary, I suggest that they are not sufficient for geriatric research. I therefore propose the following fourth condition: that the elderly research subject's actual understanding of the experiment be accurate and complete to the satisfaction of the researcher, or IRB, or other monitor.

Voluntariness and Autonomy. Voluntariness, the first element of a truly informed consent, raises the larger issue of autonomy. The elderly patient, whether institutionalized or not, often leads a dependent life. Dependence on social services, relatives, neighbors, federal monies in the form of health insurance and social security—this pervasive web of dependence creates one of the characteristic Catch-22s in clinical geriatric research. Succinctly stated: "The aged cannot be singled out for special advantages without also being stigmatized as being incompetent or needy."[22]

The loss of autonomy for elderly people is usually the result of the simultaneous physical, mental, and environmental forces of attrition, which necessitate the assistance of others. Such age-related dependence may be due, in part, to the subtle adoption of specific role expectations and age-appropriate norms, that is, changes in attitudes and roles that occur as a function of, and simultaneously with, successive life-stages. Bernice Neugarten, a sociologist, has pointed out that as they go from middle to old age people often become passive, in part because they think they are supposed to act that way. Their willing compliance, reinforced by society's expectations about behavior in the elderly, further complicates the problem of voluntariness.

This age-related behavior may explain, along with approaching death, the apathy frequently encountered in the elderly. As Father Luke, age seventy-five, in *The View in Winter* puts it, "I care less .... In fact I'm just about to fly out to South Africa, and I don't much mind whether the aeroplane crashes or it doesn't."[23] The obvious implications for acquiescing to research rather than volunteering for it require special consideration, especially in institutions.

Institutionalization usually leads to less, not more autonomy with important psychological consequences. There is, for example, a marked diminution in patients' sense of wellbeing when they are told that their nurses, not they, will make decisions about themselves and their environment. In addition, the institutionalized elderly must deal with a heightened interdependency—what may be called the "dining room effect." Peer pressures exerted by communal eating and social gathering in institutions can be enormous. One study concluded, "Influences of environment and peer group seem to have more bearing on the decision to volunteer than explanations of the experiment itself. The decision to participate is made within a social context."[24] Peer pressure; institutionalization; and physical, mental, and financial vulnerabilities often subtly erode elderly subjects' autonomy to the degree that they need special protection—not so much from their vulnerabilities but from the loss of liberty which is a consequence of their vulnerabilities.

No specific legal guidelines recognize the unique status of elderly research subjects, but relevant case law may provide some help. According to one such case, *Wyatt* v. *Stickney*, mentally ill and mentally retarded patients involuntarily confined in institutions have a constitutional right to treatment. Included in this right to treatment is an institutionalized mentally ill patient's "right not to be subjected to experimental research without the express and informed consent of the patient, if the patient is able to give such consent, and of his guardian or next-of-kin, after opportunities for consultation with independent specialists and with legal counsel."[25]

Wyatt v. *Stickney* concerns research intended primarily for therapy and only that research performed on institutionalized subjects and only those institutionalized subjects who are confined involuntarily.

The strictures of *Wyatt* v. *Stickney* apply only to a very small subset of clinical geriatric research, namely, the elderly, involuntarily confined person who is involved in research primarily for therapy.

Many elderly persons are institutionalized involuntarily, albeit de facto rather than de jure in most instances. This closet institutionalization makes their research status undefined, leaving them, therefore, at greater risk since they fall in between the federal regulations and the court cases. Rushing in to protect the elderly, especially the institutionalized elderly, is the angel of paternalism.

Paternalism. The most insidious loss of liberty for an elderly subject, the one least likely to be detected and corrected, is paternalism. The elderly often *do* need help in providing for themselves and thereby set the stage for what Lionel Trilling called "the dangers which lie in our most generous wishes ... to go on to make them [our fellow men] the objects of our pity, then of our wisdom, ultimately of our coercion."[26]

Such paternalist coercion may be protective or intrusive. The protective paternalists no doubt share the concept, popularized by Sir Isaiah Berlin, of a "negative" sense of personal liberty, and the intrusive paternalists a "positive" sense. "Negative" liberty embodies the notion that personal freedom is freedom from intervention. "Positive" liberty is based on man's concept of self-mastery—the freedom to assert one's individuality. Whereas the intrusive paternalists were the rule in geriatrics (e.g., the JCDH case) in the 1960s and 70s, the advent of medical ethics has witnessed the ascendancy of a new breed of paternalists, the custodial protectors of the elderly.

In clinical geriatrics, three negative effects of such custodial protection of subjects from research have been identified: harm to the subject, exclusion of the subject from research, and limitation of research in general.[27] Harm to the subject is a consequence of the subject's making a choice that is based on incomplete or selected information in an attempt to protect him or her. This protection presupposes the inability of *all* elderly subjects to possess information and arrive at a decision. Marcia Leader and Elizabeth Neuwirth warn researchers not to "fall into the trap of underestimating the older person's capacities to act with as much enlightened self-interest as any other adult citizen in deciding whether a particular research project is something which is desirable for him or her."[28]

The second negative effect of paternalism is the revocation of what many elderly subjects desire and feel is their right to volunteer, to help others, to participate. Exactly when to allow a subject of limited competence to exert this right, even at the possible risk of his or her own health, is indeed complex. Joseph Goldstein argues in a paper prepared for the National Commission that "to deny such persons the right to decide whether to participate in research because he or she is incompetent is to reduce that person's individual autonomy beyond that which can be justified by the designation or the incarceration."[29] In a study examining two approaches to elderly subject recruitment for clinical research, Leader and Neuwirth found that their "first obstacle was anxiety about experimental research among those who direct senior citizens programs."[30] They learned that previous researchers had already discovered that a successful strategy for thwarting paternalistic protectors was to seek approval from "highest administrative levels first."

The third danger of overprotection, limitation of research, represents still another paradox in geriatric research. If we can only perform senile dementia research using demented patients, but should not allow them to participate because they are incompetent, then we are left in a quandary. We cannot ethically conduct senile dementia research using demented subjects because they are incompetent; but we cannot technically perform it using competent subjects because they are not demented. Consequently, as Neil Chayet, a lawyer, rightly complains, "If prohibition of research continues to be the protective device that is utilized, we may well "protect" thousands of institutionalized mentally ill persons to death or to lives of misery."[31]

To complicate matters, paternalists of the intrusive sort are still extant. In a survey of eighty-three investigators conducting research at institutions for the mentally disabled and sixty-eight investigators at other institutions, Arnold Tannenbaum and Robert Cooke found that 23 percent of the former (compared to 18 percent of the latter) admitted that they

did not divulge certain information to their research subjects.[32] If such research was felt, by the investigators, to be in the best interest of the mentally disabled, the elderly, and mankind in general, even if not beneficial to the particular elderly subject participating in it, we have an example of paternalism in the "positive" sense of liberty. That is, this altruistic volunteering represents a "better" choice for them to make than refusal, at least in the minds of the researchers. Whether it is the protective or the intrusive sort, paternalism is a dilemma for anyone taking care of the elderly. As Thomas Halper asks, "Granting the utility of limited paternalism for the aged," how do we "confine it within its proper bounds?"[33]

The answer to Halper's question is that it is difficult, requires experience, good faith, and constant reassessment. One solution might be to apply B. F. Skinner's "principle of making the controller a member of the group he controls,"[34] which for geriatrics would mean having elderly people help make most of the research policies for elderly people, a situation that certainly does not exist now.

Another solution would be to consider Gerald Dworkin's suggestion that paternalism is permissible in certain instances.[35] He views paternalism as acceptable if it "preserves and enhances for the individual his ability rationally to consider and carry out his own decisions," that is, a kind of volitional insurance policy. It is exactly this type of paternalism that the elderly need. They are often debilitated, needing help and asking for it. To do good in this setting is to restore only that which necessitated their requesting help, that is, their lost autonomy.

The only paternalism acceptable for the elderly is one that places them in a protected milieu of autonomy, a milieu over which they may exercise as much control as is consistent with our objective assessment of their deficits and their subjective perception of their benefits, not vice versa.

Competence. Mental competence, the second condition of an informed consent, is often assumed rather than objectively tested. Indeed, there is considerable controversy over whether or not it can be tested, ought to be tested, and by whom. Legally, competence for a specific capability—such as being able to participate in one's defense in a trial—is strictly judged as present or absent without gradations. As Lance Tribbles states, however, the all-or-none judgment of competency is "inappropriate" for the gradations of competency found in clinical geriatric practice. He suggests alternatives such as power of attorney.[36]

Several tests used to determine competency include evidencing a choice, reasonable outcome of choice, choice based on rational reasons, ability to understand, and actual understanding. What then are the implications for informed consent in clinical geriatric research when using these different criteria for competence? First, there is much evidence for a decline in cognitive abilities with normal aging; thus any elderly subject's comprehension of the proposed research becomes problematic. Researchers have substantiated significant differences, and often a decline, in the memory and learning of older subjects when compared to younger ones.[37] The effects of aging on intellectual ability are more controversial but also suggestive of deterioration.[38] Many of the experiments testing cognition in the elderly repeatedly found that novelty of information, rate of response, complexity of tasks to be performed, and organizational strategies were all important factors apparently responsible for the decreased performances of normal older subjects. Indeed, some of the older persons with decreased cognitive abilities were well-educated professionals of high socioeconomic status. Some researchers have found that bright, aged normals, when compared to young normals, manifested a conceptual deficit comparable to that found in a group of neurologically impaired patients.[39]

Problem-solving ability, which is what the giving of informed consent is all about in a true volunteer, also seems to change with normal aging, and often for the worse. A "vicious spiral" retards and undermines the problem-solving process in some aged subjects: when faced with the increased memory load of a new problem, a weakened elderly memory gets slower and makes more mistakes, leading to decisions that require extra operations, slowing memory down even more, leading to more mistakes, and so on.[40] An analysis of the problem-solving performance of 100 successful professional people suggests that there is a *different*, rather than an impaired, performance.[41] Some of the differences were: how the older subject

defined the problem to be solved; the relation of the problem to new goals; the self-recognized necessity for greater discipline; and a tolerance toward people around them. These observations suggest that, in this research group at least, there was not only an approach to problem-solving different from that found in younger subjects but that it was consciously different. It may be that the differences in this group of older subjects are adaptations to aging, not intellectual deterioration. In any case, as Patrick Rabbitt points out, it would be naive merely to "regard them as passive victims of a cognitive degeneration of which they are helplessly unaware."[42]

A second consideration in the obtaining of informed consent from an apparently competent elderly subject is the increased likelihood of occult, that is, latent dementia, especially senile dementia of the Alzheimer's type, which is often clinically latent in its early stages. The clinical spectrum of senile dementia and its definition are sufficiently varied and problematic that the detection of minimally but definitely impaired elderly persons can be difficult when attempted and nearly impossible when not. The implications for obtaining informed consent from possibly demented subjects over the age of sixty-five are obvious.

Another aspect of early senile dementia that affects informed consent is the frequent fluctuation of its severity. The interplay between the effects of senile dementia itself, associated psychiatric illness, and the influence of medication can cause swings in mental ability such that competence to understand a problem may be fair on Monday, yet hopeless on Tuesday. Consequently, it seems unwise to obtain informed consent from an elderly person in whom there is the question of even minimal senile dementia using the same process one would for a younger one. Robert Veatch, a philosopher, argues that the problem of intermittent competence requires that a "formerly competent patient's wishes clearly expressed while competent should be determinative when the patient is no longer competent."[43] In theory, this is a good suggestion, though primarily for therapeutic decisions. However, for some future, unspecified research primarily intended for knowledge, no matter how unobtrusive or benign, this plan is obviously not tenable.

A related problem is the question of who determines competency. Legally, it has traditionally been a physician, usually a psychiatrist. If all the parties involved agree to having a psychiatrist establish the competency of an elderly subject, which psychiatrist will it be? Many large institutions have salaried or fee-for-service psychiatrists. If one of these evaluates the competency of an elderly subject for an institutional research project, a "double-agent" problem emerges. This conflict of interest becomes especially dangerous since the subject, by virtue of his or her possible incompetency and the dependency of institutionalization, is not likely to have the option—or having it, to exercise it—of selecting a different psychiatrist. If a psychiatrist other than the resident one is mandated, the establishment of competency may become a cumbersome routine.

Finally, it is imperative for anyone judging the competency of an elderly subject to remember the differences in goals and values that many older subjects integrate into problem solving (for our discussion, the giving of informed consent). Tibbles makes the point clearly: "A long life of frugality followed at 65 years of age by the spending of large sums on pleasures foregone in the past may not be a sign of incompetence. It may be a recognition of mortality."[44]

Information. The third condition of informed consent is that the subject be provided with information about the experiment. But, how much information? Who provides it? The recent trend has been to give the patient more information. This shift is due mainly to a closer scrutiny of the medical profession by lay critics and the general movement over the past fifteen years toward judicial and legislative protection of consumers' and individuals' rights. Part of this trend has been the emphasis on disclosure of material information.

Materiality of information is one of the most dramatic issues distinguishing clinical geriatric research from that in other age groups. The widespread alterations in function and decreased reserve of most organ systems in the elderly dictate a reorientation of emphasis when describing possible consequences of a particular experiment. If an experimental drug has a 1 percent chance of leaving the subject with impaired hearing, that information is "more" material for the subject to know if she is an eighty-three-year-old wearing a hearing aid than a healthy thirty-nine-year-old.

Another issue in informed consent relevant to geriatrics is the format of the explanation and consent form. Lynn Epstein and Louis Lasagna showed quite clearly that "comprehension and consent to volunteer were inversely related to length of form."[45] Ralph Alfidi compared two forms, an inclusive one and a less detailed one.[46] Both offered more information if desired. He found no appreciable difference in consent rates. In conjunction with these studies and the literature on problem-solving (that is, complexity of tasks and novel information), I suggest that consent forms for the elderly resemble Alfidi's less detailed one.

Of practical importance for clinical geriatric researchers, no matter which consent form is used, is the question of how much information we *can* give the geriatric subject. For example, if anything, the growing literature on pharmacokinetics in the elderly reveals to us just how much we do not know.[47] Much of the experimental data concerning the differences between young and old subjects with cardiovascular disease, malnutrition, and surgery of all types lie buried in a literature antedating the advent of geriatrics as a discipline, with the result that all adults, both under and over sixty-five, are lumped together simply as "adults."

Perhaps the most controversial aspect of how much information should be provided to a subject is the question of intentional selection of information by the researcher or physician, commonly referred to as the therapeutic privilege. Although *Canterbury* v. *Spence*[48] and *Cobbs* v. *Grant,*[49] the 1972 cases that helped define the role of information in informed consent, involved mentally competent patients, some writers have stated that therapeutic privilege is no less inappropriate for mentally incompetent subjects. Goldstein argues that the patient's right of self-decision "is effectively safeguarded if the authorities provide him with a real opportunity (not with an obligation) to possess what information he and a reasonable person might require in order to exercise a choice."[50]

The real risk of therapeutic privilege, and therefore at the heart of the controversy, is manipulation. Such persuasion is usually toward therapy or participation. However, a physician can also manipulate the subject toward refusal by exaggerating risks or understating benefits. Whether motivated by paternalism or not, the physician-as-manipulator with his or her specialized knowledge is an almost insuperable adversary when invested with the respect and power usually imputed him or her, especially by elderly subjects. And if, as one recent study has found, older women react more positively to persuasive information despite their understanding less of it, such manipulation can become a science with almost guaranteed results.[51]

Assessment. I propose that a fourth stipulation be added for the obtaining of informed consent in clinical geriatric research, that is, the assessment of the subject's actual understanding of the experiment. One method proposed for assessing actual understanding is the two-part consent form. Such a consent form has been proposed for all subjects of human research, the second part being a "questionnaire to check how well they understand the information that has been presented to them."[52] This questionnaire, it was proposed, would be an integral part of the consent process. It would be the embodiment, in practice, of the "actual understanding" criterion for informed consent.[53]

There is certainly ample evidence for the need of such a process. One useful paper demonstrated that prisoners volunteering to participate in a malaria experiment understood its risk "no better or worse" than those who did not volunteer.[54] Bradford Gray has shown that although they signed an informed consent form, 39 percent of the pregnant women in an experiment concerning labor induction said they only learned of their status as research subjects from Gray's interview after the experiment had already begun.[55]

There is also evidence for the efficacy of a two-part process. Roger L. Williams and his colleagues discovered an improvement in potential subjects' understanding of the experiment after a discussion of it with a physician for twenty minutes as compared to those subjects whose knowledge of the experiment consisted of details gleaned only from the hearsay of previous participants.[56]

However, the range of correct answers for both groups was wide and the informed group did "better" than the hearsay group in that only twelve of twenty informed subjects (as compared to seven of twenty hearsay subjects) answered correctly the question: "Is it possible that you could develop a serious and even permanent illness as a result of participating in a study at this project?" When subjects scored less than fourteen (of twenty questions), they were not accepted for participation. Moreover, those who scored between fourteen and nineteen were reinformed until "the physician was satisfied that comprehension of the material was complete."

In addition to assessing the comprehension and informing the subject of those areas he or she misunderstood, the two-part consent form helps protect the investigator. It also furnishes the investigator with responses concerning the perception of the experiment by the subjects, their perception of the explanation, and thus possible ways to improve both. Finally, it allows the subjects more time to make an important decision.

Although dividing the consent process for elderly subjects into two or more interviews, held at different times, would improve the likelihood of a valid informed consent, it also allows more occasion for influence by private physicians, family, and other peer members who have already been approached by the interviewer. Interaction among subjects may lead to support during participation.[57] However, in the setting of an institution, such support would probably most often take the form of subtle peer pressures to refuse to participate. In a sense, that first moment of privacy in the first interview may be the institutionalized elderly subject's freest moment, the first and last chance to make a truly autonomous decision.

Some mechanism like the two-part consent form is essential for geriatric subjects. Their comprehension may be different, if not lessened, because of age. A deficient recent memory may convert a valid consent on Monday into a fiction on Tuesday; and a fluctuating mental status due to senile dementia or medication, or both, may make unethical an experiment that is separated from the consent process by more than an hour. Although older subjects have less time to live, they often need more time to consent.

Proxy Consent. The difficult problem of proxy consent when a subject is unable, for whatever reason, to make decisions about care, experimental or otherwise, has been extensively reviewed. The question of proxy consent for elderly subjects suffering from a clinically wide range of significant cognitive deficits has not, unfortunately, received the same attention.

The proxies for elderly subjects are often their grown children or other close relatives. Such a proxy may have a lifetime of emotions invested in the subject or, worse, a hope of inheriting material goods. If there are no close relatives, there is frequently no one at all. Like his or her cardiac reserve, the elderly person's reserve of interested others grows small with age.

It is therefore especially important, when considering proxy consent for an elderly subject, to avoid the protective paternalism of a relative (prohibiting what in fact the subject might have willed), and the exploitative paternalism of a researcher convincing an apathetic guardian or all-too-eager heir of the subject's noble role as martyr. What are some of the possible solutions to this problem?

One is to have the still competent subject appoint an agent who will be empowered with the authority to make any future medical decisions that occur after the subject is no longer able to decide them. Such is the gist of Leslie Libow's penultimate will[58] and the much publicized Michigan House Bill No. 4058.[59]

Another solution would be to appoint as proxy a consent auditor—a suggestion proposed by the National Commission. Unfortunately there are problems both with the consent auditor's assuming this role and with the very concept. First, who exactly is the consent auditor and who would it be for the institutionalized elderly? The National Commission is vague about his or her identity, how the person would be selected, and who would pay his or her salary. If salaried by the institution, the person would again face the double-agent problem. If salaried by the government, is this agreeable to all? If the consent auditor does become a federal employee, what would be the relationship to Veterans Administration institutions, one of the largest potential research sources of those institutionalized elderly most often needing a proxy? And most important, what would be the consent auditor's real power in the consent process—a vote or a veto? Should he or she be old, that is, a peer of the research subject? If so, who will assess his or her competence tactfully? These questions need answers before the consent auditor audits anything.

Of further interest is the almost complete lack of discussion in the proxy consent literature about the proxy. Proxy consent, so often equated with the decision that a reasonable, competent subject would have made, or with the decision that someone (usually a relative) who knows the subject predicts he or she would have made, is merely shifting all the informed consent issues one step back, still begging all the fundamental questions of informed consent. Is the proxy informed? Has his or her actual understanding of the information been assessed? What is his or her motivation, a prime consideration for the proxy of many geriatric subjects?

SUGGESTED RESEARCH ON ETHICAL PROBLEMS

There are major ethical problems in performing clinical geriatric research which may, or may not, be unique. There may, or may not, be the need for what Donald Marquis calls "an ethics of the elderly." However, there are very special questions concerning informed consent and autonomy in clinical geriatric research that require more data. Some possible areas of research that may help answer these questions are the following:

1. Who volunteers, or will volunteer, for experiments in the elderly population, and why?

The psychopathology found in "normal volunteers" is well described. Samuel I. Shuman sums up the problem well: "If a volunteer comes forward out of neurotic desire to satisfy masochistic drives to subject himself to pain or discomfort, is it appropriate to call him a volunteer?"[60] What are the attitudes of the elderly toward research? Is the rate of volunteering a function of senile dementia? These are relevant questions with some data available, though mainly from British populations.[61]

The information we do have is fragmentary and inferential. Daniel Martin showed definite sex differences in volunteers and, of particular relevance to geriatrics, he discovered a "significantly greater willingness to volunteer when the potential volunteer is not obligated to others.... When the subjects have only themselves to be concerned about, volunteering is relatively frequent."[62] Should we therefore place on Jonas's "descending order" of consent the now numerous deinstitutionalized geriatric subjects living alone in resident hotels, realizing they may be more willing to volunteer?

We need data on elderly research subjects—their attitudes toward research; their problem-solving abilities using research protocols and not anagrams; their interpretation of risk, intrusiveness, and autonomy; and their idea of proportional participation vs. the burden of institutionalization. We certainly need more data on the elderly research subjects already participating in experiments. For example, none of the National Commission's data on those institutionalized as mentally disabled are broken down by age.

2. Should we act on Goldstein's suggestion that "serious consideration should be given to making the failures to abide by the proscribed standards of conduct" in research on those institutionalized as mentally disabled "a matter of strict liability in criminal law?"

In a "Report on the Mentally Infirm," a survey of experiments involving the institutionalized mentally disabled, many infractions of DHEW regulations for the protection of human subjects were found.[63] For example, at least 20 percent of the investigators polled felt that the proxy consent used did not protect adequately the mentally disabled subject. Fully 45 percent of the forms had no mention of risks. Bradford Gray's recent study indicates a less than reassuring efficacy of institutional review committees in safeguarding subjects' rights.[64]

3. Can there or should there be a screening test when obtaining informed consent in the elderly?

There are several short bedside tests commonly used in clinical geriatrics to assess cognitive abilities and the presence of organic brain disease. Many of them have been found to correlate with the more cumbersome but more informative psychometric tests.[65] It seems unlikely, however, that any test can accurately gauge the older subject's competency for a particular experiment more precisely than the assessment of his or her understanding of that particular experiment itself.

RECOMMENDATIONS

The elderly research subject often has cognitive abilities, attitudes, and values that are different from those of younger subjects. These cognitive abilities,

whether less or different, make the problem-solving process of informed consent a radically different one for many elderly subjects. It is often a slower, more arduous process—more dependent on the format, amount, and kind of information involved, and one less likely to arrive at a solution considered "rational" by younger investigators and IRB members. Yet the traditional picture of a wise man being old, like Nestor or Samuel Johnson, supports the idea that the elderly's manner of problem-solving is not only different, but often of value. As J.B. Priestley observed, "Grandfather was not a problem but a solver of problems."[66]

The heightened dependence of elderly research subjects on physical, mental and environmental supports makes them more vulnerable to institutionalization, further usurpation of their autonomy, and possible exploitation for research purposes. The excessively altruistic attempt to protect their "negative" sense of freedom and the equally excessive attempt by researchers to further their "positive" sense of freedom by contributing their services to society's medical progress represent a paternalistic rack on which elderly research subjects may be helplessly stretched unless we provide them with the protection they need—the exact amount necessary to require no further protection.

I recommend the following proposals for the conduct of clinical geriatric research:

1. Since the National Commission no longer exists, the President's Commission for the Study of Ethical Problems in Medicine and Biomedical and Behavioral Research should request a Report and Recommendations Concerning Research Involving Elderly Research Subjects. Such a report should have the contributions of ethicists, geriatricians, the National Institute on Aging, interested citizens, and certainly a generous representation of the elderly—the "young" elderly (ages sixty-five to seventy-five), the very elderly, the poor elderly, the minimally demented elderly, black elderly, Hispanic elderly, Jewish elderly, and so on.

2. I suggest that the consent process for the elderly take place in more than one interview, with a shorter consent form in larger type face, using simply worded, ordinary language. In addition,

the objective assessment of the subject's actual understanding should be documented before initiation of the experiment, and, if deemed appropriate by a consent auditor, during the experiment as well. If this assessment reveals less than a satisfactory understanding of the experiment by the subject, the research should be delayed until the subject's understanding can be improved. Corroborative techniques like video-taping should be tried to monitor the consent process.

3. The DHHS should be more specific about the proposed consent auditor's power in auditing research on those institutionalized as mentally disabled. Such a better-defined consent auditor could perform a valuable function in clinical geriatric research and is recommended for the institutionalized elderly subject.

4. Recommendation (4) of the National Commmissions's Report concerning research involving those institutionalized as mentally disabled should be amended in the final regulations to protect the elderly research subject from research involving greater than minimal risk.

5. Consideration of measures such as power of attorney or the penultimate will should be more actively pursued by nursing homes, elderly interest groups, and bar associations.

As Mrs. Robins, matron of the county council home, states in *The View in Winter,* "Being old makes you different, whatever they say, just as being young makes you different."[67] Insofar as the elderly do have different values, strengths, and weaknesses from those of younger adults, these differences must be considered and respected when the elderly are asked to volunteer for research. And if these differences significantly alter methods of recruitment and safeguards for autonomy and respect which are necessary in order to ensure that elderly persons are treated as ends and not as means, then we must pursue such methods and safeguards.

Author's Note

I would like to acknowledge the indispensable contributions to this paper of Stuart Spicker, Ph.D., Joseph M. Healey, J.D., and Ian R. Lawson, M.D., F.R.C.P.E. I would also like to thank Fran Bernstein and the Mt. Sinai Hospital Library staff for research assistance and Joan Epstein for help in preparation of the manuscript.

Notes

1. "The Jewish Chronic Disease Hospital Case," in *Experimentation With Human Beings,* edited by Jay Katz (New York: Russell Sage Foundation, 1973), pp. 9-65.

2. E.W.D. Young, "Health Care and Research in the Aged," in *Encyclopedia of Bioethics,* edited by Warren T. Reich (New York: Free Press, 1978), I, 68-69

3. The five articles are: J.E. Bernstein and F.K. Nelson, "Medical Experimentation in the Elderly," *Journal of the American Geriatric Society* 23 (1975), 327-29; S. Berkowitz, "Informed Consent, Research and the Elderly," *Gerontologist* 18 (1978), 237-43; J.B. Wales and D.L. Treybig, "Recent Legislative Trends Toward Protection of Human Subjects: Implication for Gerontologists," *Gerontologist* 18 (1978), 244-49; J.L. Makarushka and R.D. McDonald, "Informed Consent, Research, and Geriatric Patients: The Responsibility of Institutional Review Committees," *Gerontologist* 19 (1979), 61-66; W.T. Reich, "Ethical Issues Related to Research Involving Elderly Subjects," *Gerontologist* 18 (1978), 326-37.

    Furthermore, the topic is absent from two of the leading texts in geriatrics; and, in a sample of eighteen recent clinical research papers in geriatrics, only half stated that informed consent was obtained from either the patient or proxy, whereas in the rest consent was either not mentioned, or was ethically questionable (e.g., volunteers were paid to ensure participation; unnecessary invasive procedures were called a routine part of diagnosis). In no instance were the procedures for obtaining informed consent stated to have been different from those customarily used for younger subjects.

4. National Commission for the Protection of Human Subjects of Biomedical and Behavioral Research, *Report and Recommendations: Research Involving Those Institutionalized as Mentally Infirm.* DHEW Publication No. (OS) 78-0006, Washington, 1978.

5. DHEW, "Protection of Human Subjects: Proposed Regulations on Research Involving Those Institutionalized as Mentally Disabled," *Federal Register* 43 (No. 223) (November 17, 1978), 53950-56.

6. D.G. Fowles, *Some Prospects For the Future Elderly Population,* Washington, DC: DHEW Publication No. (OHDS) 78-20288, January 1978.

7. R. Goldman, "The Social Impact of the Organic Dementias of the Aged," in *Senile Dementia: A Biomedical Approach*, edited by K. Nandy (New York: Elsevier North-Holland Inc., 1978), pp. 3-17.

8. W. Reichel, "Demographic Aspects of Aging," in *Clinical Aspects of Aging,* edited by W. Reichel (Baltimore: Willliams and Wilkins Co., 1978), pp. 435-37.

9. United States Bureau of the Census, *Current Population Reports*, Series P 25, No. 704, July 1977.

10. R.M. Gibson and C.R. Fisher, "Age Differences in Health Care Spending, Fiscal Year 1977," *Social Security Bulletin* 42 (1979), 3-14.

11. "Jewish Chronic Disease Hospital Case," pp. 31-32.

12. D.C. Martin, J.D. Arnold, T.F. Zimmerman, et al. "Human Subjects in Clinical Research: A Report of Three Studies," *New England Journal of Medicine* 279 (1968), 1426-31.

13. Hans Jonas, "Philosophical Reflections on Experimenting With Human Subjects," in *Experimenting With Human Subjects,* edited by Paul A. Freund (New York: George Braziller, 1969), pp. 1-32

14. Joseph Goldstein, "On the Right of the 'Institutionalized Mentally Infirm' to Consent to or Refuse to Participate as Subjects in Biomedical and Behavioral Research," prepared for the National Commission, Appendix to *Research Involving Those Institutionalized as Mentally Infirm*. DHEW Publication No. (OS) 78-0007, Washington, 1978, p. 2-38.

15. Reich, "Ethical Issues Related to Research Involving Elderly Subject."

16. B.M. Ashley, "Ethics of Experimenting with Persons," in *Research and the Psychiatric Patient,* edited by Joseph C. Schoolar and Charles M. Gaitz (New York: Brunner/Mazel, 1975), pp. 15-27.

17. Jonas, "Philosophical Reflections."

18. A.S. Tannenbaum and R.A. Cooke, "Report on the Mentally Infirm," prepared for the National Commission, Appendix to *Research Involving Those Institutionalized as Mentally Infirm*. DHEW Publication No. (OS) 78-0007; B.H. Gray, R.A. Cooke, and A.S. Tannenbaum, "Research Involving Human Subjects," *Science* 201 (1978), 1094-1101.

19. DHEW, "Proposed Regulations of Research Involving Those Institutionalized as Mentally Disabled," p. 53956.

20. L.E. Hollister, "The Use of Psychiatric Patients as Experimental Subjects," in *Medical, Moral and Legal Issues in Mental Health Care,* edited by Frank J. Ayd, Jr. (Baltimore: Williams and Wilkins Co., 1974), pp. 28-36.

21. Jonas, "Philosophical Reflections."

22. T. Halper, "Paternalism and the Elderly," in *Aging and the Elderly,* edited by S.F. Spicker, K.M. Woodward, and D.D. Van Tassel (Atlantic Highlands, N.J.: Humanities Press, 1978), pp. 321-39.

23. R. Blythe, *The View in Winter: Reflections on Old Age* (New York: Harcourt Brace Jovanovich, 1979), p. 252.

24. Martin et al., "Human Subjects in Clinical Research"; see also E.M. Brody, "Environmental Factors in Dependency," in *Care of the Elderly: Meeting the Challenge of Dependency,* edited by A.N. Exton-Smith and J.G. Evans (New York: Grune and Stratton, 1977), pp. 81-95.

25. Wyatt v. Stickney, 344, F Supp. 373, 380, (1972).

26. Lionel Trilling, "Manners, Morals, and the Novel," in *The Liberal Imagination* (London: Secker and Warburg, 1951), p. 221.

27. Makarushka and McDonald, "Informed Consent, Research, and Geriatric Patients."

28. M.A. Leader and E. Neuwirth, "Clinical Research and the Noninstitutional Elderly: A Model for Subject Recruitment," *Journal of the American Geriatric Society* 26 (1978), 27-31.

29. Goldstein, "On the Right of the Institutionalized Mentally Infirm...."

30. Leader and Neuwirth, "Clinical Research and the Noninstitutionalized Elderly."

31. Neil L. Chayet, "Informed Consent on the Mentally Disabled: A Failing Fiction," *Psychiatric Annals* 6 (1976), 82-89.

32. Tannenbaum and Cooke, "Report on the Mentally Infirm."

33. Halper, "Paternalism and the Elderly," p. 332.

34. B.F. Skinner, *Beyond Freedom and Dignity* (New York: Bantam Books, 1971), p. 164.

35. Gerald Dworkin, "Paternalism," *Monist* 56 (1972), 64-84.

36. Lance Tibbles, "Medical and Legal Aspects of Competency as Affected by Old Age," in *Aging and the Elderly,* pp. 127-51.

37. F.I.M. Craik, "Age Differences in Human Memory," in *Handbook of the Psychology of Aging,* edited by J.E. Birren and K.W. Schaie (New York: Van Nostrand Reinhold Co., 1977), pp. 384-420; D. Arenberg and E.A. Robertson-Tchabo, "Learning and Aging," in *Handbook of the Psychology of Aging,* pp. 421-49.

38. J. Botwinick, "Intellectual Abilities," in *Handbook of the Psychology of Aging,* pp. 580-605.

39. J.L. Mack and N.J. Carlson, "Conceptual Deficits and Aging: The Category Test," *Perception and Motor Skills* 46 (1978), 123-28.

40. P. Rabbitt, "Change in Problem Solving Ability in Old Age," in *Handbook of the Psychology of Aging,* pp. 606-25.

41. J.E. Birren, "Age and Decision Strategies," in *Decision Making and Age: Interdisciplinary Topics in Gerontology,* edited by A.T. Welford and J.E. Birren (Basel and New York: S. Karger, 1969), IV, 23-36.

42. Rabbitt, "Change in Problem Solving Ability in Old Age."

43. Robert M. Veatch, "Three Theories of Informed Consent: Philosophical Foundations and Policy Implications," submitted to the National Commission (February 3, 1976), Recommendation 13.

44. Tibbles, "Medical and Legal Aspects of Competency...."

45. L.C. Epstein and L. Lasagna, "Obtaining Informed Consent: Form or Substance," *Archives of Internal Medicine* 123 (1969), 682-88.

46. R.J. Alfidi, "Informed Consent: A Study of Patient Reaction," *JAMA* 216 (1971), 1325-29.

47. *Pharmacological Intervention on the Aging Process,* edited by J. Roberts, R.C. Adelman, and V.J. Cristofalo (New York and London: Plenum Press, 1978).

48. Canterbury v. Spence, 464 F 2nd 722 (D. C. Cir. 1972).

49. Cobbs v. Grant, 8 Cal. 3d 229, 502 P. 2d 1, 104 Cal. Rptr. 505 (1972).

50. Goldstein, "On the Right of the Institutionalized Mentally Infirm...."

51. A.R. Herzog, "Attitude Change in Older Age: An Experimental Study," *Journal of Geronotology* 34 (1979), 697-703.

52. R. Miller and H.S. Willner, "The Two-Part Consent Form: A Suggestion for Promoting Free and Informed Consent," *New England Journal of Medicine* 290 (1974), 964-66.

53. Loren H. Roth, Alan Meisel, and Charles W. Lidz, "Tests of Competency to Consent to Treatment," *American Journal of Psychiatry* 134 (1977), 279-84.

54. Martin et al., "Human Subjects in Clinical Research."

55. Bradford H. Gray, "An Assessment of Institutional Review Committees in Human Experimentation," *Medical Care* 13 (1975), 318-28.

56. R.L. Williams, K.H. Rieckmann, G.M. Trenholme, et al., "The Use of a Test to Determine That Consent is Informed," *Military Medicine* 142 (1977), 542-45.

57. D. Axelsen and R.A. Wiggins, "An Application of Moral Guidelines in Human Clinical Trials to a Study of Benzodiazepine Compound as a Hypnotic Agent Among the Elderly," *Clinical Research* 25 (1977), 1-7.

58. L.S. Libow and R. Zicklin, "The Penultimate Will: Its Potential as an Instrument to Protect the Mentally Deteriorated Patient," *Gerontologist* 13 (1973), 440-42.

59. Arnold S. Relman, "Michigan's Sensible 'Living Will,'" *New England Journal of Medicine* 300 (1979), 1270-71.

60. Samuel I. Shuman, "Patients, Subjects and Voluntariness," in *Research and the Psychiatric Patient,* pp. 50-66.

61. *Textbook of Geriatric Medicine and Gerontology,* second ed., edited by J.C. Brocklehurst (Edinburgh, London and New York: Churchill Livingstone, 1978).

62. Martin et al., "Human Subjects in Clinical Research."

63. Tannenbaum and Cooke, "Report on the Mentally Infirm."

64. Gray, Cooke, and Tannenbaum, "Research Involving Human Subjects."

65. R.L. Kahn, A.L. Goldfarb, M. Pollack et al., "Brief Objective Measures for the Determination of Mental Status in the Aged," *American Journal of Psychiatry* 117 (1960), 326-28.

66. J.B. Priestley, "Growing Old," in *Essays of Five Decades* (Boston: Little Brown & Co., 1968), p. 309.

67. Blythe, *The View in Winter,* p. 111.

39.
THE ETHICS OF GENETIC RESEARCH ON SEXUAL ORIENTATION

Udo Schüklenk, Edward Stein, Jacinta Kerin, and William Byne

Research on the origins of sexual orientation has received much public attention in recent years, especially findings consistent with the notion of relatively simple links between genes and sexual orientation. Investigation into the causes of same-sex attraction has, however, been ongoing for more than one hundred years.[1] Claims that such inquiry is dangerous, especially in certain social and political climates, are as old as the research itself. In this paper, we show that such genetic research in particular gives rise to serious ethical issues.

GENETIC RESEARCH

Scientific research on sexual orientation has taken many forms. One early idea was to find evidence of a person's sexual orientation in such bodily features as amount of facial hair, size of external genitalia, and the ratio of shoulder width to hip width. Today's seemingly more sophisticated morphological research looks instead at neuroanatomical structures. Such inquiry usually assumes sexual orientation is a trait with two forms, one typically associated with males and the other typically associated with females. Researchers who accept this assumption expect particular aspects of an individual's brain or physiology to conform to either a male type that causes sexual attraction to women (shared by heterosexual men and lesbians) or a female type that causes sexual attraction to men (shared by heterosexual women and gay men). This assumption is scientifically unsupported and there are alternatives to it.

Another early approach was to find evidence of a person's sexual orientation in his or her endocrine system. The idea was that gay men would have less androgenic hormones (the so-called male-typical hormones) or more estrogenic hormones (the so-called female-typical sex hormones) than straight

men and that lesbians would have more androgenic and less estrogenic sex hormones than straight women. However, an overwhelming majority of studies failed to demonstrate any correlation between sexual orientation and adult hormonal constitution.[2] According to current hormonal theories of sexual orientation, lesbians and gay men were exposed to atypical hormone levels early in their development. Such theories draw heavily on the observation that, in rodents, hormonal exposure in early development exerts organizational influences on the brain that determine the balance between male and female patterns of mating behaviors in adulthood. Extrapolating from behaviors in rodents to psychological phenomena in humans is, however, quite problematic. In rodents, a male who allows himself to be mounted by another male is counted as homosexual, while a male that mounts another male is considered heterosexual. This model defines sexual orientation in terms of specific postures and behaviors. In contrast, in the human case, sexual orientation is defined not by what "position" one takes in sexual intercourse but by one's pattern of erotic responsiveness and the sex of one's preferred sex partner.

Although early sex researchers reported that homosexuality runs in families, careful studies of this hypothesis are only beginning to be done. Several studies suggest that male homosexuality runs in families,[3] but they are not helpful in distinguishing between genetic and environmental influences because most related individuals share both genes and environmental variables. Further disentanglement of genetic and environmental influences requires adoption studies.

The only heritability study of male homosexuality that includes an adoption component is the highly publicized study of Bailey and Pillard.[4] The study suggests a significant environmental contribution to the development of sexual orientation in men in addition to a moderate generic influence. This study assessed sexual orientation not only in the identical and fraternal twins, but also in the nontwin biological brothers and the unrelated adopted brothers of the gay men who volunteered for the study. The concordance rate for identical twins (52 percent) was much higher than the concordance rate for the fraternal twins (22 percent). These concordance rates show that the environment must play a significant role in sex orientation because approximately half of the monozygotic twin pairs were discordant for sexual orientation despite sharing both their genes and familial environments. The higher concordance rate in the identical twins is *consistent* with a genetic effect because identical twins share all of their genes while fraternal twins, on average, share only half. Genes cannot, however, explain the remaining results of this study. In the absence of a significant environmental influence, the incidence of homosexuality among the adopted brothers of gay men should be equal to the rate of homosexuality in the general population, which recent studies place at somewhere between 2 and 5 percent. The observed concordance rate was 11 percent (two and five times higher than expected given the estimates); this suggests a major environmental contribution. Further, no genetic explanation can account for the fact that the concordance rate for homosexuality among nontwin brothers was about the same whether or not they were genetically related (the rate for homosexuality among nontwin biological brothers was 9 percent; among adopted brothers it was 11 percent.).

When all the data from the twin study are considered, it appears that sexual orientation is the result of a combination of both genetic and environmental influences. Further, the combined effect of genetic and environmental influences might not simply be their sum; these factors could interact in a nonadditive or synergistic manner. In fact, recent heritability studies consistently find that almost half of the identical twin pairs are discordant for sexual orientations even though they share the same genes and similar familial environments. This finding underscores how little we know about the origins of sexual orientation.

Of all the recent biological studies, the genetic linkage study by Dean Hamer's group is the most conceptually complex. This study presents statistical evidence that genes influencing sexual orientation may reside in the q28 region of the X chromosome.[5] Females have two X chromosomes, but they pass a copy of only one to a son. The theoretical probability of two sons receiving a copy of the same Xq28 from their mother is thus 50 percent. Hamer found that of forty pairs of gay siblings, thirty-three instead of the expected twenty had received the same Xq28 region from their mother. Hamer's finding is often misinterpreted as showing that all sixty-six men from these thirty-three pairs shared the same Xq28 sequence. In fact, all he showed was that each member of the thirty-three concordant pairs shared his Xq28 region with his brother but not with any of the other sixty-four men. No single specific Xq28 sequence was common to all sixty-six men.

There are several problems with Hamer's study. First, a Canadian research team has been unable to duplicate the finding using a comparable experimental design.[6] Second, Hamer confined his search to the X-chromosome on the basis of family interviews, which seems to reveal a disproportionately high number of male homosexuals on the mothers' side of the family. Women might, however, be more likely to know details of family medical history, rendering these interviews less than objective in terms of directing experimental design.[7] Third, one of Hamer's coauthors has expressed serious concerns about the methodology of the study.[8] Fourth, there is some question about whether Hamer's results, correctly interpreted, are statistically significant. His conclusions rest on the assumption that the rate of homosexuality in the population at large (the base rate of homosexuality) is 2 percent. If the base rate is actually 4 percent or higher, then Hamer's results are not statistically significant. A leading geneticist argues that Hamer's own data support the four percent estimate.[9]

To understand what is at issue here, it is useful to contrast three models of the role genes might play in sexual orientation.[10] According to the "permissive effect model," genes or other biological factors influence the neural substrate on which sexual orientation is inscribed by formative experience. On this view, genetic factors might also delimit the period during which experience can affect a person's sexual orientation. According to the "indirect effect model," genes code for (or other biological factors influence) temperamental or personality factors that influence how one interacts with and shapes one's environment and formative experiences. On this view, the same gene (or set of genes) might predispose to homosexuality in some environments, to heterosexuality in others, and have no effect on sexual orientation in others. Finally, according to the "direct effect model," genes (or other biological factors) influence the brain structures that mediate sexual orientation. Hamer, LeVay, and most other researchers seem to favor the direct model.

One version of the direct model involves talk of "gay genes." It is important to remember that genes in themselves cannot directly specify any behaviors or psychological phenomena; rather, a gene directs a particular pattern of RNA synthesis that in turn specifies the amino acid sequence of a particular protein that may influence behavior. There are necessarily many intervening pathways between a gene and a behavior and even more between a gene and a pattern that involves both thinking and behaving. For the term "gay gene" to have a clear meaning, one needs to propose that a particular gene, perhaps through a hormonal mechanism, organizes the brain specifically to support the desire to have sex with people of the same sex. No one has, however, presented evidence in support of such a simple and direct link between genes and sexual orientation.

Importantly, "gay genes" are not required for homosexuality to be heritable. This is because heritability has a precise technical meaning; it refers to the ratio of genetic variation to total (phenotypic) variation. As such, heritability merely reflects the degree to which a given outcome is linked to genetic factors; it says nothing about the nature of those factors nor about their mechanism of action. Homosexuality would be heritable if genes worked through a very indirect mechanism. For example, if the indirect model is right and genes act on temperamental variables that influence how we perceive and interact with our environment, then temperament could play an important role from the moment of birth in shaping the relationships and experience that influence

how sexual orientation develops. The moral is that any genetic influence on sexual orientation might prove to be very indirect. In general, there is no convincing evidence to support the direct model; current biological evidence is equally compatible with both the direct and the indirect model.

ETHICAL CONCERNS

We have several ethical concerns about genetic research on sexual orientation. Underlying these concerns is the fact that even in our contemporary societies, lesbians, gay men, and bisexuals are subject to widespread discrimination and social disapprobation. Against this background, we are concerned about the particularly gruesome history of the use of such research. Many homosexual people have been forced to undergo "treatments" to change their sexual orientation, while others have "chosen" to undergo them in order to escape societal homophobia. All too often, scientifically questionable "therapeutic" approaches destroyed the lives of perfectly healthy people. "Conversion therapies" have included electroshock treatment, hormonal therapies, genital mutilation, and brain surgery.[11] We are concerned about the negative ramifications of biological research on sexual orientation, especially in homophobic societies. In Germany, some scholars have warned of the potential for abuse of such genetic research, while others have called for a moratorium on such research to prevent the possible abuse of its results in homophobic societies. These warnings should be taken seriously.

We are concerned that people conducting research on sexual orientation work within homophobic frameworks, despite their occasional claims to the contrary. A prime example is the German obstetrician Günter Dörner, whose descriptions of homosexuality ill-conceal his heterosexism. Dörner writes about homosexuality as a "dysfunction" or "disease" based on "abnormal brain development." He postulates that it can be prevented by *"optimizing"* natural conditions or by *"correcting* abnormal hormonal concentrations prenatally"* (emphasis added).[12] Another example is provided by psychoanalyst Richard Friedman, who engages in speculation about nongay outcome given proper therapeutic intervention.[13] Research influenced by homophobia is likely to result in significantly biased accounts of human sexuality; further, such work is more likely to strengthen and perpetuate the homophobic attitudes on which it is based.

SEXUAL ORIENTATION RESEARCH IS NOT VALUE NEUTRAL

Furthermore, we question whether those who research sexual orientation can ever conduct their work in a value-neutral manner. One might think that the majority of American sex researchers treat homosexuality not as a disease, but rather as a variation analogous to a neutral polymorphism. To consider whether or not this is the case, one must look at the context in which interest in sexual orientation arises. Homophobia still exists to some degree in all societies within which sexual orientation research is conducted. The cultures in which scientists live and work influence both the questions they ask and the hypotheses they imagine and explore. Given this, we believe it is unlikely that the sexual orientation research of any scientist (even one who is homosexual) will escape some taint of homophobia. This argument is importantly different from one which claims that objective research can be used unethically in discriminatory societies. The latter logic implies that what should be questioned is the regulation of the application of technology, not the development of the technology in the first place. While we do provide arguments for questioning the efficacy of such regulations should they be developed, our deeper concerns are directed toward the institutional and social structures that constrain sex research. Attention to these contextual details shows that research into sexual orientation is different from research into most other physical/behavioral variations. Since sexual orientation is the focus of intense private and public interest, relevant inquiry cannot be studied independently of societal investment. It is naive to suggest that individual researchers might suddenly find themselves in the position of neutral inquirers. Social mores both constrain and enable the ways in which an individual's research is focused.

We are not claiming that all researchers are homophobic to some degree whether or not they are aware of it. Nor are we talking about the implicit or explicit intentions of individual sexual orientation researchers. Rather we are seeking to highlight that the very motivation for seeking the "origin" of homosexuality has its source within social frameworks that are pervasively homophobic. Recognition that scientific projects are constituted by, and to some degree complicit in, social structures does not necessarily entail that all such science should cease. At the very least, however, it follows that sexual orientation research and its use should be subject to critique. Such a critique will call into question the claim that, by treating homosexuality as a mere variation of human behavior, researchers are conducting neutral investigations into sexual orientation.

PREDICTING SEXUAL ORIENTATION IN UTERO

We are also worried that an amniocentesis-like test will be developed that claims to detect genes or hormonal levels that might predispose for homosexuality. This concern may seem paradoxical, since the development of such a test seems to rely on the truth of the direct model of sexual orientation, which we describe as scientifically unsupported. Yet the development of such a test is, in principle, compatible with either the direct or indirect genetic model of sexual orientation. While current scientific results favor neither model, it is conceivable that future studies might clarify this impasse. Even evidence for the indirect model might inform the creation of a genetic screening technique that purports to influence sexual orientation in a given environment. Thus we are concerned that tests which do no more than suggest a predisposition for homosexuality would be favorably received in homophobic societies. If prospective parents believe they are able to predict the sexual orientation of a fetus by using a prenatal screening technique, it is possible that they would choose to abort a fetus that seemed to be "homosexually predisposed." In many countries, the preference for male versus female offspring leads to the abortion of female fetuses. This preference is clearly connected to sexism operating at a societal level. In such instances, science is subverted to serve the interests of discriminatory societies. Thus, discrimination can be institutionalized through genetic screening techniques.

Moreover, tests can be both developed and well received even if they are based on bad science. People might make use of genetic screening procedures that are supposed to select for heterosexual children even if such procedures did not work. This is partly for the general reason that the public can, in various ways, be lead to accept unsound scientific procedures. More specifically, potential users of sexual-orientation-selection procedures will have a difficult time assessing the efficacy of such procedures for at least three reasons. First, since some children turn out to be heterosexual even without the use of such a procedure, many parents who make use of it will believe that the procedure has worked, even though the procedure has done nothing. Second, many people take a long time to come to grips with their sexual orientation. Parents who made use of such a procedure might think that it had been successful, but only because their child had not yet figured out her or his sexual orientation. Third, because some lesbians, gay men, and bisexuals hide their sexual orientation, many parents will think that their attempt at selecting their child's sexual orientation has worked when in fact it has not. Further, if a lesbian, gay man, or bisexual knows that his or her parents used such a procedure, this would increase the likelihood that the person would hide his or her sexual orientation from them. For these reasons, such a procedure is likely to appear to work even if it does not. Given the appearance that such procedures work, as well as the widespread prejudice and discrimination against lesbians, gay men, and bisexuals, some people will attempt to select the sexual orientation of their children. This would likely engender and perpetuate attitudes that lesbians and gay men are undesirable and not valuable, policies that discriminate against lesbians and gay men, and the very conditions that give rise to such attitudes and policies.[14]

REPLIES TO THESE CONCERNS

Given the wide-ranging abuse of the results of biological research on sexual orientation in the past, it is not surprising that people realize that ethical justifications for this work are needed. Some researchers say their work can provide answers to century-old questions surrounding religious propositions that homosexuality is abnormal or unnatural.[15] However, biological research on the causes of sexual orientation cannot possibly provide answers to questions

concerning the nature and normality of homosexuality. As we will go on to illustrate, the only senses in which homosexuality can be said to be, or fail to be, natural or normal are of no ethical relevance. Given that some scientists claim their *empirical* research can provide answers to *normative* questions, the danger of committing a naturalistic fallacy in this context is very real.

Normativity of Naturalness and Normality. Why is there a dispute as to whether homosexuality is natural or normal? We suggest it is because many people seem to think that nature has a prescriptive normative force such that what is deemed natural or normal is necessarily good and therefore *ought* to be. Everything that falls outside these terms is constructed as unnatural and abnormal, and it has been argued that this constitutes sufficient reason to consider homosexuality worth avoiding.[16] Arguments that appeal to "normality" to provide us with moral guidelines also risk committing the naturalistic fallacy. The naturalistic fallacy is committed when one mistakenly deduces from the way things are to the way they ought to be. For instance, Dean Hamer and colleagues commit this error in their *Science* article when they state that "it would be fundamentally unethical to use such information to try to assess or alter a person's current or future sexual orientation, either heterosexual or homosexual, or other normal attributes of human behavior."[17] Hamer and colleagues believe that there is a major genetic factor contributing to sexual orientation. From this they think it follows that homosexuality is normal, and thus worthy of preservation. Thus they believe that genetics can tell us what is normal, and that the content of what is normal tells us what ought to be. This is a typical example of a naturalistic fallacy.

Normality can be defined in a number of ways, but none of them direct us in the making of moral judgments. First, normality can be reasonably defined in a *descriptive* sense as a statistical average. Appeals to what is usual, regular, and/or conforming to existing standards ultimately collapse into statistical statements. For an ethical evaluation of homosexuality, it is irrelevant whether homosexuality is normal or abnormal in this sense. All sorts of human traits and behaviors are abnormal in a statistical sense, but this is not a sufficient justification for a negative ethical judgment about them. Second, "normality" might be defined in a functional sense, where what is normal is something that has served an adaptive function from an evolutionary perspective. This definition of normality can be found in sociobiology, which seeks biological explanations for social behavior. There are a number of serious problems with the sociobiological project.[18] For the purposes of this argument, however, suffice it to say that even if sociobiology could establish that certain behavioral traits were the direct result of biological evolution, no moral assessment of these traits would follow. To illustrate our point, suppose any trait that can be reasonably believed to have served an adaptive function at some evolutionary stage is normal. Some questions arise that exemplify the problems with deriving normative conclusions from descriptive science. Are traits that are perpetuated simply through linkage to selectively advantageous loci less "normal" than those for which selection was direct? Given that social contexts now exert "selective pressure" in a way that nature once did, how are we to decide which traits are to be intentionally fostered?

Positions holding the view that homosexuality is unnatural, and therefore wrong, also inevitably develop incoherencies. They often fail to explicate the basis upon which the line between natural and unnatural is drawn. More importantly, they fail to explain why we should consider all human-made or artificial things as immoral or wrong. These views are usually firmly based in a nonempirical, *prescriptive* interpretation of nature rather than a scientific *descriptive* approach. They define arbitrarily what is natural and have to import other normative assumptions and premises to build a basis for their conclusions. For instance, they often claim that an entity called "God" has declared homosexuality to be unnatural and sinful.[19] Unfortunately, these analyses have real-world consequences. In Singapore, "unnatural acts" are considered a criminal offence, and "natural intercourse" is arbitrarily defined as "the coitus of the male and female organs." A recent High Court decision there declared oral sex "unnatural," and therefore a criminal offence, unless it leads to subsequent reproductive intercourse.

Historical Evidence. In response to some of the ethical concerns about biological research on sexual

orientation, some people have appealed to previous research on homosexuality that has *not* been used to the detriment of homosexuals. For example, Timothy Murphy invokes the work of Evelyn Hooker, which arguably provided evidence for the "normality" of homosexuals.[20] However, historical examples are often disanalogous to present-day biological research. Hooker's small-scale study, in fact, had nothing to do with the origins of sexual orientation. Rather, she sought to discover whether or or not homosexual people were "well-adapted" (by assessing the degree to which their daily practices conformed with that of "normal"Americans). Showing that nonbiological research has not been used unethically does not show that biological research will be used ethically. It is important to discern which *sorts* of historical events can be considered relevant to the debate concerning the implications and applications of research on sexual orientation.

Another defense of genetic research on sexual orientation, offered by Simon LeVay, suggests that psychological and sociological research is even more dangerous. LeVay bases his argument on the assertion that, for ideological reasons, the Nazis did not generally consider homosexuality to be innate or a sign of degeneracy, but rather that they thought homosexuality was spread by seduction.[21] This is historically not true. The Nazis were as supportive of genetic research as they were of any other type of research designed to support the elimination of homosexuality.[22] Even if LeVay's assertions were historically correct, however, they would not provide any support (ethical or otherwise) for genetic research. Arguing that one type of research is ethically problematic does not legitimize the other; indeed, it only provides further reason to question the whole enterprise.

U.S.-Specific Arguments. In the United States, several scholars and lesbian and gay activists have argued that establishing a genetic basis for sexual orientation will help make the case for lesbian and gay rights. The idea is that scientific research will show that people do not choose their sexual orientations and therefore they should not be punished or discriminated against in virtue of them. This general argument is flawed in several ways.[23] First, we do not need to show that a trait is genetically determined to argue that it is not amenable to change at will. This is clearly shown by the failure rates of conversion "therapies."[24] These failures establish that sexual orientation is resistant to change, but they do not say anything about its ontogeny or etiology. Sexual orientation can be unchangeable without being genetically determined. There is strong observational evidence to support the claim that sexual orientation is difficult to change, but this evidence is perfectly compatible with nongenetic accounts of the origins of sexual orientations. More importantly, we should not embrace arguments that seek to legitimate homosexuality by denying that there is any choice in sexual preference because the implicit premise of such arguments is that if there *was* a choice, then homosexuals would be blameworthy.

Relatedly, arguments for lesbian and gay rights based on scientific evidence run the risk of leading to impoverished forms of lesbian and gay rights. Regardless of what causes homosexuality, a person has to decide to publicly identify as a lesbian, to engage in sexual acts with another woman, to raise children with her same-sex lover, or to be active in the lesbian and gay community. It is when people make such decisions that they are likely to face discrimination, arrest, or physical violence. It is decisions like these that need legal protection. An argument for lesbian and gay rights based on genetic evidence is impotent with respect to protecting such decisions because it focuses exclusively on the very aspects of sexuality that might not involve choices.

Another version of this argument focuses on the specifics of U.S. law. According to this version, scientific evidence will establish the immutability of sexual orientation, which, according to one current interpretation of the Equal Protection Clause of the Fourteenth Amendment of the U.S. Constitution, is one of three criteria required of a classification if it is to evoke heightened judicial scrutiny. While this line of argument has serious internal problems, [25] such an argument, like a good deal of American bioethical reasoning, has limited or no relevance to the global context. Since the results of the scientific research are not confined within American borders, justifications that go beyond U.S. legislation are required.

The same sort of problem occurs in other defenses of sexual orientation research that discuss possible ramifications in U.S.-specific legislative terms. For instance, Timothy Murphy claims that, even if a genetic probe predictive of sexual orientation were available, mandatory testing would be unlikely.[26] He bases this claim on the fact that in some states employment and housing discrimination against homosexual people is illegal. In many countries, however, the political climate is vastly different, and legal anti-gay discrimination is widespread. And there is evidence that scientific research would be used in a manner that discriminates against homosexuals.[27] As already mentioned, in Singapore, homosexual sex acts are a criminal offense. The Singapore Penal Code sections 377 and 377A threaten sentences ranging from two years to life imprisonment for homosexual people engaging in same-sex acts. Not coincidentally, in light of our concerns, a National University of Singapore psychiatrist recently implied that "pre-symptomatic testing for homosexuality should be offered in the absence of treatment,"[28] thereby accepting the idea that homosexuality is something in need of a cure.

Genetic Screening. Several attempts to defend sexual orientation research against ethical concerns related to the selective abortion of "pre-homosexual" fetuses have been made. It has been claimed that this sort of genetic screening will not become commonplace because "diagnostic genetic testing is at present the exception rather than the rule."[29] While this may indeed be true in the U.S., it has far more to do with the types of tests currently offered than with a reluctance on the part of either the medical profession or the reproducing public to partake of such technology. For example, the types of tests available are diagnostic for diseases and are offered on the basis of family history or specific risk factors. The possibility of tests that are supposed to be (however vaguely) predictive of behavioral traits opens genetic technology to a far greater population, especially when the traits in question are undesired by a largely prejudiced society.

Furthermore, it has been claimed that the medical profession would not advocate such a test that does not serve "important state interests" (p. 341). This argument not only ignores the existence of homophobia among individuals within medicine,[30] it assumes also that public demand for genetic testing varies predominantly according to medical advice. However, should such a test become available, the media hype surrounding its market arrival would render its existence common knowledge, which, coupled with homophobic bias, would create a demand for the test irrespective of its accuracy and of any kind of state interest. Furthermore, this argument ignores the fact that genetic screening for a socially undesirable characteristic has already been greeted with great public demand in countries such as India, where abortion on the basis of female sex is commonplace, irrespective of its legality.[31] Techniques to select the sexual orientation of children, if made available, might well be widely utilized.[32]

Some have argued that orientation-selection techniques involving genetic screening will not succeed because environmental factors influencing sexual orientation would elude genetic screening.[33] While there are such environmental factors, we are still concerned about the potential effects of the availability of orientation-selection techniques, even if they fail to work. Further, if environmental factors are identified, their modification could be defended on the same grounds as the elimination of "gay genes." In fact, behavior modification techniques have been, and continue to be, used to prevent homosexuality in children with "gender identity disorder" (that is, "sissies" and "tom boys").[34]

It has also been claimed that if homosexual people themselves made use of orientation-selection techniques (whether to ensure homosexual or heterosexual offspring), the charge that such testing is inherently homophobic becomes "paradoxical."[35] However, just as the fact that homosexual people conduct scientific research on sexual orientation does not show that such research is ethically justifiable, the fact that some homosexuals might use such techniques would not prove that the technology does not serve to discriminate. To illustrate this point, consider that in a society like India in which widespread discrimination against women exists, there are many pragmatic reasons why one might prefer a male child. We would not argue, however, that prenatal sex selection is no longer discriminatory against females because women sometimes seek abortions for the purpose of having male offspring. Similarly, in societies with entrenched homophobia,

a heterosexual child might be preferable for reasons that might appear most salient to homosexuals themselves in lieu of the discrimination they have encountered. The use of a technology by people against whom it may discriminate (even if they attempt to use it to their benefit) does not establish its neutrality. It does, however, highlight the pervasive biases within a given society that should be addressed directly rather than be fostered with enabling technology. Discriminated-against users of discriminatory technology might have a variety of motives, none of which necessarily diffuse the charge of bias.

The Value of Knowing the Truth. Finally, various scholars appeal to the value of the truth to defend research on sexual orientation in the face of ethical concerns. Scientific research does, however, have its costs and not every research program is of equal importance. Even granting that, in general, knowledge is better than ignorance, not all risks for the sake of knowledge are worth taking. With respect to sexual orientation, historically, almost every hypothesis about the causes of homosexuality led to attempts to "cure" healthy people. History indicates that current genetic research is likely to have negative effects on lesbians and gay men, particularly those living in homophobic societies.[36]

A GLOBAL PERSPECTIVE

Homosexual people have in the past suffered greatly from societal discrimination. Historically, the results of biological research on sexual orientation have been used against them. We have analyzed the arguments offered by well-intentioned defenders of such work and concluded that none survive philosophical scrutiny. It is true that in some countries in Scandinavia, North America, and most parts of Western Europe the legal situation of homosexual people has improved, but an adequate ethical analysis of the implications of genetic inquiry into the causes of sexual orientation must operate from a global perspective. Sexual orientation researchers should be aware that their work may harm homosexuals in countries other than their own. It is difficult to imagine any good that could come of genetic research on sexual orientation in homophobic societies. Such work faces serious ethical concerns so long as homophobic societies continue to exist. Insofar as a socially responsible genetic research on sexual orientation is possible, it must begin with the awareness that it will not be a cure for homophobia and that the ethical status of lesbians and gay men does not in any way hinge on its results.

Notes

1. Rüdiger Lautmann, ed., *Homosexualität: Handbuch der Theorie und Forschungsgeschichte* (Campus Verlag: Frankfurt am Main, 1993); Vern Bullough, *Science in the Bedroom: The History of Sex Research* (Basic Books: New York, 1994).

2. Heino Meyer-Bahlburg, "Psychoendocrine Research on Sexual Orientation: Current Status and Future Options," *Progress in Brain Research* 71 (1984): 375-97.

3. For example, Richard Pillard and James Weinrich, "Evidence for a Familial Nature of Male Homosexuality," *Archives of General Psychiatry* 43 (1986): 808-12

4. J. Michael Bailey and Richard Pillard, "A Genetic Study of Male Sexual Orientation," *Archives of General Psychiatry* 48 (1991): 1089-96.

5. Dean Hamer et al., " A Linkage Between DNA Markers on the X Chromosome and Male Sexual Orientation," *Science* 261 (1993): 321-27.

6. G. Rice, C. Anderson, N. Risch, and G. Ebers, "Male Homosexuality: Absence of Linkage to Microsatellite Markers on the X Chromosome in a Canadian Study," presented at the 21st Annual Meeting of the International Academy of Sex Research 1995, Provincetown. Mass. This presentation is discussed in E. Marshall, "NIH 'Gay Gene' Study Questioned," *Science* 268 (1995):1841.

7. Evan Balaban, quoted in V. D'Alessio, "Born to be Gay?" *New Scientist* (28 September 1996):32-35.

8. Marshall, "NIH's 'Gay Gene' Study Questioned," p. 1841.

9. Neil Risch, Elizabeth Squires-Wheeler, and Bronya Keats, "Male Sexual Orientation and Genetic Evidence," *Science* 262 (1993): 2063-65.

10. William Byne, "Biology and Sexual Orientation: Implications of Endocronological and Neuroanatomical Research," in *Comprehensive Textbook of Homosexuality*, ed. R. Labaj and T. Stein (Washington, D. C.: American Psychiatric Press, 1996), pp. 129-46.

11. Jonathan Ned Katz, *Gay American History* (New York: Thomas Crowell, 1976), pp. 197-422.

12. Günter Dörner, "Hormone-dependent Brain Development and Neuroendocrine Prophylaxis," *Experimental and Clinical Endocrinology* 94 (1989):4-22.

13. Richard C. Friedman, *Male Homosexuality: A Contemporary Psychoanalytic Perspective* (New Haven: Yale University Press, 1988), p. 20.

14. Edward Stein, "Choosing the Sexual Orientation of Children," *Bioethics* (1998), forthcoming.

15. Udo Schüklenk and Michael Ristow, "The Ethics of Research into the Causes of Homosexuality," *Journal of Homosexuality* 31, nos. 3, 4 (1996):5-30.

16. Michael Levin, "Why Homosexuality is Abnormal," *Monist* 67 (1984: 251-83.

17. Hamer et al., "A Linkage Between DNA Markers on the X Chromosome and Male Sexual Orientation," p. 326.

18. Philip Kitcher, *Vaulting Ambition: Sociobiology and the Quest for Human Nature* (Cambridge, Mass.: MIT Press, 1985).

19. Udo Schüklenk and David Mertz, "Christliche Kirchen und AIDS," in *Die Lehre des Unheils,* ed. Edgar Dahl. (Hamburg: Carlsen, 1993), pp. 263-79 and 309-12.

20. Timothy Murphy, "Abortion and the Ethics of Genetic Sexual Orientation Research," *Cambridge Quarterly of Healthcare Ethics* 4 (1995): 340-50, especially p. 347.

21. Simon LeVay, *Queer Science: The Use and Abuse of Research on Homosexuality* (Cambridge, Mass: MIT Press, 1996), pp. 38 and 113.

22. See, for example, Julius Deussen, "Sexualpathologie," in *Fortschritte der Erbpathologie, Rassenhygiene und ihrer Grenzgebiete* 2 (1939): 67-102. Interestingly, the British Eugenics Society showed a keen interest in the outcome of this research. Matthias Weber, Ernst Rüdin. *Eine kritische Biographie* (Berlin: Springer, 1993). See also Pauline M. H. Mazumdar, *Eugenics, Human Genetics and Human Failings: The Eugenics Society, Its Sources and Its Critics in Britain* (London: Routledge 1992). We thank Professor Hans-Peter Kröner, Institute for Theory and History of Medicine Westfälische Wilhelms-Universität Münster, for bringing this information to our attention.

23. Edward Stein, "The Relevance of Scientific Research Concerning Sexual Orientation to Lesbian and Gay Rights," *Journal of Homosexuality* 27 (1994): 269-308.

24. Charles Silverstein, "Psychological and Medical Treatments of Homosexuality," in *Homosexuality: Research Implications for Public Policy,* ed. J.C. Gonsiorek and J.D. Weinrich (Newbury Park, Calif.: Sage, 1991), pp. 101-14.

25. Janet Halley, "Sexual Orientation and the Politics of Biology: A Critique of the New Argument from Immutability," *Stanford Law Review* 46 (1994): 503-68.

26. Murphy, "Abortion and the Ethics of Genetic Sexual Orientation Research," p. 341.

27. Paul Billings, "Genetic Discrimination and Behavioural Genetics: The Analysis of Sexual Orientation," in *Intractable Neurological Disorders, Human Genome, Research and Society,* ed. Norio Fujiki and Darryl Macer (Christchurch and Tsukuba: Eubios Ethics Institute, 1993), p. 37; Paul Billings, "International Aspects of Genetic Discrimination," in *Human Genome Research and Society,* ed. Norio Fujiki and Darryl Macer (Christchurch and Tsukuba: Eubios Ethics Institute, 1992), pp. 114-17.

28. L.C.C. Lim, "Present Controversies in the Genetics of Male Homosexuality," *Annals of the Academy of Medicine Singapore* 24 (1995): 759-62.

29. Murphy, "Abortion and the Ethics of Genetic Sexual Orientation Research," p. 341.

30. Kevin Speight, "Homophobia Is a Health Issue," *Health Care Analysis* 3 (1995): 143-48.

31. Kusum, "The Use of Prenatal Diagnostic Techniques for Sex Selection: The Indian Scene," *Bioethics* 7 (1993): 149-65.

32. Richard Posner, *Sex and Reason* (Cambridge, Mass.: Harvard University Press, 1992), p. 308

33. Murphy, "Abortion and the Ethics of Genetic Sexual Orientation Research," p. 346. Indeed, the recently announced Environmental Genome Project launched by the NIH has begun with research on the interaction of genes and the environment.

34. See Richard Green, *The "Sissy Boy" Syndrome and the Development of Homosexuality* (New Haven: Yale University Press, 1987); Phyllis Burke, *Gender Shock: Exploding the Myths of Male and Female* (New York: Anchor Books, 1996).

35. Murphy, "Abortion and the Ethics of Genetic Sexual Orientation Research," p. 343.

36. For further elaborations on this argument see Edward Stein, Udo Schüklenk, and Jacinta Kerin, "Scientific Research on Sexual Orientation," in *Encyclopedia of Applied Ethics,* ed. Ruth Chadwick (San Diego: Academic Press, 1997).

40.
DECLARATION OF HELSINKI

World Medical Association

INTRODUCTION

It is the mission of the medical doctor to safeguard the health of the people. His or her knowledge and conscience are dedicated to the fulfillment of this mission.

The Declaration of Geneva of The World Medical Association binds the doctor with the words "The health of my patient will be my first consideration," and the International Code of Medical Ethics declares that, "Any act or advice which could weaken physical or mental resistance of a human being may be used only in his interest."

The purpose of biomedical research involving human subjects must be to improve diagnostic, therapeutic and prophylactic procedures and the understanding of the aetiology and pathogenesis of disease.

In current medical practice most diagnostic, therapeutic or prophylactic procedures involve hazards. This applies *a fortiori* to biomedical research.

Medical progress is based on research which ultimately must rest in part on experimentation involving human subjects.

In the field of biomedical research a fundamental distinction must be recognized between medical research in which the aim is essentially diagnostic or therapeutic for a patient, and medical research, the essential object of which is purely scientific and without direct diagnostic or therapeutic value to the person subjected to the research.

Special caution must be exercised in the conduct of research which may affect the environment, and the welfare of animals used for research must be respected.

Because it is essential that the results of laboratory experiments be applied to human beings to further scientific knowledge and to help suffering humanity, The World Medical Association has prepared the following recommendations as a guide to every doctor in biomedical research involving human subjects. They should be kept under review in the future. It must be stressed that the standards as drafted are only a guide to physicians all over the world. Doctors are not relieved from criminal, civil and ethical responsibilities under the laws of their own countries.

I. BASIC PRINCIPLES

1. Biomedical research involving human subjects must conform to generally accepted scientific principles and should be based on adequately performed laboratory and animal experimentation and on a thorough knowledge of the scientific literature.

2. The design and performance of each experimental procedure involving human subjects should be clearly formulated in an experimental protocol which should be transmitted to a specially appointed independent committee for consideration, comment and guidance.

3. Biomedical research involving human subjects should be conducted only by scientifically qualified persons and under the supervision of a clinically competent medical person. The responsibility for the human subject must always rest with a medically qualified person and never rest on the subject of research, even though the subject has given his or her consent.

4. Biomedical research involving human subjects cannot legitimately be carried out unless the importance of the objective is in proportion to the inherent risk to the subject.

5. Every biomedical research project involving human subjects should be preceded by careful assessment of predictable risks in comparison with foreseeable benefits to the subject or to others. Concern for the interests of the subject must always prevail over the interests of science and society.

6. The right of the research subject to safeguard his or her integrity must always be respected. Every precaution should be taken to respect the privacy of the subject and to minimize the impact of the study on the subject's physical and mental integrity and on the personality of the subject.

7. Doctors should abstain from engaging in research projects involving human subjects unless they are satisfied that the hazards involved are believed to be predictable. Doctors should cease any investigation if the hazards are found to outweigh the potential benefits.

8. In publication of the results of his or her research, the doctor is obliged to preserve the accuracy of the results. Reports of experimentation not in accordance with the principles laid down in the Declaration should not be accepted for publication.

9. In any research on human beings, each potential subject must be adequately informed of the aims, methods, anticipated benefits and potential hazards of the study and the discomfort it may entail. He or she should be informed that he or she is at liberty to abstain from participation in the study and that he or she is free to withdraw his or her consent to participation at any time. The doctor should then obtain the subject's freely given informed consent, preferably in writing.

10. When obtaining informed consent for the research project the doctor should be particularly cautious if the subject is in a dependent relationship to him or her or may consent under duress. In that case the informed consent should be obtained by a doctor who is not engaged in the investigation and who is completely independent of this official relationship.

11. In case of legal incompetence, informed consent should be obtained from the legal guardian in accordance with national legislation. Where physical or mental incapacity makes it impossible to obtain informed consent, or when the subject is a minor, permission from the responsible relative replaces that of the subject in accordance with national legislation.

12. The research protocol should always contain a statement of the ethical considerations involved and should indicate that the principles enunciated in the present Declaration are complied with.

II. Medical Research Combined with Professional Care (Clinical Research)

1. In the treatment of the sick person, the doctor must be free to use a new diagnostic and therapeutic measure, if in his or her judgment it offers hope of saving life, reestablishing health or alleviating suffering.

2. The potential benefits, hazards and discomfort of a new method should be weighed against the advantages of the best current diagnostic and therapeutic methods.

3. In any medical study, every patient–including those of a control group, if any–should be assured of the best proven diagnostic and therapeutic method.

4. The refusal of the patient to participate in a study must never interfere with the doctor-patient relationship.

5. If the doctor considers it essential not to obtain informed consent, the specific reasons for this proposal should be stated in the experimental protocol for transmission to the independent committee (I, 2).

6. The doctor can combine medical research with professional care, the objective being the acquisition of new medical knowledge, only to the extent that medical research is justified by its potential diagnostic or therapeutic value for the patient.

III. Non-Therapeutic Biomedical Research Involving Human Subjects (Non-Clinical Biomedical Research)

1. In the purely scientific application of medical research carried out on a human being, it is the duty of the doctor to remain the protector of the life and health of that person on whom biomedical research is being carried out.

2. The subjects should be volunteers–either healthy persons or patients for whom the experimental design is not related to the patient's illness.

3. The investigator or the investigating team should discontinue the research if in his/her or their judgment it may, if continued, be harmful to the individual.

4. In research on man, the interest of science and society should never take precedence over considerations related to the well-being of the subject.

41.
TRI-COUNCIL POLICY STATEMENT: ETHICAL CONDUCT FOR RESEARCH INVOLVING HUMANS

Medical Research Council of Canada, Social Sciences and Humanities Research Council of Canada, and Public Works and Government Services Canada

C. GUIDING ETHICAL PRINCIPLES

The approach taken in this framework is to guide and evoke thoughtful actions based on principles. The principles that follow are based on the guidelines of the Councils over the last decades,[1] on more recent statements by other Canadian agencies,[2] and on statements from the international community.[3] The principles have been widely adopted by diverse research disciplines. As such, they express common standards, values and aspirations of the research community.

Respect for Human Dignity: The cardinal principle of modern research ethics, as discussed above, is respect for human dignity. This principle aspires to protecting the multiple and interdependent interests of the person—from bodily to psychological to cultural integrity. This principle forms the basis of the ethical obligations in research that are listed below.

In certain situations, conflicts may arise from application of these principles in isolation from one other. Researchers and REBs must carefully weigh all the principles and circumstances involved to reach a reasoned and defensible conclusion.

Respect for Free and Informed Consent:[4] Individuals are generally presumed to have the capacity and right to make free and informed decisions. Respect for persons thus means respecting the exercise of individual consent. In practical terms within the ethics review process, the principle of respect for persons translates into the dialogue, process, rights, duties and requirements for free and informed consent by the research subject.

Respect for Vulnerable Persons: Respect for human dignity entails high ethical obligations towards vulnerable persons—to those whose diminished competence and/or decision-making capacity make them vulnerable. Children, institutionalized persons or others who are vulnerable are entitled, on grounds of human dignity, caring, solidarity and fairness, to special protection against abuse, exploitation or discrimination. Ethical obligations to vulnerable individuals in the research enterprise will often translate into special procedures to protect their interests.

Respect for Privacy and Confidentiality: Respect for human dignity also implies the principles of respect for privacy and confidentiality. In many cultures, privacy and confidentiality are considered fundamental to human dignity. Thus, standards of privacy and confidentiality protect the access, control and dissemination of personal information. In doing so, such standards help to protect mental or psychological integrity. They are thus consonant with values underlying privacy, confidentiality and anonymity respected.

Respect for Justice and Inclusiveness: Justice connotes fairness and equity. Procedural justice requires that the ethics review process have fair methods, standards and procedures for reviewing research protocols, and that the process be effectively independent. Justice also concerns the distribution of benefits and burdens of research. On the one hand, distributive justice means that no segment of the population should be unfairly burdened with the harms of research. It thus imposes particular obligations toward individuals who are vulnerable and unable to protect their own interests in order to ensure that they are not exploited for the advancement of knowledge. History has many chapters of such exploitation. On the other hand, distributive justice also imposes duties neither to neglect nor discriminate against individuals and groups who may benefit from advances in research.

Balancing Harms and Benefits: The analysis, balance and distribution of harms and benefits are critical to the ethics of human research. Modern research ethics, for instance, require a favourable harms-benefit balance—that is, that the foreseeable harms should not outweigh anticipated benefits. Harms-benefits analysis thus affects the welfare and rights of research subjects, the informed assumption of harms and benefits, and the ethical justifications for competing research paths. Because research involves advancing the frontiers of knowledge, its undertaking often involves uncertainty about the precise magnitude and kind of benefits or harms that attend proposed research. These realities and the principle of respect for human dignity impose ethical obligations on the prerequisites, scientific validity, design and conduct of research. These concerns are particularly evident in biomedical and health research; in research they need to be tempered in areas such as political science, economics or modern history (including biographies), areas in which research may ethically result in the harming of the reputations of organizations or individuals in public life.

Minimizing Harm: A principle directly related to harms-benefits analysis is non-maleficence, or the duty to avoid, prevent or minimize harms to others. Research subjects must not be subjected to unnecessary risks of harm, and their participation in research must be essential to achieving scientifically and societally important aims that cannot be realized without the participation of human subjects. In addition, it should be kept in mind that the principle of minimizing harm requires that the research involve the smallest number of human subjects and the smallest number of tests on these subjects that will ensure scientifically valid data.

Maximizing Benefit: Another principle related to the harms and benefits of research is beneficence. The principle of beneficence imposes a duty to benefit others and, in research ethics, a duty to maximize net benefits. The principle has particular relevance for

researchers in professions such as social work, education, health care and applied psychology. As noted earlier, human research is intended to produce benefits for subjects themselves, for other individuals or society as a whole, or for the advancement of knowledge. In most research, the primary benefits produced are for society and for the advancement of knowledge.

D. A SUBJECT-CENTRED PERSPECTIVE

Research subjects contribute enormously to the progress and promise of research in advancing the human condition. In many areas of research, subjects are participants in the development of a research project and collaboration between them and the researcher in such circumstances is vital and requires nurturing. Such collaboration entails an active involvement by research subjects, and ensures both that their interests are central to the project or study, and that they will not be treated simply as objects. Especially in certain areas of the humanities and social sciences this collaborative approach is essential, and the research could not be conducted in any other way. For example, a study on how a theatrical company developed its approach to a particular play would be difficult without the participation of the theatre company in question. Nevertheless, some research will require a more formal separation between subject and researcher because of the nature of the research design.

A subject-centred approach should, however, also recognize that researchers and research subjects may not always see the harms and benefits of a research project in the same way. Indeed, individual subjects within the same study may respond very differently to the information provided in the free and informed consent process. Hence, researchers and REBs must strive to understand the views of the potential or actual research subjects.

In this context, researchers should take into account that potential subjects who are asked to participate in research by, for example, their caregiver, teacher or supervisor may be overly influenced by such factors as trust in the researcher or the hope for other goals, more than by assessment of the pros and cons of participation in the research. A patient may hope for a cure from an experimental drug, an employee for better working conditions, a student for better marks. This places extra demands on the researcher for accuracy, candour, objectivity and sensitivity in forming potential subjects about proposed research.

However, researchers and REB should also be aware that some research may be deliberately and legitimately opposed to the interests of the research subjects. This is particularly true of research in the social sciences and the humanities that may be critical of public personalities or organizations. Such research should, of course, be carried out according to professional standards, but it should not be blocked through the use of harms/benefits analysis or because it may not involve collaboration with the research subjects.

Notes

1. Medical Research Council of Canada, Guidelines for Research Involving Human Subjects, 1987, Ottawa 1988; Social Sciences and Humanities Research Council, Ethics in Human Experimentation, Ottawa, 1978.

2. See, e.g., National Research Council of Canada, *Ethical Guidelines for Research*, Ottawa, 1993; Royal Commission on New Reproductive Technologies, *Proceed With Care: Final Reports of the Royal Commission on New Reproductive Technologies*, Ottawa: Minister of Government Services Canada, 1993; vol 1.: 53-66.

3. See, e.g., The National Commission for the Protection of Human Subjects of Biomedical and Behav-

ioural Research, The Belmont Report: Ethical Principles and Guidelines for the Protection of Human Subjects of Research, Washington, DC, 1979; council for International Organizations of Medical Sciences, International Ethical Guidelines for Biomedical Research Involving Human Subjects, Geneva, 1993; UNESCO, Ethical Guidelines for International Comparative Social Science Research in the Framework of M.O.S.T. (Management of Social Transformation), Paris, 1994; The Research Council of Norway, Guidelines for Research Ethics in the Social Sciences, Law and the Humanities, Oslo, 1994.

4. During preparation of this Policy Statement, there was extensive discussion of the optimal way to refer to the decision made by the potential research subject on whether to participate in the research. The frequently used phrase "obtain informed consent" was rejected early in the discussion because "obtain" implies that getting the consent is the goal, whereas ethically the goal must be to enable the potential subject to choose freely, and with full information, on whether to agree to participate in the research. Though earlier drafts used both "choice" and "consent," it was often difficult to be certain which was the most appropriate in the various contexts. Hence, a brief means of expressing this concept was sought.

"Free and informed consent" was decided upon for a number of reasons: it states the requirement for voluntariness and information; it was felt to include the idea that consent is the act of deciding, perhaps as a result of balancing a number of choices; it retains the traditional word "consent"; and the phrase has unambiguous meaning in the law.

CHAPTER NINE

SCARCE MEDICAL RESOURCES

42.
PURPOSE AND FUNCTION IN GOVERNMENT-FUNDED HEALTH COVERAGE

Benjamin Freedman and Françoise Baylis

Government-funded health insurance schemes are under increasing pressure to reconcile finite medical resources with seemingly infinite demands for medical services. Consequently, problems regarding the macroallocation of available resources must constantly be readdressed. The substantive macroallocational questions are familiar: What portions of health care funding should be directed toward acute, chronic, or preventive care, or toward research in these respective areas? What, if any, provision should be made for the funding of novel therapies? When more than one approach to a disorder is available (e.g., medical or surgical treatment of angina pectoris), should the insurance program reward the use of the cheapest option (one assumption underlying the DRG system; see Wasserman 1983), the option which the physician believes is clinically preferable, or that which the patient prefers, perhaps on grounds of compatibility with lifestyle?

Questions such as these underline the need for a demarcation principle which government-funded health insurance programs could use to determine what should not be funded. The usefulness of such a principle is obvious, particularly from the government's perspective, when one considers how quickly new approaches to health care are adopted by health care providers (creating a demand for insurance reimbursement on their behalf). Current examples would include transportation, advanced diagnostic and imaging equipment, and expensive techniques for the treatment of infertility (most notoriously, *in vitro* fertilization). A demarcation principle would serve to limit the constantly expanding claims for health insurance coverage which feed upon (and, when successful, fuel) the unrealistic expectation that the government-funded health care system can guarantee everyone a long, happy, and productive life.

At present, the approach to funding adopted by government health care programs is eclectic. Aside from strictly medical concerns, attention is given to factors deriving from economics, politics, and public policy. Even within the mélange of compromise that constitutes health insurance, however, we may discern a basic theme of demarcation; absent special considerations, a purposive (deductive) approach is commonly used in deciding whether a specific service should be a covered benefit. The results of this theme may be reconstructed in almost syllogistic terms: the insurance scheme should fund that which yields, or leads to, health (major premise); the proposed service does (or does not) yield or lead to health (minor premise); therefore the proposed service should (should not) be reimbursed. Presented in this way, the deductive approach is, of course, an artificial reconstruction of a more complicated reality. In the cases that we will be presenting, however, it plausibly captures an important theme in insurance decision making as that is publicly presented.

The Preamble to the Ontario Health Insurance Plan's *Schedule of Benefits* (1983), for example, states at the outset that "Insured medical services are limited to the services which are medically necessary ..." (p. 1). This we understand to mean that only those services designed to restore health ("medically necessary") are to be funded. The purposive concept of medical necessity is therefore ostensibly an *exclusive* criterion of demarcation—that is, a necessary but not sufficient condition for coverage. However, medical necessity also serves as an *inclusive* criterion of demarcation. The fitting of contact lenses, for example, is not a covered benefit unless it is being done to correct aphakia, myopia greater than nine diopters, irregular astigmatism, or keratoconus (p. 20). Similarly, other services commonly sought for reasons of vanity or convenience are not covered benefits unless they are called for by some substantial degree of medical necessity. A case in point is cosmetic surgery, which is not an insured benefit "except where medically required" (p. 19).

The deductive model, idealized as it is, is a plausible—sometimes, the *only* plausible—reconstruction of a number of specific decisions on insurance coverage. Although it is initially appealing, we shall argue that this form of reasoning results in some obvious inequalities and distortions in government coverage practice. An alternative approach, which may be termed functional or inductive, will be suggested. The functional approach would have us resolve the problem of demarcation by asking whether the specific service in question represents a demand which the health care system may efficiently satisfy. The question of whether the funded service supplies "health" or "health care" is thereby intentionally finessed.

The examples we shall be using are drawn largely from Canadian (and predominantly Ontarian) experiences. They are intended to serve for purposes of illustration alone. If successful, they point to problems and approaches generally prevalent among any government-funded insurance scheme which claims to comprehensively fund the health demands of the serviced population.

THE PURPOSIVE APPROACH

In ordinary language, "purpose" broadly refers to the end one has in view in acting in a certain way (i.e., "purposively"). The use of the term implies the conscious choice of both a goal and an action designed to achieve the stated goal. By extension, we may think of objects as purposively designed. For example, a television receiver is built with the end of it serving as a decoder of electronic impulses. In designing it, a certain size and shape are chosen on the grounds of fitness toward that end (Turkel 1984); any components which prove unreliable in achieving that end are either discarded or redesigned. Social institutions, such as traffic regulation, can also be construed as purposive. A panoply of elements (road markings, rules, etc.) are chosen subordinate to the primary goal of the swift and accident-free motion of traffic.

Similarly, some view medical practice as a purposive enterprise. It is usual to distinguish medical

from nonmedical interventions—to demarcate medical practice—by referring to current beliefs concerning what promotes or conserves health; in theory new forms of medical treatment are accepted into practice and old ones discarded on the basis of their fitness to serve the purpose of health. It is on this basis alone that physicians, in the course of their daily practice, "may, unquestioned and with impunity, slice, puncture, bind, grind, inject, and extract various organic and inorganic substances into and from" their patients (Freedman 1984, 5).

As health is the organizing principle and rule of demarcation for medical practice, it is natural to assume that this concept should apply as well to that system which funds medical practice. That is, it seems natural to assume that problems of demarcation in health care funding cannot be decided unless prior agreement has been arrived at concerning the definition of health, so that the nature of "medically necessary" services may be ascertained. By extension, a government-funded health insurance program may be purposively understood as an institution designed to secure health, although it is constrained by economic and political factors.

If the purpose of the government-funded insurance system is to promote health, and if that purpose is to serve as its rule of demarcation, a definition of health must be presented. However, the definition of health and related concepts (such as illness and disease) has resisted numerous scholarly efforts. Those definitions which have gained favorable attention have succeeded by stipulating a definition which could then be explicated or operationalized (Boorse 1975). But this approach will not serve the purposes of a government-funded health insurance scheme, since these purposes require a definition or an understanding of health with a basis in social consensus and usage.

The most widely known and most frequently criticized definition of health is found in the Preamble to the Constitution of the World Health Organization: "Health is a state of complete physical, mental and social well-being and not merely the absence of disease or infirmity" (WHO 1976). Daniel Callahan, a relatively sympathetic commentator on the WHO definition, notes nonetheless that this definition fosters "the cultural tendency to define all social problems, from war to crime on the streets, as 'health' problems" (Callahan 1973, 78). It "makes the medical profession the gate-keeper for happiness and social well-being ... the final magic-healer of human misery" (p. 81).

These eloquent criticisms relate to the one point that makes the WHO definition of health inadequate for the purposes of our discussion: it provides a government-funded health insurance scheme with no rule of demarcation whatsoever....

Mindful of the need for demarcation, Callahan offered the following definition of health as a counterproposal: "Health is a state of physical well-being," a state which need not be "complete" but must be "at least adequate, i.e., without significant impairment of function" (Callahan 1973, 87). With this narrow definition of health, mental illness would qualify as "ill health," if at all, only if it substantially interfered with functioning.

Would Callahan's definition, or one equally narrow, represent a satisfactory rule of demarcation for government-funded health insurance schemes? It is important to examine this question at some length, because the narrowness of the definition as well as its common-sense roots make it attractive to economically pressed governments. Therefore, even if Callahan would not use his definition of health as a rule of demarcation, governments faced with competing priorities might be tempted to do so.

In judging the adequacy of any proposed rule of demarcation, two different kinds of questions may be asked. First, *could* the rule serve (i.e., would it clearly distinguish between those services to be included and those to be excluded from the funding system)? Second, *should* the rule serve (i.e., if applied, would it yield satisfactory results)? The first question concerns the formal adequacy of the rule; the second, its substantive adequacy.

The notion of "well-being" and of "impairment of function" are two crucial elements of Callahan's definition which are unavoidably ambiguous; these ambiguities speak to the issue of formal adequacy. To revert to the example introduced earlier, consider a patient suffering from exercise-onset angina pectoris. Two types of treatment are available. One option is medical management, which requires of the patient a commitment to control of diet, a modifica-

tion of activity, and the tolerance of some degree of continued pain. The alternative is surgical intervention, which avoids the above problems at the expense of discrete surgical risk and substantial surgical and hospitalization costs. An appeal to "well-being" and "functioning" fails to indicate which of these forms of treatment should appropriately be funded. The problem is further complicated when one considers that the judgments of the patient and of the physician may differ; and, whereas people tend to think of "health" or "therapy" as technical concepts whose application is in the hands of professionals, they tend to define other concepts like "well-being" and "functioning" for themselves. The formal adequacy of Callahan's definition is therefore in question.

What about the substantive adequacy of the definition as a demarcation rule? This may seem to beg the question. We need a demarcation rule because we don't know what should and what should not be funded; therefore, how can we question such a rule by saying that it includes the wrong items? But this point presumes a false dichotomy, as often occurs when applying deductive approaches to social questions. We may (we almost certainly do) have some idea of the results desired from a rule of demarcation. We likely wish to develop a demarcation rule to sharpen an initially hazy understanding, rather than to fill a total vacuum.

Substantively, a rule may be faulty because it is either overinclusive, underinclusive, or both. It would be overinconclusive because it fails to account for the quantity of resources expended in marginal improvements in well-being or functioning. It does not tell us when the game is no longer worth the candle; and, as was noted at the outset, it is because medicine continues to yield improvements in these parameters, albeit at ever-increasing expense, that the problem we are discussing arises.

Callahan's definition would be underinclusive as well, because if it were applied rigorously benign and worthwhile services would be excluded from coverage. In his concern to combat the view that medicine should be held responsible to deliver perfect happiness, Callahan eliminates any role medicine might legitimately satisfy in this direction. Sometimes medical expertise is necessary to provide a modicum of happiness; if the costs thereby incurred are trivial enough, and the benefits (even in mere happiness) great enough, why should the required service not be funded?

Consider the following. The removal of tattoos is not usually necessary to restore function; nor, strictly speaking, is it a necessary component of well-being. Yet, the safe eradication of tattoos may require medical expertise. In Ontario, in most cases the provincial health insurance scheme does not cover the cost of tattoo removal. However, an exception is made for the eradication of prisoner-of-war or concentration camp tattoos. In some isolated instances well-being or functioning might require the removal of such tattoos, and to these cases Callahan's principle would extend. But in the usual case physical well-being and functioning are not impaired by these offensive tattoos. Is it wrong to fund this service simply out of consideration for the victims' feelings, in a situation where practical concern for these feelings requires medical expertise?

Evidently a definition of health from either end of the continuum—the relatively inclusive WHO definition, and the rather exclusive definition proposed by Callahan—will not serve as a satisfactory demarcation principle. However, quite apart from the specific problems arising from any particular definition of health, a further obstacle confronts the definitional approach to health care funding in that no definition of health has garnered general agreement. This lack of consensus is no mere accident. While on the surface the debate concerning the definition of health is technical in nature, it is clear in the writings of Szasz (1961), Kass (1975), and others that this debate serves an ideological role as well. Often the definitions advocated reflect broad views concerning such disparate issues as technocracy, nature versus nurture, and the allowable limits of eccentricity in liberal societies. Unhappily, therefore, it may be the case that consensus regarding the definition of health will have to wait for prior consensus on political and social ideology.

Also, the economic facts of health care may be another source of dissent regarding the definition of health and disease. Consider a study by Campbell, Scadding, and Roberts (1979), in which subjects were presented with a number of conditions and asked whether these represented "disease." The con-

ditions ranged from malaria and tuberculosis to drowning and starvation. Physicians, and especially general practitioners, were more likely to characterize a condition as "disease" than were lay respondents. The authors suggest that the operational equivalents of "disease" are different in the two groups. For the layman, "disease" means "Do I need a doctor?" For the physician, it means "Is it useful for me to use this label?" An alternative suggestion compatible with the observed differences is that physicians, especially family practitioners, have a vested economic interest in broadening the scope of the term "disease."

We have been arguing that reliance upon the definition of health for the purposive elucidation of a government-funded insurance program is unlikely to result in a consensual, usable, and fair system. To this one might object that the preceding argument has erred in identifying the purpose of a government-funded health insurance system as the provision of "health." A health insurance system cannot provide *health*, but at best can only provide *health care*.

This amended purposive description is not, however, immune from the criticism noted above. The objection purports to take a realistic look at what the government-funded insurance system actually does: it funds "health care." This is presumed to be a less ambiguous concept than "health." However, the definition of health care itself is crucially dependent upon prior agreement on the definition of health, so the objection only succeeds in pushing the problems we have noted one step back.

Others will object that the health care system provides neither "health" nor "health care" but "medical care" *tout court*. This, however, is no more serious an objection, for although the term "medical care" is perhaps even less ambiguous than the term "health care," the problem remains in that "medical care" is commonly understood to require that a physician's expertise be applied on behalf of restoring or preserving the health of patients. Furthermore, if we were to be fully realistic, we would have to admit that government-funded health insurance systems do not fund medical care or health care any more than they fund health. Rather, they fund health care providers, as public monies are made available precisely to pay for medical services rendered.

STRUCTURAL DEFICIENCIES OF THE PURPOSIVE APPROACH

As noted above, the two definitions of health drawn from either end of the continuum fail to adequately demarcate insurable services. It does not necessarily follow from this, however, that a definition in between these extremes would not serve.

Allowing for the remote possibility that a consensual definition of health were to be adopted, some important structural problems would remain to confront any purposive system of government-funded health insurance. These problems derive from the approach's top-down, deductive fashion of reasoning, and therefore would not be solved by any improvement in the formulation of the premises. In particular, they would persist despite changes in the definition of health or health care.

An inherent problem with the purposive-deductive approach is its rationalization of the issue of demarcation. In principle, once the premises have been adopted, all of the solutions are present; as logicians say, deductive reasoning produces no new knowledge not already embedded in the premises. Two difficulties follow from this. The purposive approach does not in principle allow for an incremental solution to the issues, within which some procedures might be funded on a trial basis while other relevantly similar procedures await the lessons of experience. Furthermore, this rationalized approach does not permit any wisdom of quantification, a problem noted earlier in reference to Callahan. It does not allow us by its premises to say that some procedure does not fall on the "fundable" side of the demarcation line, but that it is still worthy of funding (e.g., tattoo removal), or alternatively that some procedure might fall on the "fundable" side of the demarcation line, but that it is nonetheless too expensive a proposition to fund (e.g., heart transplants).

A further problem is who decides whether some service is fundable under the definition consensually adopted. He almost certainly will be some professional: possibly the individual health care provider, but more likely some government official. Thus, control of the health insurance system passes into the hands of the technocracy, and the patient is lost in the shuffle, as is indeed lay input in general (which currently may be provided through political representa-tion and control). How is the technocracy to resolve these problems? In the deductive mode of reasoning, issues of application are reduced to a search for semantic clarity and consensus. Practical issues of whether it is useful, fair, or right to cover a given treatment for a given condition are converted into an obsessive contemplation of the definition of health.

PROBLEMS OF THE PURPOSIVE APPROACH IN PRACTICE

The purposive-deductive approach is necessarily obsessed with determining whether a condition is "really" an illness. Two representative cases illustrate this point, though many other examples could be cited if space permitted. Jane Smith (a real case, though not her real name) approached an endocrinologist with a presenting complaint of excessive growth of facial and body hair. After an extensive workup (covered, incidentally, by the provincial health plan) in which no endocrinological disorder was established, she was diagnosed as suffering from "essential hirsutism." Mrs. Smith then requested of the physician a referral to an electrolysist, in the belief that the health care plan would then cover the cost of treatment. This request was refused. She was told that if the condition was causing her acute discomfort or embarrassment, she could be referred to a psychiatrist, who could then make the referral for hair removal. The kinds of questions the psychiatrist would be likely to ask could equally well have been asked by the endocrinologist. However, he felt constrained by the purposive nature of the system to validate the electrolytic referral by means of special expertise (into mental illness) which he did not feel he possessed. Thus, inappropriate gatekeeping mechanisms which are both costly and inefficient were introduced. This case illustrates one way in which the technocratic and logomachistic tendencies of the purposive approach reinforce one another.

To further illustrate this point, consider the treatment of infertility, which might include hormonal therapy or surgery as well as counselling. These therapies ordinarily are thought to fall within the boundaries of medical care. But the purposive approach must question whether infertility itself is really a "disease." If we look to an American example, Great Southern Life of Houston, a private insurance company, is reported as having denied coverage for *in vitro* fertilization on the grounds that it is "not a treatment of an illness" (*Surrogate Parenting News* 1983). Presumably a government-funded health care system similarly concerned with purposive considerations might apply the same reasoning.

Another distinction covertly used is that of the internal versus the external. There is a vague feeling that health care is a concept that relates to the individual rather than to the environment, and that fundable, fee-for-service health care interventions may be demarcated in part as those which represent internal adjustments to the human organism rather than modifications of the organism's environment. When a malnourished patient is nursed back to health through intravenous infusions, that is health care; when he or she is given money or remunerative employment supplying the wherewithal for self-nourishment, that is not health care.

The distinction makes less sense in other contexts. What of a patient suffering from a definable illness whose comprehensive treatment would include environmental modification? A major and growing current example are those patients suffering from pan-allergic syndromes. It is sometimes claimed that the alleviation of the symptoms from this disorder requires a total readjustment of the patient's living arrangements, such as moving into a cabin tiled with ceramics and discarding a wardrobe laced with allergens. Although this is asserted to be the treatment of choice, it is "external" and therefore not a covered benefit under the government health insurance scheme. Similarly, prosthetics that are implanted, like heart pacemakers, are covered benefits under Ontario's health insurance scheme, whereas externally attached prosthetics, like limbs, generally are not paid for by the Ontario Health Insurance Plan (OHIP).

THE FUNCTIONAL APPROACH: AN ALTERNATIVE

Most social institutions are established with a purpose in view. When a government-funded health insurance program is initiated, the purpose is vaguely understood to contribute to the provision of health or health care. This original purpose is in fact critical to the establishment of a government health insurance program, which is often given higher priority than comparable welfare schemes dealing in less

critical services and commodities. But once an insurance scheme is in place, it would be foolish to freeze the system in its embryonic state. With the continuing development of a health insurance plan, as it confronts issues of macroallocation and demarcation, there is no need to restrict it to the a priori wisdom that went into its establishment. On these grounds we advocate a functional approach to government health care funding.

In accordance with common usage, we define a "function" as any output of a system which is positively evaluated, whether that output was intentional or not.[1] Purposes are therefore a subset of functions, the latter including happy surprises in addition to anticipated outcomes. To revert to our earlier example, the purpose of a television set is to decode electronic signals. In most homes, however, it will also service a variety of additional functions: conversation piece, plant stand, and so on.

What would be distinctive about a functional approach to a government-funded health insurance plan? Three main differences stand between a purposive and a functional approach. These differences have to do with the characterization of those conditions which the government health insurance program should ameliorate, the demarcation of reimbursable from nonreimbursable services, and the relationship between the health plan and other government services.

With the purposive approach to the question of health care funding, funding decisions turn on whether a condition represents ill health, a disease, an illness. With a functional approach, in contrast, questions outside the realm of health are also considered. For example, has the condition resulted in impaired occupational performance? (In the infamous words of an anonymous Polish public health official, "Tuberculosis slows production.") Does the person afflicted with the condition experience disturbed functioning in other areas as a result? Is he severely distressed or depressed as a result of the condition? Is he experiencing pain? These types of considerations do sometimes appear in the purposive conception, but in a distorted, Procrustean way, as questions concerning "mental health" or "adjustment."

To illustrate this point, consider how the different approaches would deal with a difficult case of demarcation like sex-reassignment surgery. The purposive approach would need to discover whether the surgery represented the treatment of a genuine disease. In this context, the neologism "gender dysphoria" has been introduced, and psychiatrists continue to battle over its propriety and etiology. With a functional approach the questions considered in reaching a funding decision on a macro level (by bureaucrats) and in implementing the decision at the micro level (by physicians) are more straightforward. How seriously has the applicant's life been affected ? How likely is it that he/she will improve with the treatment? Is the cost justified by these benefits? Admittedly, similar questions might be asked by psychiatrists in the gender dysphoria debate. We suggest, however, that such questions are both clearer and more realistic when not filtered through the prism of a definition of disease.

The second contrast between the purposive and the functional approach is evident when deciding about the funding of discrete services. Whereas with the purposive approach one asks whether some service represents health care, with the functional approach one would ask if the service or procedure is good, worthwhile, and desired.

Consider fertility interventions. For the vast majority of women, tubal ligation per se has almost no discrete medical justification (although it certainly will "cure" the "disorder" of fecundity). On these grounds, Kass (1975) has suggested that tubal ligation or vasectomy not be included within the medical orbit. But clearly, tubal ligation is a much-desired intervention; it has recently become the most popular form of female contraception in Canada. And clearly, medical expertise is necessary to provide ligations. Also, from the economic point of view of the insurance plan, sterilization is one of the most efficient interventions available, obviating both medical costs of parturition and costs of care of the (forever-to-remain) unborn. Whereas the purposive conception forces government health care officials to conceptualize health matters in futile and disingenuous ways, the functional conception allows one to examine the real underlying concerns. Does a requested procedure—for example, tubal ligation—represent a treatment whose cost is rationally proportionate to the need it serves?

When the issue is phrased in this way, we are required to confront questions which are never raised

by the purposive approach. For example: Does the procedure in question address a human want or need, or perhaps something people ought to want or need? As difficult as these questions are, they seem to us to be the right ones to address. Among their advantages is the fact that their solution demands of us that we understand and respect the patient's perceptions of health care.

A recent study (Freedman 1983) yielded some suggestive data on this very point. The study included interviews of Canadian women applying for microsurgical attempts at reversing a prior ligation (tubal reanatomosis). During the interview, the women were asked "Do you see the reversal of the sterilization as a health procedure (like an appendectomy) or as a social procedure requiring medical assistance (like cosmetic surgery)? Most of these women, both in questionnaires and during the subsequent interviews, classified the procedure they requested as medical, but the interview responses of some of the women revealed ambivalence stemming from a variety of considerations. The following representative statements are worthy of careful consideration as they encapsulate a lay response to the issue of demarcation: " I think for my mental and emotional well-being it is necessary. It is not like cosmetic surgery, like something I could do. It is something that is inside of me. I never thought I'd feel as strongly about [it]." "No [it's not a social procedure] ... I don't feel that having a tubal done is the same thing as having a reversal done. I'm having it [the reversal] done so that we can have children ... So I really don't see it as being something that you do just to fit in. It's hard to explain but that's the way I feel about it."

How did these laypeople go about resolving this critical question of demarcation? What themes emerge from their responses? Hints are found of a variety of approaches, including the "internal/external" approach. However, their major point of consensus was the belief that because the procedure was so important to them personally, and because a doctor was needed to perform it, the procedure *must* be medical.

The population from which these responses were drawn would be expected to provide tendentious replies. It is in these women's interest to argue that the procedure they are requesting is medical in nature, and hence reimbursable. However, this fact only sharpens the point, because we would expect that they would be choosing the most persuasive demarcation principle available to support their claim.

The third divergence between the two approaches concerns the relationship between the health care system (and its public funding agent) and other elements of society. The purposive approach makes of the health care system a hermetically sealed enterprise, self-directed in terms of its original purpose and resistant to other legitimate social concerns and institutionalized values. On the other hand, with the functional approach, other social interests and resources are taken into account in deciding whether to supply a particular benefit when its request is justified in terms of health.

A functionalist perspective also allows one to consider whether the health care system is the best institution to respond to demands for particular needs. Needs (or wants) and the associated goods and services that have traditionally been seen as medical in nature may be better served by some other social institution. Alcoholism, obesity , and other diseases of lifestyle are notoriously resistant to treatment by the medical model. For the purposive approach, however, provided that these conditions are diseases and that a physician is prepared to "treat" them, such treatment would be insured. The fact that other social institutions could better deal with these conditions is irrelevant from a purposive perspective. With a functional approach one questions whether we might not be better served by "divestiture" of these conditions from medicine, at least at this point in time. Conversely, the health care system may be better suited to providing some needs which traditionally have been served outside the medical model. One such possibility might be the care of the families of dying patients by physicians, nurses, or medical social workers, a role traditionally relegated to pastors and family support systems. The funding of such a service should not wait upon the discovery of a new "disease" ("impending grief syndrome"), but should proceed immediately upon the recognition that these forms of care are valid, useful, and best accomplished within the institutions of the health care system.

QUESTIONS FOR THE FUNCTIONAL APPROACH

It might seem that the functional approach is necessarily heir to all of the criticisms presented above concerning the WHO definition of health. Under a functional approach, as under the WHO definition, the full range of human suffering and discontent become potential targets of a government-supported health care system. In fact, some might even argue that the functional approach is even more latitudinous than WHO, although it is hard to imagine what has been left out once "a complete state of physical, mental and social well-being" has been included.

This criticism, however, dissolves in the face of a critical distinction. The problem with the WHO definition, which is that it fails to exclude anything from coverage, arises in the context of a purposive system. In contrast, with a functional approach to health care funding, demarcation does not end with the recognition of a need or demand for services, but rather only begins at this point. It must then be determined whether the health care system, with its particular expertise and modalities of intervention, may redress that need efficiently; whether another social program or practice would better serve; or whether the need is so difficult to satisfy or so at odds with other values that it should not be served at all.

The whole point of the functional approach is the recognition that decisions regarding coverage involve more than semantics. In a purposive approach, once we know that a procedure serves health, we have an argument (which, to be sure, might need to be tempered by political or economic realities) that it should be funded. In a functional approach, when we know that a procedure satisfies a demand, we simply know that it is *potentially* fundable—not that it should be funded, let alone that it should be funded by the health care system.

A further point worth noting is that since functionalism contains no single decision rule for demarcation, it must address new problems which do not trouble a purposive system. However, the fact that a theory raises new questions does not necessarily count as a strike against it, provided that the questions are ones which are worth confronting. In fact, a theory might be deficient precisely because it fails to raise questions which should be answered, as at times the purposive approach slurs over the complications faced by the functional approach. In general the new problems which the functional approach must address are actually complications which arise due to the fact that patient choice is allowed, and that services traditionally considered nonmedical may be included within the boundaries of health care; therefore, a greater range of alternatives must be considered. For example, a possible negative consequence of allowing patient choice is that the costs involved might be greater. This criticism, however, also applies to the purposive approach, as the following examples will serve to illustrate.

Under the Ontario Health Insurance Plan postmastectomy breast reconstruction surgery is a covered service. This type of procedure fits comfortably within the naive notion of health services, since it involves a direct "internal" procedure on a patient's behalf. On the other hand, prosthetic devices, being "external," have not been a covered benefit for adults and have represented a repeated source of political contention. A system which proceeds under the strong purposive principle of demarcation does not recognize the need to fund environmental adjustments, since these would fall under the rubric of social welfare rather than health care. Ontario, therefore, has long refused to cover the costs of breast prostheses and surgical brassieres for victims of breast cancer, while still funding surgical breast reconstruction for those interested in pursuing that course.

A complicated situation arose in Ontario when a woman eligible for a breast reconstruction procedure offered to exchange this service for a Tucker valve set (a prosthetic device needed for "normal" speech after she had undergone a tracheotomy). The trade would have been cost-effective for the Ministry of Health, and might have saved $1000 or more. The insurance plan declined the offer as there was no apt bureaucratic means of accepting it, given that the health insurance plan funds "services" and not "goods" (*London Free Press* 1982).

Another Ontario woman suffering from a lung condition lived at home, using a mobile oxygen cart. Eventually her monthly oxygen bills—which the public health insurance program would not cover— rose to over $700. At this point, entering the hospital became, for her, the only practical economic move,

because then the insurance plan would supply her with oxygen gratis. The average cost of inpatient hospital care was estimated at approximately ten times the cost of the oxygen alone (*London Free Press* 1984). This situation similarly indicates the unreasoning prejudice a purposive system may have against environmental adjustment.

A functional approach would deal with such situations differently since patient choice would be independently relevant (if not necessarily decisive) in determining fundability. The implications of this are obviously quite serious, particularly as patients persist in expressing individual preferences on this issue, a fact which must be taken seriously by a system concerned with lay input. Honoring the choice of patients will at times be far more expensive than acceding to the choice dictated by a purposive demarcation rule. Patient autonomy in relation to funding decisions has not been an issue; but, without presuming any particular resolution, we suggest that it should be.

A functional conception would need to reexamine funding of the diverse forms of health care practice. In Ontario's quasi-purposive system, all reimbursements flow directly to, or indirectly from, physicians. Doctors may perform a service directly, or engage another professional (e.g., psychologist, physiotherapist) on a salaried basis to work under their direction, with the physician billing the government insurance program. Since physicians are certified specialists in "health," this arrangement is acceptable (although certainly not inevitable) under a purposive system. Similarly, although a physician may bill for consultation with a patient, parent, or other physician, he or she may not bill for consultation with nonphysician providers of health care. If a child is experiencing behavioral problems in school which have concerned the school psychologist, the physician may charge the government insurance plan for consultation with the parents, who may serve as middlemen between the school psychologist and the physician; but if the physician wishes to discuss the matter with the psychologist directly, he must do so on his own account. A functional system would necessarily call such arrangements into question.

As a result, in implementing a functional approach, a comprehensive government health plan would face bureaucratic dislocation. How serious would this be? To this, three points can be made: some dislocation has already occurred; some dislocation is good; and remaining dislocations need not all be faced at once.

SOME DISLOCATION HAS ALREADY OCCURRED

In Ontario, a system of psychiatric hospitals is run by the Ministry of Health. A system of facilities for the developmentally disabled is run by the Ministry of Community and Social Services (COMSOC). This kind of division would be preserved if a consistently functional approach were adopted. The facilities for the developmentally handicapped require a high level of expertise in development and programming, but the specific forms required—training of various sorts, behavioral techniques, and custodial care—are not specifically medical or nursing in nature (although both of these disciplines perform an important ancillary function). Indeed, because developmental handicap constitutes an "illness" under almost any definition, the division that currently exists between psychiatric and COMSOC facilities is inexplicable under a purposive conception.

SOME DISLOCATION IS GOOD

Many of the decisions noted above (e.g., concerning prostheses and oxygen) would be inappropriate given a functionalist perspective. Their reversal involves dislocation in itself; but in the cases noted, that seems to be all to the good. Also, some bureaucratic awkwardness, intrinsic to a purposive system, would be resolved under a functional approach. While a physician may recover from the Ontario Health Insurance Plan on behalf of the examination of a patient carried out for investigation, confirmation, or documentation of an alleged sexual assault, a portion of its outlays on this behalf are then recovered from the Ministries of the Attorney General and the Solicitor General. Similar cumbersome paper shuffling may be involved in other instances which require medical expertise, albeit outside of medical treatment (e.g., in assessments of insurance or for the purpose of establishing workmen's compensation). It would seem that the only reason the money needs to be shuffled at present is to keep the accounts clear on behalf of a system that is purposively designed to fund health care.

NOT ALL DISLOCATIONS NEED BE FUNDED AT ONCE

The saving grace of the functional approach is that it may, consistent with its own logic, be activated in an incrementalist fashion. The facts of bureaucratic life are, as are the facts of economic, political and medical life, all to be included within the calculation that should precede a decision on inclusion of a service within coverage.

In general, then, new questions of the division between medical and social services and of the cost-effectiveness of different modes of health care would directly arise under a functional system. Quantitative concerns would also need to be directly confronted: How serious is the need or desire? What value should be assigned to the honoring of the preferences of the patient? These questions need not be raised at all in a purposive system, which deals instead with questions concerning the nuances of the definitions of "health" and "health care." We will leave to others the task of parsing the seriousness of these questions. In choosing between these two approaches, however, we ought to consider which kinds of questions we want to contemplate, as well as which results we wish to achieve.

Notes

1. " ... functional analysis seeks to understand a behavior pattern or a sociocultural institution by determining the role it plays in keeping the given system in proper working order or maintaining it as a going concern" (Hempel 1985). For a general discussion of the functional approach see the chapter "The Logic of Functional Analysis," pp. 297-330, in Hempel (1985).

References

Boorse, C. 1975. On The Distinction Between Disease and Illness. *Philosophy and Public Affairs* 5 (Fall): 49-68.

Callahan, D. 1973. The WHO Definition of "Health." *The Hastings Center Studies* 1:77-87.

Campbell, E.J.M., J.G. Scadding, and R.S. Roberts. 1979. The Concept of Disease. *British Medical Journal* 2 (September): 757-62.

Freedman, B. 1983-85. Study of Ethical Issues In Infertility (unpublished material).

—. 1985. Ethical Issues in Clinical Obstetrics and Gynecology. *Current Problems in Obstetrics, Gynecology and Fertility* 7 (March): 1-47.

Hempel, C.G. 1985. *Aspects of Scientific Explanation.* New York: The Free Press.

Kass, L.R. 1975. Regarding the End of Medicine and the Pursuit of Health. *The Public Interest* 40 (Summer): 11-42.

London Free Press. 1982. OHIP won't pay for vocal device it calls luxury. 5 June: 2.

London Free Press. 1984. Woman needing pure oxygen may be forced into hospital. 3 August: 12.

Ontario Health Insurance Plan. 1983. Ministry of Health of the Province of Ontario. *Schedule of Benefits: Physician Services.* 1 January.

Surrogate Parenting News. 1983. Insurance Coverage of In Vitro. 1 (October/November):71-72.

Szasz, T. 1961. *The Myth of Mental Illness.* New York: Dell Publishing Co.

Taylor, F.K. 1971. A Logical Analysis of the Medico-Psychological Concepts of Disease. *Psychological Medicine* 1:356-64.

Turkel, Sherry. 1984. *The Second Self.* New York: Simon and Schuster.

Wasserman, J. 1983. How DRGs Work. *The Hastings Center Report* 13 (October): 24.

World Health Organization.1976. Constitution of the World Health Organization. In *World Health Organization: Basic Documents*, ed. 26. Geneva: WHO.

43.
THE PROSTITUTE, THE PLAYBOY, AND THE POET: RATIONING SCHEMES FOR ORGAN TRANSPLANTATION

George J. Annas

In the public debate about the availability of heart and liver transplants, the issue of rationing on a massive scale has been credibly raised for the first time in United States medical care. In an era of scarce resources, the eventual arrival of such a discussion was, of course, inevitable.[1] Unless we decide to ban heart and liver transplantation, or make them available to everyone, some rationing scheme must be used to choose among potential transplant candidates. The debate has existed throughout the history of medical ethics. Traditionally it has been stated as a choice between saving one of two patients, both of whom require the immediate assistance of the only available physician to survive.

National attention was focused on decisions regarding the rationing of kidney dialysis machines when they were first used on a limited basis in the late 1960s. As one commentator described the debate within the medical profession:

> Shall machines or organs go to the sickest, or to the ones with most promise of recovery; on a first-come, first-served basis; to the most "valuable" patient (based on wealth, education, position, what?); to the one with the most dependents; to women and children first; to those who can pay; to whom? Or should lots be cast, impersonally and uncritically?[2]

In Seattle, Washington, an anonymous screening committee was set up to pick who among competing candidates would receive the life-saving technology. One lay member of the screening committee is quoted as saying:

> The choices were hard ... I remember voting against a young woman who was a known prostitute. I found I couldn't vote for her, rather than another candidate, a young wife and mother. I also voted against a young man who, until he learned he had renal failure, had been a ne'er do-well, a real playboy. He promised he would reform his character, go back to school and so on, if only he were selected for treatment. But I felt I'd lived long enough to know that a person like that won't do what he was promising at the time.[3]

When the biases and selection criteria of the committee were made public, there was a general negative reaction against this type of arbitrary device. Two experts reacted to the "numbing accounts of how close to the surface lie the prejudices and mindless clichés that pollute the committee's deliberations," by concluding that the committee was "measuring persons in accordance with its own middle-class values." The committee process, they noted, ruled out "creative nonconformists" and made the Pacific Northwest "no place for a Henry David Thoreau with bad kidneys."[4]

There are four major approaches to rationing scarce medical resources: the market approach; the selection committee approach; the lottery approach; and the "customary" approach.[5]

THE MARKET APPROACH

The market approach would provide an organ to everyone who could pay for it with their own funds or private insurance. It puts a very high value on individual rights, and a very low value on equality and fairness. It has properly been criticized on a number of bases, including that the transplant technologies have been developed and are supported with public funds, that medical resources used for transplantation will not be available for higher priority care, and that financial success alone is an insufficient justification for demanding a medical procedure. Most telling is its complete lack of concern for fairness and equity.[6]

A "bake sale" or charity approach that requires the less financially fortunate to make public appeals for funding is demeaning to the individuals involved, and to society as a whole. Rationing by financial ability says we do not believe in equality, but believe that a price can and should be placed on human life and that it should be paid by the individual whose life is at stake. Neither belief is tolerable in a society in which income is inequitably distributed.

THE COMMITTEE SELECTION PROCESS

The Seattle Selection Committee is a model of the committee process. Ethic committees set up in some hospitals to decide whether or not certain handicapped newborn infants should be given medical care may represent another.[7] These committees have developed because it was seen as unworkable or unwise to explicitly set forth the criteria on which selection decisions would be made. But only two results are possible, as Professor Guido Calabrezi has pointed out: either a pattern of decision-making will develop or it will not. If a pattern does develop (e.g., in Seattle, the imposition of middle-class values), then it can be articulated and those decision "rules" codified and used directly, without resort to the committee. If a pattern does not develop, the committee is vulnerable to the charge that it is acting arbitrarily, or dishonestly, and therefore cannot be permitted to continue to make such important decision.[8]

In the end, public designation of a committee to make selection decisions on vague criteria will fail because it too closely involves the state and all members of society in explicitly preferring specific individuals over others, and in devaluing the interests those others have in living. It thus directly undermines, as surely as the market system does, society's view of equality and the value of human life.

THE LOTTERY APPROACH

The lottery approach is the ultimate equalizer which puts equality ahead of every other value. This makes it extremely attractive, since all comers have an equal chance at selection regardless of race, color, creed, or financial status. On the other hand, it offends our notions of efficiency and fairness since it makes no distinctions among such things as the strength of the desires of the candidates, their poten-

tial survival, and their quality of life. In this sense it is a mindless method of trying to solve society's dilemma which is caused by its unwillingness or inability to spend enough resources to make a lottery unnecessary. By making this macro spending decision evident to all, it also undermines society's view of the pricelessness of human life. A first-come, first-served system is a type of natural lottery since referral to a transplant program is generally random in time. Nonetheless, higher income groups have quicker access to referral networks and thus have an inherent advantage over the poor in a strict first-come, first-served system.[9]

THE CUSTOMARY APPROACH

Society has traditionally attempted to avoid explicitly recognizing that we are making a choice not to save individual lives because it is too expensive to do so. As long as such decisions are not explicitly acknowledged, they can be tolerated by society. For example, until recently there was said to be a general understanding among general practitioners in Britain that individuals over age 55 suffering from end-stage kidney disease not be referred for dialysis or transplant. In 1984, however, this unwritten practice became highly publicized, with figures that showed a rate of new cases of end-stage kidney disease treated in Britain at 40 per million (versus the US figure of 80 per million) resulting in 1500-3000 "unnecessary deaths" annually.[10] This has, predictably, led to movements to enlarge the National Health Service budget to expand dialysis to meet this need, a more socially acceptable solution than permitting the now publicly recognized situation to continue.

In the US, the customary approach permits individual physicians to select their patients on the basis of medical criteria or clinical suitability. This, however, contains much hidden social worth criteria. For example, one criterion, common in the transplant literature, requires an individual to have sufficient family support for successful aftercare. This discriminates against individuals without families and those who have become alienated from their families. The criterion may be relevant, but it is hardly medical.

Similar observations can be made about medical criteria that include IQ, mental illness, criminal records, employment, indigency, alcoholism, drug addiction, or geographical location. Age is perhaps more difficult, since it may be impressionistically related to outcome. But it is not medically logical to assume that an individual who is 49 years old is necessarily a better medical candidate for a transplant than one who is 50 years old. Unless specific examination of the characteristics of older persons that make them less desirable candidates is undertaken, such a cut off is arbitrary, and thus devalues the lives of older citizens. The same can be said of blanket exclusions of alcoholics and drug addicts.

In short, the customary approach has one great advantage for society and one great disadvantage: it gives us the illusion that we do not have to make choices; but the cost is mass deception, and when this deception is uncovered, we must deal with it either by universal entitlement or by choosing another method of patient selection.

A Combination of Approaches

A socially acceptable approach must be fair, efficient, and reflective of important social values. The most important values at stake in organ transplantation are fairness itself, equity in the sense of equality, and the value of life. To promote efficiency, it is important that no one receive a transplant unless they want one and are likely to obtain significant benefit from it in the sense of years of life at a reasonable level of functioning.

Accordingly, it is appropriate for there to be an initial screening process that is based *exclusively* on medical criteria designed to measure the probability of a successful transplant, i.e., one in which the patient survives for at least a number of years and is rehabilitated. There is room in medical criteria for social worth judgments, but there is probably no way to avoid this completely. For example, it has been noted that "in many respects social and medical criteria are inextricably intertwined" and that therefore medical criteria might "exclude the poor and disadvantaged because health and socioeconomic status are highly interdependent."[11] Roger Evans gives an example. In the End Stage Renal Disease Program, "those of lower socioeconomic status are likely to have multiple comorbid health conditions such as diabetes, hepatitis, and hypertension" making them both less desirable candidates and more expensive to treat.[12]

To prevent the gulf between the haves and have nots from widening, we must make every reasonable attempt to develop medical criteria that are objective and independent of social worth categories. One minimal way to approach this is to require that medical screening be reviewed and approved by an ethics committee with significant public representation, filed with a public agency, and made readily available to the public for comment. In the event that more than one hospital in a state is offering a particular transplant service, it would be most fair and efficient for the individual hospitals to perform the initial medical screening themselves (based on the uniform, objective criteria), but to have all subsequent non-medical selection done by a method approved by a single selection committee composed of representatives of all hospitals engaged in the particular transplant procedure, as well as significant representation of the public at large.

As this implies, after the medical screening is performed, there may be more acceptable candidates in the "pool" than there are organs or surgical teams to go around. Selection among waiting candidates will then be necessary. This situation occurs now in kidney transplantation, but since the organ matching is much more sophisticated than in hearts and livers (permitting much more precise matching of organ and recipient), and since dialysis permits individuals to wait almost indefinitely for an organ without risking death, the situations are not close enough to permit use of the same matching criteria. On the other hand, to the extent that organs are specifically tissue- and size-matched and fairly distributed to the best matched candidate, the organ distribution system itself will resemble a natural lottery.

When a pool of acceptable candidates is developed, a decision about who gets the next available, suitable organ must be made. We must choose between using a conscious, value-laden, social worth selection criterion (including a committee to make the actual choice), or some type of random device. In view of the unacceptability and arbitrariness of social worth criteria being applied, implicitly or explicitly, by committee, this method is neither viable nor proper. On the other hand, strict adherence to a lottery might create a situation where an individual who has only a one-in-four chance of living five years with a transplant (but who could survive another six months without one) would get an organ before an individual who could survive as long or longer, but who will die within days or hours if he or she is not immediately transplanted. Accordingly, the most reasonable approach seems to be to allocate organs on a first-come, first-served basis to members of the pool but permit individuals to "jump" the queue if the second level selection committee believes they are in immediate danger of death (but still have a reasonable prospect for long-term survival with a transplant) and the person who would otherwise get the organ can survive long enough to be reasonably assured that he or she will be able to get another organ.

The first-come, first-served method of basic selection (after a medical screen) seems the preferred method because it most closely approximates the randomness of a straight lottery without the obviousness of making equity the only promoted value. Some unfairness is introduced by the fact that the more wealthy and medically astute will likely get into the pool first, and thus be ahead in line, but this advantage should decrease sharply as public awareness of the system grows. The possibility of unfairness is also inherent in permitting individuals to jump the queue, but some flexibility needs to be retained in the system to permit it to respond to reasonable contingencies.

We will have to face the fact that should the resources devoted to organ transplantation be limited (as they are now and are likely to be in the future), at some point it is likely that significant numbers of individuals will die in the pool waiting for a transplant. Three things can be done to avoid this: 1) medical criteria can be made stricter, perhaps by adding a more rigorous notion of "quality" of life to longevity and prospects for rehabilitation; 2) resources devoted to transplantation and organ procurement can be increased; or 3) individuals can be persuaded not to attempt to join the pool.

Of these three options, only the third has the promise of both conserving resources and promoting autonomy. While most persons medically eligible for a transplant would probably want one, some would not—at least if they understood all that was

involved, including the need for a lifetime commitment to daily immunosuppression medications, and periodic medical monitoring for rejection symptoms. Accordingly, it makes public policy sense to publicize the risks and side effects of transplantation, and to require careful explanations of the procedure be given to prospective patients before they undergo medical screening. It is likely that by the time patients come to the transplant center they have made up their minds and would do almost anything to get the transplant. Nonetheless, if there are patients who, when confronted with all the facts, would voluntarily elect not to proceed, we enhance both their own freedom and the efficiency and cost-effectiveness of the transplantation system by screening them out as early as possible.

CONCLUSION

Choices among patients that seem to condemn some to death and give others an opportunity to survive will always be tragic. Society has developed a number of mechanisms to make such decisions more acceptable by camouflaging them. In an era of scarce resources and conscious cost containment, such mechanism will become public, and they will be usable only if they are fair and efficient. If they are not so perceived, we will shift from one mechanism to another in an effort to continue the illusion that tragic choices really don't have to be made, and that we can simultaneously move toward equity of access, quality of services, and cost containment without any challenges to our values. Along with the prostitute, the playboy, and the poet, we all need to be involved in the development of an access model to extreme and expensive medical technologies with which we can live.

Notes

1. Calabresi G, Bobbit P: *Tragic Choices*. New York: Norton, 1978.
2. Fletcher J: Our shameful waste of human tissue. *In* : Cutler DR. (ed): The Religious Situation. Boston: Beacon Press, 1969; 223-252.
3. Quoted in Fox R, Swazey J: The Courage to Fail. Chicago: Univ of Chicago Press, 1974; 232.

4. Sanders and Dukeminier: Medical advance and legal lag: hemodialysis and kidney transplantation. UCLA L Rev 1968: 15: 357.

5. See note 1.

6. President's Commission for the Study of Ethical Problems in Medicine: *Securing Access to Health Care.* US Govt Printing Office, 1983; 25.

7. Annas GJ: Ethics committees on neonatal care: substantive protection or procedural diversion? Am J Public Health 1984; 74: 843-845.

8. See note 1.

9. Bayer R: Justice and health care in an era of cost containment: allocating scarce medical resources. Soc Responsibility 1984; 9:37-52; Annas GJ: Allocation of artificial hearts in the year 2002: *Minerva v. National Health Agency.* Am J Law Med 1977; 3:59-76.

10. Commentary: UK's poor record in treatment of renal failure. Lancet July 7, 1984; 53.

11. Evans R: Health care technology and the inevitability of resource allocation and rationing decisions, Part II. JAMA 1983; 249:2208, 2217.

12. See note 11.

44.
IN VITRO FERTILIZATION AND THE JUST USE OF HEALTH CARE RESOURCES

Leonard J. Weber

INTRODUCTION

One of the ethical questions raised by the development of new human reproductive technologies is the social justice question of the circumstances under which these techniques should be services that are provided in health care plans. In a just and caring society, when would these services be available to whom?

Presuming that there are patients and physicians who find a new procedure for fertility enhancement ethically acceptable and who think that it may be of value to try it in a particular case, there still remains the question of how central or fundamental to the provision of health care it should be considered. Is it to be considered necessary care? Is it even appropriate use of health care resources?

The reproductive technology considered in this chapter is in vitro fertilization. Before turning the specific question of what justice requires in regard to access to IVF, however, it is important to reflect more generally on patient rights and on the appropriate criteria for allocating limited health care resources.

PATIENT RIGHTS

Much of the emphasis in health care ethics during the last generation has been focused on patient rights. The emphasis on patient rights has led to a more extended understanding of some patient prerogatives than previously acknowledged. It has become widely accepted, for example, that, except in unusual circumstances, an informed patient's refusal of unwanted medical treatment should be respected, even if the treatment is likely to be quite beneficial and even if the patient may die as a result of refusing the treatment. A patient's right to informed consent means that she or he should not be treated without permission. This is much more clearly recognized now than it was a generation ago.

Not every claim to a right is of the same sort, however. It is one thing to claim that we all have a basic right to refuse unwanted medical treatment. It is something quite different to claim that we all have a basic right to a medical treatment or technology simply because we think it would meet our needs or wants. These are very different claims about rights.

The right to consent to, or to refuse, proposed treatment is best understood as a negative right. It is a right to be left alone, a claim not to be coerced or compelled or interfered with as one lives according to his or her beliefs and values. A physician may not agree with my decision to refuse treatment. She or he may, in fact, think that I am doing myself great harm and may try to persuade me to change my mind. But, if I am not harming someone else and understand the consequences of my decision, I have a justifiable claim that others let me act according to my understanding of what is best for me. This right is closely related to the right to freedom of worship or to freedom of speech. The claim is that others should let me live and express myself according to my own values.

The recognition that we have basic negative rights does not take us very far in understanding the legitimate claim that patients can make on society to have certain health care services available. This is a different sort of claim. Negative rights are based on the need that we all have for self-determination and for privacy. Positive rights are claims that we legitimately make on society that certain needs be met or certain services be available for our use. To claim a positive right is to claim that others have a responsibility to facilitate one's claim, not simply to leave one alone. These rights are based on the recognition that social goods should be distributed in a way that meets everyone's basic needs. They are based on the principle of justice rather than on the principle of self-determination.

To claim that everyone with a certain condition has a right to medical treatment (or a particular type of medical treatment) is to assert a positive right. It is to say that, if society is to be just, it has a responsibility to make that treatment available. The emphasis given in medical ethics on a patient's negative rights, such as the right to refuse proposed treatment, has no implications whatsoever for the question of whether society has an ethical responsibility to make a certain type of medical technology available.

John Robertson has argued that there is a close connection between traditional concepts of reproductive freedom and the right to assisted reproduction. He says, for example, that infertile couples have "the same right to have and rear offspring through the assistance of medical technology that fertile couples have through sexual intercourse."[1] This comparison confuses rather than helps to understand the issue, it seems to me. The right to procreate should primarily be recognized as a negative right, the right to make one's own decisions regarding whether or not to reproduce. That is very different from a right to medical assistance in reproduction or the right to have a baby. It is confusing a negative right with a positive right. If we come to recognize that persons do, in fact, have a legitimate claim (a right) to demand medical assistance in human reproduction, it would be because we have determined that the right to reproduce is a positive right. That recognition does follow automatically, however, from the traditional recognition of the negative right to reproduction.

No Consumer Sovereignty

Justice does require that certain health care services be made available to those who can benefit from them (even if they may not be able to purchase these services). In this sense, there is a positive right to a level or type of health care. There will be further discussion of this a little later, but first it may be helpful to try to address another potential source of confusion.

Although market mechanisms are often used in the provision of health care, the model of a private economic exchange is not very helpful for understanding what are appropriate claims that patients can make. Patient claims for services should not be confused with "consumer sovereignty." The concept of consumer sovereignty suggests that customers are always right; they can have whatever they want, provided, of course, they can arrange payment. Consumer sovereignty may make good sense when talking about private marketplace purchases of commodities. It does not serve as an adequate principle, however, when individuals seek services from professionals or when we as a society determine what sorts of professional services should be available to the public, or when decisions are made about what services should be covered in a health care plan. I can choose a blazer that the salesperson thinks will not "do anything" for me. I cannot (and should not be able to) choose a surgery that the surgeon thinks will not "do anything" for me.[2]

Respect for patient rights does not mean that patients should be able to get whatever health care services they want or are convinced that they need. It does not mean the recognition of a right to demand and get what is not considered medically appropriate or what is judged contrary to professional ethics. It does not mean that one has a right to demand "everything" and get it. A just health care system is one that seeks to base decision-making on need, on benefit, and on a consideration of alternative uses of resources. George Annas has claimed that professional associations have failed in their responsibility to establish criteria for the appropriate use of assisted reproduction techniques and that this failure is the result, in large part, of the acceptance of a market-consumer model:

> Current practice is to provide consumer-patients whatever they want (and can pay for), rather than to attempt to develop a professional model that sets meaningful practice and ethical standards or that takes the welfare of resulting children seriously.[3]

Whether Anna's judgment about current practice is correct or not, the concern is very much to the point. There is a problem when professional services are provided as though they are simply consumer items.

Health care is best thought of as a social or public good that should be used to meet the health care needs of the community. Even in the United States, where there is a strong effort to maintain a private dimension to health care, many practices reflect this public dimension. The government invests in and subsidizes health care extensively (in medical education, research, and facilities, for example); the state licenses those who are permitted to practice in the health professions; the public provides health care for (some of) those who are unable to meet their own needs. What should be available to individuals in the health care system is, at least in part, a question of the appropriate use of public resources. The market model of simple exchange between private parties is not adequate.[4]

If patients are not consumers who can have whatever they want and are able to pay for, what are the legitimate demands that patients can make? In a just and caring society, individual patients:

1. Have a legitimate claim to a basic level of health care; and
2. Have a legitimate claim to their fair share of limited resources; but
3. Have no legitimate claim to treatment judged by professionals to be nonbeneficial; and
4. Have no legitimate claim to treatment that is being withheld as part of a just rationing or allocation system.

This formulation is proposed as one way of expressing the nature and limits of the patient's positive rights in health care. It provides a framework for reflecting on the question of whether justice requires that a particular medical procedure be available to those who find it ethically acceptable.

ALLOCATION OF LIMITED HEALTH CARE RESOURCES

Society is not able or willing to invest all the resources necessary to provide everyone with all potentially beneficial treatment. Furthermore, there are limits on what we as a society ought to spend on health care, given other social goods (like education, safety, recreation, economic security). We cannot have everything; we must make some choices. Health care rationing, the policy of limiting the availability of potentially beneficial treatment, is a necessity. It is both a practical necessity and a moral necessity.

Once we acknowledge that everyone cannot have all potentially beneficial treatment, we are faced with the question of how to decide who gets what. This is the question of the just allocation of limited health care resources or the question of just rationing. One method is to let the market make this determination: Those who are able to pay the market price have access to particular treatments, those who cannot do not.

A market-based allocation of limited health care resources is usually not referred to as rationing, but it is clearly a method of deciding who gets what limited resources. I think that we can find a better approach to rationing, one that meets justice standards more satisfactorily.

Respect for the dignity of each individual is the essential foundation of a just and caring society. Respect for human dignity means that all of us, regardless of our power, our race, our abilities, our achievements, or our financial resources can make binding claims on others and on the society in which we live. We can make a legitimate claim that our fundamental freedoms be respected (negative rights), and that our most basic and essential needs be met (positive rights). There is something fundamentally and morally wrong when they are not.

As a society, we have a responsibility to assure that persons do not starve or suffer serious malnutrition simply because they are unable to buy food, that they do not freeze to death or live without shelter simply because they cannot pay rent, and that they have an opportunity for basic education even if they cannot buy education. Meeting these needs is indispensable to the protection of human dignity. So also, I think, is access to a basic level of health care. A just society assures access to a basic level of medical care and to a basic level of public health services, even if one cannot afford to buy health care.

The very first principle of just allocation is, therefore, that *a basic level of health care must be provided for everyone.* The requirement that everyone be assured access to a basic level of health care does not mean, of course, that everyone must have access to all potentially beneficial treatments or all the treatments that he or she wants, just as the right to education does not mean a right to unlimited education or to whatever type of education one desires.

The second principle is a response to a different concern. Before withholding any treatment that has a reasonable expectation of some benefit, it is important that limited resources not be wasted on nonbeneficial treatments. Justice requires that *no one be provided treatment that is expected to be futile or nonbeneficial*. Where research and experience indicate that a patient at a certain stage of a particular condition is, in the best medical judgment, not going to benefit from a particular intervention, it should not be done, even if the patient or family insists that it be done. Professional standards should clearly not permit such health care delivery and a just health insurance should not include it as a covered service.

JUST RATIONING

Basic health care should be provided for everyone; nonbeneficial health care should be provided for no one. The third category is treatment that is not required as basic health care (essential to minimal respect for human dignity), but may provide benefit. Limited health care resources are not so limited that none of the potentially beneficial treatment that goes beyond the basic level can be provided. On the other hand, the limited resources are not so vast that nearly all of the potential beneficial treatments can be provided for everyone. It is in this third category that we must make the hard decisions regarding what should be available for whom.

The third principle of just allocation is that *allocation criteria for potentially beneficial treatment should be established in a public and democratic (open) process*. There are a variety of possible methods to be used to determine who gets what when not everyone can get everything. It is essential that the decisions be made as policy decisions and not by individuals "at the bedside." It is also essential that the process of setting policy be one that permits all those affected to have the opportunity to know what is at issue and the opportunity to have their points of view considered.

This is a requirement for a fair or just procedure. What is ethically unacceptable is what is sometimes referred to as implicit or invisible rationing. Fair policies and practices are ones in which nothing needs to be hidden.[5]

A good rationing policy requires the determination of how high a particular treatment is in a priority listing. As a caring society or as a group of caring persons joined together in a common health care plan, we would like to have as many potentially beneficial treatments available as possible. Since we cannot provide all treatments for everyone, however, it makes sense to cover first those that have a higher priority.

A statement of proposed priority principles may be helpful in identifying the kinds of questions that need to be answered when making decisions about how high a priority a particular treatment should have in the allocation of limited health care resources. Such principles might include the following:

1. Treatment that, if successful, provides a significant benefit to the patient takes priority over treatment that, if successful, provides only marginal benefit.
2. A treatment that can benefit many persons generally takes priority over a treatment that can benefit only a few.
3. A treatment that is less expensive generally takes priority over a treatment that is more expensive.

These first three principles are simply different expressions of the belief that it makes good ethical sense to try to get as much benefit as possible out of limited resources. It is reasonable to try to achieve as much good as possible.

It is also important to include priority principles that help to minimize bias and the influence of the powerful in the determination of who should get what. For example:

4. Allocation decisions should not be made on the basis of who personally "merits" or "deserves" treatment.
5. Special consideration should be given to prevent a major negative impact of allocation decisions on persons with disabilities or on those who are the least powerful members of the society.

These last principles are necessary to reduce the likelihood that efforts at democratic decision making will lead to the implementation of widely shared negative biases or to decision making simply for the majority. True democracy protects the interests of all the people, including those who are not vocal in speaking for themselves.

There is no guarantee, of course, that an open and public process for establishing rationing policy will adopt principles or guidelines like the ones that I have just proposed. The discussion that follows regarding coverage of in vitro fertilization in a just allocation system is, however, based on these principles as well as on the understanding of patient rights outlined in the preceding.

IVF AND A BASIC LEVEL OF HEALTH CARE

Whether the in vitro fertilization process, as used, is so ethically questionable and so filled with serious negative social implications that it should not be permitted at all is a question that is beyond the parameters of this chapter. The assumption here is that it will not be prohibited in all cases and that there will continue to be infertile couples who personally find this an ethically acceptable method to use in trying to achieve parenthood. In these circumstances, when should it be an insured service?

Applying the general approach to just allocation of health care resources outlined earlier, the first question that must be asked about IVF is whether it should be understood to be part of the basic level of health care that should be provided for everyone.

If the right to have a baby is a positive human right, then society has a responsibility to provide services like IVF to all those who desire them and could benefit from them. I do not think, however, that a convincing case can be made that becoming a parent is necessary in order to meet basic human needs. It is certainly very important to many individuals and couples, but it does not rate as essential to human dignity in the same way that food and shelter do. As was suggested earlier, and as Mary Mahowald concludes, it "seems clear that the right to have a baby is at most a ... negative right of individuals."[6]

To say that there is no basic right to medical assistance to have a baby is not to say that such medical assistance should not be available at all. It is simply to say that a health-care allocation plan without guaranteed access to this service for everyone is not, by that fact, unjust.

Sometimes the term "medically necessary" is used to describe the procedures that should be included in a basic health insurance plan. The problem with the concept of medical necessity is that it can be a very elastic term. Physicians sometimes say that a patient "needs" a particular treatment when they mean that the patient will suffer serious harm without the treatment and that, with the treatment, there is a good possibility of preventing the harm. They sometimes say that a patient "needs" a particular treatment when they mean that the treatment may or may not help, but is the only medical intervention available. For "medical necessity" to be a useful term for what types of medical treatments should be provided for everyone, we need greater clarity and precision regarding the meaning of the term.

In an article focusing on the meaning of "medical necessity" in mental health care, Sabin and Daniels consider different ways of understanding the concept.[7] Although their focus is on mental health care, their discussion may be helpful in reflecting on a condition like infertility. In particular, I find the distinction made between the "normal function model" and the "capability model" of medical necessity an important one.

> In the normal function model, the central purpose of health care is to maintain, restore, or compensate for the restricted opportunity and loss of function caused by disease and disability. Successful health care restores people to the range of capabilities that they would have had without the pathological condition or prevents further deterioration.[8]

It is not the fundamental purpose of health care to try to correct all disadvantages, according to this view. Thus, health care insurance coverage should be focused primarily on those disadvantages caused by disease or a specifically diagnosed disability.

In the capability model, health care should strive to give greater opportunity to people of diminished capacity, whatever the cause of the diminished capacity. "The capability model makes no moral dis-

tinction between treatment of illness and enhancement of disadvantageous personal capabilities."[9] The
very fact that one is disadvantaged in the ability to
function is sufficient reason to say that treatment is
medically necessary.

Sabin and Daniels argue that a well-grounded
understanding of medical necessity is essential for
the development of a just and practical system of
health insurance in an age of limited resources. They
conclude, and I agree, that the normal function model
provides for a better understanding of medical necessity. Although there are important moral considerations in the capability model (society should be concerned about assisting those with disadvantages), the
concept is too broad to distinguish between what
health insurance should necessarily cover and what
might be considered optional. Enhancing human
capabilities is an important social goal, but health
care is not the only way in which society should
respond to the disadvantages of individuals.

There may well be situations in which health care
technology can and should be used to enhance fertility. The point here is simply that the fact of infertility does not itself make such treatment medically
necessary or one that should be covered as a basic
service. As George Annas has noted, new technologies can quickly get perceived as medically necessary: "Thus it was not surprising to see the indication
for IVF expand quickly from an initial indication of
blocked fallopian tubes to a point where idiopathic
infertility is a sufficient indication."[10] When we are
unable to make a distinction between what is necessary and what is desirable, it is very difficult to place
any reasonable limits on the kind of health care that
must be provided to everyone in order to provide
necessary care.

There is no basic right to assisted reproduction. It
is not medically necessary to provide IVF in every
case where it might be considered an option for infertile couples seeking parenthood. Society's responsibility to meet everyone's essential and basic heath
care needs does not require guaranteed access to IVF.

IVF AND THE RATIONING OF HEALTH CARE

To recommend that IVF not be part of basic health
care guaranteed to everyone who can benefit from
the treatment is not to say that IVF should never be
available for anyone. I agree with the conviction
expressed by the Canadian Royal Commission on
New Reproductive Technologies: "if ethical, safe,
and effective medical procedures are available to
assist people to have children, a caring society
should provide them through the health care system."[11] I would add an additional qualifier that the
Commission also uses in its work: provided these
medical procedures are not overly costly.

Infertility is a serious misfortune for those who
would like to have children. Although it is essential
to evaluate the ethical nature and the social effects of
the methods used to assist those who are or appear to
be infertile, the goal of improving their chances of
having children is a highly desirable one.

IVF was originally used to assist in reproduction
for women who have fallopian tube blockage resulting from disease. Over the years it has come to be
applied in a much wider variety of indications (such
as unexplained infertility, ovulation defects,
endometriosis, and menopause). The Canadian
Royal Commission researched the effectiveness of
IVF and concluded that: "despite the proliferation of
its use for other diagnoses, we found that IVF has
been demonstrated to be effective only for the indication it was originally developed to treat—fallopian
tube blockage."[12] The criterion for effectiveness
used was that IVF should be considered effective if
couples with IVF had a greater likelihood of having
a live birth than infertile couples who did not undergo IVF.[13]

The Commission adopted the concept of "evi-
dence-based medicine" for its work. Medical practice should be based on knowledge gained from evaluation of treatments and their results. It is not
enough that there is a problem that a particular intervention "might" help. The Commission took a strong
stand in regard to the use of procedures that have not
been proven effective:

It would be unethical ... to offer services or assistance in
the form of unproven procedures or treatment. It would
be irresponsible to devote public resources to such procedures in the absence of knowledge about their risks
and effectiveness, and about their costs and benefits relative to other approaches to solving the problem and
other calls on available resources.[14]

Applying this principle to IVF, the Commission concluded that it is "unethical and unsafe to permit IVF to be used as a treatment for indications for which it has not been found effective."[15] The use of IVF for other diagnoses than complete fallopian tube blockage should be restricted to research trials to determine effectiveness and safety. In the future, there may be reason to expand the number of approved uses of IVF as a treatment, but not at this time. The Commission recommended that IVF as a treatment for complete fallopian tube blockage be covered by provincial health insurance plans.

Although the Canadian Royal Commission is making its recommendations in a health care system that is very different from the one in effect in the United States, it might well be followed in determining when health care plans in the US should cover IVF. The Commission's principles and criteria for the allocation of health care resources are quite similar to those advocated in this chapter. Treatment that does not provide a reasonable expectation of benefit should ordinarily not be provided. Treatment that does have a reasonable likelihood of providing a significant benefit should be quite high in priority listing.

If the Commission's findings on the effectiveness of IVF are accurate, it seems reasonable to conclude that a just allocation of health care resources would include IVF in cases of complete fallopian tube blockage as a covered treatment, if possible. That is, it would be covered unless available resources are such that, when compared with other desired health care treatments for other problems in terms of cost, benefits, effectiveness, and number of persons affected, it cannot be afforded. Although it is desirable to cover IVF in these cases, no one's rights are being violated if it is not.

If the Commission's findings on the effectiveness of IVF are accurate, IVF as a treatment for the other indications for which it is sometimes used would not be covered as a just health care plan at this time. Until there is evidence that IVF is truly effective for some other indication, it would be extremely hard to justify using limited health care plan resources for its use.

There remains, of course, one other option available to some infertile couples who are considering IVF for noncovered indications: the private pay/private clinic option. This remains an option, but not, it seems, one to be enthusiastically promoted. Reasons to hesitate regarding the use of IVF as a privately paid option, outside the health care plan, include the lack of evidence regarding the effectiveness of IVF for most diagnoses of infertility and the commercialization of reproduction that may result from purchasing IVF outside shared health care plans.

CONCLUSION

A just and caring society would make medical assistance available through the health care system to infertile persons who want to have a baby, if the methods used do not undermine important social and ethical values, the methods used are safe and effective achieving their goals, and this use of health care has a high enough priority when compared with other types of safe and effective medical treatments.

The question of the social and ethical impact of IVF technique and the actual ways in which the procedure is used has not been addressed here. The conclusion proposed here is that, even if we are satisfied that ethical and social considerations should not lead to the prohibition of the use of the technique, IVF can claim a relatively high priority only as a treatment for complete fallopian tube blockage.

Notes

1. Robertson, John (1994) Liberty and assisted reproduction. *Trial* (August), 49-53.
2. Weber, Leonard (1990) Consumer sovereignty vs. informed consent: saying no to requests to "do everything" for dying patients. *Bus. Prof. Ethics J.* (Fall-Winter), 95-102.
3. Annas, George (1994) Regulatory models for human embryo cloning: the free market, professional guidelines, and government restrictions. *Kennedy Inst. Ethics J.* 4, 235-249.
4. Fleck, Leonard (1992) Just health care rationing: a democratic decisionmaking approach. *U. Penn. Law Rev.* 140, 1597-1636.
5. *Idem.*
6. Mahowald, Mary (1993) *Women and Children in Health Care: An Unequal Majority.* Oxford University Press, New York.

7. Sabin, James and Daniels, Norman (1994) Determining "medical necessity" in mental health practice. *Hastings Ctr. Rep.* (November-December) 5-13.

8. *Idem.*

9. *Idem.*

10. See note 3.

11. Royal Commission on New Reproductive Technologies (1993) *Proceed with Care,* 2 vols, Minister of Government Services, Ottawa.

12. *Idem.*

13. *Idem.*

14. *Idem.*

15. *Idem.*

45

EQUALITY AND EFFICIENCY AS BASIC SOCIAL VALUES

Michael Stingl

SOCIAL VALUES AND POLITICAL CHOICES

Equality and efficiency are two key terms in the growing national debate over reforming the Canadian health system. Both are widely understood to refer to values basic in the structure and identity of Canadian society. But this is true only on a loose understanding of both terms; in the debate over health reform, both terms mean different things to different people. As long as equality and efficiency remain widely but only loosely understood, the likelihood increases that this debate will become politically intractable and socially divisive.

In this paper, I examine some of the different things that those participating in the debate often mean by equality and efficiency. Taking stock of these different meanings, I distinguish several points of potential reform where we can expect the two values to coincide, as well as several where we can expect them to collide. It is this latter possibility, of course, that is the more ethically interesting and troubling: the fact that in reforming the health system, having more of the one value will sometimes mean having less of the other.

Basic social values guide public policy, and more generally, determine the conditions and limits of social interaction between individuals, groups, and institutions within Canada. They provide the shared social framework within which each of us defines his or her own life. When such values collide, we are individually and collectively faced with a social choice. On the one hand, we might allow our social values to shift in ways that, at least on the surface, avoid conflict; on the other hand, we might simply accept the fact that social values will sometimes collide, and when this happens, face the difficult choice of which value ought to give way to which. In either case, we need to be clear about who the "we" is that is determining the course of social change. Choices regarding basic social values must not be hidden away within governmental bureaucracies, but debated publicly and openly within the larger political context of Canadian society as a whole. In a modern liberal society, determining the basic conditions of our social network with one another is an important right and an important responsibility, for again, basic social values not only determine the structure and identity of Canadian society, but as well, the structure and identity of our lives as individual Canadians.

Determining which basic social value should give way to which is thus a political choice in the broadest sense of the term. What is required to make such choices is public debate and government action. And this is what we are now seeing in varying degrees across Canada: public debate about the importance and possible limits of the Canadian health system and Canadian social services more generally, and government initiatives to make these services more responsive to deficit and debt as well as the needs of all Canadians. To evaluate these initiatives, and to make the social choices they represent wisely, we need a clear public understanding of what terms equality and efficiency really mean.

TWO DIFFERENT MEANINGS OF EQUALITY

In the debate over health reform it is necessary to distinguish between two very different ways of thinking about human society. On the one hand, we might see society as providing nothing more than the institutional framework necessary for humans to organize the individual pursuit of their own separate ends, as they personally choose to define them. On this picture of society, it is the individual who is of fundamental value; society exists only as a set of formalized arrangements to better enable each individual to pursue his or her own personal good. This is the libertarian view of society.

On the other hand, we might see society as a joint, cooperative venture, participation in which creates the sense of a greater, social good that grounds and gives context to everyone's own personal good. On this second picture of human society individuals will still be fundamentally important, but so too will society. Personal goods may be pursued, but only as part of a larger, cooperative enterprise that works fairly and equally for the good of everyone. This second sort of view might be called liberal egalitarianism, "liberal" because it values the liberty to pursue one's own personal good, but "egalitarian" because it is prepared to limit such liberty for the good of others.[1]

Each of the two different ways of thinking about human society leads to its own idea of what it means to treat persons equally. To understand these two different meanings of equality, we need to examine more fully the views of society on which they are based.[2]

Let us start with what is common between the two views: the value of individual liberty. What makes human beings the interesting, valuable creatures that they are is the fact that they are able to think about and choose the ends towards which they will act. At the most general level, these ends may include such diverse things as material wealth, love and friendship, knowledge, or social power and prestige. Whatever particular mix of such ends a person might choose to pursue, the important thing about people is that they are able to make such choices; they are able, that is, to determine the goals and aims that give structure and meaning to their individual lives.

Acting alone, however, no one individual is likely to get very far towards any of the more interesting or complex ends that make our lives richly or fully human. For the goods that matter most to us, like having children or embarking on a career, we need the help of other people, or at the very least, their non-interference. This, then, is one minimal role that society might play in human life: to insure that no one individual unfairly interferes with the independent choices of another.

This libertarian view of society is developed at length by the philosopher Robert Nozick in his book *Anarchy, State and Utopia*.[3] According to Nozick, legitimate state authority exists only to enforce rules of non-interference between individual citizens, rules that outlaw things like lying, cheating, stealing, or reneging on promises. Regulating such actions allows a free market to develop between individuals

that enables them to trade goods and service in ways that are mutually beneficial. On this free market view of human society, any trade that is consented to is fair, as long as the consent is not the result of coercion; as long, that is, as it is not the result of anything like lying, cheating, or any of the other forms of illicit interference in the life of another. The function of the state is not to create a market of exchanges, but rather to create the social conditions that freely allow such markets to develop and flourish. The markets themselves are nothing more than the separately motivated choices of individuals to enter into trading arrangements with one another.

According to this first view of society, people are ultimately separate from one another, and relationships of interchange and benefit require mutual agreement. Beyond non-interference, no one owes anyone anything. Each may enter into a free market of exchanges to derive whatever goods or services others agree to trade, but no one is obliged to participate in whatever markets might otherwise develop between others, nor to benefit in any way those who are for some reason unable to participate in such markets. Out of charity one might choose to help such a person, but no one is in any way morally obliged to render aid. The motto of this view is that I have my life, and you have yours: and just as I might choose to enter freely into an exchange of goods or services with you, I might just as freely choose not to.

The second way of thinking about human society and human life is not a simple reversal of libertarianism. It does not move to the opposite extreme of declaring that it is society that is of fundamental or primary importance, and individuals of mere derivative value. Liberal egalitarianism, like libertarianism, values individual choice. But unlike libertarianism, it gives independent value to the ongoing social relationships that link the choices of one person to those of the next. It recognizes that although each of us may choose the course of our own life, none of us chooses the background of ongoing social cooperation that makes such a choice possible. Where libertarianism sees society as nothing more than a series of individual agreements, the second conception sees society as having an independent existence and value of its own.

This second view of society is developed at length by the philosopher John Rawls in his book *A Theory of Justice.*[4] According to Rawls, a society is fairly arranged only when it is reasonable for any and all its members to consent to being part of it. Because the rich, full lives that matter most to humans require the shared cooperation of others, some social arrangement will be preferable to no social arrangement in all but the most dire circumstances. The problem is that different arrangements will offer different benefits to different people. A social arrangement that benefits some individuals more will benefit others less, depending on whose natural talents are in greater demand and generate greater social and individual rewards. Moreover, just as some individuals will suffer accidents that diminish whatever opportunities they would have had for developing their talents or lives in ways they might otherwise have chosen, some individuals will be born in ways that similarly limit the range of opportunities available to them.

So the question is, what sort of social arrangement would it be reasonable to enter into, regardless of one's plans, talents, or infirmities? According to Rawls, the only society it would be reasonable for each of us to enter into is one that guarantees every individual the same equal chance to pursue whatever life plan he or she might choose. People being people, such plans will of course vary greatly, some plans requiring more social resources, some fewer. But Rawls's idea is that whatever sort of life we might choose to lead, two basic sorts of goods will be important to us: civil liberties, like freedom of speech, association, and conscience, and material resources, like income and wealth. Since there is no way that those with fewer civil liberties could ever be advantaged by a social system that distributed such liberties unequally, the first principle of a just society is equal liberty for all. But with regard to material resources, Rawls claims that the situation is markedly different: if more productive individuals are allowed economic incentives, the social pie as a whole will be greater, and so those with lower incomes will have more material resources than they would under a system which distributed income and wealth in a strictly egalitarian fashion. To the extent that those with less material wealth are more advantaged than they otherwise would be, unequal levels of material wealth will be reasonable in a fair and just society.

We will return to Rawls' two principles in the next section, the first governing the fair distribution of basic liberties, and the second governing the fair distribution of material wealth. The question there will be whether health care, or health more generally, is a good more like liberty or more like wealth.

The point here is that just as there are two different ideals of modern society, there are also two different conceptions of equality. For the libertarian, each individual is treated equally by a state that guarantees no more than non-interference between individuals. The state itself treats individuals unequally when it interferes in the lives of its citizens to transfer between them material resources that were initially acquired through free exchange. Enforced charity, by means of a taxation scheme, for example, that transfers resources from those with more to those with less, is not fair or just according to the libertarian view of human life and society. Again, those with more may freely choose to help those with less, but they may just as freely choose not to.

For Rawls, on the other hand, transfers between individuals are required to ensure that each has an equal opportunity to lead whatever life he or she might choose. Since more productive individuals are allowed greater material resources only so far as this is required as an economic incentive to produce more goods and services overall, taxation is just up to the point that the social product as a whole would begin to diminish. Taxation is fair, that is, up to the point that the economic incentives for the better off would cease to motivate them to be more productive.

Something like this second notion of equality is arguably behind the single-tiered structure of the current Canadian health system.[5] The general form of the argument would be that because our health is equally important to all of us regardless of what sort of life we might choose to pursue, taxation schemes that provide equal health benefits to everyone represent a fair and just social arrangement, one that it would be reasonable for all individuals to enter into no matter what their talents of infirmities. Because of the kind of good that health is, each of us is treated as a moral equal only if we are each given an equal amount of health insurance.

In contrast, the current health system of the United States is more nearly libertarian, since individuals are guaranteed only as much health insurance as they are able to purchase in the free market of private insurance plans. This system is not perfectly libertarian, however, because public insurance is provided for people falling below a certain economic baseline or over a certain age limit. Even so, public insurance plans in the U.S. are extremely limited in their coverage, and there are a significant number of Americans above the economic baseline for public insurance who can nevertheless afford little or no private insurance.[6] It is thus unclear to what extent public insurance plans in the U.S. represent charity or justice for those unable to afford adequate private insurance.

More interesting than the U.S. system, and more conceptually problematic, is the sort of hybrid, two-tiered system of health insurance advocated by some Canadian health reformers.[7] Unlike public insurance plans in the United States, all medically necessary services would be covered for all Canadians, but for services deemed not necessary, or for faster or better quality service, access would be available only to people able to afford additional insurance or direct payment. As we shall see in the next section, it is hard to determine whether the idea of equality presupposed by this sort of two-tiered health system is a coherent one.

HEALTH AS A BASIC GOOD

Just as there are two importantly different ways in which we might think about society, and hence equality, there are two importantly different ways in which we might think about the value of health services.

On the one hand, we might think of health services as services like any other: just as we might avail ourselves of the services of a travel agent or hair dresser, we might also avail ourselves of the services of a doctor, nurse, or any other health professional. On the other hand we might think of health services as having a direct tie to health, which alongside political liberty and material wealth we might consider a basic social good.[8]

If we follow Rawls in defining basic goods as those things that are likely to matter to us whatever our life plan might be, health seems an obvious addi-

tion to the list. Some people, however, seem entirely prepared to trade off at least portions of their health for other goods, such as the pleasures of smoking or high cholesterol diets. Although this does not change the fact that certain levels of health are needed to lead human lives however they might be defined by the individuals leading them, it does raise the possibility of a mixed understanding of the good of health, and hence, of health services. Perhaps only some health services, but not all, need to be understood as integral to the basic good of health. The health services that are not tied directly to the level of health needed to lead a good life, however one might define it, might then be understood as service like any other, commodities to be sought out and paid for by those who desire them.

Let us return here to Rawls' two principles for distributing basic goods. The first principle, the one regarding liberty, is strictly egalitarian. Because of the kind of basic good civil liberties represent, people are treated equally only if they receive equal amounts of this particular good. Here we need to remember the leading idea of Rawls' two principles, that it is equally reasonable for all to participate in a given social arrangement only if that arrangement gives everyone an equal opportunity to pursue their life plans however they might choose to define them. In general, this conception of society requires basic social goods to be distributed equally; the only exception is when distributing a good unequally means more of that same good for all. This is the situation, Rawls says, with material wealth: all do better than they otherwise would if some are given economic incentives to be more productive.

Considered alongside the basic goods of liberty and material wealth, health would seem to be a good more like the former than the latter. Allowing different levels of health does not in any immediate sort of way make those with less health better off than they would otherwise be, and so in this important respect, health seems to have more in common with political liberty than material wealth. If there are no other important differences between them, then it would seem that health ought to be distributed like liberty: in a strictly egalitarian way.

But there are a number of important differences between health services and the sorts of social arrangements needed to guarantee our civil liberties. First, health services can increase in number, kind, and cost. Civil liberties, on the other hand, are limited in number, and tend to be all or nothing. Were a state, for example, to guarantee political but not religious freedom, we would not think it a state that guaranteed freedom of speech, association, and conscience. But it does not seem in principle wrong that a state might provide antibiotics for everyone who needed them but not artificial hearts. Moreover, certain choices of what sort of a life one is going to lead seem legitimately to require or to allow trade-offs involving increased health risks. So while a state can guarantee through its laws and political institutions equal liberty, it cannot through its health services guarantee anything approaching equal health, whatever technologies might be available to it.

Finally, it may be that by allowing a second tier of health services to develop, those with only publicly provided, first-tier services available to them will do better than they otherwise might. There are several ways this might happen, such as less waiting time or innovative treatment options that are developed at and filter down from the more expensive privately purchased second tier of services. But there are also reasons for supposing that things will not be better for those who find themselves limited to first-tier services, as resources, personnel, and finally funding are increasingly drawn away from the first tier to the second. What would in fact happen were the Canadian system to go from one tier to two is far from clear.

Taken together, these differences between liberty and health suggest that health services might be more appropriately distributed in accord with something like Rawl's second principle of justice, the one regarding material wealth. The most straightforward way of doing this would be to incorporate their distribution directly into the second principle's distribution of material wealth. Assume, that is, that income and wealth were distributed in such a way that whatever inequalities existed made those with less as well off as they could be. To give those with less any more would be to decrease the incentives to the more productive members of society below the level at which they will continue to be as productive as they are.[9] It might then seem to be fair to allow

people to purchase as much or as little as they wanted. What rankles about this suggestion given the current free market method of distributing health services in the U.S. is that material wealth is clearly not distributed in accord with Rawls' second principle in either the U.S. or Canada; one result in the U.S., of course, is that a significant number of Americans are unable to purchase health insurance that would be considered in any way adequate or affordable by Canadian standards. But suppose wealth were distributed in a more equal fashion; why not let people spend their money on as much or as little as they wanted?

One practical problem with this market approach to the distribution of health services is that it would seem to require private insurance schemes, which are economically inefficient.[10] A second problem is that preventative services are in some ways more efficient than curative services, and it is not immediately clear how or why people would choose to insure themselves in ways that might allow full realization of the advantages of preventative medicine.[11]

These sorts of practical problems might be resolved with the right sort of public insurance plan, and the right sort of political will to establish and maintain such a plan. But this suggests an even more insurmountable problem for any proposal tying the distribution of health services to a more equal distribution of material wealth: to the extent that the struggle in both Canada and the U.S. for more egalitarian health systems has been uphill, the struggle for greater economic equality has faced a more nearly vertical climb.

This being so, we might wonder whether Rawls' theory of justice has any relevance for the current debate over Canadian health reform. Whatever we might want to say about the overall distribution of material wealth in Canada, all health services are currently available to all Canadians, at least in principle. But this very principle is itself one significant aspect of the Canadian health system that is now being threatened by governmental responses to increasing deficits and debts. Thinking about universality in the context of Rawls' two principles of justice may yet help clarify some of the larger social issues that are at stake in initiatives to trim deficits by trimming health services.

For example, one direct response to the problems involved in tying health services to the principle for distributing material wealth is to insist that health is ultimately more like liberty than not; despite the differences listed above, health services, like liberty, ought to be distributed in a strictly equal fashion. This would respond well to the idea that like liberty, having a certain level of health is central to our having any life plans at all. But we must still recognize at least this one important difference between the two goods: health services can escalate in cost and number in a way that the institutional arrangements guaranteeing equal liberty cannot. This difference could be met, however, by limiting the comprehensiveness of services provided rather than their universal provision. That cost containment should be focused on comprehensiveness rather than universality is suggested by the idea that health is more like liberty than material wealth.

Limiting the comprehensiveness of the public health plan raises a second interesting question regarding current proposals for reforming the health system. Would it be fair to all Canadians to tie basic, medically necessary services to the strictly egalitarian sort of principle appropriate to liberty, and then, in addition, piggyback the accessibility of all other services onto something like Rawls' second principle? This would preserve universal medical coverage for those services determined to be medially necessary, and allow people with more income or wealth to purchase whatever additional services they wanted to. The underlying idea would be that it is only basic health services that are like liberty; whatever life a person might choose to lead, certain basic health services, like liberty, are equally important to everyone . Additional health services, though, are like material wealth: some people will want to pursue more, some people less, depending on the different kinds of lives they choose to lead. Unequal access to additional health services, like unequal levels of material wealth, will be a fair social arrangement just so long as those who have less benefit more than they otherwise would have given a completely equal arrangement.

Arguments of precisely this kind were aired at the 1995 annual general meeting of the Canadian Medical Association.[12] Some doctors, agreeing that

equality requires all basic health services be provided to all Canadians, suggested that there was nothing wrong with providing additional services to those who were willing to pay for them. They argued that in allowing this second tier of services to develop, the first tier of basic services would in fact be strengthened.

Again, it is an open question whether this last claim is true. But even ignoring the question of how a second tier of health services might in fact impact on the quality of the first tier of publicly funded services, and ignoring, as well, the question of whether material wealth is itself fairly distributed in Canadian society, there is a deeper conceptual problem with this two-tiered sort of approach to reforming the health system. How are we to distinguish between basic and non-basic services? In some few cases, the distinction may appear to be quite clear: face lifts are not a medical necessity, however much one might plan one's life around the availability of such a service. But this is hardly the sort of service that is causing any cost problems for the health system, especially since it is not now included in any public health insurance plan. More relevant in this regard are newly developing life-saving technologies, many of which are costly and publicly available. For the individuals directly affected by them, such technologies will certainly appear to be medically necessary. The problem facing a publicly funded health system, however, is what happens when services of this kind begin to overreach the public's ability to pay for them? What happens when we can't afford to provide life-saving technologies to all those whose lives could thus be saved? Talking about basic versus non-basic services does nothing to resolve this problem.

We might, of course, try to avoid the problem by reinterpreting basic to refer only the those services that could be provided to all who need them, given the limitations of an antecedently determined budget, one that balanced the costs of the health against those of other public goods, such as defense, education, social assistance, and economic development. But what this means is that some individuals with the life-threatening conditions will be saved, while other individuals, with other life-threatening conditions, will not. Are those who are not saved treated equally to those who are? Even in a single tiered system, one which accepts the economic necessity of limitations on comprehensiveness, this is a question that would have to be faced. But it is an even more difficult question if we allow those who can afford it to purchase life-saving treatments privately. The problem of what it means to call some services but not others part of the basic package of health insurance owed equally to every member of Canadian society is exacerbated by the fact that in a two-tiered system, those who would find themselves unable to purchase the additional treatments available to the economically advantaged would be even more disadvantaged by the advent of their ill health than they already are. Worse yet, those individuals least able to afford to purchase additional services would be the same ones most likely to need to.[13]

It is thus far from clear whether any proposal for two-tiered health reform based on a distinction between basic and non-basic services is workable or coherent. What this suggests, from the perspective of a liberal egalitarian theory of justice, is that the only fair health system is one that is single-tiered.

CONFLICTS BETWEEN EQUALITY AND EFFICIENCY

Complicating questions about equality is the ambiguity of its companion term in the health reform debate, efficiency. Everyone seems to agree, in a vague, general sort of way, that the health system can and should be more efficiently organized and operated. The differences of opinion are over what exactly this means.

In its simplest use, pursuing greater efficiency means doing what we now do better. Better utilization of the services now available, it is claimed, will cost governments less and at the same time respond more fully to the actual health needs of all Canadians. The argument is that many tests, treatments, and services are currently being provided to those who do not need them or in ways that have not been proven to be generally effective and that may be even harmful.[14]

Regardless of the extent to which this is in fact true, problems regarding equality arise on even this simplest understanding of efficiency. For example, while the current system overtreats individuals consulting their doctors with nothing more than a common cold, other individuals, such as pregnant women who are economically or otherwise disadvantaged, go without appropriate medical care. Merely eliminating the waste in the health system as it currently exists will do nothing by itself to respond to this second sort of problem, which bears directly on the question of the extent to which the current system is responding equally to the health needs of all Canadians. Achieving better treatment for disadvantaged individuals is, however, one important area of health reform where equality and efficiency might coincide, were the right sorts of reforms to be pursued. Current data suggests that a great many costly medical conditions arise out of early deficiencies in prenatal and childhood nutrition and care. Thus, ensuring that all Canadian fetuses and children receive sufficient nutrition and care is not just a question of greater social equality, but greater economic efficiency as well.

This leads us to a second meaning of efficiency, one that emphasizes preventative over curative health services. The argument here is that it is cheaper to prevent illness rather than to treat it once it has arisen. So far as those who are the most economically disadvantaged are also among the sickest, this is a second important area of health reform where considerations of equality and efficiency might coincide. The extent to which this is so, however, will depend on the extent to which the health statuses of those who are economically less advantaged are tied to social conditions that go beyond the purview of the health system. If a low income job, for example, is bad for your health, it is not clear what the health system can or should do about this fact.

Equality and efficiency are also less clearly connected in a third sense of efficiency, the one at issue in the discussion of the preceding sections. Given the ever expanding horizon of medical possibility, we will soon be at that point, if we are not indeed already there, of not being able to afford to provide every possible medical service to every Canadian who might benefit from it. If we can't provide every service to everyone who might need it, what might it mean to provide as many services to as many people as we can? How are we to measure the efficiency of responding to the health needs of some Canadians, but not others?[15] Even supposing we felt able to answer such questions about efficiency, there is no reason to assume that the most efficient use of services would necessarily be the most equal.

Suppose, for example, that considerations regarding the most efficient use of health services led us to offer hip surgery to those younger than seventy-five but not to those over seventy-five. Would such a policy represent equal treatment for younger and older people, or is it in some sense ageist? Or suppose we were to treat less serious but more prevalent conditions at the expense of more serious but less prevalent conditions; are those affected by the more serious conditions and those affected by the less serious conditions treated as true equals? These sorts of questions are again exacerbated by the data that suggest that those individuals with less advantaged economic backgrounds are likely to experience more, and more serious, medical conditions.

A fourth and final meaning of efficiency involves reforms to the health system that reduce the cost to governments of providing services, but increase the cost to consumers of these services in either time or money. One example of such a reform is shortened hospital stays, which cost the hospital and hence the government less, but cost the consumer more in paying for home care or in relying on the time and energy of family members or friends. Assuming the current tax system to be more or less equal, the question is whether transferring such costs from the citizen as taxpayer to the citizen as consumer of health services introduces more or less equality into Canadian society. Looking back to the discussion of the second section of this paper, we might say, if we were libertarians, that those who are healthy have no social obligation to pay for those who are not. If some people get sick, this is their problem, those of us who are healthy might choose to help those of us who are sick out of charity, but the state should not compel such help by transferring money from the healthy to the sick through taxation.

On the liberal egalitarian conception of society, however, we must ask ourselves whether it would be reasonable to enter into a society that does not provide equal care for its sick and injured, regardless of their individual ability to pay for health services. For just as any one of us might find ourselves sick or injured, any one of us might experience a dramatic change in our ability to pay for whatever health we might need. This sort of situation is prevalent in the United States, where for many people, losing either their jobs or their health means losing their health insurance.[16]

One way of responding to this problem is the health system adopted by Canada, universally available to all and publicly funded through taxation. Compared to the European Union, taxes in both Canada and the U.S. are low; yet in the U.S., and increasingly in Canada, there is much concern that taxes are too high. There is also concern in the European Union over high taxes, but it exists alongside concern for preserving the basic structure of the egalitarian sort of society that these taxes support. One German, a corporate manager facing a tax rate of nearly 60 percent, put the point this way:

> The European knows that if he gets sick he can go to a good hospital and it won't bankrupt him ... he knows that if his old parents get sick ... they're protected. To Americans, these can be financially disastrous. But we don't fear them. That is why we keep paying. That is why we say we don't like it but the taxes are necessary.[17]

This point returns us the idea that the current health reform debate in Canada is not just about the kind of health system we want for ourselves and our family members. At a deeper and more far-reaching level, it is about the kind of society we want to live in, one that feels an obligation to care for its sick and injured or one that does not. Economic inequalities may be part of a fair and reasonable society, as both libertarians and liberal egalitarians seem to agree. But unless we are willing to adopt the libertarian view of what a modern, liberal society should be, introducing additional inequalities into our health system does not appear to be either reasonable or fair.

Notes

1. This is the term used, for example, by Will Kymlicka in *Contemporary Political Philosophy: An Introduction* (Oxford University Press, 1990). Some commen-

tators on the health reform debate call the second view of society communitarianism, but this term has quite a different meaning in contemporary political debate. For a thorough discussion of the main differences between communitarianism and liberal egalitarianism, see Kymlicka, Chapter 6.

2. For further discussion of these different approaches to equality, as well as some of their implications for the just distribution of health care services, see Allen Buchanan, "Justice: A Philosophical Review," in *Justice and Health Care*, ed. Earl Shelp (Dordrecth: Reidel, 1981), 3-21.

3. Robert Nozick, *Anarchy, State, and Utopia*n (New York: Basic Books, 1974).

4. John Rawls, *A Theory of Justice* (Cambridge: Harvard University Press, 1971).

5. For such an argument see Kai Nielsen, "Autonomy, Equality and a Just Health Care System," *The International Journal of Applied Philosophy* 4 (Spring 1989): 39-44.

6. Robert G. Evans, "Less is More: Contrasting Styles in Health Care," in *Canada and the United States: Differences that Count*, ed. David Thomas (Peterborough: Broadview, 1993), 21-41. For a glimpse into what the statistics mean for the everyday lives of affected Americans, see Eleanor D. Kinney and Suzanne K. Steinmetz, "Note from the Insurance Underground: How the Chronically Ill Cope," *Journal of Health Politics, Policy and Law* 19, 3 (1994): 633-642.

7. Patrick Sullivan, "Private Health Care Dominates Meeting as General Council Calls for National Debate on Issue," *Canadian Medical Association Journal* 153, 6 (1995): 801-803.

8. For a more extended effort to include health in Rawls' theory of justice, see Norman Daniels, *Just Health Care* (Cambridge: Cambridge University Press, 1985). An interesting alternative to Daniels approach, closer to the one suggested here, is provided in Ronald M. Green, "The Priority of Health Care," *Journal of Medicine and Philosophy* 9 (1983): 373-379. Recent work on the social determinants of health (see note 13) suggests, however, that we might regard health itself, and not just health care services or health more generally, as a primary social good; this is the view I begin to develop here.

9. Again, the idea here is that if the general level of productivity in a society goes down there is less for every-

body, those who are less advantaged together with those who are more advantaged. The underlying assumption is that financial incentives, and hence inequalities in the distribution of wealth, are necessary for high levels of productivity in any modern, industrial society. Social programs whose costs cut too deeply into these incentives will thus have less funding available to them than they otherwise might due to a diminished GDP in the society in question. True or not, the underlying assumption of this line of thought is generally accepted among liberal egalitarians.

10. Evans.

11. One important option here is the idea of health maintenance organizations. For the preventative and health promotional potential of this sort of insurance and delivery arrangement, see Michael Rachlis and Carl Kushner, *Strong Medicine: How to Save Canada's Health Care System* (Toronto: Harper Collins 1994), 248-252, and H.H. Schauffler and T. Rodriguez, "The Availability and Utilization of Health Promotion Programs and Satisfaction with Health Plan," *Medical Care* 32, 12 (1994): 1182-1196. But for concomitant problems relating to equal access to all provided services, see H.B. Fox, L.B. Wicks, and P.W. Newacheck, "Health Maintenance Organizations and Children with Special Health Needs: A Suitable Match?" *American Journal of Diseases of Children* 147, 5 (1993): 546-552.

12. Sullivan.

13. There is a fast-growing literature on the linkages between health and social position. An early work is Michael Marmot and Tores Theorell, "Social Class and Cardiovascular Disease: The Contribution of Work," *International Journal of Health Science* 18, 4 (1988): 659-674. Recent collections are Robert G. Evans, M. L. Barer, and T. R. Marmor, eds., *Why are Some People Healthy and Others Not? The Determinants of Health of Populations* (New York: Aldine de Gruyter, 1994) together with the fall 1994 issue of *Daedalus*. Especially interesting with regard to the version of liberal egalitarianism explored above is Richard G. Wilkinson, "National Mortality Rates: the Impact of Inequality?" *American Journal of Public Health* 82, 8 (1992): 1082-1084, and Richard G. Wilkinson, "Income Distribution and Life Expectancy," *British Medial Journal* 304, 6820 (1992): 165-168.

14. Rachlis and Kushner.

15. Health economists have, of course, developed an extensive literature devoted to the question of how we might measure the efficiency of different treatment or service options. But whether such precise, technical definitions of efficiency capture what we really ought to mean by the term remains an open question, depending, in part, on how acceptable we find the simplifying assumptions that are necessary to produce precise, technical definitions of such a multifaceted and complex idea. In the debate over health reform, efficiency is in many ways a much more slippery term than equality. For a recent challenge to economic notions of efficiency as they relate to health reform, see Erik Nord, Jeff Richardson, Andrew Street, Helga Kuhse, and Peter Singer, "Who Cares about Cost? Does Economic Analysis Impose or Reflect Social Values?" *Health Policy* 34, 2 (1995): 79-94, and Alastair V. Campbell, "Defining Core Health Services: The New Zealand Experience," *Bioethics* 9, 3/4 (1995): 252-258.

16. Evans.

17. Nathaniel C. Nash, "Europeans Brace Themselves for Higher Taxes," *Globe and Mail*, 25 February 1995, 4 (D).

46.
FOUR UNSOLVED RATIONING PROBLEMS: A CHALLENGE

Norman Daniels

Faced with limited resources, medical providers and planners often ask bioethicists how to limit or ration the delivery of beneficial services in a fair or just way. What advice should we give them? To focus our thinking on the problems they face, I offer a friendly challenge to the field: solve the four rationing problems described here.

We have generally ignored these problems because we think rationing an unusual phenomenon, associated with gas lines, butter coupons, or organ registries. But rationing is pervasive, not peripheral, since we simply cannot afford, for example, to educate, treat medically, or protect legally people in all the ways that their needs for these goods require or that accepted distributive principles seem to demand. Whenever we design institutions that distribute these goods, and whenever we operate those institutions, we are involved in rationing.

Rationing decisions, both at the micro and macro levels, share three key features. First, the goods we often must provide—legal services, health care, educational benefits—are not sufficiently divisible (unlike money) to avoid unequal or "lumpy" distributions. Meeting the educational, health care, or legal needs of some people, for example, will mean that the requirements of others will go unsatisfied. Second, when we ration, we deny benefits to some individuals who can plausibly claim they are *owed them in principle;* losers as well as winners have plausible claims to have their needs met. Third, the general distributive principles appealed to by claimants as well as by rationers do not by themselves provide adequate reasons for choosing among claimants. They are too schematic; like my "fair equality of opportunity" account of just health care, they fail to yield specific solutions to these rationing problems. Solving these problems thus bridges the gap between principles of distributive justice and problems of institutional design.

THE FAIR CHANCES/BEST OUTCOMES PROBLEM

How much should we favor producing the best outcome with our limited resources?

Like the other problems, the fair chances/best outcomes problem arises in both micro and macro contexts. Consider first its more familiar macrorationing form: which of several equally needy individuals should get a scarce resource, such as a heart transplant? Suppose that Alice and Betty are the same age, have waited on queue the same length of time, and will each live only one week without a transplant. With the transplant, however, Alice is expected to live two years and Betty twenty. Who should get the transplant?[1] Giving priority to producing best outcomes, as in some point systems for awarding organs, would mean that Betty gets the organ and Alice dies (assuming persistent scarcity of organs, as Dan Brock notes).[2] But Alice might complain, "Why should I give up my only chance at survival—and two years of survival is not insignificant—just because Betty has a chance to live longer?" Alice demands a lottery that gives her an equal chance with Betty.

To see the problem in its macroallocation version, suppose our health care budget allows us to introduce one of two treatments, T1 and T2, which can be given to comparable but different groups. Because T1 restores patients to a higher level of functioning than T2, it has a higher net benefit. We could produce the best outcomes by putting all our resources into T1; then patients treatable by T2 might, like Alice, complain that they are being asked to forgo any chance at a significant benefit.

The problem has no satisfactory solution at either the intuitive or theoretical level. Few would agree with Alice, for example, if she had very little chance at survival; more would agree if her outcomes were only somewhat worse than Betty's. At the level of intuitions, there is much disagreement about when and how much to favor best outcomes, though we reject the extreme positions of giving full priority to fair chances or best outcomes. Brock proposes breaking this deadlock by giving Alice and Betty chances proportional to the benefits they can get (e.g., by assigning Alice one side of a ten-sided die). Frances Kamm proposes a more complex assignment of multiplicative weights.[3] Both suggestions seem ad hoc, adding an element of precision our intuitions lack. But theoretical considerations also fall short of solving the problem. For example, we might respond to Alice that she already has lost a "natural" lottery; she might have been the one with twenty years expected survival, but it turned out to be Betty instead. After the fact, however, Alice is unlikely to agree that there has already been a fair "natural" lottery. We might try to persuade her to decide behind a veil of ignorance, but even then there is controversy about what kinds of gambling are permissible.

THE PRIORITIES PROBLEM

How much priority should we give to treating the sickest or most disabled patients?

Suppose Xs are much sicker or more disabled patients than Ys and suppose that we can measure the units of benefit that can be given each patient, for example, in QUALYs or some other unit. Most people believe that if a treatment can deliver equal benefit to Xs or Ys, we should give priority to helping Xs, who are worse off to start with. This intuition is ignored by some uses of cost-effectiveness or cost-benefit methodologies, which may be neutral between Xs and Ys if the benefits and costs are the same. Similarly, we may be willing to forgo some extra benefits for Ys in order to provide lesser benefits to Xs. We favor Xs in more than tie-breaking cases, though we intuitively reject giving full priority to them. How much priority we give to Xs rather than Ys may also depend on whether Xs end up much better than Ys after treatment.

As in the previous problem, we intuitively reject extreme positions but we have no satisfactory theoretical characterization of an intermediary position.

THE AGGREGATION PROBLEM

When should we allow an aggregation of modest benefits to larger numbers of people to outweigh more significant benefits to fewer people?

In June of 1990, the Oregon Health Services Commission released a list of treatment-condition pairs ranked by a cost-benefit calculation. Critics were quick to seize on rankings that seemed completely counterintuitive. For example, as David Hadorn noted, tooth capping was ranked higher than appendectomy.[4] The reason was simple: an appendectomy cost about $4000, many times the cost of capping a tooth. Simply aggregating the net medical benefit of many capped teeth yielded a net benefit greater than that produced by one appendectomy.

As David Eddy pointed out, our intuitions in these cases are largely based on comparing treatment-condition pairs for their importance on a one-to-one basis.[5] One appendectomy is more important than one tooth capping because it saves a life rather than merely reducing pain and preserving dental function. Our intuitions are much less well developed when it comes to making one-to-many comparisons, though economists have used standard techniques to measure them.[6] Kamm shows that we are not straightforward aggregators of all benefits, though we do permit some forms of aggregation. Nevertheless, our moral views are both complex and difficult to explicate in terms of well-ordered principles. While we are not aggregate maximizers, as presupposed by the dominant methodologies derived from welfare economics, we do permit or require some forms of aggregation. Are there principles that govern the aggregation we accept? Failing to find justifiable principles would give us strong reason to rely instead on fair procedures.

THE DEMOCRACY PROBLEM

When must we rely on a fair democratic process as the only way to determine what constitutes a fair rationing outcome?

There is much that is appealing about relying on people's preferences and values in deciding how it is fair to ration medical services. Which preferences and values must we take at face value, however, regardless of the outcomes they imply? In Oregon, for example, people's attitudes were included in the process of ranking medical services in several ways. Adapting Kaplan's "quality of well-being" scale for use in measuring the benefit of medical treatments, Oregon surveyed residents, asking them to judge on a scale of 0 (death) to 100 (perfect health) what the impact would be of having to live the rest of one's life with some physical or mental impairment or symptom; for example, wearing eyeglasses was rated 95 out of 100, for a weighting of -0.05, which is about the same as the weight assigned to not being able to drive a car or use public transportation and to having to stay at a hospital or nursing home. Are these weightings the result of poor methodology? If they represent real attitudes, must we accept them at face value? Whose attitudes should we rely on, the public as a whole or the people who have experienced the condition in question? Those who do not have a disabling condition may suffer from cultural biases, overestimating the impact of disability. But those who have the condition may rate it as less serious because they have modified their preferences, goals, and values in order to make a "healthy adjustment" to their condition. Their overall dissatisfaction—tapped by these methodologies—may not reflect the impact that would be captured by a measure more directly attuned to the range of capabilities they retain. Insisting on the more objective measure has a high political cost and may even seem paternalistic.

The democracy problem arises at another level in procedures that purport to be directly democratic. The Oregon plan called for the OHSC to respect "community values" in its ranking of services. Because prevention and family planning services were frequently discussed in community meetings, the OHSC assigned the categories that included those services very high ranking. Consequently, in Oregon, vasectomies are ranked more important than hip replacements. Remember the priority and aggregation problems: it would seem more important to restore mobility to someone who cannot walk than to improve the convenience of birth control though vasectomy in several people. But, assuming that the commissioners properly interpreted the

wishes of Oregonians, that is not what Oregonians wanted the rankings to be. Should we treat this as error? Or must we abide by whatever the democratic process yields?

Thus far I have characterized the problem of democracy as a problem of error: a fair democratic process, or a methodology that rests in part on expressions of preferences, leads to judgments that deviate from either intuitive or theoretically based judgments about the relative importance of certain health outcomes or services. The problem is how much weight to give the intuitive or theoretically based judgments as opposed to the expressed preferences. The point should be put in another way as well. Should we in the end think of the democratic process as a matter of pure procedural justice? If so, then we have no way to correct the judgment made through that process, for what it determines to be fair is what counts as fair. Or should we really consider the democratic process as an impure and imperfect form of procedural justice? Then it is one that can be corrected by appeal to some prior notion of what constitutes a fair outcome of rationing. I suggest that we do not yet know the answer to this question, and we will not be able to answer it until we work harder at providing a theory of rationing.

––––––––––

Acknowledgments

This work was generously supported by the National Endowment for the Humanities (RH 20917) and the National Library of Medicine (1R01LM05005). This paper is adapted from my "Rationing Fairly: Programmatic Considerations," *Bioethics* 7 nos. 2/3 (1993): 224-33.

Notes

Norman Daniels is Goldthwaite Professor and professor of biomedical ethics and community medicine in the philosophy department at Tufts University, Medford, Mass.

1. Francis M. Kamm, "The Report of the U.S. Task Force on Organ Transplantation: Criticisms and Alternatives," *Mt. Sinai Journal of Medicine* (June 1989):207-20.

2. Dan Brock, "Ethical Issues in Recipient Selection for Organ Transplantation," in *Organ Substitution Technology: Ethical, Legal, and Public Policy Issues,* ed. Deborah Mathieu (Boulder: Westview, 1988), pp. 86-99.

3. Frances M. Kamm, *Morality, Mortality*, vol. 1., *Death and Whom to Save from It* (New York: Oxford University Press, 1993); see also Kamm, "Report of the U.S. Task Force."

4. David Hadorn, "Setting Health Care Priorities in Oregon: Cost-Effectiveness Meets the Rule of Rescue," *JAMA* 265, no. 17 (1991): 2218-25.

5. David Eddy, "Oregon's Methods: Did Cost-Effectiveness Analysis Fail?" *JAMA* 266, no. 15 (1991): 2135-41.

6. Eric Nord, "The Relevance of Health State after Treatment in Priorities between Different Patients," unpublished manuscript in author's possession.

CHAPTER TEN

ACQUIRING AND DISTRIBUTING BODY PARTS

47.
ANENCEPHALIC NEWBORNS AS ORGAN DONORS: A CRITIQUE

John D. Arras and Shlomo Shinnar

THE ISSUES

The case for taking hearts, paired kidneys, and other vital organs from anencephalic newborns is based on two distinct needs. First, there are many chronically ill infants, children, and adults who may benefit from organ transplant, and there is a relative scarcity of available donors. Second, there is the need of the parents of an anencephalic infant to salvage some good from a tragic situation. Allowing the infant to be used as an organ donor may help satisfy this need.

An important feature of anencephaly is the relative certitude of diagnosis and prognosis. Ultrasonography can now detect anencephaly in utero with relative certainty. The prognosis for these infants is death within hours, days, or weeks from birth, although there is some controversy over their exact life span. In view of the need for organs and the alleged uniqueness of anencephaly, it has been proposed that society consider such infants as persons who are born "brain absent." Anencephaly would be declared the *only* legitimate exception to our current insistence that all vital organ donors meet the criteria for whole-brain death. This would be useful in procuring neonatal organs, especially since the diagnosis of whole-brain death in the neonate is extremely difficult and fraught with uncertainty. The lack of established brain death criteria in the first week of life also poses additional problems for those who would use "brain dead" neonates as organ donors (*New York Times*, Oct 19, 1987, p A1).

Advocates of the brain absent approach specifically decline to view anencephalic newborns as "nonpersons" and insist that these infants are "persons" deserving of respect. However, they state that since they are also brain absent, they should be functionally equivalent to brain dead insofar as vital organs might be harvested from them. Another approach for justifying the use of anencephalic newborns as organ donors would be to regard them as nonpersons—ie, as biologically human entities that nevertheless lack the prerequisites of "personal" life and thus lack full moral status. This perspective provides the most direct route to salvaging their organs at the expense of redefining society's views of "personhood."

Despite the manifest importance of the "gift of life" to organ recipients and the laudable desire to help parents salvage some good from a tragedy, society must consider whether allowing anencephalic infants to be used as organ donors before they meet the traditional criteria for brain death is a morally acceptable and legitimate act. We believe it is not.

BRAIN ABSENT THEORY

Let us first address the issues posed by the brain absent theory. By insisting on the personhood of these infants, proponents of this scheme commit themselves to treat the anencephalic infant as a full member of the moral community, ie, one who has rights and is worthy of respect. The question is whether prolonging the infant's life by mechanical ventilation and then abruptly terminating it by harvesting vital organs is compatible with the minimum respect due to all persons. In Kantian philosophy, which is the source of many contemporary moral theories based on the concept of personhood, using one person merely as a means to benefit another constitutes a paradigmatic violation of moral law. As "ends in themselves," persons have an intrinsic worth that cannot be reduced to their instrumental value to others. The investigators' claims notwithstanding, it is difficult to reconcile the treatment of anencephalic newborns outlined in the ... reports (*New York Times,* Oct 19, 1987, p A1) with the notion of respect for personhood.

One response to this objection is to claim that if the anencephalic infant could (miraculously) reflect on his plight, he would consent to organ donation, since losing vital organs would not deprive him of anything he would desire. Similar arguments can be made using the social contract theory of Rawls, in which the decision maker is unbiased because he does not know what role (parent, recipient, anencephalic infant, or physician) he would have in the societal drama and therefore tries to minimize the worst outcome, which may be a person in need of an organ with no available donor. However, these arguments are by no means unique to anencephalic newborns. They are equally applicable to other severely damaged infants as well as to adults in permanent vegetative states. We do not believe society is willing to harvest organs from living patients who have permanently lost the capacity for intelligent thought.

PERSONHOOD THEORY

Justifying the use of anencephalic newborns as organ donors by labeling them "nonpersons" creates the same uniqueness problem. In this philosophical theory, only beings capable of sapient life, whatever that means, have the rights and privileges of "personhood." If anencephalic newborns are nonpersons, one could perhaps justify using them as a mere means for the benefit of persons. Again, if the theory is carried out to its logical conclusion, other infants with conditions such as holoprosencephaly, hydranencephaly, and certain trisomies as well as adults in permanent vegetative states should be considered as potential organ donors.

Those who justify using anencephalic newborns as organ donors based on the fact that they will all die soon after birth must deal with two objections. First, even a dying person is still a person and is entitled to a full measure of dignity and respect as discussed above. Second, there is nothing special in this respect about anencephaly. If the crucial issue is uniform early mortality, then a number of other conditions, such as Potter's syndrome and trisomy 13, would qualify.

The availability of reliable prenatal diagnosis has led some authors to conclude that abortion of anencephalic fetuses is justified even in the third trimester. If we are willing to terminate a viable fetus just prior to term, why not terminate life just after delivery? However, the moral justification for third-trimester abortion is based on the certitude of both diagnosis and prognosis and not on any inherently unique feature of anencephaly. Many other conditions would meet the authors' criteria if reliable antenatal diagnosis were available.

BRAIN DEATH

Another fundamental objection to the proposals for amending the brain death statutes to define anencephalic infants as "dead" or "brain absent" is that this violates the spirit of our present brain death statutes regarding the definition of death. Although anencephalic infants lack a cerebral cortex, they certainly have a brain stem that sustains and regulates a wide variety of vital bodily functions, including spontaneous respiration. Thus, it would be more accurate to describe them as "higher-brain absent" than as "brain absent." According to the present definition of brain death, ie, complete and irreversible cessation of all brain functions, including those of the brain stem, anencephalic infants are indisputably living human beings. Indeed, no one with spontaneous respirations meets the current criteria for brain death. Permitting the use of anencephalic newborns as organ donors by defining them as legally dead requires a radical reformulation of our current definition of death.

One way to accomplish this would be to reinterpret the original intent of the whole-brain definition of death. One advocate of this approach has argued that the stringent safeguards built into the current brain death statutes were put there to protect comatose patients who might eventually recover some higher cortical functions. Since anencephalic infants lack the capacity ever to achieve such a level of existence, there is no need to protect them with such rigorous definitions of brain death. Consequently, it is argued that taking organs from brain absent anencephalic newborns is ethically compatible with the spirit if not the letter of the laws governing brain death. Although the argument sounds plausible, it confuses a necessary condition for the definition of brain death with a sufficient condition. Of course, any adequate definition of brain death must preclude the possibility of meaningful recovery. However, it is one thing to note that a person is incapable of recovery of higher cortical functions and/or is imminently dying but quite another to say that he or she is dead.

Why should irreversible cessation of activity of the entire brain be necessary for a definition of death? According to the President's Commission, the brain, including the brain stem, performs an irreplaceable function in sustaining and regulating the physiological systems that keep us alive. Once it ceases to perform these vital tasks, modern technology can continue to oxygenate other organs, for a time creating a simulacrum of life, but cannot substitute for the spontaneous integrative functions that the Commission identified as the sine qua non of human life. The Commission insisted on a rigorous definition of brain death not solely to protect comatose patients, but because it believed that anything short of whole-brain death was not equivalent to the death of the human being. The Commission also specifically insisted that organ donors be *dead*, not just irrevocably brain damaged or imminently dying. This position has been cogently reiterated ... by the former executive director of the Commission. Thus, the attempt to reconcile the use of anencephalic newborns as organ donors with current principles of brain death founders on a flawed account of the rationale for accepting whole-brain death as death of the human being.

CONCLUSIONS

Current public policy and practice embody two fundamental principles: first, that vital organs may not be taken from the living for the benefit of others and, second, that for brain death to be considered the moral and legal equivalent of the death of the person, the strict criteria for whole-brain death must be satisfied. The second principle is accepted as sound public policy even by many, including one of us (J.D.A), who do not fully agree with the President's Commission's philosophical rationale for choosing whole-brain death. The use of anencephalic newborns as organ donors is incompatible with both of these generally accepted principles. Advocates of using these infants as organ donors can invoke the more controversial "higher brain" definitions of either death or personhood to justify their proposal. However, to be consistent, infants with other severe brain malformations as well as adults in chronic vegetative states should then also be candidates for use as organ donors. We believe that the current principles of the strict definition of brain death are sound public policy and good ethics. We hope that, after careful scrutiny and debate, the use of anencephalic infants as organ donors is rejected. Admirable goals should not be advanced by improper means.

48.
JOIN THE CLUB: A MODEST PROPOSAL TO INCREASE AVAILABILITY OF DONOR ORGANS

Rupert Jarvis

I.

In a health service where rationing has become a fact of life, nowhere is the problem of demand outstripping supply more obvious than in the field of organ transplants. For reasons not entirely obvious, despite the fact that the majority of Britons believe that cadaver donation of organs is both ethically acceptable and practically desirable, still only a minority actually possess donor cards, and even fewer carry them:

> a Gallup poll for the British Kidney Patient Association, quoted in *The Guardian* (9.5.90), found that 73 per cent of respondents would agree to their kidneys being used for transplantation, although only 27 per cent actually had a donor card and only seven per cent were carrying one on them at the time[1]

The problem is not that there are insufficient numbers of organs potentially suitable for transplantation, but that these organs, far from being made available for transplant, are destroyed, leaving those in need of a transplant either to improve their quality of life, as in the case of a kidney transplant, or as a life-saving measure, in the case of a heart transplant, still waiting. At one and the same time, the organs necessary to save or immeasurably improve actual, identifiable lives[2] are themselves in existence, and yet people are dying for the want of them: "Organ supply is the major limiting factor in organ transplantation."[3] That is to say, the number of lives saved as a result of transplants could—if donor organs were more readily available to transplant surgeons—be considerably higher.

Nor is the problem a medical one: since the introduction of immunosuppressive drugs such as cyclosporin, which vastly lessen the dangers of rejection, the actual process of transplantation is not a particularly unusual or dangerous one. Although the operations are long and complex, they are, at least in centres largely dedicated to such procedures, relatively routine. In the best B-movie tradition, we have the technology.

The upshot of this is clear enough: given that demand for resources exceeds the (presently available) supply, there is a need to ration the available resources by prioritising demand—to decide who is to receive the benefits offered by a transplant operation, and who is to go without. Such overt rationing, particularly when it is applied to identifiable individual patients, is often held to be highly distasteful both by health care professionals and by the lay public, since it seems to sit uneasily alongside a duty to care. It is not my present purpose to examine the interesting question of whether a health care professional can or should act as a gatekeeper to resources. Instead, I shall look briefly at some problems associated with the current parameters by reference to which transplant organ availability is rationed, and examine two suggested remedies to the current shortage of organs available for transplant. I shall then suggest some desiderata of any proposed solution to the problem, and apply them to one further possible solution.

II

There is a familiar suggestion that any finite health care resources for which there is excessive demand could be rationed by one or more of the more or less quantifiable, non-medical parameters, such as age, desert, or social utility. The latter two are, fortunately, not often suggested except in the context of a thought experiment, while the former is more usually dressed up in the guise of ability to benefit, which I discuss below. I take it that there is little doubt that it would be unjust to ration access to transplant services by such factors as desert or social utility, or any other non-medical category, such as class, ethnic origin,[4] or gender. What would be unjust about a policy that used such criteria to ration is that it would violate the Aristotelian principle of distributive justice, that only those cases that are relevantly dissimilar should be treated differently. It is abundantly clear that class or social utility are utterly irrelevant to considerations of prioritising demand for transplant services.

If such non-medical criteria are of no use in rationing, then what of the traditional concept of ability to benefit from the treatment? Even a cursory review of the literature reveals that of the various criteria, this is the one most nearly agreed upon, and it seems reasonable that this should be so: to take an extreme example, there is neither point nor justification in treating someone for a condition which is not present. More realistically, it seems reasonable to suggest that those patients whose chance of survival is significantly lower for one reason or another, for example the existence of another condition which prejudices their chance of surviving the operation, should not receive as high a priority in the queue for donor organs as those whose ability to benefit is greater. This is to say that an assessment of the relationship between a proposed transplant's risks and benefits to an individual could be used to determine access to transplant services.

The "free rider"

While this looks like an elegant and reasonable solution to the rationing problem, it is not. As a means of *ordering* a queue it has a certain merit, particularly that it takes account only of those differences which are relevant to the particular case. However, perhaps unfortunately from the point of view of finding a tool for rationing, there are still many, many more people who could benefit *somewhat* from a transplant operation than there are available donor organs for them. The problem of the inequality between supply and demand, then, is not to be resolved simply by applying the criterion of the patient's ability to benefit. It is inadequate as a tool of rationing since it allows far too many in through the gates. While it may serve to reduce the total number of those waiting for transplants by a small amount, it leaves us a long way from a satisfactory account of how to ration donor organs.

A third problem with the current system by which donor organs are rationed is that it takes no account of, indeed it encourages, the "free rider": the individual who hopes to benefit from the co-operation of others even though he does not himself contribute to the socially desired end. Although it is in each individual's interest that donor organs should be available, it is in nobody's interests to make *his/her own* organs available: the choice to donate post *mortem is* an entirely altruistic one. We therefore have the current situation where demand is not matched by supply, and individual patients who could benefit from a transplanted organ are denied that treatment owing to a lack of suitable organs available for transplant.

III

If that is the problem, what have been the suggested solutions? Two main strands have emerged, one of which has received little support. They can be labelled respectively opting-out, and cash payments for organs.

The first proposed solution has already been implemented in a number of countries, including Denmark, Austria, Sweden, France, Israel and Switzerland. It involves a "presumed consent polic[y], where physicians can take required tissues and organs unless either the deceased carries a card to prohibit this, or the next of kin object."[5] It therefore places the burden of decision on the individual, who is required to make a conscious effort to opt *out* of the scheme if s/he wishes to do so.

Hint of coercion

Mason and McCall Smith suggest that this policy "smacks of 'body-snatching' and carries with it a hint of coercion .... [and they] cannot foresee a British government risking such a major policy change."[6] Although I do not disagree with their conclusion, it is worth being clear what exactly is coercive about such a scheme.

The notion of consent, properly voluntary and adequately informed, is absolutely central to modern medical ethics, and readers of the journal will not need to be reminded of its salient features. But it is worth reminding ourselves that "the notion underlying 'giving one's consent' is 'feeling together'—that is 'agreeing' and hence 'giving approval or permission.'"[7] In the increasingly abstruse discussion of informed consent, it is easy to lose sight of the fact that underlying the whole question is the notion of agreeing—of deciding *together*. Given that the notion of agreement *between* is internal to the idea of consent, it is clear why true consent cannot go by default: we cannot assume that in the absence of any contra-indications, a brainstem dead patient would not have minded his/her organs being removed for transplant. If consent is as important to the ethical practice of medicine as it is held to be, then an opt-out scheme is not a possibility.

It may of course be that an individual's wishes are held to be irrelevant in the face of the public good, and that the general utility would be promoted by the removal of cadaveric organs without express permission, but that is another matter entirely. Utilitarian considerations of the problem of the shortage of potential donor organs, as Harris has shown, give very different—and often strikingly counterintuitive—results.[8]

Market in organs

The other solution to the drastic shortage that is conventionally proposed, usually but not exclusively as a thought experiment,[9] is to create a market in organs. The purchase of organs from live donors has yet to be legalised, although the practice is by no means unknown[10] and proposals to allow cadaveric organs to be purchased have so far failed to be realised. But once a demand among the rich has been identified and the means to satisfy that demand devised by the poor, it becomes increasingly difficult to stop the development of a market. It is therefore imperative to be absolutely clear whether that market is an acceptable one or not before it gains a foothold.

Since 1989, the sale of organs has been outlawed in Britain by the Human Organ Transplants Act, in line with the principle of English common law that the body is not to be treated as property. Abouna *et al* considered the notion of paid organ donation and found it to be

"a flawed, short-sighted, and self-defeating approach to a complex problem. Paid organ donation has a serious negative impact on many of the medical, moral, and ethical values intimately connected with organ transplanta-

tion including the donor, the recipient, the local transplant programmes, the medical profession, society, and the international community."[11]

The problems with paying live donors for organs are too well known to rehearse in any great detail here, but mainly concern danger to, and exploitation of, both donor and recipient in the face of commercial pressures, and a fall-off in voluntary donation. These undesirable consequences are in addition to the conceptual problems concerned with treating the body or its parts as property.

Paying next of kin

A variant of the policy is sometimes proposed, which advocates paying the deceased donor's next of kin.[12] Although this avoids the problem of danger to the donor, a moment's reflection reveals that it is even less attractive an option than paid donation from live donors. Not only are the same conceptual difficulties present, but

"the selling of cadaver organs is, at root, directed to the enticement of the next of kin. Put this way, the proposition can only be seen as appealing to the basest of human instincts and as something with which the medical profession should have no truck."[13]

As lawyers from the city where Burke and Hare once plied their horrid trade, Mason and McCall Smith are only too well aware of what lies at the bottom of this particular slope.

Allied to this suggestion is the notion of "required request" which has been embodied in federal law in the USA since October 1987, whereby physicians are *obliged* to ask the relatives of suitable deceased patients for permission to harvest organs for transplant. This policy seems objectionable for two reasons. Firstly, and most importantly, it makes the wishes of the surviving relatives determinative rather than those of the individual whose organs are being sought; secondly, it risks creating the impression in the minds of the relatives that a patient's ventilation is being discontinued simply because his/her organs are needed by somebody else, thus eroding trust in the intensivists.

It should also be clear that our pre-reflective notions of justice are outraged by the possibility of a market in donor organs. The NHS is founded on a principle of equity of access to care irrespective of income or wealth, and this is hardly likely to be served by establishing a means by which the already limited supply of donor organs for transplants can be further diminished by financially enabled queue-jumping.

IV

If these traditional solutions to the problem fail, then what more can we offer? Or is there nothing more that we can do except commission bigger and louder advertisements exhorting the public to carry donor cards? Before we can answer that question, we need to have an idea of the sort of answer we are looking for. I suggest that there are six desiderata of any proposed solution.

Firstly, and most obviously, any putative solution must address the problem of shortage by better matching supply of donor organs to demand for them. This might be achieved either by increasing the supply, for instance by a successful campaign to encourage donation, or by reducing the demand by, for instance, the development of acceptable alternative therapies.[14]

Secondly, the solution must satisfy the requirements of justice, which I glossed above, following Aristotle, as treating only those cases that are relevantly dissimilar in different ways.

Derived from this general condition but specific to current understandings of health care provision in Britain, no individual should be excluded from the transplant programme on the grounds of inability to pay for the treatment. As I argued above, this condition rules out the creation of a market in donor organs.

Fourth, in accordance with our conception of the individual as a rational free agent, our putative solution should be founded in an autonomous choice. Although it would be easy (in theory) to ensure an adequate supply of donor organs if no account were taken of individuals' wishes—by Harris-like selected sacrifice, for example—our basic intuitions about the place of autonomy in our lives rules out such coercive practices. It can, of course, be argued that all laws are in some measure coercive, and that therefore any legislative solution to the problem will inevitably infringe the autonomy of some. Notwithstanding this, in a liberal society coercion, particularly over a matter as important as bodily integrity, is to be shunned.

Although the fifth condition is not central in the way that the first four are, it nonetheless seems desirable in a solution that should address the problem of the free rider. Of course, if a proposal can be tabled that appears to fit the other desiderata but still allows some individuals to benefit from, without participating in, the scheme, then we would not on those grounds alone reject it. Even so, a solution that eliminates the possibility is to be preferred to one that does not, *ceteris paribus*.

Finally, and equally non-centrally, it would be desirable although in no way necessary, if the solution were to encourage altruism.

V

I now turn to another possible solution to the problem which I shall outline briefly and examine with these desiderata in mind. It is worth noting in passing that this solution relies on a decision that takes place behind a Rawlsian veil of ignorance, and might therefore be presumed to yield a *prima facie* just result.

I suggest that legislation governing organ donation be amended such that all and only those who identify themselves as potential donors (perhaps by a card similar to the one currently in use, or by registration on a central computer) are eligible themselves to receive transplant organs.[15]

It will be immediately apparent that this solution is a form of the closed, co-operative agreement beloved of social contract theorists: that is, its members receive a benefit in return for the agreed, mutual sacrifice of one or more of their interests. That is the positive side of the contract, as embodied by the principle that *all* those who participate stand to benefit. The negative aspect of exclusion is captured in the condition that *only* those who undertake to sacrifice their own interests are eligible for the benefits.

Thoroughly attractive option

This is a particularly compelling example of a social contract, however, because of an unusual feature. Many hypothetical contracts focus on the trade-off between two interests that are seen as mutually exclusive (standardly, my—presumed—wish to rape and pillage and my own desire for the security to be free from being myself raped and the victim of pillage). This contract, however, trades a—if not *the*—central interest, one's interest in remaining alive, against one's *post mortem* interest in not having one's organs removed. This latter is at best *de minimis*: my interests in my organs after death can hardly be said to be enormous. We are presented, then, with what seems to be a thoroughly attractive option: by sacrificing our minimal *post mortem* interest we guarantee our inclusion on the waiting list for the donor organ which might save or vastly improve the quality of our own life. That is, we make possible the satisfaction of our own most compelling interest by renouncing one which is of little or no concern to us.

Adoption to this scheme would, I suggest, address the problem of shortage on two fronts simultaneously. Firstly, by excluding those who do not elect to join the scheme, it will reduce legitimate demand for donor organs. It should be noted that the reduction thus effected will probably be minimal, which is surely a good thing, in that it seems preferable that supply be better matched to demand by increasing supply rather than by eliminating or reducing demand.

Secondly, and more importantly, the supply of donor organs would at the same time increase as a result of an upturn in the number of registered potential donors. It hardly seems fanciful to suggest that the vast majority of people would elect to join the scheme, since it is so clearly in their interests to do so, with the potential gain (life) being infinite and the potential loss (*post mortem* dissection which, depending on the manner of their death, they might well have to undergo anyway) being zero. Unlike the "survival lottery" proposed by Harris, nobody is going to be sacrificed in order to save others. Under this scheme, the potential for benefit and loss is separated by the moment of death: *only* benefits can accrue to the living, and losses—if it makes sense to speak of *post mortem* losses—can only occur after death.

The proposed scheme appears to satisfy the requirements of justice, in that differences in access to a particular treatment are grounded in relevant considerations, and those and only those who elect potentially to contribute to the system stand to benefit from it. In this way the problem of the free rider is eliminated by the exclusion of those who do not—at least potentially—contribute.

The contract scheme would also have the (marginal) benefit of promoting—albeit self-regarding—altruism, which is taken to be a morally desirable End in and of itself. Moreover, this alignment of the individual's self-regarding interests with the public good is a strength as far as the scheme's likely successful implementation is concerned. Given a moderate version of the social contract theorist's premise, that people tend to act in what they perceive to be their own best interests, if follows that a scheme under which acting in one's best interest is concomitant with, and necessarily entails acting in, the best interests of the population at large will be inevitably tend to promote the public good.

Conceptual, ethical and aesthetic problems arising from the commercialisation and objectification of body parts are avoided since the scheme makes no reference to money OR any market principles. Similarly, since there is no question of purchasing organs, there is no danger of individuals being excluded from a transplant programme on the grounds of their inability to pay. Nor, moreover, is there the financial inducement to sell organs as a live donor in order to alleviate financial hardship.

Finally, the proposal seems no more coercive than any other arrangement which offers a valued future goal as a reward for some sacrifice. Indeed, the coercion involved looks to be particularly thin, given that all the benefits accrue to the individual while s/he is alive while the costs are exacted exclusively after his/her death. The responsibility to register as a potential donor—and therefore as a potential recipient—rests with the individual alone. Voluntary exclusion, therefore, is a real possibility, although it would carry with it obvious costs. But the choice remains a real one.

VI

The scheme seems to me to be self-evidently in the interests of all of us jointly and each of us severally. However, it is worth pointing out that there is one possible injustice that could arise from its successful implementation. Imagine that ten years hence, the registration scheme has been adopted and has been found to be a success. Transplant specialists are now no longer restricted with respect to their choice of recipients by the availability of donor organs, but by medical criteria. In fact, so successful has the scheme been in encouraging voluntary cadaver organ donation, that there is a surplus of organs suitable for transplant: more hearts, lungs, kidneys and livers are being donated than are required to transplant into those individuals registered as potential donors, who are the only ones who have a legitimate claim on them.

Imagine also that there are a number of people *outside* the registration scheme who objected to, balked at, or simply never got around to registering as potential organ donors. A certain percentage of these people will suffer renal failure, or develop cardio-pulmonary conditions that could be alleviated by a transplant. But, because of their failure to join up, they have no legitimate claim on the—available—donor organs. They would be dying only because of an inflexibility in the law.

I think this situation would indeed offend our sense of justice. We would be right to be sickened if it were to come about. But this does not show that the scheme is at fault, merely that it may, if it is very successful, need to be flexible in its implementation. Perhaps it would be fairer to say that those who register as potential organ donors will be given *first refusal* on any organ available for transplant. Perhaps there is another proviso that could be added. That seems a matter for the legal draftsman, and not the philosopher.

But note that the kind of injustice that we are considering here arises from an *over*-supply of donated organs, rather than the shortage that is the *status quo*. If this is a kind of injustice (and I suggest that it is easily avoided in the manner I have sketched above) then it is a very different sort from the one we have presently. And it is not only different, but considerably less offensive.

Acknowledgements
I would like to thank the two anonymous reviewers for their helpful comments on an earlier draft of this paper.

Notes

1. West R. *Organ transplantation*. London: Office of Health Economics, 1991:10.

2. One of the remarkable features of transplant surgery that makes resource allocation in this field such a compelling problem is that the opportunity costs of any decision are clear and immediate. If Mr. McHenry and Mr. McTavish both need the same donor heart—which is of a particularly rare blood group and weight—in order to survive beyond the end of the year, then the surgeon knows, even as s/he is saving Mr McHenry's life in the operating theatre, that s/he is—in all likelihood—depriving Mr McTavish of his last chance. Unlike many fields of health care resource allocation, where on Positron Emission tomography (PET) scan represents an opportunity cost of so many theoretical, anonymous, hip replacements, in transplant surgery the cost can be traced to one particular individual.

3. See reference 1 : 9.

4. Ethnic origin *may* become a relevant medical factor where tissue matching is dependent on it. In such a case, however, since the difference is *a relevant* one, it justifies discrimination on those grounds.

5. See reference 1: 7.

6. Mason J, McCall Smith R. *Law and medical ethics* [3rd ed]. London: Butterworths, 1991:312.

7. Ayto J. *Bloomsbury dictionary of word origins*. London: Bloomsbury, 1990: 132.

8. Harris J. The survival lottery. *Philosophy* 1975; 50: 81-87.

9. Cohen L. The ethical virtues of a futures market in cadaveric organs. In: Land W, Dossetor J. *Organ replacement therapy: ethics, justice, commerce*. Berlin: Springer Verlag, 1991: 302-310.

10. See reference 9: 164-172.

11. See reference 9: 165.

12. Pliskin J. Cadaveric organs for transplantation: is there a need for more? *Journal of forensic sciences* 1976; 21: 83.

13. See reference 6: 313.

14. The implantation of an entirely artificial mechanical heart into Arthur Cornhill at Papworth Hospital in August 1994 provides some hope that such alternatives may no longer be the reserve of science fiction. We may be moving forward from the time when "the

artificial heart is ... only seen as a bridge until a suitable donor can be found." (See reference 1: 12.)

15. Note that "being eligible to receive" does not necessarily entail "will receive." Obviously, any eligibility will be subject to suitable organs being available. Moreover, there is a case for applying a risk/benefit assessment even *within* the contractual scheme. However, as I argued above, any such assessment would be useful only to *order* a waiting list, not to govern admittance to it. Simple application of risk/benefit analysis is inadequate to resolve rationing problems.

49

ON GIVING PREFERENCE TO PRIOR VOLUNTEERS WHEN ALLOCATING ORGANS FOR TRANSPLANTATION

Raanan Gillon

In this issue of the journal Rupert Jarvis argues for a simple idea—a "modest proposal"—that he believes will radically increase the supply of organs for transplantation.[1] Given the existing shortage of donor organs for transplantation it would be entirely just, he reasons, for our society to give priority for receipt of organs for transplantation to those patients who had previously volunteered to donate their own organs. Once such a scheme was promulgated, the incentive to volunteer as an organ donor would, he plausibly argues, become very great indeed, and thus the supply of organs would become much larger than at present.

Many positive benefits of such a scheme are claimed by Mr Jarvis. It meets, he argues, the Aristotelian criterion for distributive justice in that people are treated un-equally only if there are morally relevant differences between them; including the morally relevant differences of whether or not they themselves had been prepared to contribute to the scheme from which they wish to benefit. The scheme, he says, tends to promote altruism—"albeit self-regarding" altruism. Moreover, aligning the individual's self-interest with the public good tends to promote both the satisfaction of individual self-interest and the public good, both of which are morally desirable. The scheme respects the autonomy of donors with minimal coercion. And if sufficient organs are donated as a result of the scheme's success, it could also make possible organ transplants for those who had not previously volunteered their own organs.

If one pursues the moral analysis using the Beauchamp and Childress "four principles," along with consideration of their scope of application, Mr Jarvis's "modest proposal" certainly does seem to meet some standard moral requirements.

As he points out, respect for donors' autonomy is achieved in that donors are not coerced into volunteering their own organs,. His proposal does not even involve the element of coercion by inertia that a presumed consent law would allegedly entail. People are simply positively rewarded for volunteering their organs and thus behaving in a way that is both of potential benefit to themselves and also of potential benefit to others.

So far as the autonomy of potential recipients is concerned, all would retain their right to have their autonomy respected if they refused treatment. As for their preference to be given treatment by organ transplant should they need it, suffice it here merely to assert that this is not strictly an issue of autonomy—(literally self rule). Rather it is an issue of beneficence, and more specifically of the just distribution of scarce medical benefits, to be addressed below, in relation to justice.

So far as the scope of autonomy is concerned, familiar problems would arise in an unfamiliar context—notably the context of inadequately autonomous potential organ donors. These would comprise, for the most part, either inadequately autonomous children, or adults who are inadequately autonomous as a result of mental and or neurological disorder or immaturity. One way of resolving these problems would be to exempt all inadequately autonomous people from the proposed scheme.

Alternatively, some scheme could be devised to make possible (and easy) proxy advance donations by parents on behalf of their children, so long as the children were deemed too young to make autonomous prior donations themselves. Perhaps this could be done at the time of infant immunisations, which in developed countries, at least, almost all infants have. While any such discussion is likely to be distasteful and unpleasant to both health care workers and parents—who wants to think about an infant's possible death—the positive potential benefit to the child could be emphasised as an excellent reason for the parents to add their child to the pool of possible organ donors. (At the same time the parents might be encouraged to review their own organ donor status, again in the interests not only of concern for others but also in their own interests should they ever need an organ transplant).

Later, a routine invitation to volunteer as a potential organ donor could be sent to each young person on his or her sixteenth birthday. An additional and relatively simple method for contacting all adults from the age of sixteen upwards would be to add a question about organ donation onto the voters' registration form that all households in the UK are legally obliged to complete in order to maintain the electoral register. This would ensure that the vast majority of adults would be given regular opportunities and encouragement to "opt in" to a scheme that is of social as well as personal benefit—what current business jargon calls a "win-win situation."

More complicated would be the development of a scheme for proxy donation of their organs by adults who were deemed incompetent to make autonomous advance donations because of sufficiently severe mental and or neurological disorder or immaturity. Again, one solution would be to exempt this group from the scheme. Alternatively, health care workers, in co-operation with other carers, could be empowered to make decisions to volunteer their organs on behalf of mentally incapacitated adults. Such proxy decisions could be made, in the large majority of cases, on the straightforward grounds that they were clearly likely to be in the medical best interests of the person thus "volunteered," (by placing that person in the priority group for receipt of transplant organs should a transplant be necessary), without causing any significant harm.

So far as "substituted judgment" is concerned, unless there were valid prior directives to the contrary, it could reasonably be assumed that the person concerned, were he or she adequately autonomous, *would* probably volunteer to be an organ donor, given the existence of such a scheme. This claim is made on the assumptions (a) that such volunteering would be in the person's self-interest—it in no way relies on any assumption of altruism; and (b) that the large majority of people would autonomously

choose in their own best interests if there were no countervailing moral objections.

What about benefits and harms? So far as volunteers are concerned there seems little doubt that they would benefit from such a scheme. Furthermore, if the plausible prediction of a considerable increase in organ donors were borne out in practice, then there would be a considerable increase in overall benefits for people who could benefit from transplantation but who currently do not benefit because of the shortage of supply. Indeed, if the rejuvenated supply of organs became sufficiently augmented by the scheme, even non-volunteers of organ donation would benefit.

In the absence of such an enormous increase in organ supply, however, the non-volunteers would clearly lose out and stand to benefit less than at present, if the proposal were accepted. They would be deliberately put at the bottom of the queue for transplanted organs, even in particular situations where their need for, and the extent and probability of their potential benefit from, such transplants would be greater than the needs and benefits of the pre-volunteers who would be given priority.

Here seems to be the Achilles heel of Mr Jarvis's proposal. For even if such non-volunteers can properly be said to have only themselves to blame for their predicament; even if they can properly be said to have deliberately and autonomously made their choice and rejected the opportunity to give themselves priority for receipt of transplanted organs; even if they can properly be said to have been selfish, and or inconsiderate and or foolish, even immoral, in refusing to pre-volunteer their own organs, nonetheless there is an important countervailing moral tradition in medicine. It is that patients should be given treatment in relation to their medical need, and that scarce medical resources should not be prioritised on the basis of a patient's blameworthiness. This moral tradition of medicine is partly an aspect of the medico-moral obligation of medical beneficence—doctors have obligations to try to provide medical benefits to all their patients who are in medical need, and they should not deny such benefits on the grounds of a patient's past or present fault. It is also a matter of justice—doctors should not use fault as a criterion for just distribution of scarce medical resources.

Mr Jarvis says that his proposal accords with Aristotle's formal principle of justice, and no doubt it does, for in some moral contexts undoubtedly past fault, past decisions, past choices, do indeed justify treating people as unequals for the purposes of justice. But the Aristotelian *formal* principle of justice (equals should be treated equally, unequals unequally in proportion to the morally relevant inequality) is compatible with a variety of *substantive* principles of justice. Fault, past or present, is widely rejected as a "morally relevant inequality" by currently accepted substantive principles of distributive justice for scarce medical resources. Attractive though Mr Jarvis's proposal may otherwise be, it does seem to entail reversing this moral norm. If past or present fault thus became an accepted criterion for distributive justice for scarce medical resources, a very steep "logical slippery slope" would have been created.

If the fault and/or inconsiderateness of not previously volunteering his or her organs for transplantation were to justify withholding scarcer life-saving medical resources from a patient, then all other prior faults and inconsiderateness of equal or greater weight could, logically, also be regarded as morally relevant and potentially justificatory for withholding scarce life-saving medical resources from patients. Such a prospect hardly bears contemplation. While fault may well be an entirely "morally relevant" criterion for legal justice, it seems highly likely to create far more social harm than benefit if it is used as a criterion for distributing scarce life-saving medical resources. Alas, Mr Jarvis's otherwise apparently admirable "modest proposal" seems likely to succumb to this major objection.[2]

Notes

1. Jarvis R. Join the club: a modest proposal to increase availability of donor organs. *Journal of medical ethics* 1995; 21:199-204.
2. *Idem.*

50

AS IF THERE WERE FETUSES WITHOUT WOMEN: A REMEDIAL ESSAY

Mary B. Mahowald

As with abortion, most of the moral controversy regarding fetal tissue transplantation focuses on fetuses rather than pregnant women. In both of these related issues, that focus needs to be corrected so as to avoid the fallacy of abstraction, that is, consideration of an object as if it exists without a context. For example, "pro-life" arguments are generally based on the claim that the fetus is a person, and "pro-choice" arguments are generally based on the claim that the fetus is not a person.[1] Assuming the validity of arguments on both sides, the truth status of their conclusions depends on whether the criteria for personhood have been met by the fetus. Despite the fact that fetuses do not exist apart from women, who are inevitably affected by decisions about fetuses, women are ignored by either side so long as fetuses are the pivotal focus of the argument.

With regard to fetal tissue transplantation, women are ignored to the extent that arguments supporting and opposing it are linked with abortion as the means through which the tissue is made available. Women are also ignored where the focus is solely on commercialization of fetal tissue, the experimental status of the technique, or the needs of possible recipients. Interestingly, the important parallel between this issue and others that principally and undeniably affect women (such as contract motherhood, egg provision, and prostitution) is that women have been neglected, and in some cases, flatly ignored.

In this chapter, I want to redress the omission that prevails by reviewing the issue of fetal tissue transplantation with a focus that explicitly includes women as necessary participants in the process. In doing so, I will compare and contrast this with other issues that particularly affect women, and examine different frameworks for ethical assessment of fetal tissue transplantation. First, however, I want to say why it is wrong to focus on fetuses apart from their relationship to women.

FETUSES AS SUCH

The term "fetus" is defined as "the unborn young of an animal while still within the uterus."[2] Fortunately or unfortunately, medical technology has not yet produced an artificial uterus, and it may be biologically impossible to do so. To speak of the uterus without acknowledgment that it is within a woman is thus another example of prescinding from necessary context. According to *Stedman's Medical Dictionary*, the human fetus "represents the product of conception from the end of the eighth week to the moment of birth."[3] Human birth is understood to mean the emergence of a fetus from a woman's body. Stedman's defines the human embryo as "the developing organism from conception until approximately the end of the second month."[4] Since the advent of in vitro fertilization techniques, development of an embryo can be initiated and sustained for several days apart from a woman's body. By definition, nonviable fetuses cannot be so sustained. No matter how early the gestation, a viable fetus removed from a woman's body is no longer a fetus but a newborn. If a nonviable fetus is removed from a woman's body, it is an abortus. In other words, no fetus as such exists apart from a woman's body.

Two major (overlapping) feminist criticisms of traditional ethics are exemplified in our insistence that fetuses not be considered as if they were not present in women. First is the objection that traditional ethics calls for a deductive process through which universal principles are applied to cases.[5] Starting from different principles, whether these are a priori or a posteriori in their derivation, the process (if conducted correctly) leads inexorably to answers about what should be done in specific situations. Feminists argue that this type of deductive analysis cannot adequately attend to the complexity and uniqueness of real cases and issues. To rectify the inadequacy, attention to context is essential.[6]

Second is the objection that much of traditional ethics emphasizes the rights of individuals, neglecting the realm of relationships.[7] In fact, through its assumption that impartiality is a requirement of ethically justifiable judgments, traditional ethics eschews considerations based on particular relationships such as occur between pregnant women and their fetuses. Many of the arguments in which abortion is supported or opposed solely on grounds of the moral status of the fetus exemplify this. In contrast, feminists insist on the moral relevance of relationships, whether these are based on choice, chance, genetics, or affection.[8] The ethics of care elaborated by Carol Gilligan, Nel Noddings, and Sara Ruddick provide frameworks for understanding the essential role that relationships play in moral decision making.[9]

When it is consistently recognized that fetuses exist only in relationship to women who are inevitably affected by decisions regarding them, the above concerns are addressed. Inattention to this ongoing relationship is unscientific because it neglects an element of analysis that affects the validity of scientific interpretation. It is unethical because it ignores the interests and preferences of pregnant women, which may be at odds with the interests of the fetus.

USE OF FETAL TISSUE IN TRANSPLANTATION

An accurate understanding of reality can only be attained through analysis of the complexity of context. With regard to fetal tissue transplantation, the analysis involves at least the following variables: (1) the empirical status of fetuses or abortuses used for grafts, (2) different purposes and sites of tissue retrieval or implantation, (3) therapeutic potential for the recipient, (4) the means through which fetuses are made available for transplantation, and (5) possible motives, "donors," and recipients of fetal tissue.[10]

Regarding (1), human fetuses or abortuses used for tissue grafts may be living or dead. Living fetuses or abortuses may be viable, nonviable, nonviable, or possibly viable, and they may be sentient, nonsentient, or possibly sentient, depending in part on the duration of gestation.[11] Viability is particularly

relevant because it implies that others in addition to the pregnant woman can maintain the fetus ex utero if it is to be delivered or aborted. Sentience is relevant because the prima facie obligation to avoid inflicting pain on others applies to fetuses regardless of whether they are persons. While that obligation does not imply that killing is always wrong, it does imply that pain relief or prevention should be attempted for all sentient, or even possibly sentient, individuals.

Regarding (2), the procedure may be undertaken solely for research purposes, as experimental treatment, or (if and when the procedure becomes standard therapy) solely as therapy for recipients. Ordinarily, therapeutic reasons are more compelling than research reasons for medical procedures. Thus governmental and institutional regulations are more strict for research protocols than for therapeutic protocols.[12] Tissue may be retrieved from the brain or from other parts of a fetus, and implanted directly into a recipient's brain or into other regions of the recipient's body. Brain grafts are generally more problematic than nonbrain grafts because the brain is usually seen as, and may in fact be, the source of a person's identity as well as cognitive function. Nonetheless, the small amount and immaturity of tissue used in transplants serve to minimize this concern.

Regarding (3), non-neural fetal tissue has been transplanted for many years to treat diseases such as DeGeorge's syndrome and diabetes mellitus, without creating public controversy.[13] The prospects that have evoked public debate involve use of neural tissue for treatment of severe and previously incurable neurological disorders. Among the neurological conditions that are potentially treatable are Alzheimer's disease, Parkinson's disease, amyotrophic lateral sclerosis (Lou Gehrig's disease), Huntington's disease, multiple sclerosis, spinal-cord injury, epilepsy, and stroke.[14] The research is most advanced in treatment of Parkinson's disease, but this treatment is still experimental. Comparatively few Parkinson patients have thus far been treated.[15] One case of apparent success in treatment of Hurler's syndrome (through fetus-to-fetus transplant) has also been reported.[16] While preliminary results are promising, there are too little data as yet to generalize about the treatment's effectiveness.

Regarding (4), abortion is the means through which human fetal tissue becomes available for transplantation. Abortions may be spontaneous or induced, and induced abortions may be performed for medical or non-medical reasons. Medical reasons for induced abortion include those based on the pregnant women's health, those based on fetal anomaly, or both. While use of tissue obtained from spontaneous abortions may be less ethically controversial than use of tissue obtained from induced abortions, the tissue from spontaneously aborted fetuses is unlikely to be normal or suitable for transplantation.[17] Because of that likelihood, it may be argued that use of tissue from spontaneously aborted fetuses constitutes undue risk to the recipient. Nonetheless, the first reported human use of fetal neural tissue for treatment of Parkinson's patients involved tissue retrieved from a spontaneously aborted fetus. This work evoked criticism from researchers involved in neurografting.[18]

Regarding (5), fetal tissue may be "donated" for altruistic reasons, self-interested reasons, or both. Ordinarily, the recipient is unrelated and unknown to the pregnant woman. Anonymity has been proposed by at least two panels reviewing the issue as a requirement for donor status.[19] However, an ethic that emphasizes relationships supports a decision to donate the tissue on the part of someone such as a friend or spouse who is both known and related to the recipient. A care ethic may also support a decision to become pregnant in order to provide the tissue to someone with whom one has a special relationship.

Further, a pregnant woman might herself be the recipient, and could deliberately become pregnant in order to provide the fetal tissue that might lead to her own cure. There is one published report of a woman with severe aplastic anemia who was transplanted with the liver of her own fetus after an elective abortion.[20] Although the details of the case are sketchy, the pregnancy was probably not initiated with the intention of providing the fetal tissue for two reasons. First, pregnancy is a serious risk to women with this disease, and second, the fetus would not necessarily be an appropriate tissue match for the woman. Nonetheless, a woman's right to self-preservation supports such an attempt to provide the tissue for her own treatment.

From a feminist perspective, all of the above variables are morally relevant to determination of whether fetal tissue transplantation is justified in specific cases. Particularly important is the means through which fetal tissue is obtained, namely, abortion. In order to insure respect for women's autonomy, decisions to terminate pregnancies must be separable from decisions to provide fetal tissue for transplantation. (Note that I have used the word "separable" rather than "separate.") As we will see in the next section, however, the possibility of separating the two has been disputed.

FETAL TISSUE TRANSPLANTATION AND ABORTION

Although the connection between grafts of human fetal tissue and abortion might have triggered public controversy decades ago, this did not occur until reports circulated early in 1987 about the prospect of using the tissue for treatment of neurological disorders.[21] Apparent reasons for the shift include the fact that abortion was not the volatile issue that it is today when fetal tissue was first used for research or therapeutic purposes. Another reason is that the type of diseases that the tissue may potentially be used to treat afflict literally millions of people who are severely debilitated with otherwise incurable diseases. There seems to be little doubt that political interests were at work in establishing the moratorium on government funding in the United States for research projects involving use of fetal tissue obtained from abortions. Before the Clinton administration lifted the moratorium in 1993, researchers could only find support for use of electively aborted fetal tissue through private sources. Although the moratorium slowed progress in the United States, researchers in Colorado and Connecticut, states that permit research with electively aborted fetal tissue, pursued their projects through private funding.[22]

The problematic connection between fetal tissue transplantation and abortion was first noted by a group who met in Cleveland in 1986. In collaboration with neuroscientist Jerry Silver, I had organized the meeting to review the issue in order to facilitate informed public debate. In March 1987, a consensus statement of the group appeared in *Science*.[23] We maintained that the procedure held "the promise of great benefit to victims of serious neurological disorders." Despite the legality of abortion, fetal tissue transplantation "was acknowledged to be ethically controversial because of its association with abortion." In light of that controversy, we proposed "separation between decisions related to the acquisition of tissue and decisions regarding the transplantation of tissue into a recipient." Two years later, a panel of experts convened by the National Institutes of Health (NIH), several of whom had signed the earlier consensus statement, offered a similar recommendation.[24]

Feminist support for distinguishing between decisions about abortion and decisions about fetal tissue transplantation is mainly based on concerns about possibilities for exploiting women or pressuring them to undergo abortions, or to delay or modify abortion procedures in order to provide fetal tissue to prospective recipients. As yet, it has not been necessary to delay or modify abortion procedures in treatment by means of fetal tissue grafts. Preliminary data suggest that the gestational age optimal for successful transplants into Parkinson's patients is as early as seven weeks, using tissue obtained from abortions performed by standard clinical methods.[25]

While feminists generally support the right of women to terminate pregnancies, most see abortion as a "forced" and tragic option.[26] It is regrettable that a woman must choose between continuation and termination of her pregnancy because both alternatives involve burdens or harms. Accordingly, we would not like to see the option of providing fetal tissue for transplantation precipitate an increase in abortions. Ironically, this concern coincides with one of the concerns mentioned in minority reports of the NIH Human Fetal Tissue Transplantation Research panel (hereafter, NIH panel). Several members of the NIH panel argued against government support for the procedure on grounds that it would constitute an inducement to abortion, at least for pregnant women who had not yet decided whether to terminate their pregnancies.[27] There are no data supporting this claim.

A further concern of a minority of the NIH panel was that participation in fetal tissue transplantation constitutes complicity in, and legitimation of, abortion. According to James Bopp and James Burtchaell,

Whatever the researcher's intentions may be, by entering into an institutionalized partnership with the abortion industry as a supplier of preference, he or she becomes complicit, though after the fact, with the abortions that have expropriated the tissue for his or her purposes.[28]

They thus maintain that those who use fetal tissue from elective abortions ally themselves with the "evil" that abortion represents.

Bopp and Burtchaell further claim that legitimation occurs when pregnant women considering abortion construe the possibility of benefiting someone by donating fetal tissue as a positive endorsement of abortion. The abortion is then seen as a less tragic choice than it would otherwise be, and in some circumstances it might even be seen as virtuous. Legitimation would occur on a social level if the good of successful treatment through fetal tissue transplantation became so compelling that the means of achieving the success were never critically assessed. The end would then have justified the means, at least as perceived by those who pursue the end without scrutinizing the end in its own right.

The legitimation argument illustrates more general concerns about slippery slope reasoning. Questions such as the following are then raised: if we now approve use of fetal tissue for transplants under restrictive conditions, are we not likely in time to relax the conditions if the therapy proves highly successful or if the restrictive conditions limit its usefulness? Most people agree that some restrictions are necessary to avoid abuses that could accompany use of the technology; they disagree about where to place wedges along the slippery slope.[29]

Some have proposed less restrictive guidelines than those recommended by the NIH panel, particularly with regard to commercialization. For example, Lori Andrews argues that a woman should be allowed to sell the tissue of a fetus she has agreed to abort. Feminists, she maintains, are inconsistent with their commitment to promote women's right to control their own bodies if they oppose commercial surrogacy.[30] Most feminists, however, oppose both contract motherhood and commerce in fetal tissue because of the possibility they present for exploiting women. Unlike Andrews, we thus place greater emphasis on social equality than on individual liberty. Social equality is seen as a necessary condition for authentic choice. Until and unless general equality prevails, the liberty of individual women is inevitably curtailed.

Different views regarding abortion also give rise to different views regarding the consent necessary for fetal tissue transplantation. Those who are morally opposed to elective abortion generally deny that women who choose abortion have a right to donate fetal tissue.[31] Such women, they allege, have forfeited that right even as parents may forfeit their right to consent for their child if they abuse or abandon the child. On the other side of the issue are those who stress the importance of the pregnant woman's consent to use of fetal tissue because she has the right to abortion and because the tissue belongs to her.[32] Among those who consider abortion a separable issue from fetal tissue transplantation, some insist that the pregnant woman's consent is necessary because the timing and procedure for abortion may be altered in order to maximize the chance for a successful graft.[33] In other words, if the pregnant woman may herself be affected, her consent to use fetal tissue is morally indispensable.

On therapeutic grounds alone, a comparison of the potential advantages of using fetal tissue from electively aborted fetuses with the potential and actual disadvantages of treatment through other means provides a strong case for use of fetal tissue from elective abortions. Many of the diseases that are potentially curable with fetal tissue grafts are curable by no other known means. However, therapeutic efficacy alone doesn't constitute moral justification. This returns us, then, to the problem of whether the question of induced abortion is morally separable from the question of fetal tissue transplantation. The issue calls for reexamination of the traditional moral dilemma involving the relationship between means and ends. Does the end justify the means in transplantation of fetal tissue for cure of otherwise incurable disorders?

A simplistic version of utilitarianism supports an affirmative answer to the question. In other words, the tremendous good that might be accomplished through the new technique outweighs the harm that might be done through elective abortion. However, if

endorsement of the procedure led to widespread increase in elective abortions and to exploitation of women, such undesirable consequences might outweigh the potential benefit of the technique. So, even if ends can justify means, it is not clear that the end justifies the means in this case. Whether or not the overall consequences of treating debilitating disorders through fetal tissue transplantation will generally constitute a preponderance of harms over benefits is an empirical issue for which more data is needed to support a credible utilitarian position.

From a deontological point of view, the end does not justify means that are otherwise morally unacceptable, but this does not imply that fetal tissue transplantation is morally unjustified. The individual who knowingly and freely pursues a specific end, also knowingly and freely chooses the means to its fulfilment. Intention is thus crucial to the moral relevance of the relationship. If a woman were to deliberately become pregnant, choose abortion, or persuade another to become pregnant or choose abortion, solely for the sake of fetal tissue transplantation, she would then be responsible for both means and end because she would be intending both. As we already noted, the motive of the decision may be altruistic, self-interested, or both. Although worthy motives are morally relevant, they do not alter the fact that the intention in such cases applies to both ends and means.

In other situations involving fetal tissue transplantation, the individual who intends to use the tissue need not even be aware of the abortion through which the tissue becomes available. Presumably, she does intend the retrieval procedure. However, just as a transplant surgeon may retrieve essential organs from the brain-dead victim of a drunk-driving accident, without any implication that she thus endorses the behavior that led to the availability of the organs, so may a neurosurgeon who is totally opposed to abortion transplant neural tissue from an electively aborted fetus into a severely impaired patient, without thereby compromising her moral convictions. In fact, one may argue that a truly pro-life position favors the saving or prolonging of life that the transplantation intends, while acknowledging the negation of life that abortion implies. When the abortion decision has already been made by others, a decision not to transplant seems less in keeping with a position that is genuinely pro-life than its opposite. One opponent of abortion even found support for fetal tissue transplants in the biblical account of creation. Barbara Culliton attributed the following statement to the Baptist father whose infant had prenatally been treated with cells obtained from an aborted fetus: "God formed one human being from the tissue of another. Not only does God approve of this [transplantation], he himself performed the first one."[34]

FETAL TISSUE TRANSPLANTS AND USE OF WOMEN'S BODIES

If abortion and fetal tissue transplants are not separable issues, then the latter is parallel in important respects to at least three other practices which can only be undertaken through use of women's bodies. Contract motherhood, egg provision, and prostitution are comparable practices because they all involve both benefit to a third party and material remuneration to the woman who provides the benefit through use of her body. The rationale by which most feminists oppose these practices is also applicable to the apparent tie between abortion and fetal tissue grafts. However, this opposition does not extend to fetal tissue grafts considered as an issue distinct from abortion. From a feminist standpoint, it is possible to support a woman's right to abortion while opposing the practice of fetal tissue transplantation.

Contract motherhood necessarily involves the commodification of a woman's body: she "rents" or lends her womb, and may have contributed an egg to the embryo that develops within her. In commercial contracts, the woman accepts payment from an infertile couple for her "services." According to the final ruling in the Mary Beth Whitehead case, payment for such "services" is equivalent to baby selling.[35] This is an interesting designation because it totally ignores what pregnancy and birth meant to the woman, focusing exclusively on the baby to whom she gives birth. Adoption is the better analogue for the act through which infertile women or couples thus become parents. The woman has agreed to rent her womb and donate or sell her egg, and a child has been produced through the services rendered. Whether or not she is genetically related to the fetus, the surrogate is biologically related to it through gestation.

If contract motherhood is equivalent to baby selling, payment to pregnant women for use of their aborted fetuses may also be equivalent to baby selling.[36] In both cases, it is the use of the woman's body *before* abortion or delivery that is remunerated by someone to whom the fetus is valued. Neither case *necessarily* involves financial remuneration because both *may* be undertaken for altruistic reasons. Contract motherhood and use of fetal tissue may also be undertaken by mutual agreement prior to the establishment of pregnancy. In neither case is there an intent to keep the product of conception. In one case, however, a living infant is provided for a third party; in the other, the tissue of a dead fetus is obtained in order to provide for the health of a third party. In both situations, the intention of the pregnant women may be both self-interested and altruistic, regardless of whether payment is involved.

Egg donation may be compared with sperm "donation" because both involve the provision of gametes, usually for financial compensation. But unlike the provision of sperm, providing eggs involves considerable discomfort and risk. When the procedure was first reported in Cleveland in 1987, it required administration of superovulatory drugs and laparoscopic retrieval of ova under general anaesthesia.[37] In most centers, retrieval is now undertaken trough transvaginal aspiration with a local anaesthetic. As with sperm, the term "donation" is misleading because individuals who agree to provide ova generally do so for the money. As a student who volunteered for the world's first egg donor program put it: "I would never go through this if I were not a poor student."[38] The compensation provided to egg donors in the program in which she enrolled was $900-$1200. In 1992, compensation ranged from $1500 to $3000, depending on the clinic.[39]

The practice of egg donation is comparable to fetal tissue provision insofar as the woman in each case contributes genetic material and may receive compensation. Occasionally, the ova retrieved may simply be the product of a normal menstrual cycle, without requiring administration of superovulatory medication. When this occurs, the retrieval is comparable to retrieval of fetal tissue from women who undergo abortions to terminate unwanted pregnancies. Unlike fetuses, ova are regularly disposed of through menstruation. They may even be retrieved as a by-product of surgery undertaken for treatment purposes. In such circumstances, providing eggs for another is more like providing tissue from spontaneously aborted fetuses than providing tissue obtained from elective abortions.

As with contract motherhood and sperm donation, egg donation is oriented to the development of a new human life. Fetal tissue becomes available for transplantation only after the death of the embryo or fetus, which occurs in the context of either spontaneous or elective abortion. The tissue that thus becomes available constitutes the possibility of extending another human life. In all of these cases, therefore, another life is affirmed through birth or healing.

Prostitution is different from the other issues discussed because it does not involve a comparable goal. To some people, the very suggestion of a parallel between prostitution and egg provision or contract motherhood is offensive because the former practice is clearly illegal and immoral, while the latter two practices are not.[40] Another difference is that prostitution does not involve medical technology. Although contract motherhood through artificial insemination may be undertaken without the help of a medical expert, this is probably a rare event, and arrangements in which gestational and genetic roles are separate require *in vitro* fertilization.[41] Despite these differences, the parallel between prostitution and the other issues is valid insofar as all of them involve the use of women's bodies to satisfy the desires of another. So does fetal tissue transplantation.

By definition, prostitution is practiced for material remuneration, usually money, and not for altruistic reasons intended to benefit those who employ prostitutes.[42] In some cases, however, women sell the intimacy of their bodies in order to support their children; for many women, prostitution is a means of survival, and in some cases it is perceived as (and may in fact be) the only available means of survival.[43] From a moral point of view, prostitution to obtain funds necessary for one's own or others' survival is surely defensible. What is immoral in such a situation is the social situation that presents so tragic a limitation of alternatives to women.[44]

Because prostitution is always practiced for material gain for the prostitute, it is only comparable to fetal tissue transplantation when the latter procedure also procures material gain for the woman who provides the fetal tissue. As with prostitution, however, the material gain that is accessible through fetal tissue grafts may be sought indirectly, and the motive for providing the tissue may be altruistic rather than self-interested. It is possible, for example, for a woman to initiate and terminate a pregnancy to produce fetal tissue for someone from whom she hopes to inherit wealth because of that decision. It is also possible to sell fetal tissue that she develops through a pregnancy that is deliberately undertaken to obtain funds necessary for her own or others' sustenance. A woman could even sell a fetus conceived through intercourse as a prostitute. While there are longstanding social, moral, and religious objections to prostitution, the grounds for these objections are not substantively different from objections that may be raised to contract motherhood, at least when the woman who gives birth is not genetically related to the offspring. Both involve the use of a woman's intimate body parts for payment, and in both cases the woman is generally of considerably lower socioeconomic status than the payor.

If prostitution is practiced to promote one's own survival, it parallels the situation of a pregnant woman who wishes her fetal tissue to be used for treatment of her own devastating disease, that is, to insure her own survival. If a pregnant woman sells her fetus to obtain funds to support others, her act is comparable to that of the woman who prostitutes herself to support her children. Fetal tissue transplantation is more morally problematic than prostitution because it involves not only the use of women's bodies but also the use of human fetuses. The same argument can be made with regard to a comparison between prostitution and eggs provision or contract motherhood. The latter practices may be viewed as more problematic because they involve the use of gametes and fetuses or newborns as well as the use of women's bodies for remuneration.

PARADIGMS AND FRAMEWORKS FOR ASSESSING FETAL TISSUE TRANSPLANTATION

Different paradigms and frameworks have been invoked to defend or oppose fetal tissue transplantation. The paradigms include transplantation from living donors, as in kidney transplants; transplantation from cadaver donors, as in heart transplants; and "surrogate motherhood."[45] The first two are familiar and generally accepted means of obtaining organs from tissue, so long as consent is obtained from the donor or proxy and the retrieval does not constitute a major threat to the donor's health. Use of tissue from living fetuses has generally been rejected, but it is sometimes difficult to determine whether a fetus is dead. Traditional means of assessing brain death are not applicable to early fetuses or abortuses. Although "surrogacy" is a more controversial paradigm for fetal tissue transplantation , it captures, as the other two paradigms do not, the unique possibilities for exploitation of women that fetal tissue transplantation represents. As I have already suggested, these possibilities are also present in egg provision and prostitution, which are also comparable to fetal tissue transplantation.

Dorothy Vawter and her colleagues at the University of Minnesota have proposed three "competing frameworks" that may be related to the above paradigms.[46] The first is based on the premise that the fetus from which tissue may be retrieved should be regarded as a human research subject. On this view, either of two rationales may prevail, depending on whether the aborted fetus is construed as living or dead. If the former, use of fetal tissue "should satisfy the federal regulations for research involving living fetuses, and be reviewed and approved by an institutional review board." If the aborted fetus is regarded as a cadaver, a proxy decision-maker should be required "to base a decision regarding participation either on the basis of what the dead fetus would have wanted or on some view of what is in the dead fetus' best interests." Not surprisingly, neither of these standards is explained, and the authors acknowledge that it is "extremely difficult to see how a proxy decision-maker could base a decision on [them]."[47]

The second ethical framework proposed by the Minnesota group is a view of the dead fetus as a cadaveric organ donor. This generally means following the standards of the Uniform Anatomical Gift Act, which is applicable in all 50 states in the United States. This Act allows either parent to provide the necessary consent for use of fetal tissue so long as the other parent does not object. Moreover, because the dead fetus can hardly be accredited with wishes or interests, parents may base their decision on their own needs, concerns, and interests. The consensus statement of the 1986 forum in Cleveland utilized this framework. According to the authors,

> retrieval of tissue from fetal remains is analogous to the transplantation of organs or tissue obtained from adult human cadavers. Similarities include the fact that the donor is dead, and the expectation that there will be significant benefits for the recipient. These similarities suggest the appropriateness of using the same ethical and legal criteria now followed for cadaver transplantation.[48]

The beginning point of the published reports from both the Cleveland group and the NIH panel is that fetal tissue should only be retrieved from *dead* fetuses. Only then does the analogy with retrieval of tissue from "adult human cadavers" work. Even so, the differences between transplantation from human fetal cadavers rather than mature human cadavers are to be addressed through added requirements, such as the exclusion of familial donors and the observance of anonymity between donors and recipients. Obviously, this excludes the possibility of a woman initiating or terminating pregnancy in order to provide tissue for herself or for another with whom she has a special relationship.

The third framework proposed by Vawter and her colleagues is one in which the dead fetus or abortus is equated with discarded tissue. In that context,

> fetal remains, whether the result of elective abortion, ectopic pregnancy, or spontaneous abortion, are treated as any other bodily tissue and fluid removed during a diagnostic or surgical procedure.[49]

Aborted tissue is thus construed as a tissue specimen of the woman from whose body it was removed. Permission from those whose discarded tissue may be examined for educative, research, or future treatment purposes is routinely obtained in the clinical setting. Typically, the consent forms include "boilerplate" language requesting blanket permission for use of any biological "waste materials" or "tissue specimens" removed during surgical procedures. Similar boilerplate language could be incorporated into the consent form for abortion procedures.

Whereas the first two frameworks proposed by the Minnesota Center focus on the fetus as a separate being from the pregnant woman, the third focuses on the fact that fetal tissue is in fact the woman's tissue, and ought to be treated as such even when aborted. It is appropriate, therefore, to ask the pregnant woman for consent to use of her fetal tissue prior to the abortion, and her consent alone is morally adequate. Some might argue that consent of the man who impregnated the woman should also be required for use of fetal tissue, but this suggests an unusual concept of "discarded tissue," and a departure from the usual manner of dealing with discarded tissue. Moreover, since abortion is a decision legally made by women and not by their male partners, men cannot effectively challenge pregnant women's decisions regarding disposition of their fetuses.

Like the "surrogacy" model, the discarded tissue framework emphasizes the essential tie between fetus and pregnant woman. The latter model is a means of avoiding the abuses that we have seen associated with contract motherhood. Because the discarded tissue model gives priority to the pregnant woman's autonomy, it serves as a check on the possibilities for exploitation of women that transplantation of fetal tissue allows. Thus there are both conceptual and moral reasons for preferring this framework to the others: it takes account of the unique relationship between fetus and pregnant woman, and the practice it engenders is consistent with respect for patient autonomy in comparable situations.

CONCLUSION

Like abortion, and probably because of its association with abortion, the issue of fetal tissue transplantation is a volatile one. Ironically, both feminists and those opposed to elective abortion are concerned about its association with abortion because for the former it represents possible pressures on women to initiate or terminate pregnancies, and for the latter it expresses complicity in, and legitimation of, abortion. From a feminist standpoint, there is strong support for keeping the two issues separable, but not necessarily separate. "Separable" allows for the possibility that individual women may choose to connect their abortions

with the provision of fetal tissue. If the issues are "separate," that connection is precluded.

Because fetuses do not exist apart from women, fetal tissue transplantation raises concerns that may be seen in other troublesome issues that centrally affect women: contract motherhood, egg provision, and prostitution. Examination of the similarities and dissimilarities among these issues facilitates a better grasp of problematic aspects of the involvement of women in fetal tissue transplantation. If abortion decisions are separable from decisions about use of fetal tissue, the problematic aspects are reduced.

Of the frameworks that have been proposed for moral assessment of fetal tissue transplantation, the use of fetal remains from abortions is more like use of discarded tissue than use of tissue from research subjects or from cadaver donors. Whether the abortion through which fetal tissue becomes available is spontaneous or induced, the tissue used for grafts is discarded from the body of the pregnant woman. However, even the analogy with use of discarded tissue misses the uniqueness and complexity of the relationship between pregnant women and fetuses. The uniqueness and complexity of that relationship call for explicit attention to the fact that fetuses do not exist without women.

———

Notes

1. My use of the terms "pro-life" and "pro-choice" accords with popular usage. In another article I have noted that this usage is not fully affirmative of life and choice, respectively. See my "Abortion and Equality," in Sidney Callahan and Daniel Callahan, eds., *Abortion* (New York: Plenum Press 1984), 179-180. One notable exception to the tendency to base "pro-choice" arguments on the status of the fetus is Judith Jarvis Thomson's "A Defense of Abortion," in *Philosophy and Public Affairs* 1,1 (1971), 47-66. Thomson defends a woman's right to abortion *even if* the fetus is a person.

2. E.g., see *Webster's New World Dictionary*, 2nd college ed. (New York: Simon and Schuster, 1982), 517; cf. *Churchill's Medical Dictionary* (New York: Churchill Livingston Inc., 1989), 693.

3. *Stedman's Medical Dictionary*, 25th ed. (Baltimore: Williams and Wilkins, 1990), 573. This calculation of the duration of gestation is based on the first day of the last menstrual period rather than fertilization. If duration of gestation is calculated from fertilization, the fetal stage of development commences at six weeks. See James Knight and Joan Callahan, *Preventing Birth* (Salt Lake City: University of Utah Press, 1989), 205.

4. *Stedman's*, 501. However, Knight and Callahan note that the term "embryo" refers to the developing human organism between weeks 2 and 6 of gestation (205). Implantation in the uterus occurs about two weeks after fertilization. Between fertilization and implantation, the conceptus may be referred to as "pre-implantation embryo." The term "pre-embryo" is sometimes used by in vitro fertilization specialists to refer to the conceptus before implantation. In popular usage, however, the term "embryo" is often used to characterize the conceptus from fertilization until fetal stage.

5. Susan Sherwin develops this criticism on the part of medical ethics as well as feminist ethics. See her "Feminist and Medical Ethics: Two different Approaches to Contextual Ethics," *Hypatia* 4, 2 (Summer 1989): 57-72.

6. Marilyn Friedman, "Care and Context in Moral Reasoning," *Women and Moral Theory*, ed. by Eva F. Kittay and Diana T. Meyers (Totowa, New Jersey: Rowman and Littlefield, 1987), 190-204.

7. See Friedman; see also Christina Sommers, "Filial Morality," in Kittay and Meyers, 69-84.

8. Some feminists argue that the genetic tie is hardly relevant in defining parental relationships. See, e.g., Barbara Katz Rothman, *Recreating Motherhood* (New York: W. W. Norton 1989), 37-40. In some cases, however, the law insists on the significance of the genetic tie. For example, known (genetic) fathers are legally responsible for support of their children. It is well known that statutes requiring such support are only occasionally enforced.

9. Carol Gilligan, *In a Different Voice* (Cambridge: Harvard University Press, 1982); Nel Noddings, *Caring* (Berkeley: University of California Press, 1984); Sara Ruddick, *Maternal Thinking* (New York: Ballantine Books 1989). While developing a model of maternal thinking that is applicable to men as well as women, Ruddick refers to the work of mothering as "caring labor" (46). See also Mary Jean Larrabee, ed., *An Ethic of Care* (New York: Routledge, 1993); Joan Tronto, *Moral Boundaries* (New York: Routledge, 1993); Rita C. Manning, *Speaking from the Heart* (Lanham, MD: Rowman and Littlefield, 1992).

10. I have discussed these variables at greater length in "Neural Fetal Tissue Transplantation—Should We Do What We Can Do?" *Neurologic Clinics* 7, 4 (November 1989): 745-753.

11. Technically, a viable or even a nonviable (living) "abortus" is a newborn. What is relevant here, however, is not that technical difference but the moral significance of viability and sentience for any developing organism.

12. Although research with human subjects, including fetuses, must be reviewed by an institutional review board, no such review is necessary for established therapies.

13. Dorothy E. Vawter, Warren Kearney, Karen G. Gervais et al., *The Use of Human Fetal Tissue: Scientific, Ethical and Policy Concerns* (Minneapolis: University of Minnesota Press, January 1990), 45-67, 2128-2129.

14. Cf. U.S. Congress, Office of Technology Assessment, *Neural Grafting: Repairing the Brain and Spinal Cord*, OTA-BA- 462 (Washington, D.C.: U.S. Government Printing Office, September 1990), 93-107.

15. Stanley Fahn, "Fetal-Tissue Transplants in Parkinson's Disease," *New England Journal of Medicine* 327, 22 (Nov. 26, 1992): 1550.

16. Barbara J. Culliton, "Needed: Fetal Tissue Research," *Nature* 355 (January 23, 1992), 295.

17. Vawter et al., 136-138

18. Vawter et al., 109, 138.

19. These were the *Forum on Transplantation of Neural Tissue from Fetuses,* convened by the Case Western Reserve University School of Medicine, Cleveland, December 4-5, 1986, and the National Institutes of Health's *Human Fetal Tissue Transplantation Research Panel,* which met in Washington, D.C. late in 1988.

20. Cited in Vawter et al., 42, from E. Kelemen, "Recovery from Chronic Idiopathic Bone Marrow Aplasia of a Young Mother after Intravenous Injection of Unprocessed Cells from the Liver (and Yolk Sac) of Her 22 m CR-length Embryo. A Preliminary Report."

Scandinavian Journal of Haemotology 10 (1973), 305-308.

21. The first of these was a letter in *Science* signed by Mary B. Mahowald, Judith Areen, Barry J. Hoffer, Albert R. Jonsen, Patricia King, Jerry Silver, John R. Sladek, Jr., and LeRoy Walters, "Transplantation of Neural Tissue from Fetuses," *Science* 235 (Mar. 13, 1987), 1307-1308.

22. Cf. Curt R. Freed, Robert E. Breeze, Neil L. Rosenberg et al., "Survival of Implanted Fetal Dopamine Cells and Neurologic Improvement 12 to 46 Months after Transplantation for Parkinson's Disease," *New England Journal of Medicine* 327, 22 (Nov. 26, 1992): 1549-1555; Dennis D. Spencer, Richard J. Robbins, Frederick Naftolin et al., "Unilateral Transplantation of Human Fetal Mesencephalic Tissue into the Caudate Nucleus of Patients with Parkinson's Disease," *New England Journal of Medicine* 327, 22 (Nov. 26, 1992), 1541-1548.

23. Mahowald et al., *Science,* 1308-1309.

24. Consultants to the Advisory Committee to the Director, National Institutes of Health, *Report of the Human Fetal Tissue Transplantation Research Panel* (hereafter NIH Report), vol. 2 (December 1988), A2.

25. Freed, Breeze, Rosenberg et al., 1550.

26. It is "forced" in the sense that William James delineates one of the marks of a genuine option. In other words, choice is unavoidable. See "The Will to Believe," in William James, *Essays on Faith and Morals* (Cleveland: Meridian Books, 1962), 34.

27. In addition to its three chairs, the NIH panel consisted of 18 members, three of whom disagreed with the majority view.

28. *Report of the Human Fetal Tissue Transplantation Research Panel* (NIH Report), vol. 1 (December 1988), 70.

29. Cf. my "Placing Wedges along the Slippery Slope," *Clinical Research* 36, 3 (1988): 220-222.

30. Cf. NIH Report 1, 56 and Lori B. Andrews, "Feminism Revisited: Fallacies and Policies in the Surrogacy Debate," *Logos* 9 (1988), 81-96.

31. Cf. NIH Report 1, 47-50.

32. Cf. Lori Andrews, "My Body, My Property," *Hastings Center Report* 16, 5 (October 1986), 28-38, and John Robertson, "Rights, Symbolism, and Public Policy in Fetal Tissue Transplants," *Hastings Center Report* 18,6 (December 1988), 9-10. A key point here is whether

externalization of the fetus through birth or abortion terminates or reduces the woman's claims to ownership of the tissue. Mary Ann Warren distinguishes the rights of fetuses and infants, arguing that even late-term fetuses cannot have "the full and equal rights" to which newborns may be entitled. See her "The Moral Significance of Birth," *Hypatia* 4, 3 (Fall 1989), 63.

33. Cf. Mary B. Mahowald, Jerry Silver, and Robert A. Ratcheson, "The Ethical Options in Fetal Transplants," *Hastings Center Report* 17, 1 (February 1987), 13.

34. Culliton, 295. This statement was attributed to the Baptist father of a baby who had prenatally received grafted cells from an aborted fetus for treatment of Hurler's syndrome. Two older children had already died of the disease. Both parents were strongly opposed to abortion and remain so.

35. *In re Baby M.,* New Jersey Lexis 1, 79 (New Jersey Supreme Court No. A-39), Feb. 1988.

36. Admittedly, "baby selling" is different from sale of aborted fetuses insofar as "baby selling" involves living infants.

37. "Clinic in Ohio Starts Egg Donor Plan," *New York Times* (July 15, 1987), A16.

38. This was my student in a course on "Moral Problems in Medicine" at Case Western Reserve University in 1987.

39. Paula Monarez, "Halfway There," *Chicago Tribune* (Feb. 2, 1992), sect. 6, 4.

40. Although commercial surrogacy is illegal in some states (e.g., New Jersey), most states have no legislation regarding the practice. The morality of contract motherhood remains a matter of public debate.

41. The practice of self-insemination is not new, but there is no reliable documentation of its incidence, in part because the insemination occurs in private, and through private arrangement with a semen provider. While the desire of some women to become parents without the involvement of men may increase the practice, concerns about the status of semen (especially its HIV status) now prompt women to seek technical assistance to test semen used for insemination. For a description of self-insemination, see Mary Barton, Kenneth Walker, and B. P. Wiesner, "Artificial Insemination," *British Medical Journal* 1 (1945), pp. 40-43; Frederick E. Lane, "Artificial Insemination at Home," *Fertility and Sterility* 5 (1954), 372-

373; and *Self Insemination* (London: The Feminist Self-Insemination Group, Sept. 1980). Infants born as a result of self-insemination without medical assistance have sometimes been referred to as "turkey baster babies." The technique allows lesbian couples to obtain sperm, and have one inseminate the other. Lori B. Andrews describes a case of surrogate gestation in which a friend of the infertile couple inseminated herself with the sperm of the husband. See her *New Conceptions* (New York: St. Martin's Press, 1984), 202.

42. E.g., *Webster's New World Dictionary*, 2nd college ed., thus defines "prostitute": "to sell the services of (oneself or another) for purposes of sexual intercourse" (New York: Simon and Schuster, 1982), 1140.

43. Marriage has been compared with prostitution because it similarly involves the use of women's bodies for material remuneration. According to Esther Vilar,

> By the age of twelve at the latest, most women have decided to become prostitutes. Or, to put it another way, they have planned a future for themselves which consists of choosing a man and letting him do all the work. In return for his support, they are prepared to let him make use of their vagina at certain given moments.

See Vilar, "What Is Woman?" in Mary Briody Mahowald, ed., *Philosophy of Woman: Classical to Current Concepts,* revised ed. (Indianapolis, IN: Hackett, 1983), 30.

44. Cf. Alison M. Jaggar, *Feminist Politics and Human Nature* (Totowa, NJ: Rowman and Allanheld, 1983), 263-264. Also, cf. Laurie Shrage, "Should Feminists Oppose Prostitution?" *Ethics* 99, 2 (January 1989), 347-361.

45. Mahowald et al., *Hastings Center Report,* 11-12. Although I here use the term "surrogate motherhood," I agree with Rosemarie Tong's criticism of the term because it implies that the woman who gives birth is not the child's mother. Tong initially preferred the term "contract motherhood," which more accurately reflects the arrangement through which a woman agrees to become a biological mother so that another person may become a social parent. See Tong, "The Overdue Death of a Feminist Chameleon: Taking a Stand on Surrogacy Arrangements," *Journal of Social Philosophy* XXI, 2 (Fall/Winter 1990), 40-56. [Tong now suggests the term "gestational motherhood," since it better captures non-commercial arrangements and it leaves OUT the notion of contract. See her paper....]

46. Vawter et al., 211-231.

47. Vawter et al., 212-213.

48. Mahowald et al., *Science,* 235, 1308.

49. Vawter et al., 211.

51.
REQUESTS, GIFTS, AND OBLIGATIONS: THE ETHICS OF ORGAN PROCUREMENT

Arthur L. Caplan

THE INADEQUACY OF PRESENT METHODS OF PROCURING ORGANS

The field of organ transplantation has enjoyed remarkable progress since the 1960s. Early in the decade, the first attempt was made to transplant a kidney between identical twins. Since that initial attempt surgeons have perfected their techniques, immunologists have developed powerful new immunosuppressive drugs and tissue-matching capabilities, and health care professionals have learned how to manage the complications that often ensue once a transplant has been performed. Today it is possible to transplant many different organs and tissues using both cadaver and living sources to both related and nonrelated recipients. More than 400,000 transplants were performed in the United States in the 1980s, including kidneys, hearts, livers, corneas, skin, bone, and lungs.

As the ability to transplant organs and tissues has grown, the demand for these procedures has increased as well. In the early days of kidney transplant surgery the technique was seen as so experimental that many physicians would not even consider a transplant from a nonrelated or cadaver source.

While renal dialysis was developed primarily as an adjunct to kidney transplantation, the poor rates of success associated with transplant surgery in the early and mid-1960s led many physicians to recommend dialysis as the treatment of choice for those afflicted with renal failure who lacked a willing living donor. This was true despite the fact that dialysis itself was known to have many serious and even potentially lethal side-effects.[1]

As better surgical techniques and more powerful immunosuppressants were perfected and as success rates utilizing cadaver organs in nonrelated recipients improved, more and more individuals were viewed by their physicians as potential candidates for transplants. In the early days of the Stanford Heart Transplantation program it was unusual for someone over the age of 45 to receive a transplant. Today that age range has been extended to 55. Some centers believe that even this age restriction is merely arbitrary and have extended the pool of heart recipients to include those 60 and older.

The demand for organs and tissues from cadaver sources has grown to the point where it far exceeds the available supply. While approximately 5,500 kidneys were transplanted in the United States in 1984, the waiting lists at dialysis centers around the country included the names of more than 10,000 persons who were actively seeking a transplant. Similar shortfalls exist for those seeking corneas, livers, hearts, bone and pancreases.

The gap between the supply of cadaver organs and the demand for them is not adequately reflected by figures citing those actually on waiting lists to receive an organ or tissue. Many potential recipients are not even placed on waiting lists.

Physicians are well aware of the fact that there is an insufficient supply of organs to meet the demand for them. They cope with the shortage by denying access even to waiting lists on the grounds that some possible recipients are medically unsuitable candidates. This "scientific" judgment is often based upon a hodgepodge of physical, economic, and psychosocial factors.[2]

The reality is that the waiting lists for cadaver organs have grown so long that a quiet form of triage is currently undertaken in order not to raise false hopes among those dying of organ failure. For infants and children the lack of cadaver donors is so severe that for many organs the only viable source of a transplant appears to be other species. There is little doubt that if more organs were available the lists of those deemed "medically suitable" for various types of transplants would expand dramatically.[3]

Many difficult ethical questions arise whenever scarce resources cannot be given to all who might benefit. It is not clear what standards or criteria should be followed when not all who might be helped can be helped.

Uncertainty about the principles to utilize in allocating the inadequate supply of organs from cadaver sources is further complicated by the growing suspicion that there are gross inequities in the way organs are currently being allocated by various transplant centers both in the United States and in other countries. Heated controversies have emerged about the moral acceptability of using what might be termed a "green screen" to select who will and will not be transplanted. Other debates have swirled around the revelations that some centers have given priority on their waiting lists to wealthy foreign nationals.

Issues of what constitutes just and equitable standards of allocation and a fair distribution of the enormous costs involved in transplantation are obviously complex and important. Furthermore, since there is likely to be a scarcity in the supply of cadaver organs for the foreseeable future, there is a real need for both professional and public discussion of the kinds of policies that should prevail in allocating organs to those in need.

Nonetheless, it is difficult to know how to address the matter of social and professional responsibility with respect to the allocation of organs unless one is certain about the degree to which something might be done to diminish the gap between supply and demand as well as about the moral presuppositions that govern organ donation. In order to know whether anyone or any group has a special claim upon organs and tissues, it is necessary to know the moral circumstances under which they were originally obtained. Before any serious argument can be entertained concerning the best policy to use to distribute scarce resources such as hearts and livers, it seems reasonable to make sure that our social policies are such as to maximize the supply of organs and tissues available for transplantation. Unfortunately, there are many reasons for believing that our system of organ procurement is not as efficient as it could be in obtaining organs from cadaver sources.

Moreover, part of the reason for a lack of efficiency under the prevailing system is an inadequate examination of the moral status of organ donation.

It is generally estimated that about 100,000 persons die each year of accidents and strokes. Of this number about 20,000 are medically suitable candidates for organ or tissue donation.[4] While age and other medical criteria for acceptability severely limit the number who might serve as a donor of a heart, lung, or liver, most of this group could serve as a donor of bone, corneas, and other tissues.

Yet no more than 3,000 of this number actually served as a donor of any tissue or organ in 1984. Our present system of relying on voluntary donations as indicated on a "donor card" or living will on a driver's license, or the permission of a family member if the deceased's wishes are not known, yields no more than 15 percent to 20 percent of the available pool of donors of corneas, kidneys, and other life-saving and life-enhancing organs and tissues.[5]

The poor performance of the system is particularly disturbing in light of the enormous amount of time, money, and effort devoted to educating the American public about the importance of donation. Since recent advances and experiments in the field of transplantation have hardly been lacking in media coverage in recent years, there is little reason to assume that more time, money, and effort will significantly increase public awareness about organ donation. The fact is that the prevailing public policy established by the recommendations contained in the Uniform Anatomical Gift Act of 1968 has not worked. What I have termed elsewhere "encouraged voluntarism"—using public education to urge people to consider organ donation and to use donor cards to make their wishes known—has not been effective as a means of procuring organs from cadaver sources.[6]

WHY HAS ENCOURAGED VOLUNTARISM FAILED?
The reasons of the failure of the policy of encouraged voluntarism are many. Most people still do not carry a donor card or other written directive governing the disposition of their bodies when they die. Only 20 percent of Americans have a signed donor card. In only a few states does the percent of persons completing a checkoff box on the driver's license

exceed this figure. Some experts estimate that as few as 3 percent of all those who serve as organ donors are actually carrying a donor card at the time they are pronounced dead.

In one sense this is not surprising since most people are loath to contemplate their own deaths, much less make plans for the disposition of their property and bodies once they are gone. While it is all well and good to promote public education and awareness where organ donation is concerned, the fact remains that it is a subject that lacks intrinsic attraction for a large number of people.

Reservations and fears about death are not the only reasons for the low number of persons carrying written directives of some sort concerning organ donation. There are still some states where "brain death" has not been recognized by legislative statute as the definition of death. This leads to confusion on the part of both physicians and the public as to when and whether organ donation is appropriate.

The fact that health care has in recent years become increasingly centralized in large, impersonal, institutional facilities undercuts the trust that exists between patients and health care providers.[7] It is very difficult to trust in the good intentions of strangers, and many people are still afraid that if they carry a donor card they may not receive aggressive medical care if they need it.

The failure to secure high rates of compliance with respect to written directives and the mistrust of hospitals and health care providers are, however, only part of the explanation for low procurement rates. The reality of organ procurement in the United States today is that many hospitals fail to raise donation as a possibility when a death occurs. If hospital personnel do not wish to become involved in organ procurement for any reason—legal, economic, or simply out of laziness—they are under no obligation to do so. This means that even if a person has a donor card there is a good chance it will not be discovered since the possibility of donation is often not raised by those caring for the critically injured and the dying.[8]

The fact that many hospitals and physicians do not ask family members or legal guardians about organ donation means that the present system of encouraged voluntarism through written directives is not only ineffective in terms of obtaining organs and tis-

sues, but it is ethically suspect as well. Those who carry donor cards may not have their desire to donate respected because no one bothers to locate their donor card or to ask family members about the existence of a card or written directive. Those who have not signed a written directive but who have no objection to donation will not be utilized because their family, friends, or guardians are not given the opportunity to consent to donation.

Even those who have objections to donation for religious or personal reasons cannot be assured that their wishes will be respected after their deaths under the present system. In Florida, tissues were taken from prisoners executed at the state prison without prior consent of the prisoners or the consent of their family members or legal representatives, highlighting the fact that prevailing public policy is not always adequate either with respect to honoring desires to donate or in not harvesting organs when possible objections exist.

POSSIBLE REFORMS OF THE EXISTING POLICY FOR ORGAN PROCUREMENT

Present public policy based upon voluntary participation in organ procurement on the part of both the medical profession and potential donors and their families does not appear adequate in light of the current state of the art with respect to the successful transplantation of such organs as corneas, bones, kidneys, and hearts. These types of transplants work well, there are many persons currently in need of the procedures, and there are potentially thousands more who might benefit if the supply of organs could be increased.

It is important to realize that the prevailing policy of encouraged voluntarism utilizing written consent evolved at a time in the late 1960s when success rates for transplant utilizing cadaver donors were low, when the number of candidates awaiting such surgery was small, and when many of the potential donors of organs and tissues were alive rather than dead. Courts and legislatures were, during this period, rightly concerned with protecting the autonomy and free choice of living donors, especially children and mentally incompetent persons. The danger of coercing living donors against their will to undergo risky surgery of uncertain benefit as well as the need to guard against surreptitious removal of organs and tissue loomed large in the midst of those responsible for developing public policy with respect to organ procurement.

The Uniform Anatomical Gift Act, which was adopted in all fifty states and the District of Columbia during the early 1970s, made every effort to ensure that coercion and surreptitious harvesting of organs would be kept to a minimum. It insisted upon individual free and autonomous choice as the basis for donation from both living and cadaver sources.[9]

The question obviously arises as to whether a public policy that was formulated to cope with transplantation as it existed in the late 1960s is adequate for coping with transplantation today. Fifteen years ago most organs were obtained from living, related donors, but that is hardly true today. Fifteen years ago no form of transplantation was particularly successful. Today survival rates of cadaver grafts of hearts and kidneys have reached 50 percent at five years, a rate comparable to or better than that achieved with many other surgical and medical treatments. Fifteen years ago few persons were deemed medically able to withstand the rigors of a highly experimental surgical procedure. Today medical skills have evolved to the point where the very young, the old, the mentally ill, and those with various medical complications can be considered possible recipients of various types of transplants.

There are a number of social policy options that might be considered in seeking an alternative to the present policy of encouraged voluntarism. One is to allow a market in organs in order to encourage donations through financial incentives either to the living or to the next of kin of the dead. Another policy option is to modify public policy so that the burden of consent is shifted to those who do not wish to serve as donors. Rather than asking people to "opt in" to organ donation by carrying a written directive, we could simply require those who wish to "opt out" of donation to carry a written directive or so notify their next of kin.[10]

The problem with these alternatives is that they appear to subjugate individual autonomy and free choice to the socially useful purpose of obtaining more organs. Creating a market in organs would give incentives to the poor and disadvantaged to sell their body parts in ways that might adversely effect their health and well being. And even if markets were restricted to sales from the dead, the potential for conflict of interest among physician and patient, family members and the dying would appear to threaten the ability of individuals to do with their bodies as they wish.

Nor is there any guarantee that creating a market in organs would lead to an increase in the supply. Since some persons seeking organs are likely to be willing to pay any price in order to obtain them, the poor and the middle class might not be able to afford the huge amounts demanded by those with organs to sell. There are likely to be far fewer persons willing to give away what can in theory be sold for astronomical prices, so the overall effect of a market might actually be a decrease in the number of organs and tissues available for transplantation.

Putting the burden of proof on those with objections to organ procurement under a system of what is often termed presumed consent might yield more organs, but such a policy would be costly and difficult to administer. In order to assure the rights of every person to control his or her own body, it would be necessary to create a large and centralized registry that could be rapidly searched when a death occurred. The system would also have to be continuously updated to allow for modifications in the desires of each individual.

Most worrisome from an ethical point of view is that a policy of presumed consent can protect the rights of those opposed to transplant only by forcing them to indicate in some public manner their objections to the harvesting of organs. In order to assure that procurement is limited to only those without objections, it would be necessary to require each person with objections to record publicly their unwillingness to serve as a donor since this is the only way to assure compliance with their wishes. Ironically an approach intended to protect free choice might well hinder autonomous behavior rather than encourage it, since those with objections would have to state them and state them publicly rather than having the right to make no decision or to leave the decision to others if a tragedy were to occur.

A VIABLE POLICY ALTERNATIVE: REQUIRED REQUEST

There are many reasons, both ethical and practical, for skepticism about either a market or presumed consent as policy alternatives to the current policy of encouraged voluntarism. Perhaps the most serious of all is that neither of these policies takes seriously the fact that the low yield of organs obtained in the United States from cadaver sources is not attributable to the unwillingness of Americans to help those in need of transplants. If public opinion surveys can be trusted, most Americans still believe that transplantation is important, and they indicate a willingness to serve as a donor or to have a loved one donate. More impressive still are the figures associated with actual consent rates when family members are asked their permission for donation. In some hospitals, well over 60 percent of those families asked consent to donation. While one might raise questions about the competency of those asked to give a truly valid consent to donation in light of the terrible circumstances they face when an unexpected death occurs, the fact remains that the level of altruism on the part of the public in both theory and deed is high. The problem is that encouraged voluntarism using donor cards does not seem to be able to tap this powerful sentiment. A policy of a free market in buying and selling organs simply overlooks this valuable moral source of organs. A policy of presumed consent recognizes the prevailing desire of most people to help others upon their deaths but removes the moral dignity of donation by making it mandatory.

There is another way of modifying existing policy that would respect the dignity and value of individual choice while at the same time holding out the prospect of greatly increasing the number of organs and tissues obtained from cadaver sources for transplantation. It is a policy option that seems far more consistent with the contemporary realities of transplantation both in terms of need and efficacy.

If each state were to modify its existing law with respect to organ donation to require that family members or guardians be given the opportunity to make a donation when a death has occurred, this might go a long way toward both increasing the supply of available organs and tissues from cadaver sources as well as maximizing the opportunity for free choice where the harvesting of organs for transplantation or other purposes is concerned.

This policy option, which I have dubbed "required request,"[11] would restrict voluntarism but only on the part of hospitals and health care providers, not individual prospective donors and their families. A policy of required request would mandate that hospitals be responsible for designating an appropriately trained person to inquire about organ donation at the time death is pronounced. Such a request would be noted in writing on every death certificate in order to assure full and zealous compliance with the policy. A required request approach can permit exceptions to requests when there is reason to believe that a request would not be in the best interest of the next of kin of the deceased, but these exceptions would also have to be noted in writing on the death certificate.

A policy of legally mandating requests at the time of death addresses many of the failings of the current approach to cadaver organ procurement. It maximizes the opportunity to make a donation by way of a donor card or written directive since it ensures that some effort will be made by health professionals and family members to find a donor card if one exists. When no card exists, a required request approach allows families and guardians to make donations that now are simply lost due to a failure to ask.

Most importantly, routinizing a policy of requests for organ donation when death is pronounced will help ensure that better decisions are made about organ donation. If requests are customary and therefore routine, the public will soon come to expect such requests as a normal part of the process of death in hospital settings. By creating such an expectation, members of the public can be encouraged to discuss their wishes with family members, friends, or legal guardians in order to assure compliance with their wishes. Rather than coming as a surprise, as is now all too often the case, requests for donation would be routine. The decisions that are made would therefore be more likely to reflect the values and choices of all parties involved rather than the desperate, pressured reactions of unprepared and grief-stricken family members.

A policy of requiring requests about donation does give family members greater say in the process of organ donation if for no other reason than their greater involvement in terms of gross numbers in considering requests. However, there is no reason to assume that a required request policy will threaten or infringe upon the rights of individuals to control the disposition of their tissues and organs.

Family members would still be bound to honor the known objections of their loved ones to organ donation if such objections exist. They would also be responsible for helping to locate donor cards or call to the attention of health care providers the oral statements of the deceased about donation. Since most persons do not carry cards or complete written directives, a policy of required request places the burden of considering donation squarely on family members. Since these persons are generally responsible for the disposition of the body, there is little reason to assume that adding an additional inquiry about organ donation will constitute an undue burden when death occurs.

A final benefit of a required request policy is that it adds an additional level of protection for those with objections to organ donation. By requiring requests of family or guardians, individuals who are opposed to donation are afforded greater protection that nothing will be done to their bodies that they would not want done were they in a position to make their views known. This protection can be optimized by simply restricting donations to those cases in which family or guardians (or donor cards) can be located.

A policy of required request aims directly at the altruism that plausibly exists on the part of the public with respect to organ donation. It attempts to realize the effects of this altruism by ensuring that someone will ask about donation when a death occurs. The policy respects individual choice but also acknowledges the fact that giving will not occur unless someone remembers to ask.

ORGAN DONATION — CHARITY OR OBLIGATION?

Requiring requests about organ donation when death occurs is a policy that will help increase the supply of organs available from cadaver sources. However there is another aspect of the present system for procuring organs that merits examination if the number of organs available is to increase drastically.

For many years the rhetoric of public education in the organ procurement field has been that of charity. The public is constantly being urged through public service advertisements in magazines, in newspapers, and on radio and television to "make the gift of life."

What is interesting about the language of gifts in the area of organ donation is that the moral force of such language is not particularly strong. Gifts are a form of charity. Most moral theories recognize a strong moral obligation or duty not to harm others. But few theories posit the existence of an obligation or duty to give gifts to other people. Gift-giving behavior is viewed as morally laudable, even heroic, but it is not often seen as mandatory.[12]

The question raised by the use of the language of gifts in the context of organ donation is whether our society really wants to view donation exactly as that. Is organ donation a matter of preference and whim like some forms of gift giving? Or is it a morally supererogatory act—praiseworthy and admirable but not something we can reasonably expect people to do?

One way of answering these questions is to examine the ways in which positive obligations or duties to aid other people are usually generated. Some duties to help others arise as a result of particular roles or jobs in society. Fire fighters, parents, and nurses all have special duties to render positive aid to others even when helping requires sacrifice and even risk.

Another way in which duties to help others can arise is through the act of contracting or promising. I can voluntarily promise to help someone else if the need should arise, and I can be blamed for my failure to do so under the appropriate circumstances.

Unfortunately, neither of these positive obligations seems applicable to the situation that prevails with respect to organ donation. Unless I have promised to donate an organ to another and have reneged on my promise, there would seem to be no ground for saying that I ought to be an organ donor in any sense stronger than charity.

There is, however, another way in which duties to help others can go beyond exceptional cases of charity or gift giving. If it is possible for someone to do a great deal of good for another person without facing the prospect of a great deal of risk or even inconvenience, and if there is a strong likelihood of benefit for the recipient, most philosophers and theologians would argue that a duty to help arises that is stronger than the relatively weak obligations associated with charity and other generous acts.[13] If, for example, a strong swimmer can save the life of a drowning child merely by swimming twenty feet out into a calm lake, it would seem morally reprehensible and blameworthy for the swimmer not to do so.

Indeed, it would seem odd to describe such a rescue as a charitable act or even a gift from the swimmer to the drowning child!

Much more discussion and debate are in order with respect to organ donation. Is donation closer to an obligation of the sort described above than it is to an extraordinary act of moral beneficence or charity? If it is true that many people can be helped by an increase in the supply of organs, and if it is also true that the dead can suffer no harm through the utilization of their tissues and organs for transplantation or other educational or research purposes, then is it correct to describe a decision to donate as a gift that is praiseworthy if offered but not blameworthy if withheld or as an obligation that is both?

It is possible that different people may answer the question about the moral status of organ donation differently; however, the time has surely come for encouraging debate about whether a re-evaluation of the prevailing moral rhetoric of gift giving is in order. In order for this discussion to come about, both health care providers and other citizens will have to make every effort to reassure the general public that organs that are obtained are distributed fairly and efficiently. While it is true that allocation criteria are closely tied both to the availability of organs and to the system used to obtain them, it is also true that the connection between the ethics of procurement and allocation is reciprocal. Few people will feel obligated to help those in need if they perceive inequities in the system used to designate exactly who is most in need and most deserving.

Notes

1. Caplan, A. *J Health Politics, Policy, Law* 6:488, 1981.
2. Caplan, A. *Br Med J* 283:727, 1982.
3. Evans, R. et al. National Heart Transplantation Study. Final Report. Seattle. Battelle Human Affairs Research Centers, 1985.
4. Bart, K. et al. *Transplantation* 31:383, 1981.
5. Caplan, A., Bayer, R. Ethical, Legal and Policy Issues Pertaining to Solid Organ Procurement. New York, Empire Blue Cross/Blue Shield, 1985.
6. Caplan, A. *Hastings Center Rep* 13:23, 1983; also Caplan, A. *Hastings Center Rep* 14:6, 1984.
7. Starr, P. *The Social Transformation of American Medicine*. New York, Basic. 1984.
8. Prottas, J. Obtaining Replacements. Hearings on Organ Transplants before the Subcommittee on Investigations and Oversight of the Committee on Science and Technology. U.S. House of Representatives, April 1983, pp. 714-751.
9. Sadler, A., Sadler, B. *Hastings Center Rep* 14:6, 1984.
10. Dukeminier, J., Sanders, D. *New Engl J Med* 280:862, 1969; also Caplan, A. *Hastings Center Rep* 13:23, 1983.
11. Caplan, A. *Midwest Med Ethics* 1:2, 1985; also Caplan, A. *Hastings Center Rep* 14:6, 1984.
12. Beauchamp, T., Childress, J. *Principles of Biomedical Ethics*. New York, Oxford, 1979.
13. Beauchamp, T., Childress, J. *Principles of Biomedical Ethics*. New York, Oxford, 1979; also Goodin, R. *Protecting the Vulnerable*. Chicago, University of Chicago Press, 1985.

52.
IS IT TIME TO ABANDON BRAIN DEATH?

Robert D. Truog

Over the past several decades, the concept of brain death has become well entrenched within the practice of medicine. At a practical level, this concept has been successful in delineating widely accepted ethical and legal boundaries for the procurement of vital organs for transplantation. Despite this success, however, there have been persistent concerns over whether the concept is theoretically coherent and internally consistent.[1] Indeed, some have concluded that the concept is fundamentally flawed, and that it represents only a "superficial and fragile consensus."[2] In this analysis I will identify the sources of these inconsistencies, and suggest that the best resolution to these issues may be to abandon the concept of brain death altogether.

DEFINITIONS, CONCEPTS, AND TESTS

In its seminal work "Defining Death," the President's Commission for the Study of Ethical Problems in Medicine and Biomedical and Behavioral Research articulated a formulation of brain death that has come to be known as the "whole-brain standard."[3] In the Uniform Determination of Death Act, the President's Commission specified two criteria for determining death: (1) irreversible cessation of circulatory and respiratory functions, or (2) irreversible cessation of all functions of the entire brain, including the brainstem."

Neurologist James Bernat has been influential in defending and refining this standard. Along with others, he has recognized that analysis of the concept of brain death must begin by differentiating between three distinct levels. At the most general level, the concept must involve a *definition*. Next, *criteria* must be specified to determine when the definition has been fulfilled. Finally, *tests* must be available for evaluating whether the criteria have been satisfied.[4] As clarified by Bernat and colleagues, therefore, the concept of death under the whole-brain formulation can be outlined as follows:[5]

Definition of Death: The "permanent cessation of functioning of the organism as a whole."
Criterion for Death: The "permanent cessation of functioning of the entire brain."
Tests for Death: Two distinct sets of tests are available and acceptable for determining that the criterion is fulfilled:

(1) The cardiorespiratory standard is the traditional approach for determining death and relies upon documenting the prolonged absence of circulation or respiration. These tests fulfill the criterion, according to Bernat, since the prolonged absence of these vital signs is diagnostic for the permanent loss of all brain function.

(2) The neurological standard consists of a battery of tests and procedures, including establishment of an etiology sufficient to account for the loss of all brain functions, diagnosing the presence of coma, documenting apnea and the absence of brainstem reflexes, excluding reversible conditions, and showing the persistence of these findings over a sufficient period of time.[6]

CRITIQUE OF THE CURRENT FORMULATION OF BRAIN DEATH

Is this a coherent account of the concept of brain death? To answer this question, one must determine whether each level of analysis is consistent with the others. In other words, individuals who fulfill the tests must also fulfill the criterion, and those who satisfy the criterion must also satisfy the definition.[7]

First, regarding the tests-criterion relationship, there is evidence that many individuals who fulfill all of the tests for brain death do not have the "permanent cessation of functioning of the entire brain." In particular, many of these individuals retain clear evidence of integrated brain function at the level of the brainstem and midbrain, and may have evidence of cortical function.

For example, many patients who fulfill the tests for the diagnosis of brain death continue to exhibit intact neurohumoral function. Between 22 percent and 100 percent of brain-dead patients in different series have been found to retain free-water homeostasis through the neurologically mediated secretion of arginine vasopressin, as evidenced by serum hormonal levels and the absence of diabetes insipidus.[8] Since the brain is the only source of the regulated secretion of arginine vasopressin, patients without diabetes insipidus do not have the loss of all brain function. Neurologically regulated secretion of other hormones is also quite common.[9]

In addition, the tests for the diagnosis of brain death requires the patient not to be hypothermic.[10] This caveat is a particularly confusing Catch 22, since the absence of hypothermia generally indicates the continuation of neurologically mediated temperature homeostasis. The circularity of this reasoning can be clinically problematic, since hypothermic patients cannot be diagnosed as brain-dead but the absence of hypothermia is itself evidence of brain function.

Furthermore, studies have shown that many patients (20 percent in one series) who fulfill the tests for brain death continue to show electrical activity on their electroencephalograms.[11] While there is no way to determine how often this electrical activity represents true "function" (which would be incompatible with the criterion for brain death), in at least some cases the activity observed seems fully compatible with function.[12]

Finally, clinicians have observed that patients who fulfill the tests for brain death frequently respond to surgical incision at the time of organ procurement with a significant rise in both heart rate and blood pressure. This suggests that integrated neurological function at a supraspinal level may be present in at least some patients diagnosed a brain-dead.[13] This evidence points to the conclusion that there is a significant disparity between the standard tests used to make the diagnosis of brain death and the criterion these tests are purported to fulfill. Faced with these facts, even supporters of the current statutes acknowledge that the criterion of "whole-brain" death is only an approximation"[14]

If the tests for determining brain death are incompatible with the current criterion, then one way of solving the problem would be to require tests that always correlate with the "permanent cessation of functioning of the entire brain." Two options have been considered in this regard. The first would require tests that correlate with the actual destruction of the brain, since complete destruction would, of course, be incompatible with any degree of brain function. Only by satisfying these tests, some have argued, could we be assured that all functions of the entire brain have totally and permanently ceased.[15] But is there a constellation of clinical and laboratory tests that correlate with this degree of destruction? Unfortunately, a study of over 500 patients with both coma and apnea (including 146 autopsies for neuropathologic correlation) showed that "it was not possible to verify that a diagnosis made prior to cardiac arrest by any set or subset of criteria would invariably correlate with a diffusely destroyed brain."[16] On the basis of these data, a definition that required total brain destruction could only be confirmed at autopsy. Clearly, a condition that could only be determined after death could never be a requirement for declaring death.

Another way of modifying the tests to conform with the criterion would be to rely solely upon the cardiorespiratory standard for determining death. This standard would certainly identify the permanent cessation of all brain function (thereby fulfilling the criterion), since it is well established by common knowledge that prolonged absence of circulation and respiration results in the death of the entire brain (and every other organ). In addition, fulfillment of these tests would also convincingly demonstrate the cessation of function of the organism as a whole (thereby fulfilling the definition). Unfortunately, this approach for resolving the problem would also make it virtually impossible to obtain vital organs in a viable condition for transplantation, since under current laws it is generally necessary for these organs to be removed from a heart-beating donor.

These inconsistencies between the tests and the criterion are therefore not easily resolvable. In addition to these problems, there are also inconsistencies between the criterion and the definition. As outlined above, the whole-brain concept assumes that the "permanent cessation of functioning of the entire brain" (the criterion) necessarily implies the "permanent cessation of functioning of the organism as a whole." (the definition). Conceptually, this relationship assumes the principle that the brain is responsible for maintaining the body's homeostasis, and that without brain function the organism rapidly disintegrates. In the past, this relationship was demonstrated by showing that individuals who fulfilled the tests for the diagnosis of brain death inevitably had a cardiac arrest within a short period of time, even if they were provided with mechanical ventilation and intensive care.[17] Indeed, this assumption had been considered one of the linchpins in the ethical justification for the concept of brain death.[18] For example, in the largest empirical study of brain death ever performed, a collaborative group working under the auspices of the National Institutes of Health sought to specify the necessary tests for diagnosing brain death by attempting to identify a constellation of neurological findings that would inevitably predict the development of a cardiac arrest within three months, regardless of the level or intensity of support provided.[19]

This approach to defining brain death in terms of neurological findings that predict the development of cardiac arrest is plagued by both logical and scientific problems, however. First, it confuses a prognosis with a diagnosis. Demonstrating that a certain class of patients will suffer a cardiac arrest within a defined period of time certainly proves that they are *dying*, but it says nothing about whether they are *dead*.[20] This conceptual mistake can be clearly appreciated if one considers individuals who are dying of conditions not associated with severe neurological impairment. If a constellation of tests could identify a subgroup of patients with metastatic cancer who invariably suffered a cardiac arrest within a short period of time, for example, we would certainly be comfortable in concluding that they were dying, but we clearly could not claim that they were already dead.

Second, this view relies upon the intuitive notion that the brain is the principal organ of the body, the "integrating" organ whose functions cannot be replaced by any other organ or by artificial means. Up through the early 1980s, this view was supported by numerous studies showing that almost all patients who fulfilled the usual battery of tests for brain death suffered a cardiac arrest within several weeks.[21]

The loss of homeostatic equilibrium that is empirically observed in brain-dead patients is almost certainly the result of their progressive loss of integrated neurohumoral and autonomic function. Over the past several decades, however, intensive care units (ICUs) have become increasingly sophisticated "surrogate brainstems," replacing both the respiratory functions as well as the hormonal and other regulatory activities of the damaged neuraxis.[22] This technology is presently utilized in those tragic cases in which a pregnant woman is diagnosed as brain-dead and an attempt is made to maintain her somatic existence until the fetus reaches a viable gestation, as well as for prolonging the organ viability of brain-dead patients awaiting organ procurement.[23] Although the functions of the brainstem are considerably more complex than those of the heart or the lungs, in theory (and increasingly in practice) they are entirely replaceable by modern technology. In terms of maintaining homeostatic functions, therefore, the brain is no more irreplaceable than any of the other vital organs. A definition of death predicated upon the "inevitable" development of a cardiac arrest within a short period of time is therefore inadequate, since this empirical "fact" is no longer true. In other words, cardiac arrest is inevitable only if it is allowed to occur, just as respiratory arrest in brain-dead patients is inevitable only if they are not provided with mechanical ventilation. This gradual development in technical expertise has unwittingly undermined one of the central ethical justifications for the whole-brain criterion of death.

In summary, then, the whole brain concept is plagued by internal inconsistencies in both the test-criterion and the criterion-definition relationships, and these problems cannot be easily solved. In addition, there is evidence that this lack of conceptual clarity has contributed to misunderstandings about the concept among both clinicians and laypersons. For example, Stuart Youngner and colleagues found that only 35 percent of physicians and nurses who where likely to be involved in organ procurement for transplantation correctly identified the legal and medical criteria for determining death.[24] Indeed, most of the respondents used inconsistent concepts of death, and a substantial minority misunderstood the criterion to be the permanent loss of consciousness, which the President's Commission had specifically rejected, in part because it would have classified anencephalic newborns and patients in a vegetative state as dead. In other words, medical professionals who were otherwise knowledgeable and sophisticated were generally confused about the concept of brain death. In an editorial accompanying this study, Dan Wikler and Alan Weisbard claimed that this confusion was "appropriate," given the lack of philosophical coherence in the concept itself.[25] In another study, a survey of Swedes found that laypersons were more willing to consent to autopsies than to organ donation for themselves or a close relative. In seeking an explanation for these findings, the authors reported that "the fear of not being dead during the removal of organs, reported by 22 percent of those undecided toward organ donation, was related to the uncertainty surrounding brain death."[26]

On one hand, these difficulties with the concept might be deemed to be so esoteric and theoretical that they should play no role in driving the policy debate about how to define death and procure organs for transplantation. This has certainly been the predominant view up to now. In many other circumstances, theoretical issues have taken a back seat to practical matters when it comes to determining public policy. For example, the question of whether tomatoes should be considered a vegetable or a fruit for purposes of taxation was said to hinge little upon the biological facts of the matter, but to turn primarily upon the political and economic issues at stake.[27] If this view is applied to the concept of brain death, then the best public policy would be that which best served the public's interest, regardless of theoretical concerns.

On the other hand, medicine has a long and respected history of continually seeking to refine the theoretical and conceptual underpinnings of its practice. While the impact of scientific and philosophical views upon social policy and public perception must be taken seriously, they cannot be the sole forces driving the debate. Given the evidence demonstrating a lack of coherence in the whole-brain death formulation and the confusion that is apparent among medical professionals, there is ample reason to prompt a look at alternatives to our current approach.

ALTERNATIVE APPROACHES TO THE WHOLE-BRAIN FORMULATION

Alternatives to the whole-brain death formulation fall into two general categories. One approach is to emphasize the overriding importance of those functions of the brain that support the phenomenon of consciousness and to claim that individuals who have permanently suffered the loss of all consciousness are dead. This is known as the "higher-brain" criterion. The other approach is to return to the traditional tests for determining death, that is, the permanent loss of circulation and respiration. As noted above, this latter strategy could fit well with Bernat's formulation of the definition of death, since adoption of the cardiorespiratory standard as the test for determining death is consistent with both the criterion and the definition. The problem with this potential solution is that it would virtually eliminate the possibility of procuring vital organs from heart-beating donors under our present system of law and ethics, since current requirements insist that organs be removed only from individuals who have been declared dead (the "dead-donor rule").[28] Consideration of this later view would therefore be feasible only if it could be linked to fundamental changes in the permissible limits of organ procurement.

The Higher-Brain Formulation

The higher-brain criterion for death holds that maintaining the potential for consciousness is the critical function of the brain relevant to questions of life and death. Under this definition, all individuals who are permanently unconscious would be considered to be dead. Included in this category would be (1) patients who fulfill the cardiorespiratory standard, (2) those who fulfill the current tests for whole-brain death, (3) those diagnosed as being in a permanent vegetative state, and (4) newborns with anencephaly. Various versions of this view have been defended by many philosophers, and arguments have been advanced from moral as well as ontological perspectives.[29] In addition, this view correlates very well with many commonsense opinions about personal identity. To take a stock philosophical illustration, for example, consider the typical reaction of a person who has undergone a hypothetical "brain switch" procedure, when one's brain is transplanted into another's body, and vice versa. Virtually anyone presented with this scenario will say that "what matters" for their existence now resides in the new body, even though an outside observer would insist that it is the person's old body that "appears" to be the original person. Thought experiments like this one illustrate that we typically identify ourselves with our experience of consciousness, and this observation forms the basis of the claim that the permanent absence of consciousness should be seen as representing the death of the person.

Implementation of this standard would present certain problems, however. First, is it possible to diagnose the state of permanent unconsciousness with the high level of certainty required for the determination of death? More specifically, is it currently possible to definitively diagnose the permanent vegetative state and anencephaly? A Multi-Society Task Force recently outlined guidelines for diagnosis of permanent vegetative state and claimed that sufficient data are now available to make the diagnosis of permanent vegetative state in appropriate patients with a high degree of certainty.[30] On the other hand, case reports of patients who met these criteria but who later recovered a higher degree of neurological functioning suggest that use of the term "permanent" may be overstating the degree of diagnostic certainty that is currently possible. This would be an especially important issue in the context of diagnosing death, where false positive diagnoses would be particularly problematic.[31] Similarly, while the Medical Task Force on Anencephaly has concluded that most cases of anencephaly can be diagnosed by a competent clinician without significant uncertainly, others have emphasized the ambiguities inherent in evaluating this condition.[32]

Another line of criticism is that the higher-brain approach assumes the definition of death should reflect the death of the *person* rather than the death of the *organism*.[33] By focusing on the person, this theory does not account for what is common to the death of all organisms, such as humans, frogs, or trees. Since we do not know what it would mean to talk about the permanent loss of consciousness of frogs or trees, then this approach to death may appear to be idiosyncratic. In response, higher-brain theorists believe that it is critical to define death

within the context of the specific subject under consideration. For example, we may speak of the death of an ancient civilization, the death of a species, or the death of a particular system of belief. In each case, the definition of death will be different, and must be appropriate to the subject in order for the concept to make any sense. Following this line of reasoning, the higher-brain approach is correct precisely because it seeks to identify what is uniquely relevant to the death of a person.

Aside from these diagnostic and philosophical concerns, however, perhaps the greatest objections to the higher brain formulation emerge from the implications of treating breathing patients as if they are dead. For example, if patients in a permanent vegetative state were considered to be dead, then they should logically be considered suitable for burial. Yet all of these patients breathe, and some of them "live" for many years.[34] The thought of burying or cremating a breathing individual, even if unconscious, would be unthinkable for many people, creating a significant barrier to acceptance of this view into public policy.[35]

One way of avoiding this implication would be to utilize a "lethal injection" before cremation or burial to terminate cardiac and respiratory function. This would not be euthanasia, since the individual would be declared dead before the injection. The purpose of the injection would be purely "aesthetic." This practice could even be viewed as simply an extension of our current protocols, where the vital functions of patients diagnosed as brain-dead are terminated prior to burial, either by discontinuing mechanical ventilation or by removing their heart and/or lungs during the process of organ procurement. While this line of argumentation has a certain logical persuasiveness, it nevertheless fails to address the central fact that most people find it counterintuitive to perceive a breathing patient as "dead." Wikler has suggested that this attitude is likely to change over time, and that eventually society will come to accept that the body of a patient in a permanent vegetative state is simply that person's "living remains."[36] This optimism about higher-brain death is reminiscent of the comments by the President's Commission regarding whole-brain death: "Although undeniably disconcerting for many people, the confusion created in personal perception by a determination of 'brain-death' does not ... provide a basis for and ethical objection to discontinuing medical measures on these dead bodies any more than on other dead bodies."[37] Nevertheless, at the present time any inclination toward a higher brain death standard remains primarily in the realm of philosophers and not policymakers.

Return to the Traditional Cardiorespiratory Standard

In contrast to the higher-brain concept of death, the other main alternative to our current approach would involve moving in the opposite direction and abandoning the diagnosis of brain death altogether. This would involve returning to the traditional approach to determining death, that is, the cardiorespiratory standard. In evaluating the wisdom of "turning back the clock," it is helpful to retrace the development of the concept of brain death back to 1968 and the conclusions of the Ad Hoc Committee that developed the Harvard Criteria for the diagnosis of brain death. They began by claiming:

> There are two reasons why there is need for a definition [of brain death]: (1) Improvements in resuscitative and supportive measures have led to increased efforts to save those who are desperately injured. Sometimes these efforts have only partial success so that the result is an individual whose heart continues to beat but whose brain is irreversibly damaged. The burden is great on patients who suffer permanent loss of intellect, on their families, and on those in need of hospital beds already occupied by these comatose patients. (2) Obsolete criteria for the definition of death can lead to controversy in obtaining organs for transplantation.[38]

These two issues can be subdivided into at least four distinct questions:

1) When is it permissible to withdraw life support from patients with irreversible neurological damage for the benefit of the patient?
2) When is it permissible to withdraw life support from patients with irreversible neurological damage for the benefit of society, where the benefit is either in the form of economic sav-

ings or to make an ICU bed available for someone with a better prognosis?
3) When is it permissible to remove organs from a patient for transplantation?
4) When is a patient ready to be cremated or buried?

The Harvard Committee chose to address all of those questions with a single answer, that is, the determination of brain death. Each of these questions involves unique theoretical issues, however, and each raises a different set of concerns. By analyzing the concept of brain death in terms of the separate questions that led to its development, alternatives to brain death may be considered.

Withdrawal of life support. The Harvard Committee clearly viewed the diagnosis of brain death as a necessary condition for the withdrawal of life support: "It should be emphasized that we recommend the patient be declared dead before any effort is made to take him off a respirator ... [since] otherwise, the physicians would be turning off the respirator on a person who is, in the present strict, technical application of law, still alive" (p. 339).

The ethical and legal mandates that surround the withdrawal of life support have changed dramatically since the recommendations of the Harvard committee. Numerous court decisions and consensus statements have emphasized the rights of patients or their surrogates to demand the withdrawal of life-sustaining treatments, including mechanical ventilation. In the practice of critical care medicine today, patients are rarely diagnosed as brain-dead solely for the purpose of discontinuing mechanical ventilation. When patients are not candidates for organ transplantation, either because of medical contraindications or lack of consent, families are informed of the dismal prognosis, and artificial ventilation is withdrawn. While the diagnosis of brain death was once critical in allowing physicians to discontinue life-sustaining treatments, decisionmaking about these important questions is now appropriately centered around the patient's previously stated wishes and judgements about the patient's best interest. Questions about the definition of death have become virtually irrelevant to these deliberations.

Allocation of scarce resources. The Harvard Committee alluded to its concerns about having patients with a hopeless prognosis occupying ICU beds. In the years since that report this issue has become even more pressing. The diagnosis of brain death, however, is of little significance in helping to resolve these issues. Even considering the unusual cases where families refuse to have the ventilator removed from a brain-dead patient, the overall impact of the diagnosis of brain death upon scarce ICU resources is minimal. Much more important to the current debate over the just allocation of ICU resources are patients with less severe degrees of neurological dysfunction, such as patients in a permanent vegetative state or individuals with advanced dementia. Again, the diagnosis of brain death is of little relevance to this central concern of the Harvard Committee.

Organ transplantation. Without question, the most important reason for the continued use of brain death criteria is the need for transplantable organs. Yet even here, the requirement for brain death may be doing more harm than good. The need for organs is expanding at an ever-increasing rate, while the number of available organs has essentially plateaued. In an effort to expand the limited pool of organs, several attempts been made to circumvent the usual restrictions of brain death on organ procurement.

At the University of Pittsburgh, for example, a new protocol allows critically ill patients or their surrogates to offer their organs for donation after the withdrawal of life-support, even though the patients never meet brain death criteria.[39] Suitable patients are taken to the operating room, where intravascular monitors are placed and the patient is "prepped and draped" for surgical incision. Life-support is then withdrawn, and the patient is monitored for the development of cardiac arrest. Assuming this occurs within a short period of time, the attending physician waits until there has been two minutes of pulselessness, and then pronounces the patient dead. The transplant team then enters the operating room and immediately removes the organs for transplantation.

This novel approach has a number of problems when viewed from within the traditional framework. For example, after the patient is pronounced dead, why should the team rush to remove the organs? If the Pittsburgh team truly believes that the patient is dead, why not begin chest compressions and mechan-

ical ventilation, insert cannulae to place the patient on full cardiopulmonary bypass, and remove the organs in a more controlled fashion? Presumably, this is not done because two minutes of pulselessness is almost certainly not long enough to ensure the development of brain death.[40] It is even conceivable that patients managed in this way could regain consciousness during the process of organ procurement while supported with cardiopulmonary bypass, despite having already been diagnosed as "dead." In other words, the reluctance of the Pittsburgh team to extend their protocol in ways that would be acceptable for dead patients could be an indication that the patients may really not be dead after all.

A similar attempt to circumvent the usual restrictions on organ procurement was recently attempted with anencephalic newborns at Loma Linda University. Again, the protocol involved manipulation of the dying process, with mechanical ventilation being instituted and maintained solely for the purpose of preserving the organs until criteria for brain death could be documented. The results were disappointing, and the investigators concluded that "it is usually not feasible, with the restrictions of current law, to procure solid organs for transplantation from anencephalic infants."[41]

Why do these protocols strike many commentators as contrived and even somewhat bizarre? The motives of the individuals involved are certainly commendable: they want to offer the benefits of transplantable organs to individuals who desperately need them. In addition, they are seeking to obtain organs only from individuals who cannot be harmed by the procurement and only in those situations where the patient or a surrogate requests the donation. The problem with these protocols lies not with the motive, but with the method and justification. By manipulating both the process and the definition of death, these protocols give the appearance that the physicians involved are only too willing to draw the boundary between life and death wherever it happens to maximize the chances for organ procurement.

How can the legitimate desire to increase the supply of transplantable organs be reconciled with the need to maintain a clear and simple distinction between the living and the dead? One way would be to abandon the requirement for the death of the donor prior to organ procurement and, instead, focus upon alternative and perhaps more fundamental ethical criteria to constrain the procurement of organs, such as the principles of consent and nonmaleficence.[42]

For example, policies could be changed such that organ procurement would be permitted only with the consent of the donor or appropriate surrogate and only when doing so would not harm the donor. Individuals who could not be harmed by the procedure would include those who are permanently and irreversibly unconscious (patients in a persistent vegetative state or newborns with anencephaly) and those who are imminently and irreversibly dying.

The American Medical Association's Council on Ethical and Judicial Affairs recently proposed (but has subsequently retracted) a position consistent with this approach.[43] The council stated that, "It is ethically permissible to consider the anencephalic as a potential organ donor, although still alive under the current definition of death," if, among other requirements, the diagnosis is certain and the parents give their permission. The council concluded, "It is normally required that the donor be legally dead before removal of their life-necessary organs.... The use of the anencephalic neonate as a live donor is a limited exception to the general standard because of the fact that the infant has never experienced, and will never experience, consciousness" (pp. 1617-18).

This alternative approach to organ procurement would require substantial changes in the law. The process of organ procurement would have to be legitimated as a form of justified killing, rather than just as the dissecting of a corpse. There is certainly precedent in the law for recognizing instances of justified killing. The concept is also not an anathema to the public, as evidenced by the growing support for euthanasia, another practice that would have to be legally construed as a form of justified killing. Even now, surveys show that one-third of physicians and nurses do not believe brain-dead patients are actually dead, but feel comfortable with the process of organ procurement because the patients are permanently unconscious and/or imminently dying.[44] In other words, many clinicians already seem to justify their actions on the basis of nonmaleficence and consent, rather than with the belief that the patients are actually dead.

This alternative approach would also eliminate the need for protocols like the one being used at the University of Pittsburgh, with its contrived and perhaps questionable approach to declaring death prior to organ procurement. Under the proposed system, qualified individuals who had given their consent could simply have their organs removed under general anesthesia, without first undergoing an orchestrated withdrawal of life support. Anencephalic newborns whose parents requested organ donation could likewise have the organs removed under general anesthesia, without the need to wait for the diagnosis of brain death.

The diagnosis of death. Seen in this light, the concept of brain death may have become obsolete. Certainly the diagnosis of brain death has been extremely useful during the last several decades, as society has struggled with a myriad of issues that were never encountered before the era of mechanical ventilation and organ transplantation. As society emerges from this transitional period, and as many of these issues are more clearly understood as questions that are inherently unrelated to the distinction between life and death, then the concept of brain death may no longer be useful or relevant. If this is the case, then it may be preferable to return to the traditional standard and limit tests for the determination of death to those based solely upon the permanent cessation of respiration and circulation. Even today we uniformly regard the cessation of respiration and circulation as the standard for determining when patients are ready to be cremated or buried.

Another advantage of a return to the traditional approach is that it would represent a "common denominator" in the definition of death that virtually all cultural groups and religious traditions would find acceptable.[45] Recently both New Jersey and New York have enacted statutes that recognize the objections of particular religious views to the concept of brain death. In New Jersey, physicians are prohibited from declaring brain death in persons who come from religious traditions that do not accept the concept.[46] Return to a cardiorespiratory standard would eliminate problems with these objections.

Linda Emanuel recently proposed a "bounded zone" definition of death that shares some features with the approach outlined here.[47] Her proposal would adopt the cardiorespiratory standard as a "lower bound" for determining death that would apply to all cases, but would allow individuals to choose a definition of death that encompassed neurologic dysfunction up to the level of the permanent vegetative state (the "higher bound"). The practical implications of such a policy would be similar to some of those discussed here, in that it would (1) allow patients and surrogates to request organ donation when and if the patients were diagnosed with whole-brain death, permanent vegetative state, or anencephaly, and (2) it would permit rejection of the diagnosis of brain death by patients and surrogates opposed to the concept. Emanuel's proposal would not permit organ donation from terminal and imminently dying patients, however, prior to the diagnosis of death.

Despite these similarities, these two proposals differ markedly in the justifications used to support their conclusions. Emanuel follows the President's Commission in seeking to address several separate questions by reference to the diagnosis of death, whereas the approach suggested here would adopt a single and uniform definition of death, and then seek to resolve questions around organ donation on a different ethical and legal foundation.

Emanuel's proposal also provides another illustration of the problems encountered when a variety of diverse issues all hinge upon the definition of death. Under her scheme, some individuals would undoubtedly opt for a definition of death based on the "higher bound" of the permanent vegetative state in order to permit the donation of their vital organs if they should develop this condition. However, few of these individuals would probably agree to being cremated while still breathing, even if they were vegetative. Most likely, they would not want to be cremated until after they had sustained a cardiorespiratory arrest. Once again, this creates the awkward and confusing necessity of diagnosing death for one purpose (organ donation) but not for another (cremation). Only by abandoning the concept of brain death is it possible to adopt a definition of death that is valid for all purposes, while separating questions of organ donation from dependence upon the life/death dichotomy.

TURNING BACK

The tension between the need to maintain workable and practical standards for the procurement of trans-

plantable organs and our desire to have a conceptually coherent account of death is an issue that must be given serious attention. Resolving these inconsistencies by moving toward a higher-brain definition of death would most likely create additional practical problems regarding accurate diagnosis as well as introduce concepts that are highly counterintuitive to the general public. Uncoupling the link between organ transplantation and brain death, on the other hand, offers a number of advantages. By shifting the ethical foundations for organ donation to the principles of nonmaleficence and consent, the pool of potential donors may be substantially increased. In addition, by reverting to a simpler and more traditional definition of death, the long-standing debate over fundamental inconsistencies in the concept of brain death may finally be resolved.

The most difficult challenge for this proposal would be to gain acceptance of the view that killing may sometimes be a justifiable necessity for procuring transplantable organs. Careful attention to the principles of consent and nonmaleficence should provide an adequate bulwark against slippery slope concerns that this practice would be extended in unforeseen and unacceptable ways. Just as the euthanasia debate often seems to turn less upon abstract theoretical concerns and more upon the empirical question of whether guidelines for assisted dying would be abused, so the success of this proposal could also rest upon factual questions of societal acceptance and whether this approach would erode respect for human life and the integrity of clinicians. While the answers to these questions are not known, the potential benefits of this proposal make it worthy of continued discussion and debate.

Acknowledgments
The author thanks numerous friends and colleagues for critical readings of the manuscript, with special acknowledgments to Dan Wikler and Linda Emanuel.

Notes
1. Some of the more notable critiques include Robert M. Veatch, "The Whole-Brain-Oriented Concept of Death. An Outmoded Philosophical Formulation," *Journal of*

Thanatology 3 (1975): 13-30; Michael B. Green and Daniel Wikler, "Brain Death and Personal Identity," *Philosophy and Public Affairs* 9 (1980): 105-33; Stuart J. Youngner and Edward T. Bartlett, "Human Death and High Technology: The Failure of the Whole-Brain Formulations," *Annals of Internal Medicine* 99 (1983): 252-58; Amir Halevy and Baruch Brody, "Brain Death: Reconciling Definitions, Criteria, and Tests," *Annals of Internal Medicine* 119 (1993): 519-25.

2. Stuart J. Youngner, "Defining Death: A Superficial and Fragile Consensus," *Archives of Neurology* 49 (1992): 570-72.

3. Presidents's Commission for the Study of Ethical Problems in Medicine and Biomedical and Behavioral Research, *Defining Death* (Washington, D. C. Government Printing Office, 1981).

4. Karen Gervais has been especially articulate in defining these levels. See Karen G. Gervais, *Redefining Death* (New Haven: Yale University Press, 1986); "Advancing the Definition of Death: A Philosophical Essay," *Medical Humanities Review* 3, no. 2 (1989): 7-19.

5. James L. Bernat, Charles M. Culver, and Bernard Gert, "On the Definition and Criterion of Death," *Annals of Internal Medicine* 94 (1981): 389-94; James L. Bernat, "How Much of the Brain Must Die in Brain Death?" *Journal of Clinical Ethics* 3 (1992): 21-26.

6. Report of the Medical Consultants on the Diagnosis of Death, "Guidelines for the Determination of Death," *JAMA* 246 (1981): 2184-86.

7. Aspects of this analysis have been explored previously in, Robert D. Truog and James C. Fackler, "Rethinking Brain Death," *Critical Care Medicine* 20 (1992); 1705-13: Halevy and Brody, "Brain Death."

8. H. Schrader et al., "Changes of Pituitary Hormones in Brain Death," *Acta Neurochirurgica* 52 (1980): 239-48; Kristen M. Outwater and Mark A. Rockoff, "Diabetes Insipidus Accompanying Brain Death in Children," *Neurology* 34 (1984): 1243-46; James C. Fackler, Juan C. Troncoso, and Frank R. Gioia, "Age-Specific Characteristics of Brain Death in Children," *American Journal of Diseases of Childhood* 142 (1988): 999-1003.

9. Schrader et al., "Changes of Pituitary Hormones in Brain Death"; H.J. Gramm et al., "Acute Endocrine Failure after Brain Death," *Transplantation* 54 (1992):851-57.

10. Report of Medical Consultants on the Diagnosis of Death, "Guidelines for the Determination of Death," p. 339.

11. Madeleine M. Grigg et al., "Electroencephalographic Activity after Brain Death," *Archives of Neurology* 44 (1987): 948-54; A. Earl Walker, *Cerebral Death,* 2nd ed. (Baltimore: Urban & Schwarzenberg, 1981), pp. 89-90; and Christopher Pallis, "ABC of Brain Stem Death. The Arguments about the EEG," *British Medical Journal [Clinical Research]* 286 (1983): 284-87.

12. Ernst Rodin et al., "Brainstem Death," *Clinical Electroencephalography* 16 (1985): 63-71.

13. Randall C. Wetzel et al., "Hemodynamic Responses in Brain Dead Organ Donor Patients," *Anesthesia and Analgesia* 64(1985): 125-28; S. H. Pennefather, J. H. Dark, and R. E. Bullock, "Haemodynamic Responses to Surgery in Brain-Dead Organ Donors," *Anaesthesia* 48 (1993): 1034-38; and D. J. Hill, R. Munglani, and D. Sapsford, "Haemodynamic Responses to Surgery in Brain-Dead Organ Donors," *Anaesthesia* 49 (1994): 835-36.

14. Bernat, "How Much of the Brain Must Die in Brain Death?"

15. Paul A. Byrne, Sean O'Reilly, and Paul M. Quay, "Brain Death—An Opposing Viewpoint," *JAMA* 242 (1979): 1985-90.

16. Gaetano F. Molinari, "The NINCDS Collaborative Study of Brain Death: A Historical Perspective," in U.S. Department of Health and Human Services, *NINCDS monograph No. 24 NIH publication NO. 81-2286* (1980): 1-32.

17. Pallis, "ABC of Brain Stem Death," pp. 123-24; Bryan Jennett and Catherine Hessett, "Brain Death in Britain as Reflected in Renal Donors," *British Medical Journal* 283 (1981): 359-62; Peter M. Black, "Brain Death (first of two parts)," *NEJM* 299 (1978): 338-44.

18. President's Commission, *Defining Death.*

19. "An Appraisal of the Criteria of Cerebral Death, A Summary Statement: A Collaborative Study," *JAMA* 237 (1977): 982-86.

20. Green and Wikler, "Brain Death and Personal Identity."

21. President's Commission, *Defining Death.*

22. Green and Wikler, "Brain Death and Personal Identity"; Daniel Wikler, "Brain Death: A Durable Consensus?," *Bioethics* 7 (1993): 239-46.

23. David R. Field et al., "Maternal Brain Death During Pregnancy: Medical and Ethical Issues," *JAMA* 260 (1988): 816-22; Masanobu Washida et al., "Beneficial Effect of Combined 3, 5, 3' - Triiodothyronine and Vasopressin Administration on Hepatic Energy Status and Systemic Hemodynamics after Brain Death," *Transplantation* 54 (1992): 44-49.

24. Stuart J. Youngner et al., "'Brain Death' and Organ Retrieval: A Cross-Sectional Survey of Knowledge and Concepts among Health Professionals," *JAMA* 261 (1989): 2205-10.

25. Daniel Wikler and Alan J. Weisbard "Appropriate Confusion over 'Brain Death,'" *JAMA* 261 (1989): 2246.

26. Margareta Sanner, " A Comparison of Public Attitudes toward Autopsy, Organ Donation, and Anatomic Dissection: A Swedish Survey." *JAMA* 271 (1994): 284-88, at 287.

27. Green and Wikler, "Brain Death and Personal Identity."

28. Robert M. Arnold and Stuart J. Youngner, "The Dead Donor Rule: Should We Stretch It, Bend It, or Abandon It?" *Kennedy Institute of Ethics Journal* 3 (1993): 263-78.

29. Some of the many works defending this view include: Green and Wikler, "Brain Death and Personal Identity"; Gervais, *Redefining Death;* Truog and Fackler, "Rethinking Brain Death," and Robert M. Veatch, *Death, Dying, and the Biological Revolution* (New Haven: Yale University Press, 1989).

30. The Multi-Society Task Force on PVS, "Medical Aspects of the Persistent Vegetative State," *NEJM* 330 (1994): 1499-1508 and 1572-79; D. Alan Shewmon, "Anencephaly: Selected Medical Aspects," *Hastings Center Report* 18, no. 5 (1988):11-19.

31. Nancy L. Childs and Walt N. Mercer, "Brief Report: Late Improvement in Consciousness after Post-Traumatic Vegetative State," *NEJM* 334 (1996): 24-25; James L. Bernat, "The Boundaries of the Persistent Vegetative State," *Journal of Clinical Ethics* 3 (1992): 176-80.

32. Medical Task Force on Anencephaly, "The Infant with Anencephaly," *NEJM* 322 (1990): 669-74; Shewmon, "Anencephaly: Selected Medical Aspects."

33. Jeffery R. Botkin and Stephen G. Post, "Confusion in the Determination of Death: Distinguishing Philosophy from Physiology," *Perspectives in Biology and Medicine* 36 (1993): 129-38.

34. The Multi-Society Task Force on PVS. "Medical Aspects of the Persistent Vegetative State."

35. Marcia Angell, "After Quinlan: The Dilemma of the Persistent Vegetative State," *NEJM* 330 (1994): 1524-25.

36. Wikler, "Brain Death: A Durable Consensus"

37. President's Commission, *Defining Death*, p. 84.

38. Report of the Ad Hoc Committee of the Harvard Medical School to Examine the Definition of Brain Death, "A Definition of Irreversible Coma," *JAMA* 205 (1968): 337-40.

39. "University of Pittsburgh Medical Center Policy and Procedure Manual: Management of Terminally Ill Patients Who May Become Organ Donors after Death," *Kennedy Institute of Ethics Journal* 3 (1993): A1-A15; Stuart Youngner and Robert Arnold, "Ethical, Psychosocial, and Public Policy Implications of Procuring Organs from Non-Heart-Beating Cadaver Donors," *JAMA* 269 (1993): 2769-74. Of note, the June 1993 issue of the *Kennedy Institute of Ethics Journal* is devoted to this topic in its entirety.

40. Joanne Lynn, "Are the Patients Who Become Organ Donors Under the Pittsburgh Protocol for 'Non-Heart-Beating Donors' Really Dead?" *Kennedy Institute of Ethics Journal* 3 (1993): 167-78.

41. Joyce L. Peabody, Janet R. Emery, and Stephen Ashwal, "Experience with Anencephalic Infants as Prospective Organ Donors," *NEJM* 321 (1989): 344-50.

42. See for example, Norman Fost, "The New Body Snatchers: On Scott's 'The Body as Property,'" *American Bar Foundation Research Journal* 3 (1983): 718-32; John A. Robertson, "Relaxing the Death Standard for Organ Donation in Pediatric Situations," in *Organ Substitution Technology: Ethical, Legal, and Public Policy Issues*, ed. D. Mathieu (Boulder, Col.: Westview Press, 1988), pp . 69-76; Arnold and Youngner, "The Dead Donor Rule."

43. AMA Council on Ethical and Judicial Affairs, "The Use of Anencephalic Neonates as Organ Donors," *JAMA* 273 (1995): 1614-18. After extensive debate among AMA members, the Council retracted this position statement. See Charles W. Plows, "Reconsideration of AMA Opinion on Anencephalic Neonates as Organ Donors," *JAMA* 275 (1996): 443-44.

44. Youngner et al., "'Brain Death' and Organ Retrieval."

45. Jiro Nudeshima, "Obstacles to Brain Death and Organ Transplantation in Japan," *Lancet* 338 (1991): 1063-64.

46. Robert S. Olick, "Brain Death, Religious Freedom, and Public Policy: New Jersey's Landmark Legislative Initiative," *Kennedy Institute of Ethics Journal* 1 (1991): 275-88.

47. Linda L. Emanuel, "Reexamining Death: The Asymptotic Model and a Bounded Zone Definition," *Hastings Center Report* 25, no. 4 (1995): 27-35.

CHAPTER ELEVEN

GENETICS

53.
CLONING, ETHICS, AND RELIGION

Lee M. Silver

On Sunday morning, 23 February 1997, the world awoke to a technological advance that shook the foundations of biology and philosophy. On that day, we were introduced to Dolly, a 6-month-old lamb that had been cloned directly from a single cell taken from the breast tissue of an adult donor. Perhaps more astonished by this accomplishment than any of their neighbors were the scientists who actually worked in the field of mammalian genetics and embryology. Outside the lab where the cloning had actually taken place, most of us thought it could never happen. Oh, we would say that perhaps at some point in the distant future, cloning might become feasible through the use of sophisticated biotechnologies far beyond those available to us now. But what many of us really believed, deep in our hearts, was that this was one biological feat we could never master. New life,—in the special sense of a conscious being—must have its origins in an embryo formed through the merger of gametes from a mother and father. It was impossible, we thought for a cell from an adult mammal to become reprogrammed, to start all over again, to generate another entire animal or person in the image of the one born earlier.

How wrong we were.

Of course, it wasn't the cloning of a sheep that stirred the imaginations of hundreds of millions of people. It was the idea that humans could now be cloned as well, and many people were terrified by the prospect. Ninety percent of Americans polled within the first week after the story broke felt that human cloning should be banned.[1] And while not unanimous, the opinions of many media pundits, ethicists, and policy makers seemed to follow that of the public at large. The idea that humans might be cloned was called "morally despicable," "repugnant," "totally inappropriate," as well as "ethically wrong, socially misguided and biologically mistaken."[2]

Scientists who work directly in the field of animal genetics and embryology were dismayed by all the attention that now bore down on their research. Most unhappy of all were those associated with the biotechnology industry, which has the most to gain in the short-term from animal applications of the cloning technology.[3] Their fears were not unfounded. In the aftermath of Dolly, polls found that two out of three Americans considered the cloning of *animals* to be morally unacceptable, while 56 % said they would not eat meat from cloned animals.[4]

It should not be surprising, then, that scientists tried to play down the feasibility of human cloning. First they said that it might not be possible *at all* to transfer the technology to human cells.[5] And even if human cloning is possible in theory, they said, "it would take years of trial and error before it could be applied successfully," so that "cloning in humans is unlikely any time soon."[6] And even if it becomes possible to apply the technology successfully, they said, "there is no clinical reason why you would do this."[7] And even if a person wanted to clone him- or herself or someone else, he or she wouldn't be able to find trained medical professionals who would be willing to do it.

Really? That's not what science, history, or human nature suggest to me. The cloning of Dolly broke the technological barrier. There is no reason to expect that the technology couldn't be transferred to human cells. On the contrary, there is every reason to expect that it *can* be transferred. If nuclear transplantation works in every mammalian species in which it has been seriously tried, then nuclear transplantation *will* work with human cells as well. It requires only equipment and facilities that are already standard, or easy to obtain by biomedical laboratories and free-standing in vitro fertilization clinics across the world. Although the protocol itself demands the services of highly trained and skilled personnel, there are thousands of people with such skills in dozens of countries.

The initial horror elicited by the announcement of Dolly's birth was due in large part to a misunderstanding by the lay public and the media of what biological cloning is and is not. The science critic Jeremy Rifkin exclaimed: "It's a horrendous crime to make a Xerox (copy) of someone,"[8] and the Irvine, California, rabbi Bernard King was seriously frightened when he asked, 'Can the cloning create a soul? Can scientists create the soul that would make a being ethical, moral, caring, loving, all the things we attribute humanity to?'[9] The Catholic priest Father Saunders suggested the "cloning would only produce humanoids or androids—soulless replicas of human beings that could be used as slaves."[10] And *New York Times* writer Brent Staples warned us that "synthetic humans would be easy prey for humanity's worst instincts."[11]

Anyone reading this volume already knows that real human clones will simply be later-born identical twins—nothing more and nothing less. Cloned children will be full-fledged human beings, indistinguishable in biological terms from all other members of the species. But even with this understanding, many ethicists, scholars, and scientists are still vehemently opposed to the use of cloning as means of human reproduction under any circumstances whatsoever. Why do they feel this way? Why does this new reproductive technology upset them so?

First, they say, it's a question of "safety." The cloning procedure has not been proven safe and, as a result, its application toward the generation of newborn children could produce deformities and other types of birth defects. Second, they say that even if physical defects can be avoided, there is the psychological well-being of the cloned child to consider. And third, above and beyond each individual child, they are worried about the horrible effect that cloning will have on society as a whole.

What I will argue here is that people who voice any one or more of these concerns are—either consciously or subconsciously—hiding the real reason they oppose cloning. They have latched on to arguments about safety, psychology, and society because they are simply unable to come up with an ethical argument that is not based on the religious notion that by cloning human beings man will be playing God, and it is wrong to play God.

Let us take a look at the safety argument first. Throughout the 20th century, medical scientists have sought to develop new protocols and drugs for treating disease and alleviating human suffering. The safety of all these new medical protocols was initially unknown. But through experimental testing on animals first, and then volunteer human subjects, safety could be ascertained and governmental agencies—such as the Food and Drug Administration in the United States—could make a decision as to whether the new protocol or drug should be approved for use in standard medical practice.

It would be ludicrous to suggest the legislatures should pass laws banning the application of each newly imagined medical protocol before its safety has been determined. Professional ethics committees, institutional review boards, and the individual ethics of each medical practitioner are relied upon to make sure that hundreds of new experimental protocols are tested and used in an appropriate manner each year. And yet the question of unknown safety alone was the single rationale used by the National Bioethics Advisory Board (NBAC) to propose a ban on human cloning in the United States.

Opposition to cloning on the basis of safety alone is almost surely a losing proposition. Although the media have concocted fantasies of dozens of malformed monster lambs paving the way for the birth of Dolly, fantasy is all it was. Of the 277 fused cells created by Wilmut and his colleagues, only 29 developed into embryos. These 29 embryos were placed into 13 ewes, of which 1 become pregnant and gave birth to Dolly.[12] If safety is measured by the percentage of lambs born in good health, then the record, so far, is 100% for nuclear transplantation from an adult cell (albeit with a sample size of 1).

In fact, there is no scientific basis for the belief that cloned children will be any more prone to genetic problems than naturally conceived children. The commonest type of birth defect results from the presence of an abnormal number of chromosomes in the fertilized egg. This birth defect arises during gamete production and, as such, its frequency should be greatly reduced in embryos formed by cloning. The second most common class of birth defects results from the inheritance of two mutant copies of a gene from two parents who are silent carriers. With cloning, any silent mutation in a donor will be silent in the newly formed embryo and child as well. Finally, much less frequently, birth defects can be caused by new mutations; these will occur with the same frequency in embryos derived through conception or cloning. (Although some scientists have suggested that chromosome shortening in the donor cell will cause cloned children to have a shorter lifespan, there is every reason to expect that chromosome repair in the embryo will eliminate this problem.) . Surprisingly, what our current scientific understanding suggests is that birth defects in cloned children could occur less frequently than birth defects in naturally conceived ones.

Once safety has been eliminated as an objection to cloning, the next concern voiced is the psychological well-being of the child. Daniel Callahan, the former director of the Hastings Center, argues that "engineering someone's entire genetic makeup would compromise his or her right to a unique identity."[13] But no such "right" has been granted by nature— identical twins are born every day as natural clones of each other. Dr. Callahan would have to concede this fact, but he might still argue that just because twins occur naturally does not mean we should create them on purpose.

Dr. Callahan might ague that a cloned child is harmed by knowledge of her future condition. He might say that it's unfair to go through childhood knowing what you will look like as an adult, or being forced to consider future medical ailments that might befall you. But even in the absence of cloning, many children have some sense of the future possibilities encoded in the genes they got from their parents. Furthermore, genetic screening already provides people with the ability to learn about hundreds of disease predispositions. And as genetic knowledge and technology become more and more sophisticated, it will become possible for any human being to learn even more about his or her genetic future than a cloned child could learn from his or her progenitor's past.

It might also be argued that a cloned child will be harmed by having to live up to unrealistic expectations placed on her by her parents. But there is no reason to believe that her parents will be any more unreasonable than many other parents who expect their children to accomplish in their lives what they were unable to accomplish in their own. No one would argue that parents with such tendencies should be prohibited from having children.

But let's grant that among the many cloned children brought into this world, some *will* feel badly about the fact that their genetic constitution is not unique. Is this alone a strong enough reason to ban the practice of cloning? Before answering this question, ask yourself another: Is a child having knowledge of an older twin worse off than a child born into poverty? If we ban the former, shouldn't we ban the latter? Why is it that so many politicians seem to care so much about cloning but so little about the welfare of children in general?

Finally, there are those who argue against cloning based on the perception that it will harm society at large in some way. The *New York Times* columnist William Safire expresses the opinion of many others when he says that "cloning's identicality would restrict evolution."[14] This is bad, he argues, because "the continued interplay of genes ... is central to humankind's progress." But Mr. Safire is wrong on both practical and theoretical grounds. On practical grounds, even if human cloning became efficient, legal, and popular among those in the moneyed classes (which is itself highly unlikely), it would still only account for a fraction of a percent of all the children born onto this earth. Furthermore, each of the children born by cloning to different families would be different from each other, so where does the identicality come from?

On the theoretical grounds, Safire is wrong because humankind's progress has nothing to do with unfettered evolution, which is always unpredictable and not necessarily upward bound. H.G. Wells recognized this principle in his 1895 novel *The Time Machine*, which portrays the evolution of humankind into weak and dimwitted but cuddly little creatures. And Kurt Vonnegut follows this same theme in *Galápagos*, where he suggests that our "big brains" will be the cause of our downfall, and future humans with smaller brains and powerful flippers will be the only remnants of a once great species, a million years hence.

As is so often the case with new reproductive technologies, the real reason that people condemn cloning has nothing to do with technical feasibility, child psychology, societal well-being, or the preservation of the human species. The real reason derives from religious beliefs. It is the sense that cloning leaves God out of the process of human creation, and that man is venturing into places he does not belong. Of course, the playing God's objection only makes sense in the context of one's definition of God, as a supernatural being who plays a role in the birth of each new member of our species. And even if one holds this particular view of God, it does not necessarily follow that cloning is equivalent to playing God. Some who consider themselves to be religious have argued that if God didn't want man to clone, "he" wouldn't have made it possible.

Should public policy in a pluralist society be based on a narrow religious point of view? Most people would say no, which is why those who hold this point of view are grasping for secular reasons to support their call for an unconditional ban on the cloning of human beings. When the dust clears from the cloning debate, however, the secular reasons will almost certainly have disappeared. And then, only religious objections will remain.

Notes

1. Data extracted from a *Time*/CNN poll taken over the 26th and 27th of February 1979 and reported in Time on 10 March 1997; and an ABC Nightline poll taken over the same period, with results reported in the *Chicago Tribune* on 2 March 1997.

2. Quotes from the bioethicist Arthur Caplan in *Denver Post* 1997; Feb 24; the bioethicist Thomas Murrey in *New York Times* 1997; Mar 6; Congressman Vernon [Ehlers] in *New York Times* 1997; Mar 6; and evolutionary biologist Francisco Ayala in *Orange County Register* 1997; Feb 25.

3. James A. Geraghty, president of Genzyme Transgenics Corporation (a Massachusetts biotech company), testified before a Senate committee that "everyone in the biotechnology industry shares the unequivocal conviction that there is no place for the cloning of human beings in our society." *Washington Post* 1997; Mar 13.

4. Data obtained from a Yankelovich poll of 1,005 adults reported in *St. Louis Post-Dispatch* 1997; Mar 9 and a *Time*/CNN poll reported in *New York Times* 1997; Mar 5.

5. Leonard Bell, president and chief executive of Alexion Pharmaceuticals, is quoted as saying, "There is a healthy skepticism whether you can accomplish this efficiently in another species." *New York Times* 1997; Mar 3.

6. Interpretations of the judgments of scientists, reported by Specter M, Kolata G. *New York Times* 1997; Mar 3, and by Herbert W, Sheler JL, Watson T. *U.S. News & World Report* 1997; Mar 10.

7. Quote from Ian Wilmut, the scientist who brought forth Dolly, in Friend T. *USA Today* 1997; Feb 24.

8. Quoted in Kluger J. *Time* 1997; Mar 10.

9. Quoted in McGraw C, Kelleher S. *Orange County Register* 1997; Feb 25.

10. Quoted in the on line version of the *Arlington Catholic Herald* (http:// www. catholicherald.com /bissues.htm) 1997; May 16.

11. Staples B. [Editorial]. *New York Times* 1997; Feb 28.

12. Wilmut I, Schnieke AE, McWhir J, Kind AJ, Campbell KHS. Viable offspring derived from fetal and adult mammalian cells *Nature* 1997; 385: 810-13.

13. Callahan D. [op-ed] *New York Times* 1997; Feb 26.

14. Safire W. [op-ed]. *New York Times* 1997; Feb 27.

54.
GERM-LINE THERAPY AND THE MEDICAL IMPERATIVE

Ronald Munson and Lawrence H. Davis

... Gene therapy refers to the use of recombinant DNA techniques to treat diseases involving missing or impaired genes. It is still in the experimental stages with only a handful of patients at the National Institutes of Health currently undergoing the therapy. Within this decade, however, two types of gene therapy—gene augmentation and gene modification—are likely to become established modes of treatment (see Verma 1990). Gene augmentation, in which a normal copy of a gene is inserted into a cell to direct the synthesis of a protein that would normally be produced by the missing or defective gene, is the only approach so far attempted in humans. Gene modification, in which an impaired gene is corrected by splicing in a gene at a specific location in the cellular DNA but not otherwise altering the cell's genome, has been demonstrated in several mammalian species. Gene surgery, which involves excising an impaired gene and replacing it with a normal copy, remains a distant—although real—possibility.

Although even the experimental use of gene therapy is recent, its possibilities have been discussed extensively for more than a decade, and critics have raised a number of objections to it or some aspects of it (President's Commission 1982; OTA 1984; Nichols 1988; Walters 1991). NIH committees overseeing the research and many other observers now approve of somatic cell therapy as long as safeguards needed in any experimental procedure are followed and protocols pass appropriate review. No similar consensus has been reached, however, regarding the application of gene therapy to cells in the germ-line—ova, sperm, and cells that give rise to them. This is partly because of the enormous technical difficulties facing germ-line gene therapy. But it is also because germ-line gene therapy strikes many as involving especially difficult moral issues. In this paper we examine the most important of these. We argue that none presents an insurmountable moral obstacle to germ-line gene therapy. To the contrary, we will argue that medicine has a positive duty to proceed with its development.

THE LIMITS AND POSSIBILITIES OF SOMATIC CELL AND GERM-LINE THERAPY

Gene therapy is likely to have the most impact in treating diseases caused by single gene defects, especially autosomal recessive disorders (Nichols 1988; Anderson 1990; Holtzman 1989). This accounts for many conditions, including sickle-cell disease, Tay-Sachs disease, phenylketonuria, and cystic fibrosis. The hundreds of diseases caused by chromosomal disorders (e.g., Down syndrome) or by an interaction between genes and the environment during fetal development (e.g., neural tube defects) are not obvious prospects. But the estimated 4,000 monogenic diseases cause 7 percent of neonatal deaths, affect 1 percent of newborns, and are responsible for almost 10 percent of childhood deaths. About half of these diseases cause early death, and almost three-quarters of the rest produce severe impairments that make ordinary life virtually impossible (Nichols 1988, p. 9).

The thrust of efforts to find ways to treat these diseases so far has involved somatic cell therapy. Hence, even if the therapy can treat or eliminate a disease from an individual who has inherited a faulty gene, it will do nothing to alter the probability that the person's offspring will inherit the same defective gene. For example, someone with Huntington's disease has a 50-50 chance of passing on the gene causing the disease. Even if somatic cell therapy could eliminate the way the gene is expressed, the 50-50 chance of passing it on would remain.

Alteration of germ-line cells might change this. For dominant conditions, the aim would be to remove the defective gene from a person's gametes (ova or sperm cells) or their precursors, and replace it with one that would function normally. For recessive conditions, it might suffice to insert a gene that would function normally. Or instead of this "gametocyte therapy," the cells of an already-conceived pre-embryo might be similarly treated. ("pre-embryo transformation"). Success of either of these forms of germ-line gene therapy would mean that neither the individuals resulting from treated gametes or pre-embryo, nor their progeny, would inherit the disorder (Fowler et al. 1989).

If germ-line gene therapy were possible, practical, and widely employed, hundreds of genetic diseases might be eliminated from families. In each case, it would be possible for the disease to occur again through mutation, but the risk would be no greater than in the population at large, and the total number of cases needing somatic cell or other therapy would be greatly reduced. Horrible diseases like Lesch-Nyhan, PKU, and Tay-Sachs would simply disappear as a nightmarish heritage in certain family lines.... We would reach the goal described over a decade ago by Joseph Fletcher:

> The ultimate goal of [gene therapy] is not to ameliorate the ills of patients prenatally or postnatally, but to start people off healthy and free of disease through the practice of medicine preconceptively.... It aims to control people's initial genetic design and constitution—their genotypes—by gene surgery and by genetic design. (1974, p.56)

MORAL OBJECTIONS TO GERM-LINE GENE THERAPY

Against Fletcher's vision, some argue that there is a morally relevant distinction between somatic and germ-line therapy, and that germ-line therapy is a morally unacceptable means of achieving the goal of eradicating genetic disease.

But what wrong can be alleged about germ-line therapy? Its distinguishing feature is its impact on future generations. (In some cases, somatic cell therapy can also have an effect on future generations, but this is not the aim of the treatment—see Lappé 1991, pp. 623f, 627, 629f.) Somehow, this feature has led to a widespread feeling that the procedure is morally questionable. However, the moral doubts are often only hinted at in a rhetorical fashion and are not carefully articulated. Part of what we want to do here is to state those doubts as clearly and persuasively as we can so that we can lay them to rest definitively.

We think all the doubts about germ-line therapy express the single basic worry that it is illegitimate "tampering." The three lines of objection that have played important roles in the public debate see this as tampering with the rights of individuals, with the social order, and with the order of nature itself. We will present and examine each of these in turn, emphasizing the third. In no case will we find an insurmountable moral barrier to the development and use of germ-line therapy.

1. Germ-Line Therapy and Individual Rights

The Parliamentary Assembly of the Council of Europe (1982b) refers to a person's right to a genome that has not been "tampered" with:

> [The Assembly] recommends that the Committee of Ministers: ... provide for explicit recognition in the European Convention on Human Rights of the right to a genetic inheritance which has not been artificially interfered with, except in accordance with certain principles which are recognized as being fully compatible with respect for human rights (as, for example, in the field of therapeutic applications) ....

The basis for this alleged right is none too clear, even if we do not question (as many would) the very idea of a right possessed by as-yet-unconceived individuals. Prior to the passage quoted, the recommendation invokes the "rights to life and to human dignity protected by Articles 2 and 3 of the European Convention on Human Rights," and claims that these "imply" the right to a pristine genetic inheritance. We fail to see the "implication." For philosophers like Kant, human dignity is equated with our dignity as rational beings, and not with the whole of our biological nature as homo sapiens. Thus as rational beings, we are ends in ourselves, and have a right not to be treated as mere means to the ends of others (Kant [1785] 1959, p. 47). This may entail that others ought not to interfere (unjustifiably) with our pursuit of our own legitimate ends. It does not entail that others ought not to have interfered with our chances to have been conceived, say, with genes for hazel eye color....

Another possible basis mentioned by Mauron and Thévoz (1991) is Hans Jonas's view that we have "an ontological responsibility toward the preservation of the 'image of man.'" We reject this view, although we cannot discuss it here. We conclude then that the alleged right to an untouched genome has no basis and in fact there is no such right....

Less dramatically, germ-line therapy involves "tampering" with a person's body, so it may easily infringe on several genuine and important individual rights. Yet all forms of gene therapy—indeed, all forms of therapy—can be viewed as doing this. For example, procedures like coronary-artery bypass surgery could violate a person's autonomy and right not to be subjected to harm or to the risk of harm. We offer protection against such violation and legitimate the "tampering" by requiring the individual's "informed consent." Perhaps this would suffice for germ-line therapy as well.

A critic might object that this is a bad analogy because germ-line therapy can affect the descendants of the recipient, too. As many writers have emphasized, this feature makes it impossible to secure the informed consent of all the individuals affected (see, for example, Fletcher 1983; Lappé 1991).

This is undeniably true. However we are aware of no persuasive reasons for thinking that non-existent potential progeny or member of future generations have (as yet) any autonomy that could be tampered with. So there is nothing to protect by requiring their "informed consent." Thus, we see no point in lamenting the impossibility of our obtaining it.

We are less certain about whether those in this group of potential offspring and descendants have the right not to be harmed or subjected to risk of harm. But we are certain that insofar as they have such rights—or, more simply, insofar as we are obligated not to subject them to harm or (extra) risk of harm—neither the rights nor the obligations are absolute.

Some may claim that even if these rights and obligations are not absolute, they still are strong enough so that in practice, germ-line gene therapy would rarely if ever be permissible. This seems

implied by the "Declaration of Inuyama" adopted by the Council for International Organizations of Medical Sciences (CIOMS 1991): "There would have to be confidence that, when treatment affecting future generations is undertaken, descendants of those so treated would still agree with the decision generations later."

Similarly, Berger and Gert (1991, p. 679) would limit germ-line therapy to "cases in which the benefits to the person receiving the initial treatment is [sic] so great that it outweighs the risks not only for him but also for all of his descendants" since "the genetic make-up of an unlimited number of people" is affected. We cannot confidently predict what the conditions of life or people's values will be generations from now, so we cannot confidently predict our remote descendant's agreement with our decisions, nor can we judge precisely about benefits and risks to infinitely many of our descendants, so germ-line gene therapy would rarely if ever meet the requirements set by these statements.

But these statements are too strong. The first seems unduly influenced by the idea of informed consent, which we have already argued is irrelevant in this context. And the second views our actions as more momentous than they probably are. We should bear in mind that a remote future generation may be able to reverse a genetic change we introduce that turns out disadvantageous (Moseley 1991, p. 644). And as several authors have pointed out, we regularly make decisions that we know will affect future generations—including the very decision to have children—without acknowledging requirements as strong as these (Moseley 1991, pp. 642f; Lappé 1991, p. 631; and cf. Zimmerman 1991, p. 597). It is implausible that this practice is wrong, even if we have not been as responsible as we should be in our actions (including reproduction) affecting future generations.... Whatever exactly the rights of offspring and descendants, the promise of good enough consequences—say, the eradication of Lesch-Nyhan disease—could outweigh a sufficiently uncertain threat of harm and justify "tampering" with those rights.

If germ-line therapy involves illegitimate tampering, it is not illegitimate tampering with the rights of those directly affected or their descendants.

2. Germ-Line Therapy and Conflicts of Interest

H.J.J. Leenen (1988, p. 79) has pointed out another area of concern. The introduction of germ-line therapy as an option could lead to clashes between parental autonomy and the interests of present society or groups within society. For example, suppose a woman refused to agree to a demand by society or an insurance company that to become a parent she must have germ-line therapy to prevent her offspring from inheriting her gene for Huntington's disease. Should she be forced to submit?

Fletcher and Anderson (1992) ask about clashes of a different sort: "Can genetic diagnosis and therapy be equitably distributed, so as not primarily to benefit elites? Will germ-line therapy invest too-radical power in the hands of few?" Similarly, Zimmerman (1991, pp. 606-7) cites fears that germ-line therapy will lead to the development of nontherapeutic "enhancement" procedures, so that parents having the means will use it to guarantee themselves above-average children. "[T]he distribution of desirable biological traits among different socioeconomic and ethnic groups would become badly skewed, resulting de facto in exacerbated social and economic inequality" (Zimmerman 1991, p. 607; see also Anderson 1989).

Concerns like these suggest that germ-line therapy threatens to open a Pandora's box of new moral conflicts and dilemmas, and therefore some people would avoid it. Even making it available, would be a kind of "tampering" with the social order. But the problems are no different in kind from conflicts and dilemmas we already raise. For example, should we require those with Huntington's disease in their family history to be tested for the gene and allow them to reproduce only when the result is negative (Purdy 1988)? Or, to take a different kind of case, should we legally require a pregnant woman to act in ways that will not subject the fetus to greater than normal risks? Doing so would mean, at the least, that she should not smoke, consume alcohol, or use nonprescribed drugs (Mathieu 1991), and might also mean she should eat a proper diet and exercise regularly.

The examples could be multiplied, but these two are enough to show that Pandora's box is already open. Similarly, we should remember that problems of fair distribution of scarce resources are hardly unprecedented. We already have the kind of social and moral difficulties in our society to which germ-line therapy would give rise. Introduction of the therapy, then, would not be an illegitimate "tampering" with the social order.

3. Germ-Line Therapy as "Playing God"

The novel feature of germ-line therapy is that by it we modify the very genetic structure that as-yet-unconceived individuals are to have. This seems both more serious and potentially more sinister than any other medical therapies or public health measures. An individual's genetic structure, after all, determines the kind of being an individual will be, apart from and prior to the influence of both the biological and social environment. It determines whether the creature that develops is a bird or a beaver, a horse or a human. Hence, changing the genetic makeup of germ cells is tampering with the very order of nature. In the popular phrase, it is "playing God."

As rhetorically effective as this phrase may be in encouraging a negative attitude toward germ-line therapy, it is not at all clear just what is wrong with "playing God" in this particular way. Three attempts to explain are worth considering. (See also the President's Commission's 1982 report, *Splicing Life*, pp. 53-60.)

a. Germ-Line Therapy as a Prelude to Eugenics

Some argue that what begins as genetic "tampering" aimed at obliterating disease will lead to positive eugenics—"tampering" aimed at improving our children and the whole of humanity. As our understanding of the genetic basis of socially desirable traits like musical talent, mathematical insight, and athletic skill increases, we will be able to engineer human beings to meet our specifications. But trying to do this would be wrong (apart from the questions of fair distribution already mentioned) because, as Paul Ramsey (1970, p. 124) puts it, "Man [is not] wise enough to make himself a successful self-modifying system or wise enough to begin doctoring the species." (See also Anderson 1989.)

At least two problems weaken the force of this objection. First, the objection is only to genetic modification in the service of positive eugenics. Even if

Ramsey is right about our lacking the wisdom to turn ourselves into a "self-modifying system," it does not follow that there is anything intrinsically wrong with employing germ-line therapy to eliminate diseases. And as for the worry that negative eugenics will lead to positive eugenics, we may note that the potential for practicing positive eugenics has been with us at least since the time we recognized that there is a connection between the traits of offspring and those of their parents. We have resisted virtually all efforts and proposals to make use of selective breeding to shape the human species to satisfy an articulated ideal (Ludmerer 1972). Perhaps our experience with attempts at eugenics fits the description that Mauron and Thévoz give of the whole history of bioethical issues:

> [T]he slippery slope really looks more like a ramshackle staircase: once in a while, we trip down a few steps. This makes us wake up, take stock of ethical shortcomings and climb up the stairs by appropriate measures such as societal regulation. (1991, p. 658)

While it is true that germ-line engineering offers an easier and more effective way to exert control over the human gene pool, we have no reason to suppose that just because we possessed the technology we would employ it. It is simply not true that as a society we have always done whatever it is possible to do....

... Our second problem for Ramsey, then, is that it is not obvious that we lack the wisdom to "doctor" ourselves in the manner indicated. In truth, we do not know yet whether we have it or not. After we have had experience modifying the genome of other organisms and predicting the outcome, when we have learned the possible drawbacks and the chances of success in modifications performed on humans, then perhaps we can judge our wisdom. We can imagine ways of making ourselves better than we are now, but the unanswered questions concern how much and what kinds of risk we will be willing to take and what sort of price we will be willing to pay to improve ourselves. These questions cannot be answered usefully in a vacuum. (For other discussion of the acceptability of positive eugenics, see Mauron and Thévoz 1991, pp. 651-52.)

b. Germ-Line Therapy and Unpredictable Losses

Even if gene therapy remains confined to therapeutic applications, some raise the question "whether something important may be lost as disease genes are eliminated" (Cavalieri 1983, p. 473). On one interpretation, this worry is illustrated by the following sort of case. Suppose we are successful in eliminating sickle-cell disease from the human population by removing the disease causing gene and substituting a gene producing normal red blood cells. As it happens, those with sickle-cell trait (i.e., those who are heterozygous for the gene) are more resistant to falciparum malaria. Hence, if we eliminate the gene, we would also be eliminating potential benefits its possession bestows.

The objection takes it for granted that eliminating this potential benefit would be obviously wrong. Yet what it fails to consider is that, since we know about the connection between sickle-cell disease and resistance to malaria, we might decide that eliminating a lethal disease like sickle-cell is worth the loss of a relative immunity to malaria. This would be a reasonable decision, especially since we have effective ways of controlling and treating malaria, but lack adequate treatments for sickle-cell disease.

However, a critic might ask, "How many other connections might there be between diseases and important biological capacities that we don't even realize we have but would be lost forever if we rushed to eradicate the diseases by germ-line therapy?" It would be better not to "tamper" with something whose full significance we cannot hope to appreciate in advance.

Critics who invoke the hazard of an unforeseen disaster cannot be satisfied completely. No one can guarantee that an unexpected hazard might not result from germ-line therapy. However, we are not totally ignorant of the nature of genes and of the evolutionary process, and there is no reason to fear that germ-line therapy is more likely to produce an unanticipated disaster than is somatic cell therapy or any other use of recombinant DNA technology. These matters must be assessed in individual cases on the basis of acquired knowledge and experience. When the potential benefits of germ-line therapy are considered, rejecting its use on the basis of potential but unknown hazards is not justifiable.

c. Germ-Line Therapy as Threatening "Humanity"
The previous question about "whether something important may be lost" by the use of germ-line therapy refers to specific biological capacities. However, the question may be understood as having to do with the impossible-to-specify cluster of capacities and features that make us human. Thus, germ-line therapy might be said to be wrong because "tampering" with our humanity is wrong.

As we observed in our discussion of eugenics, germ-line gene therapy is unlikely to compromise the humanity of its products. "Humanity" may be understood just as membership in our biological species, or it may be interpreted as something more subtle, perhaps as our distinctive kind of consciousness or capacities to think and feel. Either way, it is unreasonable to think that the possession of the defective genes that would be eliminated by germ-line therapy—or the absence of genes that would be added—is essential to being human.

Even straightforward examples of nontherapeutic enhancement would not endanger the humanity of its products (cf. Anderson 1989, p. 685). By operating on a person's gametocytes so that her or his descendants would be prone to low cholesterol levels or unusual musical talent, we would not render these descendants nonhuman. Even if such a procedure tended to have genetic effects beyond those specifically planned and desired this would not alter matters. After all, mutations have been occurring throughout human history without compromising the humanity of those in whom they occurred. The human species, like any other, is not a fixed Platonic idea, but an ever-changing population of genes.

Nonetheless, the human species might change. First, it is possible that over many generations genetic changes, some introduced by gene therapy and some occurring by mutation, might accumulate in the gene pool of the human population. Alone, each change might be relatively unimportant, yet the total impact might be that the population embodying these changes is no longer human. In biological terms, phyletic evolution would have occurred. A second possibility is that genetic intervention, by accident or design, might produce immediate and wholesale changes in the progeny of some individuals.

Leon Kass evidently has the first possibility in mind:

> It may ... mark the end of *human* life as we and all other humans have known it. It is possible that the non-human life which may take our place will be superior, but I think it most unlikely and certainly not demonstrable. In either case, we are ourselves human beings; therefore, we have a proprietary interest in our survival, and our survival *as human beings.* (1972, p. 61)

We can call this the homo superior objection to germ-like gene therapy.

H.J.J. Leenen is concerned with a variant of the second possibility, which we can call the cyborg objection:

> In my opinion ... the science of genetics with human cells has to remain within human boundaries.... the creation of animal-human creatures and of plant-human combinations is inadmissible. This is not to say that the same holds for hybrids, which cannot develop. When scientists transgress the boundaries of what is human, they place themselves outside human society. (1988, p. 75)

Each of these authors views the production of nonhumans from humans with evident dismay. What is striking in these passages is that neither gives a cogent explanation why he feels this way, or why the feeling is justified.

Leenen perhaps is thinking of cyborgs, the monsters of ancient mythology or modern science fiction. Bringing such creatures into existence would be a great evil—to others, to the unhappy creatures themselves, or to both. But that is because these creatures are depicted as subhuman, and/or active enemies of humans. If animal- or plant-human combinations remain favorably disposed toward their human ancestors, and are superior to those ancestors, why should the scientist who originally produce them be considered "outside human society"? (cf. President's Commission (1982, pp. 57-60), which also considers "hybrids," and assumes they would be inferior to us.) Suppose for example that through genetic modifications our offspring and their descendants were equipped with chlorophyll-bearing patches on their skin and the capacity for photosynthesis. The resulting partial or complete independence of the usual food chain might be a good thing on the whole, even if we had to classify them all as nonhuman.

Kass's position is that even if our nonhuman descendants are superior to us, their existence would be contrary to our "proprietary interest" in our "survival as human beings." He claims the existence of this interest is a consequence simply of the fact that we are human. But this claim is a blatant nonsequitur. From the fact that we are human, it does not follow that we have an interest in our survival as humans, nor that we have any interest in survival at all. Compare: we (the authors) are Missourians and Americans. We have some interest in our survival as Americans, but none to speak of in our survival as Missourians. Of course Kass is speaking of collective survival. But we have no strong feeling about the survival of Missouri, nor of our descendants (or anyone else's) as Missourians. We do care about the survival of the United States, but we could accept its replacement by something "superior," to use Kass's term. By the same token, we would accept our descendants being citizens of this replacement.

In short, for Kass's argument to work, he needs a premise articulating just what it is about being human that he thinks gives us all a "proprietary interest" in survival as such. This he has conspicuously failed to supply.

Perhaps the thought underlying the objections of Kass, Leenen, and others to tampering with our humanity is something like this. We are Americans and Missourians contingently but humans necessarily. To have a sense of self-worth, then, we need to feel that being humans is a good thing to be, that a life lived within the limits of what is humanly possible is (potentially) a good kind of life to lead. There may be "superior" things actual or possible, but there is nothing unsatisfactory about being human. If our offspring will ultimately be nonhuman, then something of value which we exemplify will cease to be. If we choose to bring it about that our offspring are nonhuman, then we seem to be rendering a final negative judgment on our humanity. Tampering with the genetic structure that makes us human is wrong, then, because it conflicts with our sense of our own value.

In reply to this argument, it may be denied that a sense of self-worth requires such an attitude towards one's humanity. Nonetheless such attitudes are common, and may often play the role described. One further example may be the view of Hans Ruh as presented by Mauron and Thévoz (1991, p. 656), "that we ought to transmit to future generations ... the capability to live a genuinely human life (with its ups and downs)." What is wrong with transmitting the capability to live a superior kind of life, with more "ups" and fewer "downs"?

We concede that people like Leenen and Kass, on our analysis of their position, do have a legitimate concern. But we insist that this attachment to our humanity cannot be adequate grounds for opposition to germ-line gene therapy. First, both of the scenarios described whereby nonhumans would result from the procedure are exceedingly remote. Especially if applications of the techniques are limited to the therapeutic for the foreseeable future, the "end of human life as we know it" that worries Kass could not be a serious threat for thousands of years, if ever (cf. OTA 1984, p. 32). Nor is there any reason to think a clearly nonhuman being could or would be produced deliberately by even the most enthusiastic advocates of positive eugenics. The bare conceivability of these disasters surely does not warrant refusing to develop the techniques for eliminating genetic diseases. Second, if we imagine future circumstances in which the end of humanity because of these techniques was an immediate threat, we might find that alternatives were worse. Being remembered by whatever nonhumans succeed us may be better than simple extinction without a trace. In any case, this sort of concern need affect our values and present day practical reasoning no more than speculation about the ultimate "cosmic crunch" or heat death of the universe.

This completes our examination of reasons for thinking it wrong to tamper with our genetic structure by performing germ-line therapy. We have found no cogent objection. The claim that "we are not wise enough" is at best premature. The worry that something of great value depends on the genes that we would remove is without foundations. The concern that germ-line therapy, or nontherapeutic use of the techniques employed in it, may pose a threat to our humanity or our feelings about our humanity, cannot be taken seriously as offsetting the value of eliminating genetic disease.

In sum, all three objections are open to the same counterobjection: It may be wrong for us not to tamper with our genetic structure. Faced with the reality of genetic diseases, how can we justify not developing and employing a promising remedy? Are we wise enough to see a compelling reason for not doing so? Can we be sure that we will never face even worse dangers, against which skill in manipulating genes in germ-line cells would be our only protection? Conceivably, a day might come when our very survival as humans would depend on our ability to use complex techniques for which germ-line gene therapy is only the beginning. Why are the objections any more plausible than this counterobjection? (Mauron and Thévoz (1991, p. 660) point out that if we had foresworn recombinant DNA research since the Berg Moratorium, we would know less about AIDS today than we do; perhaps we would not even have been able to identify the HIV virus as the agent of AIDS.)

The objections take for granted that by tampering with our genetic natures, we are likely to cause more trouble than we prevent. What evidence supports this rather than its exact opposite? Occasionally, mention is made of the "wisdom of evolution" (see, for example, Cavalieri 1983, p. 472; President's Commission 1982, p. 62). But even if some "wisdom" can be found in the mechanism by which natural selection has left us susceptible to genetic diseases, it cannot be supposed that this "wisdom" is a reliable guide for us (cf. President's Commission 1982, pp. 62-63).

A more likely support for the objections is the common belief that our genetic nature is the design of a good and wise Being. His wisdom can be relied upon; if our design permits genetic diseases, there must be a good reason, which we cannot expect to fathom. Moreover, common belief also suggests that He has a right and an interest in our survival as humans which would be violated if we engineered our eventual replacement by another species. On this analysis, all the objections reduce to the claim: Germ-line gene therapy is wrong because it is tampering with His handiwork.

None of the objectors cited express themselves in these terms, and none would, not even the ones who share the belief in a good and wise Designer of humanity. The parallel to "if God wanted us to fly He would have given us wings" is too obvious and unanswerable. This sort of theological appeal cannot be correct, whether or not God exists. But we have seen that the objections as actually expressed do not work either. Germ-line gene therapy cannot be branded as illegitimate "tampering" with the order of nature.

MEDICINE AND THE THERAPEUTIC IMPERATIVE

We wish now to go beyond the moral legitimacy of this therapy and argue—still on the assumptions noted—that medicine itself has a prima facie duty to pursue and employ germ-line gene therapy. Sometimes, a certain course of action is morally right, although no one has an obligation to take it. For example, it would be right for physicians to work one day a month without fees in community clinics, but they have no moral duty to do so, either individually or collectively. However, in contrast, we want to claim that members of the medical professions would be collectively derelict if research aimed at the therapeutic use of germ-line gene therapy were neglected without good reason.

We should stress that our claim is only for the existence of a collective obligation, a duty falling on medicine as an enterprise. Very likely, if we are right and our assumptions are correct, then this collective obligation will entail some individual obligations on specific person or groups of persons. But without a detailed examination of the structure, membership, and existing practices of the medical enterprise, these individual obligations cannot be determined. For a somewhat parallel example, suppose it were argued that the American people had a collective obligation to provide shelter for its homeless; exactly which members of the "American people" had precisely which specific obligations toward this end would be a matter for a wholly different argument, depending on the structure and existing practices of our governmental and other bodies, and many other factors. We shall not attempt this "wholly different argument" for the case of medicine, and so shall not say how the collective obligation differentially affects physicians, medical researchers, public health officials, and others affiliated with the medical enterprise. Our interest is rather in the prima facie duty itself, and its basis in the nature of medicine.

Many assume unreflectively that medicine is a science, and many also think that science is "value-neutral" in some sense. These views may lead one to conclude that "medicine" cannot have any duty at all, prima facie or actual. At most, individual physicians or researchers have obligations to heal or develop therapies because of general moral principles, such as beneficence. (The arguments of Zimmerman (1991, p. 591) and Fletcher and Anderson (1992) may be read this way.) We believe that medicine itself has an obligation.

We escape the reasoning of the preceding paragraph by denying that medicine is a science. (For a detailed defense of this position, see Munson 1981.) We begin our argument by contrasting medicine with science in the respect most relevant here, the idea of what it is most concerned with....

Medicine, like science, pursues knowledge, but not in a disinterested way. Indeed, it is antithetical to the character of medicine as an enterprise to seek knowledge as an inherent or self-justifying good. Medicine's concern with knowledge is unequivocally instrumental or conditional. Medicine is joined so closely with science in inquiry and experiment, because it is by means of scientific understanding that medicine can most effectively secure its end of promoting human health.

Not all aspects of medicine involve the basic theories and concepts of the natural sciences. Clinical medicine, in particular, involves complicated human interactions, and part of the "art" of medicine involves "taking care" of patients without the guidance of established theories and proven rules. Nevertheless, science is one of contemporary medicine's major means of working to promote the welfare of patients as a population.

An enterprise is successful when it achieves its aims. Loosely speaking, science does its job when it provides persuasive reasons for accepting empirical theories about nature and character of the world. The success of medicine cannot be judged by any comparable epistemic criterion. Rather, the basic standard of evaluation must be practical or instrumental success with respect to its specific aim.

In seeking to meet health needs, medicine can be described as a quest for control over the factors affecting health. Understanding (knowledge) is important to medicine because it leads to control. Yet where understanding is lacking, medicine will seek control by relying on low-level empirical rules validated by practical success.

A consequence of medicine's aim of meeting health needs is that medicine possesses a therapeutic obligation imposed by its own character. That is, basic to medicine as an enterprise is the prima facie duty to treat those who are ill in ways that will help them achieve the degree of health of which they are capable.

Treatment by drugs or surgery, diet or exercise, is one way in which medicine exercises control over disease, but the therapeutic obligation can also be regarded as involving an obligation to prevent the occurrence of disease. Although the success of treatment might be most dramatic, preventing a disease altogether might be seen as the most effective form of control. Medicine aims at promoting human health by exercising control over disease, and since elimination is the most effective form of control, elimination of disease is the ultimate aim of medicine.

The eradication of smallpox from the world's population exemplifies the realization of this aim in a particular instance. The elimination of the disease was announced by the World Health Organization in 1979, and certainly the disappearance of the disease is to be preferred over all forms of therapy, no matter how effective. To our knowledge, no one argued that it would be morally wrong to eradicate smallpox through vaccination and other public health measures.

What is true of infectious diseases like smallpox is, of course, also true of genetic diseases. Somatic cell therapy promises to become a valuable means of controlling them and minimizing the suffering they cause. Once again, however, complete control would go beyond prevention or effective treatment in individual cases.

Germ-line gene therapy offers us the chance to rid ourselves completely (except for new mutation) of many serious genetic diseases for which there is no effective treatment. Given medicine's aim of seeing to the health of people and its instrumental character, it is this ideal that medicine is obligated to pursue. Social circumstances (such as a lack of resources to conduct research) and unavoidable difficulties (such as not being able to solve the technical problems of safety and effectively altering sex cells) may make the road leading to germ-line gene therapy a long one. Nevertheless, the prima facie duty to pursue this ideal remains.

CONCLUSION

The more than 4,000 genetic diseases involving a defect in a single gene cause thousands of deaths, an incalculable amount of suffering, and staggering economic costs. We have shown that the objections most often raised to germ-line gene therapy are not so persuasive as to stand in the way of using it to treat diseases. And we have shown that the character of medicine imposes on medical professionals a prima facie duty to pursue the development and use of germ-line gene therapy.

The diseases are so serious and the promise of the therapy so great, that it would be wrong to give in to the objections that have been raised to gene therapy. If they are allowed to prevail, then the social and scientific support needed to realize the therapeutic possibilities of gene therapy may never materialize. This outcome would be as wrong and almost as serious as if we had failed to develop and use antibiotics or vaccines.

Acknowledgements

We thank Robert Cook-Deegan and LeRoy Walters for extremely valuable comments on an earlier version of this paper. Ronald Munson gratefully acknowledges the support of a University of Missouri-St. Louis Faculty Research Fellowship.

References

Anderson, W. French. 1989. Human Gene Therapy: Why Draw a Line. *The Journal of Medicine and Philosophy* 14:681-93.

—. 1990. Genetics and Human Malleability. *Hastings Center Report* 20(1): 21-24.

Berger, Edward M., and Gert, Bernard M. 1991. Genetic Disorders and the Ethical Status of Germ-line Gene Therapy. *The Journal of Medicine and Philosophy* 16: 667-83.

Cavalieri, Liebe F. 1983. Testimony at a Hearing before the Sub-committee and Oversight Committee on Science and Technology. U.S. House of Representatives, 16-18 November 1982. In *Human Genetic Engineering,* Committee Print No. 170, pp. 470-76. Washington, DC: U.S. Government Printing Office.

CIOMS [Council for International Organizations of Medical Sciences]. 1991. *Human Genome Mapping, Genetic Screening and Gene Therapy: Ethical Issues.* Proceedings of the XXIVth CIOMS Conference: Human Genome Mapping, Genetic Screening and Therapy, ed. Z. Bankowski and A, M. Capron, Geneva.

Council of Europe, Parliamentary Assembly. 1982a. Report on genetic engineering presented by the Legal Affairs Committee, J.P. Elmquist, rapporteur. Document 4832 of the 33rd Ordinary Session, 18 January. Strasbourg, France.

—. 1982b. Recommendation 934 "On Genetic Engineering." Strasbourg, France.

Fletcher, John C. 1983. Moral Problems and Ethical Issues in Prospective Human Gene Therapy. *Virginia Law Review* 69: 538-40.

Fletcher, John C., and Anderson, W. French. 1992. Germ-Line Gene Therapy: A New Stage of Debate. *Law, Medicine, and Health Care* 20 (1-2). forthcoming.

Fletcher, Joseph. 1974. The Ethics of Genetic Control. New York: Doubleday.

Fowler, Gregory Juengst, Eric T., and Zimmerman, Burke K. 1989. Germ-Line Gene Therapy and the Clinical Ethos of Medical Genetics. *Theoretical Medicine* 10: 151-65.

Holtzman, Neil A. 1989. *Proceed with Caution.* Baltimore, MD: The Johns Hopkins University Press.

Kant, Immanuel. [1785] 1959. *Foundations of the Metaphysics of Morals.* Trans. Lewis White Beck. Indianapolis: The Bobbs Merrill Company, Inc.

Kass, Leon. 1972. New Beginings in Life. In *The New Genetics,* ed. Michael Hamilton, pp. 15-63. Grand Rapids, MI: Eerdmans.

Lappé, Marc. 1991. Ethical Issues in Manipulating The Human Germ Line. *The Journal of Medicine and Philosophy* 16: 621-39.

Leenen, H.J.J. 1988. Genetic Manipulation with Human Beings. *Medicine and Law* 7:71-79.

Ludmerer, Kenneth M. 1972. *Genetics and Ameri-*

can Society: A Historical Appraisal. Baltimore, MD: The Johns Hopkins University Press.

Mathieu, Deborah. 1991. *Preventing Prenatal Harm: Should the State Intervene?* Dordrecht, Holland: Kluwer Academic Publishers.

Mauron, Alex, and Thévoz, Jean-Marie. 1991. Germ-line Engineering: A Few European Voices. *The Journal of Medicine and Philosophy* 16: 649-66.

Moseley, Ray. 1991. Commentary: Maintaining the Somatic/Germ-line Distinction: Some Ethical Drawbacks. *The Journal of Medicine and Philosophy* 16: 641-47.

Munson, Ronald. 1981. Why Medicine Cannot Be a Science. *The Journal of Medicine and Philosophy* 6: 183-208.

Nichols, Eve K. 1988. Human Gene Therapy. Cambridge, MA: Harvard University Press.

OTA. 1984. *Human Gene Therapy—A Background Paper.* Washington, DC: Office of Technology Assessment.

President's Commission for the Study of Ethical Problems in Medicine and Biomedical and Behavioral Research. 1982. *Splicing Life: A Report on the Social and Ethical Issues of Genetic Engineering with Human Beings.* Washington, DC: U. S. Government Printing Office.

Purdy, L.M. 1988. Genetic Diseases: Can Having Children Be Immoral? In *Intervention and Reflection: Basic Issues in Medical Ethics*, ed. Ronald Munson, pp. 364-71. Belmont, CA: Wadsworth Publishing Co.

Ramsey, Paul. 1970. *Fabricated Man.* New Haven: Yale University Press.

Walters, LeRoy. 1991. Human Gene Therapy: Ethics and Public Policy. *Human Gene Therapy* 2: 115-22.

Verma, Inder M. 1990. Gene Therapy. *Scientific American* 172: 68-72.

Zimmerman, Burke K. 1991. Human Germ-line Therapy: The Case for its Development and Use. *The Journal of Medicine and Philosophy* 16: 593-612.

55.
MULTIPLEX GENETIC TESTING

The Council on Ethical and Judicial Affairs, American Medical Association

Among the most significant advances in the development of genetic medicine is the ability to test for genetic origins of specific conditions. In previous reports, the American Medical Association's Council on Ethical and Judicial Affairs has addressed many ethical issues associated with the application of the growing body of genetic information and accompanying technologies.[1]

Here, analysis is offered regarding testing for multiple genetic conditions simultaneously, or "multiplex genetic testing."

The term *multiplex genetic testing* can mean different things. It commonly refers to testing for multiple mutations that give rise to a single disorder, such as cystic fibrosis or phenylketonuria. This report deals instead with multiplex genetic testing where tests for completely different conditions are offered in a single session. As the mapping of the human genome progresses and tests for newly discovered genes are developed, the possibility has arisen that many different testing "packages" could be administered simultaneously. This latter kind of multiplex testing creates a new level of complexity because the modes of heredity, social implications, and availability of treatment can differ greatly among the conditions tested.

Existing tests can be divided into three broad categories: first, tests can be performed to find genetic conditions that will lead to future inevitable disease onset as in the case of Huntington disease. Second, tests can be designed to find specific genetic information that indicates a heightened risk to possible disease onset. Often referred to as "susceptibility testing," this type of test can be used to provide information about the possibility of contracting specific cancers, such as colon or breast cancer. Finally, genetic tests can be used to determine a patient's carrier status, providing information about the existence of a gene or gene mutation that is not necessarily manifested in an individual's phenotype, but that may be passed to children. The implications of the information conveyed by each test are different and are best addressed in separate ethical analyses.

The implications of genetic tests also differ depending on the population targeted for testing. For instance, genetic information provided to couples in the process of making reproductive decisions will likely have a different impact from information provided to an individual who has no intentions of having children. Similarly, providing genetic tests to children at the request of their parents may have different ramifications from providing the same test to consenting adults.[2] These differences are crucial to any analysis of genetic testing and must be given careful consideration as the availability of genetic medicine continues to grow.

Multiplex testing may compound the ethical complexities associated with single genetic tests rather than simply combining them. It should not be concluded that safeguards designed to limit the ethical risks associated with single genetic tests will be sufficient to meet the challenges that arise when tests are offered in combination. While this may be true in limited circumstances, in general the clinical application of multiplex testing should not proceed without a careful examination of the associated regulatory and ethical issues. Marketing of multiplex testing, both directly to consumers and through physicians' offices, could provide appealing financial returns to the biotechnology industry as well as to genetic testing centers.[3] In the face of these incentives encouraging rapid development and distribution of multiplex tests, it is critical to confront the relevant ethical issues before these tests are widely conducted without necessary safeguards. As a response to this need and as a part of its continued efforts to address the ethical implications of genetic medicine, the Council presents the following analysis of multiplex genetic testing.

SENSITIVITY, SPECIFICITY, AND PREDICTIVE VALUE

Among the variety of genetic tests, some yield high rates of false-positive and false-negative results, while others are characterized by the findings that are precise but of uncertain clinical or predictive value.[4] These problems with current genetic testing technology are complicated rather than reduced when single tests are combined to form a multiplex test.

Any single test's clinical validity is determined by three factors: the test's sensitivity, its specificity, and its positive predictive value. Sensitivity measures the test's ability to register true-positive results, while specificity measures its ability to provide true-negative results. The positive predictive value of a test is the probability that a person with a true positive will get the disease. A key determinant of the total number of false positive results is the frequency of the trait in the tested population. As an example, if a test that yields false positives 10 percent of the time is used to screen a population of 100 people in which 90 people actually have the disease, then of the ten people who are actually negative we can expect that one of them will test positive. In this case, the number of false positives would be one in 100. Thus, when high-risk groups are tested, positive results can be interpreted with greater confidence than when general populations of unknown risk are tested. Conversely, if low-risk groups are tested, the likelihood of false-positive results is correspondingly higher.

Consider the BRCA1 mutation and its relative predominance among Ashkenazi Jews. It is estimated that approximately 1 percent of all women of Ashkenazi Jewish descent carry the mutation, while approximately 0.1 percent of women in the population at large carry a mutated gene.[5] If only Ashkenazi Jewish women were tested for the trait, the rate and number of false-positives would be much lower than if all women were tested for the BRCA1 mutation. If, on the other hand, BRCA1 were tested as part of a multiplex test that targeted populations without an elevated risk for the BRCA1 mutation, the rate of false-positives would be high.

Multiplex testing contributes to the problem of false results by combining several tests, each of which carries its own risks of producing a false result. The chance that the multiplex test will yield a false-positive result increases as the number of tests included in the panel increases. For example, consider a single test that produces accurate results, in 90 percent of cases. If five tests with similar rates of accuracy are conducted at once, the laws of probability suggest that the chance that they will all yield accurate results falls just below 60 percent.

The real clinical value or utility of a panel is also questionable in multiplex genetic testing. Even when tests are accurate, providing a meaningful interpretation of the results is often complicated.[6] Genetic tests can only provide information about the state of genetic material (genotype) without saying much about physical manifestation (phenotype). In some cases where the gene mutation is manifested phenotypically in all patients who inherit the gene, a genetic test can provide results that are entirely predictive, as in the case of Huntington disease. In many cases, however, genetic tests attempt to assess presymptomatic risk for developing a disease. With these susceptibility tests, a positive result does not ensure that the individual will develop the disease, and a negative result does not preclude one from risk. Tests for the BRCA1 mutation are helpful in illustrating this point. By age seventy, the risk of breast cancer among carriers of the BRCA1 mutation has been shown to be 56 percent and the risk of ovarian cancer, 16 percent.[7] It is important to recognize, however, that those identified as having the BRCA1 mutation may not actually develop either form of cancer. Furthermore, it has been shown that only 7 percent of women with a family history of breast cancer had this specific genetic mutation. Thus even individuals with supposed risk over 90 percent would gain no predictive advantage from being tested for BRCA1.[8] In fact, obtaining the negative results of a BRCA1 test might provide false reassurance and discourage the use of important screening techniques such a breast self-examination and mammography.

INFORMED CONSENT AND COUNSELING

It is critical to assess the degree to which the nature of current genetic tests could affect the ability of patients to give informed consent. Patient autonomy is given its clearest voice in the process of consent, and the ethical community has established conditions that must be met to ensure that patients' freedom to make decisions is protected. One of the most crucial of these conditions is disclosure by the physician of all relevant information. Without such disclosure, the patient cannot reasonably be expected to make a decision that represents a clear analysis of available options and possible outcomes. The nature of genetic information, however, provides several challenges to this requirement.

As with many laboratory tests, results from genetic testing are typically assumed by patients to be correct. Many genetic tests do not validate these assumptions of near-perfect performance.[9] Communicating the problems of sensitivity and predictive value—and the need for caution when interpreting test results—to patients (who may believe that tests are by their very nature conclusive) is a difficult task. This difficulty is amplified when factors such as specificity vary for each of the different tests of the multiplex package.

Moreover, tests conducted for diagnostic purposes, susceptibility, and carrier status have different implications and counseling needs. While tests for diagnosis are associated with near-certain predictions of disease development, susceptibility tests provide information only about illness risks. Counseling in the latter cases must, for instance, include interpretation of the risks associated with particular mutations. Carrier screening is designed to provide information to potential parents about the possibility of passing a gene mutation to children. Although a carrier test itself may be fairly straightforward, assessing the implications of the test requires, for instance, an understanding of reproductive genetics. In cases involving a single genetic mutation that is either dominant or recessive, a basic discussion of Mendelian inheritance may be sufficient. However, in more complicated cases of polygenic traits or linked genes, a substantially more sophisticated understanding of biology may be required. If tests for all three purposes were combined to form a single multiplex test, substantially more counseling would be required in order to convey all the information relevant to a patient's final decision.

Not only does each type of test require different, unique information backgrounds, the tests trigger different social or personal contextual concerns.

For instance, different susceptibility tests have different implications for patients, and the information required for meaningful interpretation of the results may vary substantially.[10] As a result, grouping tests by general category will not necessarily alleviate the problems associated with counseling for multiplex tests.

The third principle challenge to obtaining informed consent lies in the nature of the information resulting from many genetic tests, particularly those designed to determine susceptibility. In many cases, receiving a positive test result for a genetic mutation does not provide any conclusive predictive evidence that one will eventually develop the disease. There may also be instances in which test results can provide insight into actual future disease onset, but in which no preventive measures or treatments exist with which to stave off or mitigate the inevitable condition. In still other cases, such as tests for cystic fibrosis, patients may be asked to consider that certain tests may predict disease onset but cannot distinguish between the often vastly disparate levels of severity. When these uncertainties are coupled with the possibilities of false results, providing patients with the information necessary to consider a multiplex test appears difficult at best.

Some will argue that clinicians can overcome these difficulties by carefully counseling patients and working through the complexities with those considering testing. Behind this position is the view that physicians should not assume that there is anything their patients cannot understand and consider in the process of giving informed consent. Furthermore, it would be paternalistic to deny patients access to tests simply because the profession recognizes the possibility that appropriate information might be lost in the process of disclosure. These are certainly compelling points; however, it is also important to examine how closely our current medical system can approximate the conditions under which adequate counseling could occur. A Human Genome Project survey found that only 54 percent of the physicians surveyed had even one course in basic genetics.[11] Experts in medical genetics concur with this finding, arguing that there currently exists a shortage of clinicians trained in genetic counseling and interpreting genetic tests. In sum, many physicians who will be asked to provide patients with tests and information about genetics will not have the background necessary to meet the challenges of that task.

Another possible solution is to refer patients to genetic counselors. Again, however, the feasibility of this solution must be evaluated in terms of currently available resources. Counseling a patient about a genetic condition is a time-consuming process consisting of pre-test information sessions, informed consent sessions, and post-test counseling sessions. Many of these sessions last over three hours, and as a result some counselors see as few as 300 new patients a year.[12] Even without the availability of the multiplex test, trained genetic counselors are under strain to meet the increasing demand for genetic services. The time demanded of these professionals will only increase with the combination of several tests conveying different information and implications with varying levels of accuracy. This poses a problem. Despite the fact that multiplex testing will require genetic clinicians to spend significantly more time with each patient, no systemic change has been proposed to handle this potentially overwhelming shift in practice. This raises profound questions about the profession's ability realistically to meet the information needs of patients attempting to make decisions about multiplex tests.

It should also be noted that the increase in time demanded of counseling physicians by multiplex testing would come at a time when physicians are often under considerable pressure to economize their interactions with patients. Incentives currently in place often have the intended or secondary effect of requiring physicians to see more patients in the course of their practice rather than fewer. In this environment, it is unlikely that physicians will be able to meet the counseling requirements presented by multiplex testing. Even if the burden of conveying strictly genetic information is shifted to non-physicians, the process of counseling must include the consideration of clinical implications that can only be conveyed by physicians.

Such concerns are only compounded by questions of whether insurers will reimburse for appropriate—and expensive—counseling services.

PHYSICIAN RESPONSIBILITY TO INDIVIDUAL PATIENTS

Past council opinions on genetic testing have assumed a link between testing and risk, addressing those circumstances in which individuals considered "at risk" for a specific conditions are offered testing for genetic status. Yet as more conditions are included in a multiplex test, a wider group of the general population becomes at-risk for at least one of the included genetic traits. It is likely that these patients would be offered the entire panel of tests rather than the single, clinically relevant test. As genome research continues, the genetic root of an increasing number of conditions will be established, thereby expanding the pool of patients considered eligible for genetic tests. It seems safe to predict that eventually virtually all patients will be shown to have a genetic disposition for some trait and that might be encouraging a trend toward a large proportion of the population seeking evaluative genetic testing. If these tests are grouped in multiplex packages without concern for the relevant risks of the individual, a substantial number of patients would receive results from evaluations that are not clinically indicated.

Experience with laboratory tests panels (often referred to as "chem 7," "chem 12," etc.) supports the assertion that multiplex testing would lead to a breakdown in the link between clinical indication and genetic evaluation. In daily practice, it is often less expensive and equally convenient to order a fixed battery of laboratory tests rather than each individual test suggested by the patient's condition. It may not be readily apparent, especially to a busy practitioner, why genetic tests should be treated differently, particularly if multiplex tests could provide a less expensive alternative to single trait testing.

This prospect is cause for some concern. Abnormal results from specific tests in laboratory panels are routinely provided to patients even if the test in question was not clinically indicated. In some instance, the information may be benign, or there may be treatments available that can be of material benefit to the patient. In other cases, however, information provided by nonindicated testing may result in unnecessary psychological distress, lifestyle modifications that negatively affect quality of life with no resulting benefit, or requests for treatment that are founded on misconceptions rather than medical science. While these problems may be resolved in cases where communication of information is unimpeded and straightforward, they are significantly more serious when associated with those tests, including genetic tests, that convey information that is difficult to explain and to understand.

The challenges facing physicians who attempt to help patients deal with fears and to clarify misconceptions by providing sufficient information about many genetic tests are not limited to scientific and personal contextual uncertainties, however. Current popular conceptions regarding the information contained in a genetic test also complicate significantly the task of patient communication. There is a substantial body of misleading information relayed to the public almost daily about the implications of genetics. Stories in the media repeatedly claim that science has uncovered an inheritable gene responsible for a wide variety of conditions and behaviors, often implying that a cure is not far behind. The response among many members of the general public is to believe that genetic information is the key to understanding future disease onset and to establishing the immutability of certain traits ad characteristics. In short, genes are often portrayed as the source of inevitable outcomes and predetermined conditions. To many, genes are even thought to represent the essence of human beings. Providing accurate information in the face of these powerful assumptions is extremely difficult.

In general terms, many patients perceive genetic information to be an indicator of their fundamental health. Despite the fact that diseases and traits cannot be reduced solely to their genetic components and that environmental and behavioral influences are critical components to the development of most conditions, current social conceptions of self place tremendous significance on genetic composition. Physicians have a responsibility to appreciate the power of genetic information and to exercise appropriate caution when providing access to tests than may be interpreted by patients as evaluations of their basic "wellness."

The far-reaching, conceptual impact genetic information may have on patients strengthens the claim that only those tests that are clinically indicated should be offered. Providing general access to testing in the clinical setting validates misconceptions that genetic information is inherently valuable and the surveying genes is a legitimate assessment of overall health. Furthermore, even seemingly benign tests that provide information about genetic status but that have no bearing on phenotype expression or reproductive decisions may have a psychological impact on the patient who interprets the presence of a mutation as a deep-seated flaw.

Given the significance of genetic information, it is also critical to ensure that test results are accurate. It has already been established that providing access to tests that are not justified by the clinical evidence may substantially compromise the clinical validity of a multiplex test. The increased risk of false-positive results inherent in expanding the pool of tested patients beyond those with a personal or family history outweighs the benefits gained by those patients who seek genetic tests to provide a survey of their genes, even if there is a small chance the test could provide information valuable to the patient. It is critical to recognize the limitations of testing as well as the potential impacts of affording access to genetic information that may be incorrect.

POPULATION TARGETING AND MULTIPLEX TESTS

Targeting of genetic testing to individuals who have an elevated risk for a specific condition has many merits. The challenge is to define and find those patients who are eligible for a given test according to this approach. One possibility is to design multiplex packages based on patterns of risk found in different populations. These populations could be identified by rates of disease incidence, and multiplex tests could be constructed that target the conditions found in a particular population. This method has been explored by a group of practitioners within the Department of Human Genetics at the Mount Sinai School of Medicine, who developed a multi-disease carrier screening program consisting of a multiplex test designed to target diseases found in an Ashkenazi Jewish population.[13] Their multiplex test encompassed individual tests for Tay-Sachs disease, cystic fibrosis, and Type I Gaucher disease.

But there are a number of potential problems with designing multiplex tests on the basis of incidence patterns in defined populations. The assumption of such testing is that elevated rates of risk are distributed throughout the selected population, such that every individual within the population presents a history that supports the need for testing. However, this assumption relies upon a history of reproductive isolation that is not evident in many socially defined populations. Individuals tend to associate according to cultural features; these may not be representative of gene pools that track with targeted mutations. The reproductive overlap between populations may be extensive. Programs that rely upon the patient's self-identification with a population to determine eligibility for testing risk targeting cultural features rather than appropriate genetic inheritance. If tests are provided to those who are not in fact members of highrisk groups, the number of false-positive results will increase and possible harm could result. These problems, both with defining a broad population that actually represents a pool of patients each having elevated risk and with selecting patients whose membership in that group is established biologically, present compelling arguments against designing multiplex tests on the basis of populations.

Proceeding with programs to test socially defined populations for multiple genetic mutations using specifically designed multiplex tests could result in different forms of discrimination. Because of the problems in defining "at risk" populations that should in fact be eligible for multiplex testing, it is likely that any such testing programs will disproportionately subject one group of patients to the negative impacts either of false results of forms of genetic discrimination. Patients who are tested according to actual risk based on clinical evaluation will benefit from more accurate test results than those given tests because of their membership in an inevitably ill-defined genetic population.

Moreover, multiplex tests that attempt to group individuals into broader populations could disrupt the patient-physician relationship by introducing an element of perceived discrimination into the clinical setting. One of the primary duties of physicians is to treat each patient according to his or her individual medical needs. To the extent that ethnic heritage may contribute to particular health concerns, it is clinically relevant and should be considered. Offering multiplex tests that are bundled according to race or ethnicity, however, serves to categorize patients rather than to address their distinct needs. Furthermore, the criteria upon which this categorization is based are the genetic mutations and diseases prevalent in a population. The profession can ill afford the perception that science is being used to bring attention to the genetic flaws present in lines of inheritance.

Perhaps the most troubling potential application of multiplex tests would be the construction of test panels explicitly designed to discriminate against specific ethnic groups. For instance a multiplex test could be built around a single test for which elevated risk exists in a particular population. The other tests in the multiplex bundle could be any tests for which reasonable risk exists in the general population. By using the one race-related trait to target the population, the remainder of the tests could point to mutations that exist in other populations but which go unnoticed for lack of testing. The insidious implication of such testing would be that one ethnic group had an abundance of mutations and must therefore be considered inferior. While this possibility might seem improbable, history provides many examples of such discrimination in other contexts, and society must not discount the possibility of such unprincipled actions.

POTENTIAL FOR DISCRIMINATION

In any discussion of genetic tests, one of the fears most commonly expressed by patients and society is the possibility that this private information might be used in discriminatory practices. Safeguards and regulations must be put in place to prevent insurers and health care service organizations from denying coverage for or discriminating against people who have tested positive for a genetic trait.[14] This basic premise should also be extended to employers, especially self-insured employers, who could use genetic information in their hiring and promotion decisions.

Potential discrimination by insurance companies and employers could be further complicated by multiplex tests designed to target specific groups. For example, a test that coupled BRCA1 and Tay-Sachs could be used to discriminate disproportionately against Ashkenazi Jews. A similar test coupling sickle-cell anemia and prostrate cancer could discriminate against African-American males. The formulation of the test itself and the determination by society, industry, and health care providers of conditions to be tested could become a powerful means of social control.

USING MULTIPLEX TESTS WISELY

Increasingly, genetic science is helping to characterize the etiology of illnesses. Genes are inherited and passed on to future generations. Viewed by many as fundamental to conceptions of self, knowledge of their genes may influence many important decisions and options in peoples' lives. However, the impact of environmental factors and behaviors on health should not be ignored, and diseases should not be reduced to their genetic components only.

Multiplex testing presents a series of challenges to adequate communication between the patient and the physician. It increases the total number of marginally indicated or non-indicated tests, thereby bolstering the rate of false results. These results may lead to psychological stress and misinformed life-altering decisions, and may also affect the ability of a physician to obtain informed consent. The inherently uncertain nature of genetic information as well as the lack of clinical geneticists and counselors available to provide adequate information also suggest that standards of disclosure will be difficult if not impossible to maintain.

Finally, multiplex testing and its resultant information may have widespread societal implications. When coupled with society's emphasis on the primary role of genetics in pathology and suffering, expanded provision of genetic tests might lead to varied forms of discrimination against those with genetic conditions. Furthermore, multiplex tests could be constructed specifically to target defined populations, which could lead to selective discrimination against particular populations.

Although multiplex tests have not reached the general health care market, the potential for their widespread application is readily apparent. Before such tests reach health care providers, clinics, and drugstores, the ethical and social implications of these tests must be well understood, and careful restrictions and regulations must be established.

The Council offers the following recommendations on the future possibilities of multiplex genetic testing:

1) Physicians should not routinely order tests for multiple genetic conditions.
2) Tests for more than one genetic condition should be ordered only when clinically relevant and after the patient has had full counseling and has given informed consent for each test included in the panel.
3) Efforts should be made to educate clinicians and society about the uncertainty surrounding genetic testing.

This report was adopted by the House of Delegates of the American Medical Association in December 1996 and has been subsequently revised in response to comments from peer reviewers.

Acknowledgments
Members of the Council on Ethical and Judicial Affairs include the following: Charles W. Plows, MD, Santa Ana, Calif. (chair); Robert M. Tenery, Jr., MD, Dallas, Tex. (vice chair); Alan Hartford, MD, PhD, Boston, Mass.; Dwight Miller, University Park, Md.; Leonard J. Morse, MD, Worcester, Mass.; Herbert Rakatansky, MD, Providence, RI.; Frank A. Riddick, Jr., MD, New Orleans, La.; Victoria Ruff, MD, Columbus, Ohio; George T. Wilkins, Jr., MD, Culver, Ind.; Linda L. Emanuel, MD, PhD, Chicago, Ill. (vice president, ethics standards); Michael Ile, JD, Chicago, Ill. (council secretary); Stephen R. Latham, JD, PhD ,Chicago, Ill. (director, ethics division); Jeffrey C. Munson, Chicago, Ill, (senior staff associate and staff author); Jessica Berg, JD, Chicago, Ill. (staff consultant); Eric Nadler, Chicago, Ill. (intern and staff author).

The Council on Ethical and Judicial Affairs acknowledges the helpful comments of Pilar Ossorio, section leader for genetics at the Institute for Ethics at the American Medical Association, and anonymous editorial reviewers.

Notes

1. Council on Ethical and Judicial Affairs, American Medical Association, "Prenatal Genetic Screening," *Archives of Family Medicine* 3 (1994): 633-42; "Genetic Testing by Employers," *Jama* 266 (1991): 1827-30; *Physician Participation in Genetic Testing by Health Insurance Companies Reports of the Council on Ethical and Judicial Affairs* (Chicago: American Medical Association, 1993); *Ethical Issues in Carrier Screening of Cystic Fibrosis and other Genetic Disorders. Reports of the Council on Ethical and Judicial Affairs* (Chicago: American Medical Association 1991); *Testing Children for Genetic Status Reports of the Council on Ethical and Judicial Affairs* (Chicago: American Medical Association, 1996).

2. Council on Ethical and Judicial Affairs, *Testing Children*.

3. Committee on Assessing Genetic Risks, Institute of Medicine, *Assessing Genetic Risks: Implications for Health and Social Policy, Executive Summary* (Washington, D.C.: National Academy Press, 1994), p. 2.

4. Committee on Assessing Genetic Risks, *Assessing Genetic Risks*.

5. Frances Collins, "BRCA1—Lots of Mutations, Lots of Dilemmas," *NEJM* 334 (1995):186-88.

6. Philip Kitcher, *The Lives to Come* (New York: Simon and Schuster, 1996). See in general pages 65-86.

7. Jeffrey P. Struewing, Patricia Hartge, Sholom Wacholder et al., "The Risk of Cancer Associated with Specific Mutations of BRCA1 and BRCA2 among Ashkenazi Jews," *NEJM* 336 (1997):1401-8.

8. Fergus J. Couch, Michelle L. DeShano, M. Anne Blackwood et al., "BRCA1 Mutations in Women Attending Clinics That Evaluate the Risk of Breast Cancer," *NEJM* 336 (1997): 1409-15.

9. Kitcher, *The Lives To Come*.

10. See, for example, Sherman Elias and George Annas, "Generic Consent For Genetic Screening" [Sounding Board], *NEJM* 330 (1994): 1611-13.

11. Ethical, Legal and Social Implication of the Human Genome Project: Education of Interdisciplinary Profession. Funded by Office of Health and Environmental Research at the Department of Energy and National Institute of Health (ELSI). Georgetown University, 10 June 1996.

12. Neil A. Holtzman, *Proceed with Caution: Predicting Genetic Risks in the Recombinant DNA Era* (Baltimore, Md.: Johns Hopkins University Press, 1989).

13. Christine M. Eng, Brynn Levy, Tania S. Burgert et al., "Evaluation of a Model Program for Multi-Disease Carrier Screening in a Target Population" [Abstract], *Pediatric Research* 35 (1995): 151A.

14. Over half of the states have enacted laws prohibiting insurers and employers from the adverse use of information derived from genetic testing.

56.
A GERM-LINE GENETIC ALTERATION

The National Reproductive Technologies Commission

POTENTIAL USES OF GERM-LINE GENETIC ALTERATION

The term "germ-line gene therapy," although widely used, is in fact misleading. "Therapy" implies treatment of an individual (a person or a developing fetus) for a disease that has been identified. Genetic alteration aimed specifically at the gonads to alter the gametes is therefore not therapy—there are no existing affected individuals. It is quite incorrect, therefore, to refer to genetic alteration done in adults with the aim of altering the germ cells as "therapy"—it is a "preventive" strategy. For purposes of analysis, it is important not to describe this, misleadingly, as "therapy," as there is much less willingness to undertake risk (both individually and societally) in order to prevent disease than to do so for therapeutic purposes.

It is possible, however, to consider genetic therapy involving the zygote or the fetus—that is, genetic alteration aimed at curing disease in that zygote or fetus. If done very early in development during the zygote stage, this could affect the germ-line. There are two windows of opportunity during which the developing entity is theoretically accessible for genetic therapy before birth. The first is after IVF and preimplantation diagnosis have shown that the zygote is affected. If gene insertion were done at this stage, before the process of cell differentiation and the development of body organs (organogenesis), then the genetic change would be present in most or all cells—and could thus affect the germ-line of the resulting fetus as well. Some have argued that this not only would treat that particular zygote but might prevent the transmission of the gene to future generations. However, rather than taking the risk of altering genes that will be passed on to the next generation, there is the less risky option of simply not transferring affected zygotes.

The next window of opportunity (before birth) is much later, after organogenesis; treatment of an affected fetus at that time would be unlikely to affect its germ-line. A major reason for interest in gene therapy before birth is that it might be able to treat certain genetic diseases that are not amenable to therapy after birth—for example, diseases that cause irreparable harm early in fetal development or that affect multiple body systems.

Germ-line genetic alteration has also been discussed (under the misnomer "germ-line therapy") in terms of relevance to adults who either have, or are carriers of, a genetic disorder. But if an adult manifests a genetic disease, then altering his or her germ cells would not treat that disease, which would continue to affect the body cells; it would mean simply that the disease gene would not be passed on to offspring. It is incorrect to call this therapy—the aim is preventive, not therapeutic. The difficulties associated with altering the gametes or gonads of adults are enormous, to the point where few proponents of germ-line alteration consider this a viable option. Germ-line genetic alteration is much more complicated than somatic cell gene therapy. Whereas somatic cell gene therapy uses gene insertion, germ-line therapy would require gene replacement (which is not feasible in human beings at present) of all the germ cells affected. If a normal gene were simply inserted, without removing the defective gene, then the genetic disease could still be passed on to future generations.

Research with animals has demonstrated that intergenerational transmission of genetic information inserted into zygotes (so the gonads contain the altered gene) is possible. However, the failure rate of insertion and transmission to offspring is high. Moreover, animal germ-line alteration is done for different purposes than human germ-line alteration would be. Germ-line genetic alteration in animal zygotes is not done to treat disease, but to create "transgenic" breeding lines of animals, either to establish an animal model of a human disease that will be inherited, enabling the production of animals that can be used in research, or to produce animals that make commercially valuable proteins. Neither of these purposes applies to human beings. At present, therefore, genetic alteration in human beings that affects the germ-line is a wholly untested procedure. Moreover, as discussed in the next section, genetic alteration intended to affect the germ-line is both unnecessary and unwise.

ISSUES IN THE USE OF GERM-LINE GENETIC ALTERATION

Many of the issues raised by somatic cell gene therapy would also apply to germ-line genetic alteration—for example, requirements for informed consent and confidentiality. However, in addition, several unique and very troubling aspects of germ-line genetic alteration distinguish it from somatic cell gene therapy.

First, the risks associated with germ-line alteration are much greater than those surrounding somatic cell gene therapy. As we have seen, it is not possible to target an inserted gene precisely to a specific chromosomal site, raising the possibility that an inserted gene could interfere with other vital gene functions or even activate genes related to cancer development. The consequences of random insertion, while serious, are less severe in the case of somatic cell gene therapy, since a "mistake" would affect only a single target cell or tissue. In genetic alteration of the zygote, however, this "mistake" would be incorporated into most or all its cells.

Moreover, there is no reason to risk these consequences, for there is an easier and less risky alternative to treatment of the zygote. Treating a zygote at a stage when the germ-line would be affected first requires determining which zygotes have a genetic disorder, which means that preimplantation diagnosis would have to be performed. It would therefore be possible not to transfer the zygote found to be affected and to transfer only those found to be unaffected. Couples who are at risk of passing on a genetic disorder have a very good chance that at least one of their zygotes will not have the defective gene, although the exact odds depend on the kind of genetic disorder. (Recall that

preimplantation diagnosis would be done on more than one zygote a time, since multiple eggs would normally be retrieved for fertilization and preimplantation diagnosis during *in vitro* fertilization procedures.)

For example, if four eggs have been retrieved and fertilized *in vitro*, and if both parents are carriers of a recessive gene, then the odds are that three of the four zygotes tested by preimplantation diagnosis will turn out to be healthy and unaffected by the genetic disease. On average, one of the four zygotes will be diagnosed as having the genetic disease, but it does not have to be transferred to the woman's uterus; three healthy zygotes can be transferred, without any need for gene therapy. There is therefore no justification for performing gene therapy on affected zygotes when healthy zygotes can be obtained for transfer.

Similarly, if one parent has a dominant disorder, the odds are that two of four zygotes tested through preimplantation diagnosis will turn out to be healthy and so can be transferred without gene therapy. Even in the very rare instance that both parents have a dominant disorder, there is still a 25 percent chance of producing a healthy zygote.

Finally, if the genetic disease is X-linked, half the zygotes with a male chromosomal complement will be affected. Preimplantation diagnosis can be used to identify the female zygotes and the unaffected male zygotes, which will be healthy and can be transferred.

In all these cases, then, preimplantation diagnosis can be used to identify healthy zygotes for transfer. Hence, it is difficult to envision the real-world situations in which genetic alteration involving a zygote at an early enough stage of development to affect the germ-line would be an appropriate response. Few couples are likely to prefer transfer of an altered zygote to not transferring those affected.

The only situation in which preimplantation diagnosis could not be used to identify normal zygotes is if both members of the couple are affected by a recessive disorder (and are not just carriers of it). In this case, it is virtually certain that all their zygotes will be affected by the disease. This would be extremely rare, however, as the average incidence of a recessive disorder is 1 in 20000. The random likelihood that two affected individuals would mate is therefore exceedingly small. Moreover, even if they do, if both are healthy and functional enough to achieve pregnancy, the condition affecting them cannot be among the most devastating of the genetic diseases. Indeed, such diseases are likely to be relatively mild (for example, deafness) and certainly not devastating enough to warrant attempting manipulation of the DNA of a zygote. Further, couples in this situation could also consider using donor gametes.

The same logic applies to the possibility, mentioned earlier, that germ-line genetic alteration could be applied to the gametes of an adult who is a carrier of a genetic disease. It is not currently feasible to perform genetic alteration of sperm or eggs. But, even if it were to become possible, in order to alter the carrier sperm the sperm carrying the disease would have to be distinguished from those that do not, or else *all* the sperm would have to be altered.

A misguided argument has been made that gene therapy on zygotes that also affects the germ-line is desirable, even if other options are available to avoid or treat affected offspring, because it has the advantage of serving a preventive function, by reducing the transmission of genetic disease to future generations. Fetuses that have been treated by somatic cell gene therapy, or zygotes from high-risk couples that have been tested by preimplantation diagnosis and found normal, do not have a genetic disease, but some are still carriers of the disease and so risk passing it on to future generations. DNA alteration of such zygotes would eliminate the risk. (The same preventive argument is make for research into germ-line genetic alteration on adult gametes or gonads.)

For example, it has been argued that "society should pursue the development of strategies for preventing or correcting, at the germ-line level, genetic features that will lead to, or enhance, pathological conditions" as a way of ensuring that present and future couples can "exercise their rights to reproductive health."[1]

The idea of eliminating the risk of transmitting genetic disease may sound attractive, but it is in fact based on a misunderstanding of human genetics. All of us are carriers of various recessive genetic disorders—that is, we all carry genetic mutations that, if found in a double dose, could be deleterious, even fatal. To set as our aim the elimination of all risk of

passing on genetic disease would involve genetic alteration of the gametes or gonads of all adults.

For example, if a recessive disorder occurs in 1 in 10000 live births, which is relatively frequent for a recessive disorder, then approximately 1 individual in 50 is a carrier for that disorder, although that individual will be quite normal and healthy. To prevent this 1 in 10000 chance of a recessive disorder, one would have to alter the DNA of 1 individual in 50—and this would have to be done for all the hundreds of recessive single-gene disorders that exist.

The fact is that all human beings carry a few genes that would be deleterious if passed on to offspring in a double dose. The risk of passing on genetic disease is inherent in the human condition; it makes no sense to try to alter this in this way. Not only is the goal of a genetically "perfect" human being impossible to achieve, but human beings in all their diversity have value in themselves.

Moreover, even if it were feasible, it is not necessarily desirable from an evolutionary perspective. The fact that we all posses a certain amount of genetic mutation is what provides the reservoir for the species to adapt to changing environmental circumstances. The risks of genetic alteration of the germ-line therefore do not affect just the individual involved. The human genome has evolved over millions of years, in complex and subtle homeostasis with the environment. For example, we know that having carriers of certain genetic disorders is beneficial to a population. The best-known example is the gene for sickle-cell anaemia, which provides greater resistance to malaria. Many other examples are suspected as well. We simply do not know enough to contemplate intentionally changing the human genome in the way required for a germ-line prevention program to have any appreciable effect.

It is important, however, not to exaggerate the possible impact of germ-line genetic alteration on the DNA of the species as a whole. Many medical treatments affect the likelihood that particular genotypes will be passed on—it can be argued that the gene pool of the next generation is altered by any medical treatment or social support that allows people with a disease with a genetic component, who would formerly have died at an early age, to survive and reproduce. We do not withhold treatment of individuals for that reason. The behaviour of humanity has always had consequences for the composition of the gene pool. For example, technological innovation and cultural change affect the human gene pool. As one observer put it,

... it seems to me that the possibilities for what can be accomplished directly through genetic engineering are being exaggerated. After all, the human gene pool is enormous; there are over three billion human beings, and a large percentage of them at any given time are fertile. To effect a really significant change in a gene pool of that size through genetic engineering would call for delicate microsurgery on a lot of people. If we wanted to introduce far-reaching and practically irreversible changes into the shape of human life, we could do so far more effectively in the old-fashioned ways, by technological innovation and cultural change.[2]

It is nonetheless important to note that germ-line genetic alteration would be unique in that it involves intentional interference in human evolution. This imposes a greater responsibility to consider the impact of decisions regarding it on our species and on the interests of future generations.

Commissioners are of the opinion that the question of the impact of technology on future generations is one that touches on gene therapy, susceptibility testing, and other new reproductive technologies, and thus should be treated in a disciplined manner over the long term by setting up a framework to clarify what is prohibited, how activities will be regulated, and how decisions will be made.

REGULATING GERM-LINE GENETIC ALTERATION
It is clear that germ-line genetic alteration is inconsistent with the Commission's guiding principles. There are many risks and potential harms, without any clear benefit to any individual. It is not an appropriate use of resources, and it jeopardizes, rather than protects, those who are vulnerable. Since any foreseeable germ-line genetic alteration would involve embryo research, it would be covered by the legislative and licensing mechanisms we propose in chapter 22. However, we believe it is important to emphasize the unacceptability of germ-line genetic alteration by including it in the licensing conditions

for infertility clinics, which in practice would be the source of human zygotes (or eggs) in Canada. The Commission therefore recommends that

269. No research involving alteration of the DNA of human zygotes be permitted or funded in Canada. This prohibition would be monitored and enforced by the Embryo Research Sub-Committee of the National Reproductive Technologies Commission.

And that

270. The Prenatal Diagnosis and Genetics Sub-Committee of the National Reproductive Technologies Commission have as part of its guidelines for centres licensed to provide PND and genetics services that no genetic alteration of a human zygote be permitted.

NON-THERAPEUTIC GENETIC ALTERATION
Genetic enhancement involves the attempt to enhance or improve an already healthy genetic structure by inserting a gene for "improvement." This non-therapeutic use of genetic technology might take the form of altering either somatic cells or germ cells.

Like gene therapy, the scope of genetic enhancement feasibility is quite narrow. Genetic alteration to improve complex human traits, such as beauty, intelligence, vigour, and longevity, is far beyond our technical capabilities and will be so for the foreseeable future. These complex traits are multifactorial in nature; that is, they are a function of complex interactions between genetic and environmental factors. As a result, enhancement of any particular gene is not likely to have the desired effect.

Genetic enhancement may be possible in principle for some simpler physical characteristics, such as height. However, the risks involved are totally disproportionate to any benefits that might be gained. These risks include not only all the risks discussed earlier with respect to somatic or germ-line gene alteration (such as inducing cancer), but others that are unique to genetic enhancement. As one scholar has commented,

Any alteration or addition [to the normal genome] is likely to have deleterious, not beneficial results. Any gene acts on the background of many other genes that also have evolved over millennia.[3]

For example, although attempts to increase the size of mice by inserting growth hormone genes have succeeded in increasing their size, they have also led to a variety of deformities and functional disturbances.

Moreover, the motivation for non-therapeutic gene alteration requires close examination. Proponents argue that genetic enhancement is really no different from cosmetic surgery, and that the desire to improve oneself is natural and commendable. However, comparing enhancement genetics to cosmetic surgery or to other ways of helping individuals "make the best of themselves" is misleading and neglects the potential harms. We see three major types of risk in connection with genetic enhancement:[4]

- *Social Risks:* A caring society values people for themselves and for their uniqueness. Our ethical principles tell us that all individuals should be valued equally. Genetic enhancement raises the prospect of a society where some people would be accepted only if they were "improved"—they would not be acceptable as themselves. This is a form of commodifying individuals—people are treated as things that can be changed according to someone else's notions of human perfection. This shows a lack of respect for human life and dignity and intolerance for human diversity, which is likely to lead to discrimination against and devaluing of certain categories of people. Any use of genetic enhancement raises troubling and potentially discriminatory judgements about what sorts of enhancement would be allowed and who would have access to them. In the case of gene therapy, the issue of who should receive the alteration is clear—those with a severe disease should be eligible or medical treatment. But in the case of genetic enhancement, the selection process, by definition, cannot be based on medical need. It must therefore be based on other, as yet unspecified, criteria. Would it be a lottery or, more likely, those most able to pay?

  As there is no therapeutic objective, the goal of such alteration would be to pursue non-medical objectives, which might be economic, social, cultural, ethnic, or other. What are these objectives, and whose objectives are they? There is also the danger that people might be pressured to undergo such a procedure and be subject to discrimination if they refused. Finally, use of technology in this way might promote a social program of eugenics or indeed change our concept of what it is to be a human being.

- *Medical risks:* Many of the risks of cosmetic surgery are documented, but we do not know the risks of inserting genetic material, such as the risk of disrupting a tumour suppressor or activating a cancer-related gene.

- *Opportunity costs:* The non-therapeutic use of genetic alteration technology would draw away needed resources and skilled personnel from real medical problems. To allow DNA alteration in healthy individuals when there are so many other pressing calls on social attention and resources would be irresponsible and unethical.

The desire to improve the longevity, talents, and vigour of ourselves and our children is not inherently objectionable. However, this can best be achieved by improving the social and environmental factors that shape our daily lives—such as improved education or a healthier environment—rather than through the risky and potentially discriminatory use of genetic enhancement by those with the money or power to gain access to the technology.

In short, Commissioners find any non-therapeutic use of gene alteration unacceptable both in principle and in practice. It is not clear who would benefit or at what cost; there is the great risk of discriminatory use; and it is unacceptable to impose serous risks on healthy individuals for unclear benefit.

Our recommendations earlier in this chapter on somatic cell gene therapy have already made clear that research on genetic alteration in human beings is appropriate only for the treatment of serious diseases when no alternative treatment exists. Any non-therapeutic use of genetic alteration technology is also inconsistent with the existing MRC guidelines, which we have endorsed and supplemented with our recommendations.

It is extremely doubtful that any use of this technology for individual enhancement would ever be proposed by a genetics centre; but, if this ever did occur, the National Reproductive Technologies Commission would be able to turn down any such proposal.

It is important to remain vigilant about the possible misuse of technology that can change DNA, and it is important for the general public to become more aware of the issues it raises. Although these areas are outside our mandate, and the uses of genetic technology in general (for example, to "improve" individuals) are outside the span of new reproductive technologies and the National Reproductive Technologies Commission, we believe that a mechanism for keeping a watching brief on this area is desirable. Hence, we conclude that the National Council on Bioethics in Human Research (NCBHR) should consider this to be an area that warrants continued attention. The Commission recommends that

271. No research involving the alteration of DNA for enhancement purposes be permitted or funded in Canada. Proposals for any such project should be refused by the Medical Research Council national review committee on gene therapy.

And that

272. The National Council on Bioethics in Human Research address the question of non-therapeutic genetic alteration and monitor developments in this field.

CONCLUSION

The widespread and intense interest in all aspects of DNA technology that can alter genetic make-up includes both ardent hopes for the development of cures for severe, often fatal, genetic diseases and equally intense concerns about the potential abuses of science's increasing capacity for genetic manipulation. Our recommendations take into account the potential uses of these technologies in the context of human reproduction. Other applications of DNA technology are outside our mandate: we believe, however, that their implications for society warrant continued vigilance and public dialogue on whether and under what circumstances such applications might be permitted. This is why we have recommended that existing bodies charged with various review responsibilities maintain a watching brief and promote the necessary dialogue through publications, discussion papers, and other public education tools. In addition, Commissioners believe that the current stage of development of DNA technology in Canada provides a unique window of opportunity for enlightened policy responses that, if adopted now, will help set the future course of how our new capacity to alter genetic make-up is used in this country.

With respect to both germ-line genetic alteration and enhancement genetics, Commissioners are of the opinion that the risks associated with any such research on human zygotes or human subjects are completely out of proportion to any potential benefits, and that publicly funded research of this type should not be conducted in Canada.

Somatic cell gene therapy in general is outside our mandate. Nevertheless, to ensure appropriate limits on those aspects of somatic cell gene therapy that are within our mandate (that is, its use in the reproductive context), and to ensure that such uses, if permitted, can be appropriately regulated, we believe that a broader approach is necessary. Only if a mechanism is in place to review all proposals for somatic cell gene therapy can we ensure that the oversight we recommend for prenatal or reproductive uses occurs. This would mean that the following division of responsibilities should be in place with respect to somatic cell gene therapy:

- The Medical Research Council would continue to regulate human gene therapy research in general and immediately establish its recommended national review committee to review all proposals for somatic cell gene therapy research involving human subjects.
- Any proposal for the application of somatic cell gene therapy to fetuses would also be subject to approval by the Prenatal Diagnosis and Genetics Sub-Committee of the National Reproductive Technologies Commission.
- As part of its regulation of research involving human zygotes, the National Reproductive Technologies Commission would prohibit any genetic alteration of human zygotes, as such alteration may affect the germ-line.

- The National Council on Bioethics in Human Research would address the question of the use of DNA technology that alters genetic make-up (for example, non-therapeutic uses or "preventive" uses) with respect to the ethical and social implications, including consideration of the interests of future generations.

We believe that this division of responsibilities will serve Canadians well, now and in the future, with regard to DNA technology that alters genetic make-up, both by overseeing present-day research and by stimulating an informed and reasoned public debate about any future uses of DNA alteration technology in health care, or indeed any other use that is proposed.

Notes

1. Zimmerman, B.K. "Human Germ-Line Therapy: The Case for Its Development and Use." *Journal of Medicine and Philosophy* 16 (1991), p. 593.
2. Porter, J. "What Is Morally Distinctive About Genetic Engineering." *Human Gene Therapy* 1 (4) (Winter 1990), p. 423.
3. Prior, L. "Somatic and Germ Line Gene Therapy: Current Status and Prospects." In Research Volumes of the Royal Commission on New Reproductive Technologies, 1993.
4. For an exploration of these issues, see Anderson, W.F. "The First Signs of Danger." *Human Gene Therapy* 3 (4) (1992): 359-60.

ACKNOWLEDGEMENTS

E. Emanuel and L. Emanuel, "Four Models of the Physician-Patient Relationship." *Journal of the American Medical Association* 267:16 (1992), 2212-26. Reprinted with permission.

Edmund D. Pellegrino, "The Virtuous Physician and the Ethics of Medicine." From *Virtue and Medicine* edited by Earl E. Shelp. Reidel, 1985: 243-55. Reprinted with kind permission of Kluwer Academic Publishers and the author.

Nancy S. Jecker and Donnie J. Self, "Separating Care and Cure." *The Journal of Medicine and Philosophy* 16:3 (1991): 285-306. Copyright © by The Journal of Medicine and Philosophy, Inc. Reprinted by permission.

Susan Sherwin, "A Relational Approach to Autonomy in Health Care." From *The Politics of Women's Health: Exploring Agency and Autonomy* by The Feminist Health Care Ethics Research Network. Reprinted by permission of Temple University Press. © 1998 by Temple University. All Rights Reserved.

Nancy S. Jecker, Joseph A. Carrese, Robert A. Pearlman, "Caring for Patients in a Cross-Cultural Setting." *Hastings Center Report* 25:1 (April 1989). © The Hastings Center. Reprinted by permission.

John Hardwig, "What About the Family?" *Hastings Center Report* 20:2 (1990). © The Hastings Center. Reprinted by permission.

Benjamin Freedman, "A Moral Theory of Consent." *Hastings Center Report* 5:4 (1975). © The Hastings Center. Reprinted with permission.

James F. Drane, "Competency to Give an Informed Consent." *Journal of the American Medical Association* 252:7 (1984) 925-27. Reprinted with permission.

John E. Thomas, "The Physician as Therapist and Investigator." From *Medical Ethics and Human Life*, by permission of Edgar Kent, Inc., Publishers.

Eike-Henner W. Kluge, "After 'Eve': Whither Proxy Decision-Making?" Reprinted by permission of the publisher from *Canadian Medical Association Journal* 137 (October 15, 1987): pp. 715-20.

Barry E. Brown, "Proxy Consent for Research on the Incompetent Elderly." Reprinted with permission of the publisher from *Ethics & Aging* edited by James E. Thornton and Earl R. Winkler © University of British Columbia Press 1988. All rights reserved by the Publisher.

Christine Harrison et al, "Bioethics for Physicians." Reprinted by permission of the author and the publisher from *Canadian Medical Association Journal* 15:6 (1997): 825-28.

John A. Robertson, "Class, Feminist, and Communitarian Critiques." From *Children of Choice: Freedom and the New Reproductive Technologies.* Copyright © 1994 Princeton University Press. Reprinted by permission of Princeton University Press.

Christine Overall, "Reflections on reproductive rights in Canada." From *Human Reproduction: Principles, Practices, Policies* by Christine Overall. Toronto: Oxford University Press, 1993. Copyright © Christine Overall 1993. Reprinted by permission of the author and Oxford University Press Canada.

Susan Sherwin, "Feminist Ethics and In Vitro Fertilization." From *Science, Morality and Feminist Theory* edited by M. Hanen and K. Nielsen. University of Calgary Press, 1987: 265-84. Reprinted by permission of the publisher.

Cynthia B. Cohen, "Give Me Children Or I Shall Die." *Hastings Center Report* 26:7 (1996). © The Hastings Center. Reprinted by permission.

Barbara J. Berg, "Listening to the Voices of the Infertile." From *Reproduction, Ethics and the Law* edited by Joan C. Callahan. Indiana University Press

1995. Reprinted with permission of Indiana University Press.

Brenda Baker, "A Case for Permitting Altruistic Surgery." From *Hypatia* 11.1. Reprinted with permission of Indiana University Press.

Don Marquis, "Why Abortion Is Immoral." *Journal of Philosophy* LXXXVI, 4 (April 1989): 183-202. Reprinted with permission of the author and the publisher.

Wayne Sumner, "A Third Way." From *Abortion and Moral Theory.* Copyright © 1981. Reprinted by permission of Princeton University Press.

Mary Anne Warren, "The Moral Significance of Birth." From *Hypatia* 4:3. Reprinted with permission of Indiana University Press.

Susan Sherwin. "Abortion Through A Feminist Lens." *Dialogue* XXX:3 (1991): 327-42. Reprinted with permission of the author and the publisher.

Thomas H. Murray, "Moral Obligations to the Not-Yet-Born." From *The Worth of A Child*, pp. 96-114. Copyright © 1996 The Regents of the University of California. Reprinted with permission of the author and the publisher.

Abby Lippman, "Prenatal Diagnosis." From *The Future of Human Reproduction* edited by Christine Overall. The Women's Press, 1989. Reprinted with permission of the author and publisher.

Laura Purdy, "Loving Future People." From *Reproduction, Ethics and the Law* edited by Joan C. Callahan. Indiana University Press 1995. Reprinted with permission of Indiana University Press.

Mary B. Mahowald, "Decisions Regarding Disabled Newborns." From *Women and Children in Health Care: An Unequal Majority* by Mary Briody Mahowald. Copyright © 1996 by Oxford University Press, Inc. Used by permission of Oxford University Press, Inc.

Helen Bequaert Holmes, "Choosing Children's Sex." From *Reproduction, Ethics and the Law* edited by Joan C. Callahan. Indiana University Press 1995. Reprinted with permission of Indiana University Press.

Margaret P. Battin, "Euthanasia: The Fundamental Issues." From *Health Care Ethics: An Introduction* edited by Donald VanDeVeer and Tom Regan. Reprinted by permission of Temple University Press. © 1987 by Temple University. All Rights Reserved.

Daniel Callahan, "When Self-Determination Runs Amok." *The Hastings Center Report* 22:2 (1992). © The Hastings Center. Reprinted with permission.

John Keown, "Voluntary Euthanasia and Physician-Assisted Suicide." *Policy Options* 18:10 (1997): 25-29. Reprinted with permission of the author and the publisher.

Susan M. Wolf, "Gender, Feminism and Death." From *Feminism and Bioethics: Beyond Reproduction* edited by Susan M. Wolf. Copyright © 1996 by The Hastings Center. Used by permission of Oxford University Press.

Tom Tomlinson and Diane Czlonka, "Futility and Hospital Policy." *The Hastings Center Report* 25:3 (1995). © The Hastings Center. Reprinted with permission.

Françoise Baylis, Jocelyn Downie, Susan Sherwin, "Reframing Research Involving Humans." From *The Politics of Women's Health: Exploring Agency and Autonomy* by The Feminist Health Care Ethics Research Network. Reprinted by permission of Temple University Press. © 1998 by Temple University. All Rights Reserved.

George J. Annas, "Baby Fae." *Hastings Center Report* 15 (February 1985). © The Hastings Center. Reprinted with permission of the publisher and the author.

Richard Ratzan, "Being Old Makes You Different." *Hastings Center Report* 10:5 (1980). © The Hasting Center. Reprinted with permission.

Udo Schüklenk, Edward Stein, Jacinte Kerin, William Byrne, "The Ethics of Genetic Research on Sexual Orientation." *The Hastings Center Report* 27:4 (1997). © The Hastings Center. Reprinted with permission.

"The Declaration of Helsinki." Reprinted with permission of the World Medical Association.

"Tri-Council Policy Statement." Public Domain.

Benjamin Freedman and Françoise Baylis, "Purpose and Function in Government-Funded Health Coverage." *Journal of Helath Politics, Policy and Law* 12:1

(Spring 1997): 97-122. © Copyright 1997, Duke University Press. All rights reserved. Reprinted with permission.

George J. Annas, "The Prostitute, The Playboy, and The Poet." *American Journal of Public Health* 75:2 (1985): 187-9. © American Journal of Public Health. Reprinted with permission.

Leonard J. Weber, "In Vitro Fertilization and the Just Use of Health Care Resources." From *Reproduction, Technology and Rights* edited by James Humber and Robert F. Almeder. Humana Press, 1996. Reprinted by permission of the publisher.

Michael Stingl, "Equality and Efficiency as Basic Social Values." From *Efficiency versus Equality*, edited by Michael Stingl. Fernwood, 1996. Reprinted by permission of the author.

Norman Daniels, "Four Unsolved Rationing Problems." *Hastings Center Report* 24:4 (1994). © The Hastings Center. Reprinted with permission of the publisher and the author.

John D. Arras and Shlomo Shinnar, "Anencephalic Newborns as Organ Donors." *Journal of the American Medical Association* 259:15 (1988): 2284-85. Reprinted with permission.

Rupert Jarvis, "Join the Club." *Journal of Medical Ethics* 21:4 (1995): 199-204. © BMJ Publishing Group. Reprinted with permission.

Raanan Gillon, "On Giving Preference to Prior Volunteers." *Journal of Medical Ethics* 21:4 (1995): 195-6. © BMJ Publishing Group. Reprinted with permission.

Mary B. Mahowald, "As If There Were Fetuses Without Women." From *Reproduction, Ethics and the Law* edited by Joan C. Callahan. Indiana University Press 1995. Reprinted with permission of Indiana University Press.

Arthur L. Caplan, "Requests, Gifts, and Obligations: The Ethics of Organ Procurement." *Transplantation Proceedings* 18:3 (1986), pp. 49-56. Reprinted with permission from Elsevier Science.

Robert D. Truog, "Is It Time To Abandon Brain Death?" *Hastings Center Report* 27: 1 (1997). Reprinted with permission of the author and publisher.

Lee M. Silver, "Cloning, Ethics, and Religion. *Cambridge Quarterly of Healthcare Ethics* 7:2 (1998): 168-72. Reprinted with the permission of Cambridge University Press.

R. Munson and L. Davis, "Germ-line Therapy and Medical Imperative." *Kennedy Institute of Ethics Journal* 2:2 (1992): 137-58. Reprinted by permission of Johns Hopkins University Press.

The Council on Ethical and Judicial Affairs, AMA, "Multiplex Genetic Testing. *Hastings Center Report* 28:4 (1998). © The Hastings Center. Reprinted with permission of the publisher and the author.

Royal Commission on New Reproductive Technologies. "Germ-Line Genetic Alteration." Privy Council Office, *Proceed With Care*, 1993: 936-47. Reproduced with the permission of the Minister of Public Works and Government Services Canada, 2000.